ADVANCES IN PROSTAGLANDIN, THROMBOXANE, AND LEUKOTRIENE RESEARCH
VOLUME 19

Taipei Conference on Prostaglandin
and Leukotriene Research

Advances in Prostaglandin, Thromboxane, and Leukotriene Research

Series Editors: Bengt Samuelsson and Rodolfo Paoletti
(Formerly *Advances in Prostaglandin and Thromboxane Research* Series)

*Out of print

Advances in Prostaglandin, Thromboxane, and Leukotriene Research

Volume 19

Taipei Conference on Prostaglandin and Leukotriene Research

Editors

Bengt Samuelsson, M.D.
Department of Physiological Chemistry
Karolinska Institute
Stockholm, Sweden

Patrick Y.-K. Wong, Ph.D.
Department of Pharmacology
New York Medical College
Valhalla, New York

Frank F. Sun, Ph.D.
Department of Hypersensitivity Diseases Research
The Upjohn Company
Kalamazoo, Michigan

Raven Press 🖋 New York

LP

Raven Press, 1185 Avenue of the Americas, New York, New York 10036

Made in the United States of America

International Standard Book Number 0-88167-496-6

9 8 7 6 5 4 3 2 1

11-10-89

Preface

This volume of the Advances in Prostaglandin, Thromboxane, and Leukotriene Research series is dedicated to developing an overall view of the state-of-the-art knowledge in the field of eicosanoids, and to exploring the nature of the major problems still facing researchers in this field. The chapters cover such diverse areas of research as biosynthesis and metabolism, receptors, phospholipases and signal transduction, renal prostaglandins and hypertension, the cardiovascular system, inflammation allergy and hypersensitivity, cellular and molecular biology of enzymes, endocrine and the central nervous system, nutritional intervention, and platelet activating factor.

Readers will find exciting advances presented, which have occurred in the area of eicosanoid research only recently. Eicosanoid research has progressed to where the molecular and cell biology aspects of the system have now taken center stage. The elucidation of gene structures of key enzymes such as 5-lipoxygenase and cyclooxygenase will lead to new insights and new approaches in the regulation of eicosanoid activity. Studies with novel enzyme inhibitors and receptor antagonists continue to reveal the mechanisms behind various biological events in which eicosanoids play a central role. Enthusiasm for the discovery of new arachidonic acid metabolites remains strong as novel structures are introduced into the field. We are convinced that this volume will be a useful reference for investigators in both basic and clinical research who are interested in the field of eicosanoid research.

The Editors

Acknowledgments

This volume contains the papers presented at the Taipei Conference on Prostaglandin and Leukotriene Research held in Taipei, Taiwan, on April 22-24, 1988. This conference continued the tradition of the Kyoto Conference in 1984 and became the second International Conference of Eicosanoid Research held in Asia. This conference was sponsored by the Institute of Biomedical Sciences, Academia Sinica, and the National Science Council, Taiwan, Republic of China, to commemorate the 60th birthday of the Academy. IBMS was established in 1987, and this was the first major international scientific conference sponsored by this young institute. We are especially indebted to Professors Paul Yu and Shu Chien, the Directors of the Institute of Biomedical Sciences in 1987 and 1988. Without their extraordinary support this conference could never have become a reality. We thank the members of international and local committees and staff members of the Institute. It was largely because of their dedicated and diligent work that this conference was a success.

We gratefully acknowledge support for this conference from the following agencies: The Ministry of Foreign Affairs and the Department of Health of Taiwan, Republic of China; China-American Foundation; The City of Taipei; Taiwan Provincial Department of Health; Upjohn International Inc. Taiwan Branch; Veterans Administration Hospital, National Taiwan University Hospital, Tri Service Hospital, Cathay Hospital and Chang-Guarg Hospital of Taiwan; Chen-Kung University Medical School, and Tien Medical Center. Many pharmaceutical companies also supported this conference. They are: American Cyanamid Co., Lederle Laboratories; Berlex Laboratories, Inc.; Cayman Chemical Co.; Ciba-Geigy Corp., U.S.A.; E. I. DuPont, Inc.; Glaxo Orient (Pte), Ltd., Taiwan Branch; Glaxo, Inc.; Giraffes Company Ltd., Taiwan; Hewlett-Packard Co., U.S.A.; Ideal Enterprise, Taipei, Taiwan; Ing-Lih Trading Co., Ltd.; Institute Henri Beaufour, Paris, France; Kyowa Hakko Kogyo, Kaiska, Co., Japan; Merck, Sharp, and Dohme Research Laboratories and Merck Frosst, Canada; Nippon Suisan Kaiska, Ltd., Japan; Ono Pharmaceutical Co., Japan; Pfizer Inc., U.S.A., Division of Immunology and Infectious Disease; Sandoz Pharmaceuticals Corp.; Sanko Co., Ltd., Biological Research Laboratories, Japan; Schering AG Berlin, F.R.G.; Shionogi Co., Ltd., Shionogi Research Laboratories, Japan; Smith Kline-Beckman Corp.; Stuart Pharmaceuticals, Division of ICI Americas, Inc.; Syntex (U.S.A.) Inc., Syntex Research Division; Taiwan Instrument Co., Ltd.; Tejin Ltd., Medical and Pharmaceutical Division, Japan; Tekeda Chemical Company, Tekeda Research Laboratories, Japan; Terumo Corp.,

Research and Development Division, Japan; The Upjohn Co., U.S.A.; Upjohn Laboratories Ltd., Wyeth-Ayerst Laboratories, Inc.; and Zu-Shing Enterprises Co., Ltd.

We particularly thank Miss Ming Chu and Miss Karren Leu for their hard work and dedication as the conference coordinators. We are grateful to Miss Gail Price, Mrs. Pamela Blank, and Mrs. Sallie McGiff for their assistance in the preparation and editing of this volume. We also would like to express our thanks for the assistance we received from the staff at the IBMS during the conference, particularly Mrs. Jenny Lin and Vivian Cheng.

The Editors

Contents

Eicosanoid Metabolism

Eicosanoid Receptors, Agonists and Antagonists

Renal Eicosanoids and Hypertension

The Cardiovascular System

Cell Growth and Differentiation

Cellular and Molecular Biology
of Eicosanoid Metabolism

Inflammation, Allergy and Hypersensitivity

Nutritional Intervention

Workshops

Conference Organizers

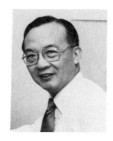

Shu Chien
Director, Institute of Biomedical Science
Academia Sinica
Taipei, Taiwan
Republic of China

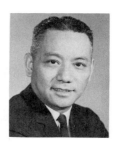

Paul Yu
President, Organizing Committee
Taipei Conference on Prostaglandin and
Leukotriene Research
Taipei, Taiwan
Republic of China

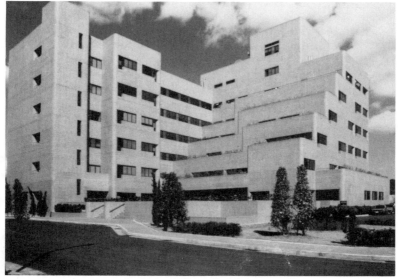

Institute of Biomedical Science
Taipei, Taiwan
Republic of China

xxvii

Nobel and Plenary Lecturers

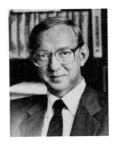

B. Samuelsson
Department of Physiological Chemistry
Karolinska Institutet
S-104 01 Stockholm, Sweden

J. R. Vane
The William Harvey Research Institute
St. Bartholomew's Hospital Medical College
London EC1 6BQ England

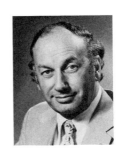

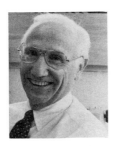

K. F. Austen
Department of Medicine
Harvard Medical School and
Department of Rheumatology and
Immunology
Brigham and Women's Hospital
Boston, Massachusetts 02115

O. Hayaishi
Hayaishi Bioinformation Transfer Project
Research Development Corporation of
Japan
Osaka Medical College
Osaka 569, Japan

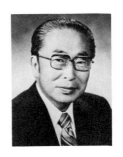

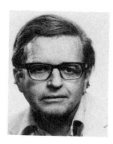

J. C. McGiff
Department of Pharmacology
New York Medical College
Valhalla, New York 10595

P. Needleman
Department of Pharmacology
Washington University School of Medicine
St. Louis, Missouri 63110

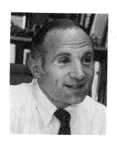

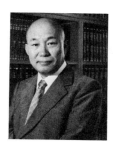

Y. Nishizuka
Department of Biochemistry
Kobe University
School of Medicine
Kobe 650, Japan

J. A. Oates
Departments of Medicine and
Pharmacology
The Vanderbilt University School of
Medicine
Nashville, Tennessee 37232

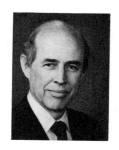

Contributors

ADVANCES IN PROSTAGLANDIN, THROMBOXANE, AND LEUKOTRIENE RESEARCH
VOLUME 19

Taipei Conference on Prostaglandin and Leukotriene Research

Advances in Prostaglandin, Thromboxane, and Leukotriene Research, Vol. 19, edited by B. Samuelsson, P. Y.-K. Wong, and F. F. Sun, Raven Press, Ltd., New York ©1989.

MOLECULAR BIOLOGY OF LEUKOTRIENE AND LIPOXIN FORMATION

Bengt Samuelsson, Colin D. Funk, Shigeru Hoshiko, Takashi Matsumoto and Olof Rådmark

Department of Physiological Chemistry
Karolinska Institutet
S-104 01 Stockholm, Sweden

The leukotrienes and lipoxins are oxygenated metabolites of arachidonic acid with biological activities indicating important roles in inflammation and immediate hypersensitivity (1,2).

This review summarizes our recent work on the characterization of the genes and the enzymes involved in leukotriene and lipoxin formation (3).

Cloning of human 5-lipoxygenase

In order to gain some insights about the structure of 5-lipoxygenase molecular cloning experiments have been undertaken (4). Human leukocyte 5-lipoxygenase was purified to near homogeneity as previously described (5) and a polyclonal antibody was prepared from immunized rabbits. The availability of a 5-lipoxygenase antibody enabled us to begin immunoscreening of a human lung cDNA library in the expression vector λgt11. Concomitantly, purified intact 5-lipoxygenase, as well as proteolytically and chemically cleaved 5-lipoxygenase peptide fragments were subjected to peptide sequence analyses.

Fourteen positive phage clones were isolated and purified to homogeneity by three successive rounds of antibody screening. One of the clones, λluS1, containing a 397 bp insert, was sequenced and was found to contain a coding sequence for a segment that was known for 17 amino acids from the peptide analyses of the lipoxygenase fragments (Fig. 1). This finding established λluS1 as part of the 5-lipoxygenase cDNA. The insert from λluS1 was nick translated and used as a probe for finding clones with longer inserts from the λgt11 human lung cDNA library and a human placenta cDNA library in the λgt11 expression vector. A clone, λpl5BS, containing a cDNA insert long enough (2.6 kbp) to encode 5-lipoxygenase was isolated from

1

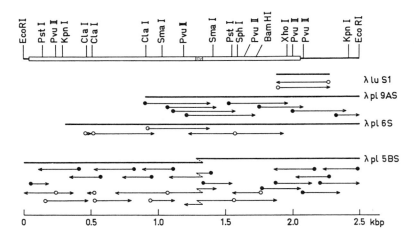

Fig. 1 Partial restriction map and sequencing strategy
for cloned cDNAs encoding human 5-lipoxygenase.
Direction and extent of sequence determinations
are indicated by arrows. The protein-coding region is shown by the open box. The cDNA insert
of λpl5BS contains a 51-bp repeat sequence that
is present only once in the other inserts. This
whole area is indicated by the stippled region
of the box and the zig-zag arrows in the sequence determinations.

the placenta cDNA library. The insert was sequenced
and was found to contain 2073 bp from the initiator
codon ATG to the stop codon TGA in a continuous open
reading frame. However, within this insert there were
two adjacent exact 51-bp repeating units. This raised
the possibility of a cloning artifact within the cDNA
insert of λpl5BS. Therefore, two additional independent clone inserts from λpl9AS and λpl6S were sequenced. These clones contained only one copy of the
51-bp unit within their inserts. Consequently, the
true 5-lipoxygenase cDNA lacks the repeat (also confirmed by genomic sequence analysis) and the open
reading frame would then encode for a mature protein
of 673 amino acids with a calculated molecular weight
of 77,856.

The structure of 5-lipoxygenase has no long segments with noticeably hydrophobic properties. A segment centered around residue 310 and, to some extent,
one after position 643 have several consecutive
hydrophobic residues but neither segment reveals
extreme properties. The protein is fairly rich in
tryptophan and aromatic residues. This also applies

to the basic residues, which often occur in pairs or small clusters.

Sequence homology of 5-lipoxygenase to other protein sequences

The amino acid sequence of 5-lipoxygenase was compared to other known protein sequences in order to investigate sequence homology. Human 5-lipoxygenase displays significant sequence homology to the soybean lipoxygenase isozymes (6-8), and to the partial amino acid sequences of several other lipoxygenases (9-11). The soybean lipoxygenase isozymes are larger (838-865 amino acids, MW ≈95,000) than human 5-lipoxygenase (673 amino acids, MW 78,000) yet common characteristic structure/function features exist between the proteins (e.g. bound non-heme iron, and the addition of dioxygen to a cis,cis-1,4-pentadiene polyunsaturated fatty acid). The homology between 5-lipoxygenase and the soybean isozymes ranges from approximately 25% when considering amino acid sequence identity to approximately 45% when taking into account amino acid similarity. Certain central regions of the proteins contain considerably higher homologies (Fig. 2). Shibata et al. (7) have proposed that a region of 40 amino acid residues containing 6 histidines and 2 tyrosines, which is highly conserved in all three soybean lipoxygenase isozymes, to be a potential iron-binding region. Interestingly, a region of 5-lipoxygenase (residues 358-401) possesses 5 of the conserved histidine residues as well as 5 of the conserved acidic and basic residues. This region could possibly comprise the iron-binding domain of 5-lipoxygenase. In addition to the sequence homologies, 5-lipoxygenase and the soybean lipoxygenase isozymes display similar overall secondary structures and hydrophobicity profiles.

Amino-terminal sequences of some other lipoxygenases have been reported. A comparison of their sequences to that of 5-lipoxygenase is made in Fig. 3. Human 5-lipoxygenase is virtually identical to RBL cell 5-lipoxygenase (2 of 30 residues differ) (9). Human 5-lipoxygenase shows 36% sequence identity (57% similarity) to the 14 amino-terminal amino acids of human leukocyte 15-lipoxygenase sequenced by Sigall et al. (10). The rabbit reticulocyte 15-lipoxygenase (11) has 39% of its amino-terminal 34 amino acids identical to human 5-lipoxygenase (48% similarity). Interestingly, a second region of homology exists between amino acids 45-88 of reticulocyte 15-lipoxygenase and amino acids 549-593 of 5-lipoxygenase. Although it is difficult to draw distinct conclusions

```
5-LX  351  K IW V RSS D FHV HQ TIT H L L R TH LVS E V F G IA MY R Q L P A V HPI F KLL VA H V
SB-1  482  K AY V IVN D SCY HQ LMS H W L N TH AAM E P F V IA TH R H L S V L HPI Y KLL TP H Y
SB-2  511  K AY V VVN D SCY HQ LMS H W L N TH AVI E P F I IA TN R H L S A L HPI Y KLL TP H Y
SB-3  502  K AY V VVN D SCY HQ LVS H W L N TH AVV E P F I IA TN R H L S V V HPI Y KLL HP H Y

5-LX  401  R F T IA IN TK AR EQ L I CEC G LFDKANAT G GGGH V Q M VQRA-M K D LTYASLCF
SB-1  532  R N N MN IN AL AR QS L I NAN  G IIETTFLP S KYS- V E M SSAV-Y K N WVFTDQAL
SB-2  561  R D T MN IN AL AR QS L I NAD  G IIEKSFLP S KHS- V E M SSAV-Y K N WVFTDQAL
SB-3  552  R D T MN IN GL AR LS L V NDG  G VIEQTFLW G RYS- V E M S-AVVY K D WVFTDQAL

5-LX  451  P EA- IK A RG M ES K ED--------- I PY Y F Y RD DGL LV W E AI R T FTA E V V DI
SB-1  581  P ADL IK - RG V AI K DPSTPHGVRLL I ED Y P Y AA DGL EI W A AI K T WVQ E Y V PL
SB-2  610  P ADL IK - RG V AI K DPSAPHGLRLL I ED Y P Y AV DGL EI W A AI K T WVQ E Y V SL
SB-3  601  P ADL IK - RG M AI E DPSCPHGIRLV I ED Y P Y AV DGL EI W D AI K T WVH E Y V FL

5-LX  492  YY EG D QV V E E D P ELQ DFVNDVYVY G MRGR K SSGF- PK SVKS R E Q L S E YLTV
SB-1  631  YY AR D DD V K N D S ELQ HWWKEAVEK G HGDL K DKPWW PK -LQT L E D L V E VCLI
SB-2  660  YY AR D DD V K P D S ELQ QWWKEAVEK G HGDL K DKPWW PK -LQT I E E L V E ICTI
SB-3  651  YY KS D DT L R E D P ELQ ACWKELVEV G HGDK K NEPWW PK -MQT R E E L V E ACAI

5-LX  542  V I F T ASA Q HAAVNFGQY DWCSW I P N A P
SB-1  681  I I W I ASA L HAAVNFGQY PYGGL I M N R P
SB-2  710  I I W T ASA L HAAVNFGQY PYGGF I L N R P
SB-3  701  I I W T ASA L HAAVNFGQY PYGGL I L N R P
```

Fig. 2 Comparison of the amino acid sequence of human 5-lipoxygenase with the sequences of the soybean lipoxygenase isozymes. Standard one-letter codes are used for amino acids. Boxed regions indicate identity to 5-lipoxygenase residues. -, spaces inserted for optimal homology. Numbers indicate the position of the amino acid within the corresponding sequence. SB, soybean.

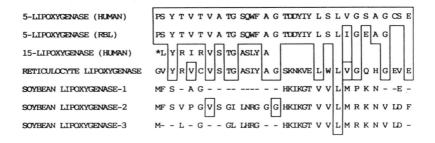

Fig. 3 Comparison of the N-terminal sequences of several lipoxygenases. Only residues identical to human 5-lipoxygenase have been boxed. Standard one-letter codes for amino acids are used. *, not determined. -, spaces added for optimal alignment of the soybean isozymes.

from the limited sequence data of some of these lipoxygenase enzymes it is becoming increasingly clear that a lipoxygenase gene family exists.

Dixon and coworkers (12) have reported the presence of a short sequence segment that is related to the interface-binding domain of the human lipoprotein lipase and the rat hepatic lipase and which is located within a region of overall hydrophobicity.

5-Lipoxygenase requires calcium and ATP for maximal activity. The amino acid sequence of 5-lipoxygenase was compared to the sequences of calcium- and ATP-binding proteins. Very limited homology was observed, however.

Human 5-lipoxygenase shows no sequence homology to either bovine cyclooxygenase (13,14) or to human LTA$_4$ hydrolase (15,16).

Characterization of the human 5-lipoxygenase gene

Since very little is known about the mechanisms controlling 5-lipoxygenase expression in various tissues we have undertaken characterization of the 5-lipoxygenase gene. Three different genomic DNA libraries were screened with several 5-lipoxygenase cDNA probes. Several overlapping clones spanning the gene were isolated and characterized by restriction endonuclease mapping and Southern blot analysis.

The human 5-lipoxygenase gene is organized into at least 13 exons (putative exon 3 has not yet been cloned) divided by 12 introns. Exons range in size from 87 bp (exon 8) to 611 bp (exon 13), whereas intron sizes range between 192 bp (intron J) and 10.5 kb (intron F). Exons 1-6, encoding the amino-terminal half of 5-lipoxygenase are spread out over more than 30 kb of DNA, while the carboxy-terminal encoding exons, 7-13 are clustered in a 6 kb segment. The total length of the gene is at least 45 kb. One particular exon (exon 6), which encodes amino acids 278-326, corresponds exactly to one of the most hydrophobic segments of 5-lipoxygenase. It is, therefore, possible that this exon represents an important functional and/or structural domain of 5-lipoxygenase.

A 270 bp region upstream of the translation initiation site, comprising the putative promoter region of the 5-lipoxygenase gene was sequenced and characterized (Fig.4). The region does not contain typical

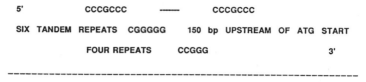

Fig. 4 Characteristics of the promoter region of the human 5-lipoxygenase gene.

TATA and CAAT box sequences, however, certain features common to housekeeping gene promoters were found. The region is very GC-rich (80 %) and contains 8 potential "GC-box" sites for binding of the transcription factor Sp1. The presence of two 11-bp inverted repeat segments in this region could possibly have some relevance to transcription factor binding and transcriptional regulation. The housekeeping genes are constitutively expressed. Since the 5-lipoxygenase gene shares similar promoter characteristics to the housekeeping genes this raises many intriguing questions about how the 5-lipoxygenase gene is regulated and expressed in a tissue-specific fashion.

Cloning of LTA$_4$-hydrolase

Screening with polyclonal antiserum

Rabbits were injected with LTA$_4$-hydrolase (purified from human neutrophils) for production of polyclonal antiserum. One clone (λluH6-1) encoded for a β-galactosidase fusion protein carrying epitopes that were recognized by the LTA$_4$-hydrolase antiserum.

Screening for additional LTA$_4$-hydrolase cDNA clones

The insert from λluH6-1a was nick-translated and used as a probe to find longer clones in the lung cDNA λgt11 library. Twenty strongly positive clones were obtained after screening $\approx$5 x 10^5 cDNA clones. These clones were purified and their EcoRI inserts ranged in size from 0.2 to 1.2 kilobases. The insert of the longest clone, λlu209-8A, was sequenced and found to contain 770 bp of cDNA encoding LTA$_4$ hydrolase, overlapping with 159 bp of the 5' end of the insert of λluH6-1a, and a 405-bp cloning artifact at the 5' end.

Since we were unable to find clones long enough to encode a full-length cDNA with the lung cDNA λgt11 library screening of additional libraries was carried out. Nineteen strongly positive clones were isolated and purified after screening ≈4 x 10^5 clones from a human placenta λgt11 library. Twelve of these clones contained a 1.1-kb/0.8-kb double-insert pattern. In DNA blot analysis ^{32}P-labeled λluH6-1a insert hybridized to the 0.8-kb insert of the 12 clones (data not shown). The pattern of these clone inserts gave strong reason to believe that an internal EcoRI site is present (Fig. 5).

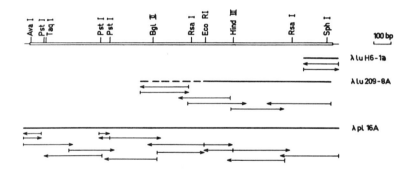

Fig. 5 Partial restriction map and sequencing strategy of cloned cDNAs encoding human LTA$_4$ hydrolase. Direction and extent of sequence determinations are indicated by arrows. The broken line indicates a cloning artifact in the cDNA of λlu209-8A. The protein-coding region is shown by the open bar.

Nucleotide sequence of cDNA and deduced amino acid sequence for LTA$_4$ hydrolase.

λp16A contains a 1910-bp insert, excluding EcoRI linkers, with a continuous open reading frame of 1830 bp terminated by a TAA stop codon. The open reading frame encodes a protein of 610 amino acids with a calculated molecular weight of 69,140.

LTA$_4$ hydrolase was analyzed by direct liquid phase sequencer degradation for 34 cycles. Results were in agreement with the deduced sequence and the

previously reported 15 N-terminal amino acids (17).
CNBr fragments of carboxyl[^{14}C]methylated LTA$_4$ hydrolase were purified. Five fragments were analyzed.
Both total compositions and amino acid sequences of
these fragments are in agreement with the structure
deduced from the cDNA sequence. Consequently, N-
terminal, internal, and near-C-terminal regions of
the deduced structure have been directly confirmed by
analysis at the protein level.

Properties of LTA$_4$ hydrolase.

The cDNA sequence of the λpl16A insert shows no
significant sequence homology with the nucleotide
sequences in the EMBL data bank (EMBL/GenBank Genetic
Sequence Database (1986) EMBL Nucleotide Sequence
Data Library (Eur. Mol. Biol. Lab., Heidelberg, Tape
Release 10), including those of rabbit and rat liver
microsomal epoxide hydrolases (18,19).
Screening of the protein sequence for internal
homologies did not reveal any consistent patterns of
long repeats (two 30 residue segments, starting at
positions 209 and 393, show some similarities - 10
identities in 29 residues). Secondary structure predictions (20) and calculations of hydropathy (21)
reveal mixed patterns, as for many proteins. However,
a segment close to position 200 displays some more
extreme properties. Thus, the segment 170-185 is the
most hydrophilic in the whole protein, 190-205 the
one most hydrophobic, and in between is one of two
strong predictions for a reverse turn (followed by a
prediction of a β-strand). One of the internal repeat
segments mentioned above is adjacent to this segment
(residues 209-238) and has a prediction for a long α-
helix (residues 220-240). Several features therefore
center around the segment 165-240, which could be related to the structure and activity of LTA$_4$ hydrolase. It was previously demonstrated that LTA^4 could
be covalently bound to the enzyme (22). The thiol
group of Cys-199 within the hydrophobic region, is
one of the possible candidates for such an interaction.

ACKNOWLEDGEMENTS

These studies were supported by a fellowship from
Fonds de la Recherche en Santé du Québec (to CDF) and
by grants from the Konung Gustav V 80-årsfond, The
Magnus Bergwall Foundation, the Scandinavian-Japan
Sasakawa Foundation and the Swedish Medical Research
Council (03X-217, 03X-3532, 03X-7467).

References

1. Samuelsson, B. (1983) Science.
2. Samuelsson, B., Dahlen, S.-E., Lindgren, J.-Å., Rouzer, C.A. and Serhan, C.N. (1987) Science 237, 1171-1176.
3. Samuelsson, B., Rouzer, C.A. and Matsumoto, T. (1987) In: Adv. in Prostaglandin, Thromboxane and Leukotriene Research (Eds. B. Samuelsson, P. Ramwell and R. Paoletti), Raven Press, N.Y. vol. 17A, pp. 1-11.
4. Matsumoto, T., Funk, C.D., Rådmark, O., Höög, J-O., Jörnvall, H. and Samuelsson, B. (1988) Proc. Natl. Acad. Sci. USA 85, 26-30.
5. Rouzer, C.A. and Samuelsson, B. (1985) Proc. Natl. Acad. Sci. USA 82, 6040-6044.
6. Shibata, D., Steczko, J., Dixon, J.E., Hermodson, M., Yazdanparast, R. and Axelrod, B. (1987) J. Biol. Chem. 262, 10080-10085.
7. Shibata, D., Steczko, J., Dixon, J.E., Andrews, P.C., Hermodson, M. and Axelrod, B. (1988) J. Biol. Chem. 262, 6816-6821.
8. Yenofsky, R.L., Fine, M. and Liu, C. (1988) Mol. Gen. Genet. 211, 215-222.
9. Hogaboom, G.K., Cook, M., Newton, J.F., Varrichio, A., Shorr, R.G.L., Sarall, H.M. and Crooke, S.T. (1986) Mol. Pharmacol. 30, 510-519.
10. Sigall, E., Grunberger, D., Craik, C.S., Caughey, G.H. and Nadel, J.A. (1988) J. Biol. Chem. 263, 5328-5332.
11. Thiele, B.J., Black, E., Fleming, J., Nack, B., Rapoport, S.M. and Harrison, P.R. (1987) Biomed. Biochim. Acta 46, 120-123.
12. Dixon, R.A.F., Jones, R.E., Diehl, R.E., Bennett, C.D., Kargman, S. and Rouzer, C.A. (1988) Proc. Natl. Acad. Sci. USA 85, 416-420.
13. Dewitt, D.L. and Smith, W.L. (1988) Proc. Natl. Acad. Sci. USA 85, 1412-1416.
14. Merlie, J.P., Fagan, D., Mudd, J. and Needleman, P. (1988) J. Biol. Chem. 263, 3550-3553.
15. Funk, C.D., Rådmark, O., Fu, J.Y., Matsumoto, T., Jörnvall, H., Shimizu, T. and Samuelsson, B. (1987) Proc. Natl. Acad. Sci. USA 84, 6677-6681.
16. Minami, M., Ohno, S., Kawasaki, H., Rådmark, O., Samuelsson, B., Jörnvall, H., Shimizu, T., Seyama, Y. and Suzuki, K. (1987) J. Biol. Chem. 262, 13873-13876.
17. Rådmark, P., Shimizu, T., Jörnvall, H. and Samuelsson, B. (1984) J. Biol. Chem. 259, 12339-12345.
18. Heinemann, F.S. and Ozols, J. (1984) J. Biol. Chem. 259, 797-804.

19. Porter, T.D., Beck, T.W. and Kasper, C.B. (1986) Arch. Biochem. Biophys. 248, 121-129.
20. Chou, P.Y. and Fasman, G.D. (1974) Biochemistry 13, 211-221.
21. Hopp, T.P. and Woods, K.R. (1981) Proc. Natl. Acad. Sci. USA, 78, 3824-3828.
22. Evans, J.F., Nathaniel, D.J., Zamboni, R.J. and Ford-Hutchinson, A.W. (1985) J. Biol. Chem. 260, 10966-10970.

Advances in Prostaglandin, Thromboxane, and Leukotriene Research, Vol. 19, edited by B. Samuelsson, P. Y.-K. Wong, and F. F. Sun, Raven Press, Ltd., New York ©1989.

CHEMICAL MEDIATORS AND THE ANTI-THROMBOTIC PROPERTIES OF ENDOTHELIAL CELLS

Regina Botting and John R. Vane

The William Harvey Research Institute, St.Bartholomew's Hospital Medical College, Charterhouse Square, London, EC1 M 6BQ, U.K.

The vascular endothelium, which envelopes the circulating blood in a continuous monolayer, is mainly responsible for maintaining the fluidity of the blood as well as the integrity and patency of blood vessels. These properties of endothelial cells (EC) have been linked with their capacity to synthesize a large number of active substances such as prostacyclin (PGI_2)(1), 13-hydroxy-9,11-octadecadienoic acid (13-HODE)(2), 15-hydroxy-5,8,11,13-eicosatetraenoic acid (15-HETE), endothelium-derived relaxing factor (EDRF)(3), von Willebrand factor (4), tissue-type plasminogen activator (t-PA), t-PA inhibitors, growth promoting factors (5), platelet-activating factor (1-alkyl-2-acetyl-sn-glycero-3-phosphocholine, PAF or PAF-acether), mucopolysaccharides, type IV collagen, a wide range of antioxidant enzymes and others. Some metabolic functions of the endothelium (especially seen in the pulmonary endothelium) include conversion of angiotensin I to angiotensin II and inactivation of bradykinin and nucleotides. In addition, pO_2 in tissues has a strong influence on the biological functions of the endothelium. Here we consider prostacyclin and EDRF as mediators which contribute to the anti-thrombotic properties of the endothelium.

PROSTACYCLIN

The discoveries of thromboxane A_2 (made by platelets) and of prostacyclin (made by the vessel wall) have led to many important new concepts in vascular pathophysiology (6).

Prostacyclin is a dienoic bicyclic eicosanoid which derives from the membrane-bound fatty acid, all-cis 5,8,11,14-eicosatetraenoic acid (arachidonic acid, AA). The chemical instability of prostacyclin at physiological pH ($t^1/_2 \sim$ 3 min) is a result of the cleavage of its furane ring with subsequent formation of the prostaglandin (PG),6-keto-PGF$_{1\alpha}$. The biosynthesis of prostacyclin by EC is initiated either through a transmembrane transference of PG endoperoxides from platelets (7) or by intra-cellular generation from AA which is liberated from endothelial phospholipids by an activated phospholipase. A haeme-containing oxygenase (cyclo-oxygenase) that requires no external source of electrons both cyclizes AA and adds the 15-hydroperoxy group to form PGG$_2$. The hydroperoxy group of PGG$_2$ is reduced to the hydroxy group of PGH$_2$ by a peroxidase that utilises a wide variety of compounds to provide the requisite pair of electrons. Both enzymes are contained in a single 71-kilodalton protein. Cyclo-oxygenase is inhibited by aspirin and aspirin-like drugs (8) and its action is modulated by lipid hydroperoxides, including PGG$_2$. The reduction of hydroperoxy- to hydroxy-lipids is associated with the generation of oxygen free radicals, and very likely of hydroxyl radicals.

Several drugs, as well as endogenous mediators, stimulate the generation of prostacyclin by cultured EC or smooth muscle cells. Endogenous prostacyclin releasers which work in several systems, include bradykinin (BK), choline esters, AA, PGH$_2$, thrombin, trypsin, platelet-derived growth factor, epidermal growth factor, interleukin-1 and adenine nucleotides. Interestingly, these same substances also stimulate the release of EDRF from EC (see later).

Glucocorticosteroids and lipocortin (9,10), cyclo-oxygenase inhibitors (11), low density lipo-proteins loaded with lipid hydroperoxides (12) and, unexpectedly, vitamin K$_1$, all inhibit the biosynthesis of prostacyclin in EC.

The capacity of vascular tissue to generate prostacyclin decreases in old and in atherosclerotic (13) animals. Indeed, it has been postulated that there is a direct link between the ability of the vascular wall to synthesize prostacyclin and its susceptibility to thrombotic or atherosclerotic episodes.

The platelet-suppressant and vasodilator actions of prostacyclin (6) are mediated by the stimulation of adenylate cyclase in platelets (14) and in vascular smooth muscle. The fibrinolytic and "cytoprotective" properties of prostacyclin do not seem to be mediated by cAMP and yet their impact on the therapeutic prospects of prostacyclin and its analogues is noteworthy. Although prostacyclin exhibits fibrinolytic action ex vivo, it shows no activity when instilled onto euglobulin clots in vitro (15). Recently, the term "cellular protection" has been proposed for the protective effects of prostacyclin in vitro and "histoprotection" for the protection of tissues in vivo. Indeed, in vitro, prostacyclin protects platelets against deterioration (16), cardiac myocytes against hypoxic damage, glial cells and neurons against anoxic injury and hepatocytes against chemical damage (17).

In man, intravenous infusion of prostacyclin for several hours on each of 4 days promotes the healing of ischaemic skin ulcers (18). Prostacyclin also protects against post-ischaemic reperfusion damage to animal brains and hearts (19). Higenbottam (20) showed that continuous infusions of prostacyclin for up to 2 years allowed patients with severe pulmonary hypertension to live independently, whilst awaiting a heart-lung transplant.

ENDOTHELIUM-DERIVED RELAXING FACTOR

EDRF is a labile vasodilator with a half life counted in seconds. It was discovered by Furchgott and Zawadzki (4) who showed that the presence of the endothelial lining is obligatory for the vaso-relaxant action of acetylcholine (ACh) on aortic and arterial strips or rings isolated from rabbits. Thus, the activation of muscarinic receptors (4) on EC triggers the generation of a diffusible and transferable substance which relaxes vascular smooth muscle; hence the name EDRF. Other substances which release EDRF from EC include BK (21), angiotensin II, histamine (via H_1 type receptors), noradrenaline (via α_2 adrenoceptors),5-hydroxytryptamine, ergometrine, calcium ionophore A23187 (22), thimerosal (a mercurial disinfectant), adenine nucleotides, thrombin, AA (23), melittin and various peptides (24). Pulsatile pressure (25), visible light and electrical field-stimulation also release EDRF and more is formed in arteries than in veins.

Vascular smooth muscle is the obvious target for the biological action of EDRF, but it also potently inhibits platelet aggregation and adhesion (26,27). Guanylate cyclase is stimulated by EDRF resulting in an increase in intracellular cGMP (28).

EDRF is also released in the iliac and epicardial arteries of conscious dogs and in arterioles on the brain surface of anaesthetised mice (29). These data obtained in vivo are in accord with the concept that endothelial production of EDRF provides the vascular wall with a shield against the vasospasm brought about by vasoconstrictors released from activated platelets.

Endothelium-dependent relaxation is impaired in arteries from hypercholestrolaemic rabbits and monkeys and from atherosclerotic humans (30). In humans, an intracoronary infusion of ACh resulted in vasodilation of healthy arteries and vasoconstriction of their stenotic atherosclerotic branches.

The chemical structure of EDRF has been intensively investigated. Activation of guanylate cyclase is common to both glyceryl trinitrate (GTN) and EDRF. EDRF is the only endogenous mediator known so far which exerts its physiological actions by activation of the soluble guanylate cyclase of smooth muscle cells. The analogy between the mechanisms of stimulation of guanylate cyclase by EDRF and GTN (31) led both Furchgott (32) and Ignarro (33) to speculate that EDRF was nitric oxide (NO).

Recent studies indeed show that EDRF released from cultured porcine EC is NO or a chemically related radical (34). EDRF released from perfused cultured EC by bradykinin or NO gas dissolved in deoxygenated water both relaxed the bioassay vascular smooth muscle in a dose dependent manner. The relaxation induced by EDRF or NO declined at the same rate ($t^{1}/_{2}$ ~ 4s) during passage down the isolated tissue cascade (35). The actions of both EDRF and NO were inhibited by haemoglobin (which binds NO) and potentiated by SOD (36). Superoxide anions must, therefore, contribute to the inactivation of both substances.

Finally, NO was assayed chemically as the chemiluminescent product of its reaction with ozone. NO was released from porcine EC by bradykinin in amounts that accounted for the actions of EDRF, showing that this EDRF was identical to NO (34). EDRF released from EC of bovine pulmonary artery and vein by ACh or bradykinin also behaved chemically like NO (37).This EDRF produced identical shifts in absorption spectrum peaks to genuine NO during its reaction with haemoglobin.

EDRF from porcine aortic EC and NO gas have also been tested on platelet aggregation. The anti-aggregatory activity of both was potentiated by SOD and the selective inhibitor of cGMP phosphodiesterase, M&B 22948 (38) and inhibited by haemoglobin and Fe^{2+}. Moreover, there was synergism between the anti-aggregatory effect of prostacyclin and subthreshold concentrations of EDRF or NO (39). As well

as inhibiting human platelet aggregation, EDRF
released from cultured bovine aortic EC by bradykinin
or NO gas reduced their adhesion to EC (26,27).

THE RELEASE OF PROSTACYCLIN AND EDRF IS COUPLED

Substances which generate PGI_2 also largely
stimulate the release of EDRF. What, then, is the
chain of events that leads to the coupled release of
PGI_2 and EDRF from EC? The first step is receptor
activation. We (40) have not attempted a rigorous
classification of the different receptors involved.
However, the fact that ADP and ATP, but not AMP or
adenosine, stimulate release of EDRF and PGI_2
suggests that ADP and ATP are acting at P_2-purinergic
receptors. Försberg et al.(41) also found that ATP
and ADP released PGI_2 from bovine adrenal medullary
EC whereas adenosine and AMP were ineffective.

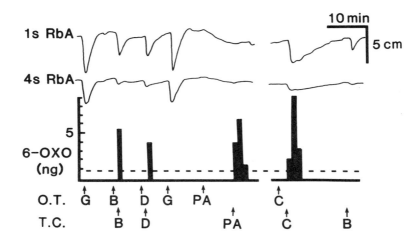

Figure 1 - Release of EDRF and PGI_2 by phospholipases. The
perfusate from the column of EC superfused a cascade of 4 rabbit
aortic strips (RbA,two not shown). Injections of agonists were
given over the tissues (O.T.) or through the endothelial cell
column (T.C.). EDRF was released from EC by 0.6 U phospholipase
C (C) but not 0.2 U phospholipase A_2 (PA). The EC were treated
with SOD (10 U/ml). G, 40 pmoles glyceryl trinitrate ; B, 10
pmoles bradykinin ; D, 2 nmoles ADP. The broken line (- - -)
indicates basal release of $6\text{-oxo-PGF}_{1\alpha}$ (6-oxo).

In our experiments (40), BK, Lys-BK, Met-Lys-BK and des-Arg-BK released EDRF and PGI_2 although the latter two analogues were less potent, des-Arg-BK being the weakest. These results suggest that BK acts on the B_2 kinin receptor proposed by Regoli et al. (42).

The formation of diacylglycerol and inositol polyphosphates by activation of phospholipase C (PLC) is now well established and our experiments suggest that release of EDRF as well as PGI_2 is due to activation of a PLC mechanism of transduction. For instance, exogenous PLC induces release of EDRF and PGI_2 (Fig.1, Table 1) whereas phospholipases B and D do not. Phospholipase A_2 released PGI_2 only (Fig.1). BK is a potent stimulus for the release of both PGI_2 and EDRF from bovine and porcine EC (37). Indeed, in porcine EC, BK activates phospholipases A_2 and C leading to rapid production of IP_3 with a subsequent mobilization of Ca^{++} and liberation of AA. In addition, ATP-stimulated PGI_2 formation is secondary to ATP-induced inositol phospholipid metabolism in adrenal medullary EC. Thus, activation of a PLC by BK or ADP provides a common transduction mechanism for the generation of both PGI_2 and EDRF in EC.

Inhibitors of phospholipase A_2 such as dexamethasone (43) or lipocortin (44) had no effect on EDRF or PGI_2 release induced by BK, ADP or AA, in agreement with the results of Föstermann et al (45).

Diacylglycerol is either hydrolyzed by lipases to monoacylglycerol and then to free arachidonate and glycerol or is phosphorylated by diacylglycerol kinase to form phosphatidic acid, which is then used in the re-synthesis of phosphoinositides. R59022 inhibits diacylglycerol kinase and should increase intracellular concentrations of diacylglycerol. R59022 had two effects: increased basal release of both EDRF and PGI_2 and thereafter, a substantially reduced release of EDRF and PGI_2 induced by BK and ADP. The release of EDRF induced by AA was also reduced as was the release of PGI_2 to a lesser extent. This enhancement in basal release of both substances, without the involvement of receptor activation reinforces our view on the coupling of EDRF and PGI_2 release. The reduction of receptor-stimulated release would follow from increased protein kinase C activity.

Diacylglycerol activates protein kinase C as does PMA. In polymorphonuclear leukocytes, PMA disrupts coupling of the G protein to PLC, suggesting a negative feedback signal induced by protein kinase C activation. This may be the mechanism by which R59022 and PMA inhibit receptor-mediated EDRF and

TABLE I. Release of PGI$_2$ from endothelial cells

Agonist	1st min	2nd min	3rd min	n
BK 10 pmol	4.1±0.5	7.1±1.2	1.6±0.1	16
ADP 10 nmol	7.5±1.8	7.5±1.5	1.5±0.2	11
ATP 10 pmol	1.2±0.2	2.3±0.6	2.3±0.8	3
AA 90 nmol	14.5±2.6	23.5±3.3	10.5±1.9	15
PLC 0.2-5 U	4.0±1	5.5±1.5	5.5±1.2	6
PLA$_2$ 0.1-1 U	6.1±4.5	8±5.4	2.8±1.6	5

[a]PGI$_2$ was measured as ng/min 6-oxo-PGF$_{1\alpha}$ during 1st, 2nd and 3rd min after injection of agonists through the endothelial cells.

[b]In all these experiments, basal release of PGI$_2$ was <1ng/min.

[c]Values represent mean±SEM. PLC, phospholipase C; PLA$_2$,phospholipase A$_2$.

PGI_2 release in our experiments and PMA inhibits EDRF release in those of others using smooth muscle strips.

The identification of EDRF as NO (34,37) accords with the fact that both are destroyed by O_2^- (36). EDRF is released from EC by a calcium ionophore, which triggers the release of O_2^- from human EC (46). Our results also point to the continuous basal release from EC of both EDRF (NO) and O_2^-, for infusions of SOD through the EC revealed a basal release of EDRF and substantially increased the amounts of EDRF detected after stimulation with agonists such as BK or ADP. The identity of the substance released by BK, ADP, AA and PLC was further confirmed as EDRF by its instability and by infusing MeB which inhibits activation of guanylate cyclase in smooth muscle. MeB completely abolished relaxations produced by EDRF (NO) released from EC.

How is the release of EDRF coupled to that of PGI_2? Clearly, ligand/receptor interactions are a common step and an increase in cytosolic Ca^{++} is needed for release of both EDRF and PGI_2 so this may also be a common trigger. We have not identified the biochemical pathway leading to EDRF (NO), but the lack of effect of inorganic nitrites or nitrates in causing its release from EC would suggest that an organic source is more likely. In this context, it is interesting that macrophages synthesize nitrite, nitrate and N-nitrosamines from L-arginine (47) and that horseradish peroxidase converts N-hydroxy-N-nitrosamines by 1-electron oxidation to nitric oxide. A possible explanation of the coupling of EDRF (NO) release with that of prostacyclin arises from the observation that prostaglandin synthetase (which includes a peroxidase) in the presence of AA can catalyze 1-electron oxidation of nitrogen-containing substrates. L-arginine can also activate soluble guanylate cyclase from neuroblastoma cells. Surprisingly, the peptides which release EDRF all seem to contain arginine.

Our conclusion that activation of the same receptors ultimately leads to release of both EDRF and PGI_2 suggests that these substances act in concord as a common mechanism of defence for the EC. The synergism already shown between EDRF (NO) and PGI_2 (39) in preventing platelet activation then takes on a new dimension, especially if there is also concerted and synergistic action against interaction of other circulating cells with the EC.

At the time of writing, another important mediator released by the EC, endothelin, has been discovered and characterised (48). It is a potent vasoconstrictor.

REFERENCES

1. Moncada S, Gryglewski RJ, Bunting S, Vane JR. Nature 1976;263:663-665.
2. Buchanan MR, Haas TA, Lagarde M, Guichardant M. J Biol Chem 1985;260:16056-16059.
3. Furchgott RF, Zawadzki JV. Nature 1980;286:373-376.
4. Jaffe EA. N Engl J Med 1977;296:377-386.
5. Ross R, Raines EW, Bowen-Pope DF. Cell 1986;46:155-169.
6. Moncada S, Vane JR. Pharmacol Rev 1979;30:293-331.
7. Bunting S, Gryglewski RJ, Moncada S, Vane JR. Prostaglandins 1976;12:897-913.
8. Vane JR. Nature (New Biol) 1971;231:232-235.
9. Gryglewski RJ, Panczenko B, Korbut R, Grodzińska L, Ocetkiewicz A. Prostaglandins 1975;10:343-355.
10. Flower RJ, Wood JM, Parente W. In: Otterness I, Capetola R, Wong S. eds, Adv Inflammation Res vol 7. New York: Raven Press, 1984;61-70.
11. Gryglewski RJ, Moncada S, Palmer RMJ. Br J Pharmacol 1986;87:685-694.
12. Szczeklik A, Gryglewski RJ. Artery 1980;7:489-491.
13. Gryglewski RJ, Dembinska-Kieć A, Żmuda A, Gryglewska T. Atherosclerosis 1978;31:385-394.
14. Tateson JE, Moncada S, Vane JR. Prostaglandins 1977; 13:389-397.
15. Gryglewski RJ, Korbut R, Radomski M. In: USA-Poland Symposium:Cardiovascular Disease. Warsaw-June 1984, NIH Publication No86-2642, 1986;9-16.
16. Blackwell GJ, Radomski M, Vargas JR, Moncada S. Biochim Biophys Acta 1982;718:60-65.
17. Bursch W, Schulte-Hermann R. In: Gryglewski RJ, Stock G, eds. Prostacyclin and Its Stable Analogue Iloprost, Berlin: Springer-Verlag, 1987;257-268.
18. Niżankowski R, Królikowski W, Bielatowicz J, Schaller J, Szczeklik A. In: Gryglewski R J, Szczeklik A, McGiff JC. eds Prostacyclin-Clinical Trials, New York: Raven Press, 1985;15-22.
19. Simpson PJ, Lucchesi BR. In: Gryglewski RJ, Stock G, eds Prostacyclin and Its Stable Analogue Iloprost, Berlin; Springer-Verlag, 1987;179-194.
20. Higgenbottam T. Am Rev Respir Dis 1987;136:782-785.
21. Cherry PD, Furchgott RF, Zawakzki JV, Jothianadan D. Proc Natl Acad Sci USA 1982;79:2106-2110.
22. Singer HA, Peach MJ. J Pharmacol Exp Ther 1983; 226:796-801.

23. De Mey JG, Claey M, Vanhoutte PM. J Pharmacol Exp Ther 1982;222:166-173.
24. Furchgott RF, Cherry PD, Zawadzki JV, Jothianandan D. J Cardiovasc Pharmacol 1984; 6: S336-S343.
25. Pohl U, Holtz J, Busse R, Bassenge E. Hypertension 1986;8:37-44.
26. Radomski MW, Palmer RMJ, Moncada S. Lancet 1987; ii:1057-1058.
27. Sneddon JM, Vane JR. Proc Natl Acad Sci USA 1988;85:(in press).
28. Griffith TM, Edwards DH, Lewis MJ, Henderson AH. Eur J Pharmacol 1985;112:195-202.
29. Watanabe M, Rosenblum WI, Nelson GH. Circ Res 1988;62:86-90.
30. Förstermann U, Mùgge A, Alheid U, Haverich A, Frölich JC. Circ Res 1988;62:185-190.
31. Murad FJ. J Clin Invest 1986;78:1-5.
32. Kahn MT, Furchgott RF. Fed Proc 1987;46:385.
33. Ignarro LJ, Byrns RE, Buga GM, Wood KS. Fed Proc 1987;46:644.
34. Palmer RMJ, Ferridge AG, Moncada S. Nature 1987; 327:524-526.
35. Vane JR. Br J Pharmacol Chemother 1964;23:360-373.
36. Gryglewski RJ, Palmer RMJ, Moncada S. Nature 1986;320:454-456.
37. Ignarro LJ, Byrns RE, Buga GM, Wood KS, Chaudhuri G. J Pharm Exp Ther 1988;244:181-189.
38. Radomski MW, Palmer RMJ, Moncada S. Br J Pharmacol 1987;92:181-187.
39. Radomski MW, Palmer RMJ, Moncada S. Br J Pharmacol 1987;92:639-646.
40. De Nucci G, Gryglewski RJ, Warner TD, Vane JR. Proc Natl Acad Sci USA 1988;85:(in press).
41. Försberg EJ, Feuerstein G, Shohami E, Pollard HB. Proc Natl Acad Sci USA 1987;84:5630-5634.
42. Regoli D, Barabé J. Pharmacol Rev 1980;32:1-46.
43. Blackwell GJ, Flower RJ, Nikjamp F, Vane JR. Br J Pharmacol 1978;62:79-89.
44. Blackwell GJ, Carnuccio R, DiRosa M, Flower RJ, Parente L, Persico P. Nature 1980;287:147-149.
45. Förstermann U, Burgwitz K, Frölich JC. J Cardiovasc Pharmacol 1987;10:356-364.
46. Matsubara T, Ziff M. J Cell Physiol 1986;127:207-210.
47. Iyengar R, Stuehr DJ, Marletta MA. Proc Natl Acad Sci USA 1987;84:6369-6373.
48. Yanagisawa M, Kurihara H, Kimura S, et al. Nature 1988; 332:411-415.

Advances in Prostaglandin, Thromboxane, and
Leukotriene Research, Vol. 19, edited by
B. Samuelsson, P. Y.-K. Wong, and F. F. Sun,
Raven Press, Ltd., New York ©1989.

THE CELL BIOLOGY AND BIOCHEMISTRY OF LEUKOTRIENE C_4 BIOSYNTHESIS

R.J. Soberman, and K.F. Austen

From the Department of Medicine, Harvard Medical School,
and the Department of Rheumatology and Immunology,
Brigham and Women's Hospital, Boston, MA 02115

This work was supported by grants AI-22531, AI-22563, AI-23401,
AR-38638, and HL-36110 from The National Institutes of Health,
and a grant-in-aid from The American Heart Association with
funds contributed in part by the Massachusetts affiliate.

Leukotrienes are biologically active oxygenated metabolites
of membrane-derived arachidonic acid (AA) which have been implicated in playing a role in the pathogenesis of a variety of
inflammatory and allergic disease states, including asthma. The
production of leukotriene C_4 (LTC_4) must be understood in terms
of a cascade of discrete enzymological reactions. Though this is
clearly true, the situation is far more complex. Not only does
LTC_4 alter the microenvironment, but the local cellular immune
response alters the amount and location of LTC_4 produced at the
tissue level. This concept will become apparent as we review the
biosynthesis of LTC_4 from this integrated perspective.
As initially stated, to understand the role of the sulfidopeptide leukotrienes in these processes, it is necessary to
understand the cell biological, biochemical, and molecular
biological control of the enzymes regulating LTC_4 biosynthesis.
AA released from the membranes of polymorphonuclear leukocytes
(PMN), human monocytes, eosinophils, and various other cell
types, is acted on by the enzyme 5-lipoxygenase (5-LO) (1-3) to
form 5-hydroperoxy-6,8,11,14-eicosatetraenoic acid (5-HPETE),
which is converted by the same enzyme to 5,6-oxido-7,9-trans-
11,14-cis-eicosatetraenoic acid (LTA_4) (4-7). In monocytes (8)
and eosinophils (9, 10), LTA_4 can be conjugated with reduced
glutathione (GSH) by the enzyme LTC_4 synthase (11) to form 5S-
hydroxy-6R-S-glutathionyl-7,9-trans-11,14-cis-eicosatetraenoic
acid (LTC_4) (12, 13). LTC_4 synthase is the microsomal enzyme
which conjugates LTA_4 with GSH to form LTC_4.

Because of our previous knowledge that sensitized guinea pig lung responds to an antigen challenge with the production of LTD_4 (14), we utilized this organ as a source for large scale purification of LTC_4 synthase. LTC_4 synthase was localized to the microsomes of lung. When LTC_4 synthase was solubilized from guinea pig microsomes (15), this enzyme demonstrated an apparent MW of 56,000, as determined by Sepharose CL-4B gel filtration chromatography, whereas the microsomal GSH-S-transferase utilizing 1-chloro-2,4-dinitrobenzene as a substrate had an apparent MW of 34,000 allowing it to be separated from LTC_4 synthase by Sepharose CL-4B gel filtration chromatography. After Sepharose CL-4B chromatography, LTC_4 synthase was purified by DEAE Sephacel ion exchange chromatography (with LTC_4 synthase appearing in the flow-through), followed by concentration on and elution from aminobutyl Sepharose and gradient elution from a DEAE 3SW anion exchange column. The final purification was 91-fold. This preparation of the enzyme demonstrates a K_m of 3 μM for LTA_4 and 16 μM for LTA_4 methyl-ester (LTA_4-Me). However, the V_{max} for LTA_4-Me was 420 nmol/3 min/mg protein, as opposed to 204 nmol/min/mg protein from LTA_4, allowing LTA_4-Me to be used as the substrate in routine assays. A known property of GSH-S-transferases is that they manifest product inhibition at product concentrations near the K_m of the enzyme for the respective xenobiotic substrate. To examine if this was the case for LTC_4 synthase, we determined the K_i of LTC_4 synthase using LTA_4-Me as the substrate and either LTC_4-Me or LTC_4 as the inhibitor. LTC_4 was found to have a K_i of 3.3 μM. At a concentration of 10 μM, LTC_4-Me inhibited the conversion of LTA_4-Me to its product by 40% (15), suggesting a potential role for product inhibition in the regulation of enzyme activity.

More significantly, this property of product inhibition suggested to us that an affinity column could be designed based on the structure of LTC_4. To accomplish this, the hydrazide of 11,12,14,15-tetrahydro-LTC_4 ("LTC_2") was prepared and covalently coupled to Affigel 10. This allowed us to modify our previous purification scheme for guinea pig lung microsome LTC_4 synthase by elimination of the agarose butylamine column and the DEAE 3SW column, and substitution with the "LTC_2" affinity column. This scheme is outlined below:

SOLUBILIZATION
v
SEPHAROSE CL-4B GEL FILTRATION CHROMATOGRAPHY
v
DEAE SEPHACEL ION EXCHANGE CHROMATOGRAPHY
v
LTC_2 AFFINITY CHROMATOGRAPHY

Specific elution of LTC_4 synthase from the affinity column with GSH yielded a preparation showing only two bands of ~17,500 MW each. Rat microsomal GSH-S-transferase has been purified and its full length amino acid sequence determined by both amino acid sequencing and cDNA cloning and found to have a MW of 17,000 (16). Whether the two bands of similar size seen on the gel of LTC_4 synthase represent two subunits of the same enzyme, isozymes of LTC_4 synthase, or two unrelated proteins remains to be determined. These data suggest that LTC_4 synthase is a novel member of the family of microsomal GSH-S-transferases. Whether LTC_4 synthase is the product of a separate gene from the GSH-S-transferase or represents alternative splicing of mRNA is not known.

Within the family of neutrophilic leukocytes, LTC_4 synthase is found predominantly in eosinophils, to a far lesser extent in monocytes, and is not present in PMN (17). Thus, in relation to many allergic diseases, what controls the recruitment, viability, and functional state of eosinophils is an important control of the production of LTC_4 at any given tissue site.

When isolated from discontinuous metrizamide or Percoll gradients, eosinophils obtained from the peripheral blood of asthmatic patients contain cells which sediment at a lighter density on metrizamide gradients, termed "hypodense", and also cells termed "normodense" which sediment at a higher density (18). Hypodense cells possess a variety of augmented biological and biochemical responses as compared to normodense cells (e.g., 19, 20). Among these is an increase in LTC_4 production in response to calcium ionophore A23187.

Recently, work in our laboratory has shown that normodense peripheral blood eosinophils cultured in the presence of either recombinant human granulocyte macrophage colony-stimulating factor (rhGM-CSF) or interleukin 3 (rhIL-3) can be converted in vitro to hypodense cells having the same augmented biological and biochemical properties as freshly isolated hypodense eosinophils (19,20). After culture for one week with 50 pM rhGM-CSF in the presence of a fibroblast monolayer, 67 ± 6% (mean ± SEM, n = 8) of eosinophils remained alive and were converted to the hypodense phenotype with augmented LTC_4 production, but virtually no eosinophils survived for >2 days in the absence of rhGM-CSF. Cells cultured in the presence of rhGM-CSF or rhIL-3 acquired an augmented ability to kill schistosomula and increased their ability to generate LTC_4 in response to calcium ionophore A23187 by 2.5-fold (19, 20). These data indicate that T cell-derived cytokines can augment both eosinophil viability and function in vitro. We have recently shown that recombinant mouse interleukin 5 (rhIL-5) can convert normodense cells to the hypodense phenotype in vitro and concomitantly augment both eosinophil viability and function in the same manner as GM-CSF (21). Eosinophils derive from bone marrow precursor cells, in the presence of IL-5, GM-CSF and IL-3 (22-24). Thus, the late stage differentiation of eosinophils is distinct from PMN and is coordinated with the expression of the LTC_4 synthase gene. The eventual cloning of the LTC$_4$ synthase cDNA will allow--coupled with the development in our laboratory of prolonged in vitro culture of eosinophils--the unique opportunity for studies of the regulation of the expression of the gene for LTC$_4$ synthase in these cells.

1. Rouzer CA, Samuelsson B. Proc Natl Acad Sci USA 1985;82: 6040.

2. Goetze A, Fayer L, Bouska J, Dommerer D, Carter GW. Prostaglandins 1985;29:689.

3. Soberman RJ, Harper TW, Betteridge D, Lewis RA, Austen KF J Biol Chem 1985;260:4508.

4. Shimizu T, Rådmark O, Samuelsson B. Proc Natl Acad Sci USA 1984;81:689.

5. Rouzer CA, Matsumoto T, Samuelsson B. Proc Natl Acad Sci USA 1984;83:857.

6. Rådmark O, Malmsten C, Samuelsson B, Goto G, Marfat A, Corey EJ. J Biol Chem 1980;255:11828.

7. Corey EJ, Arai Y, Mioskowski C. J Amer Chem Soc 1979;101: 7131.

8. Williams JD, Czop JK, Austen KF. J Immunol 1984;132:2024.

9. Weller PF, Lee CW, Foster DW, Corey EJ, Lewis RA, Austen KF. Proc Natl Acad Sci USA 1983;80:7626.

10. Owen WF Jr, Soberman RJ, Yoshimoto T, Sheffer AL, Lewis RA, Austen KF. J Immunol 1987;138:532.

11. Yoshimoto T, Soberman RJ, Lewis RA, Austen KF. Proc Natl Acad Sci USA 1985;82:8399.

12. Murphy RC, Hammarstrom S, Samuelsson B. Proc Natl Acad Sci USA 1979;76:4275.

13. Corey EJ, Barton AE, Clark DA. J Amer Chem Soc 1980;102: 4278.

14. Morris HR, Taylor GW, Piper PJ, Tippins JR. Nature 1980; 285:104.

15. Yoshimoto T, Soberman RJ, Spur B, Austen KF. J Clin Invest 1988,81:866.

16. Morganstern R, DePierre JW, Jornvall H. J Biol Chem 1985;260:13976.

17. Owen WF, Soberman RJ, Yoshimoto T, Sheffer AL, Lewis RA, Austen KF. J Immunol 1987;138:532.

18. Fukuda T, Dunnette SL, Reed CE, Ackerman SJ, Peters MS, Gleich GJ. Am Rev Respir Dis 1985;132:981.

19. Owen WF, Rothenberg ME, Silberstein DS et al. J Exp Med 1987;166:129.

20. Rothenberg ME, Owen WF, Silberstein DS et al. J Clin Invest (in press).

21. Rothenberg ME, Owen WF, Soberman RJ, Austen KF, Stevens RL. FASEB 1988;2:7563 (abstract).

22. Metcalf D, Begley CG, Johnson GR et al. Blood 1986; 67:37.

23. Lopez AF, To LB, Yang Y-C et al. Proc Natl Acad Sci USA 1987;84:2761.

24. Campbell HD, Tucker WQJ, Hort Y et al. Proc Natl Acad Sci USA 1987,84:6629.

Advances in Prostaglandin, Thromboxane, and
Leukotriene Research, Vol. 19, edited by
B. Samuelsson, P. Y.-K. Wong, and F. F. Sun,
Raven Press, Ltd., New York ©1989.

PROSTAGLANDIN D_2 AND SLEEP

Osamu Hayaishi

Hayaishi Bioinformation Transfer Project, Research Development
Corporation of Japan, c/o Osaka Medical College,
2-7 Daigakumachi, Takatsuki, Osaka 569, Japan

Prostaglandins are ubiquitously distributed in virtually
all mammalian tissues and organs and exhibit numerous and diverse
biological activities under a variety of physiological and pathological conditions. However, relatively little was known about
the presence, metabolism, and function of prostaglandins in
the central nervous system until recently. In the late 1970s
several groups of investigators including our own demonstrated
that prostaglandin D_2 is one of the major prostaglandins in
the rat brain. This particular prostaglandin had been neglected
by most investigators in this field, because the amount of PGD_2
in most other tissues is reportedly almost insignificant and
also because it had generally been considered to be biologically
inactive. Subsequently, the presence of a relatively large
amount of PGD_2 was also observed in the CNS of other mammals
including humans, indicating that prostaglandin D_2 is unique
among the prostaglandins in having a high concentration in the
mammalian brain. We therefore investigated the metabolism and
enzymes involved in the biosynthesis and degradation of prostaglandin D_2 in the CNS. Our results indicated that prostaglandin
D_2 is actively synthesized and metabolized by specific enzymes
in neurons and glia cells. We then decided to investigate the
neural functions of prostaglandin D_2 in the brain.

In order to approach this problem, we isolated, partially
purified, and characterized binding proteins, or the putative
receptors, of prostaglandins in the CNS. We also studied the
intracerebral distribution of these binding proteins by radio-
autography combined with computer-assisted image processing
with color coding (1). Our results indicated that the binding
protein for prostaglandin D_2 is found mainly in the gray matter,
namely, the neuron-rich areas, and is highly concentrated in
certain specific areas such as the olfactory bulb, cerebral
cortex, occipital cortex, hippocampus, hypothalamus, and preoptic
area, indicating that PGD_2 may be involved in certain specific
neural functions. Much less binding is seen in cerebellum,
brain stem, and midbrain.

The preoptic area has been long known as the center of regulation of sleep and body temperature. For example, in 1946, Nauta,
a Dutch anatomist, showed that when the preoptic area of a rat

was destroyed, slow-wave sleep was no longer observable (2). Then, in 1962, Stermann and Clemente reported that slow-wave sleep could be induced by electric stimulation of the preoptic area (3). However, the chemical mechanisms involved in the induction of sleep were not elucidated until now. To see if PGD_2 and/or other PG's are biochemical sleep inducers, we micro-injected PG's into the preoptic area. As a result, we found that microinjection of small amounts of PGD_2, but not of other PG's, into the preoptic area of the rat could induce sleep in a dose-dependent manner. For example, when saline was injected into the preoptic area of the control rats, under conditions of sleep depriviation, the rats were awake most of the time. However, when nanomolar amounts of PGD_2 were microinjected, the awake period was decreased almost 50% and slow-wave sleep was increased more than fivefold (Fig. 1). The site of action

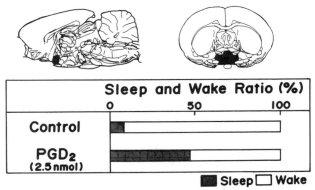

FIG. 1. MICROINJECTION OF PGD_2 INTO THE PREOPTIC AREA.

was quite specific for the preoptic area, since the injection of PGD_2 into other areas, for example, the posterior hypothalamus, was hardly effective (4). Subsequently, Garcia-Arraras and Pappenheimer of Harvard Medical School using muramyl peptide as a sleep inducing agent have confirmed that the preoptic area is the center of sleep regulation (5). Further, Kruger in Memphis showed that prostaglandin D_2 induces sleep in rabbits instead of rats (6). Roberts, Oats and coworkers in Nashville reported that patients with systemic mastocytosis go into deep sleep after the episode in which large amounts of prostaglandin D_2 is endogenously produced in mast cells, suggesting that PGD_2 induces sleep in humans, too (7).

In order to obtain more quantitative data and to critically evaluate the effect of PGD_2 on sleep, we next employed a more sophisticated continuous infusion method in collaboration with Professor Inoue of Tokyo Dental and Medical University.

Male Sprague-Dawley rats weighing about 300 gr were used for most experiments. Various electrodes and a cannula were implanted in the brain at least 7 days before the experiments. After surgery, the rat was housed in a cage placed in a sound-

proof and air-conditioned room. Lighting was controlled artificially. Food and water were available <u>ad libitum</u>. A slip ring
allowed unrestrained movement of the rat. PGD_2 was infused
through the cannula continuously for 10 hr into the third ventricle of the brain. The sleep stages were determined on the basis
of the polygraphic recordings of EEG (electroencepharogram),
EMG (electromyogram), and locomotion, and the sleep scores were
computed·by and stored in a central processing unit. The behavior of the rat was monitored by a video-recording system.

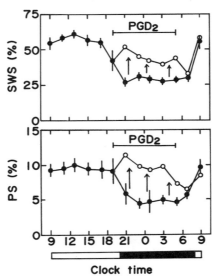

Clock time

FIG. 2. EFFECT OF PGD_2 ON SLEEP PATTERNS OF RATS.

Fig. 2 shows the effect of PGD_2 on sleep patterns, when a
small amount of PGD_2 was slowly and continuously infused into
the third ventricle. Here the vertical axis indicates the amount
of SWS (slow-wave sleep) and PS (paradoxical sleep) expressed
in % of total time of sleep; and the horizontal axis, the time
schedule. Rats are nocturnal animals and sleep during the day
but are awake most of the time during the night. When PGD_2
was infused at a rate of 0.6 pmole per minute during the night,
both slowwave sleep and paradoxical sleep increased as shown
here. The effect was dose-dependent and specific for PGD_2 (8).
As little as one femtomole (10^{-15} mol) per second was effective
in inducing excess sleep. Sleep induced by PGD_2 was indistinguishable from physiological sleep as judged by EEG, EMG, loco-
motor activities, and general behavior of the rat. Furthermore
PGD_2 is not pyrogenic and slightly decreases body temperature,
which decrease also occurs during physiological sleep. The
PGD synthetase activity exhibits a circadian fluctuation in
parallel with the sleep/wake cycle. In the light period when

rats mainly sleep, PGD_2 is more actively synthesized than in the dark period. When administered during the light period, exogenous PGD_2 fails to induce excess sleep presumably because the system has already been saturated. On the other hand, the administration of inhibitors of prostaglandin synthesis, such as indomethacin and diclofenac sodium, results in a decrease in the amount of diurnal sleep.

On the basis of these findings, we proposed in 1983 that PGD_2 is an endogenous regulator of physiological sleep in the rat. More recently, Matsumura in my laboratory has shown that intraventricular infusion of PGE_2 reduces the amount of diurnal sleep (Fig. 3). Here prostaglandin E_2 was infused at the rate of 10 pmole/min into the third ventricle of a rat during the day. The amount of slow-wave sleep was reduced to about 70% of the control and paradoxical sleep, to 37% (9).

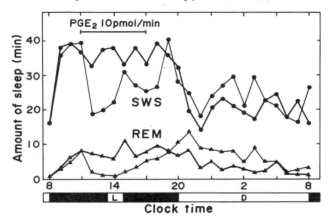

FIG. 3. EFFECT OF PGE_2 ON SLEEP PATTERNS OF RATS.

After the termination of infusion, there was a rebound and nocturnal sleep was increased to a significant extent, but the sleep pattern returned to normal during the next day. Whether or not this effect of PGE_2 on sleep is a primary effect of this particular PG is currently under investigation in our laboratory. Because the sleep pattern of rats is somewhat different from that of primates, we further extended these studies to the Rhesus monkey (Macaca Mulatta), and have shown that PGD_2 and E_2 are also sleep regulating agents in primates (10).

Adult male monkey weighing about 5-8 kg were used for the experiments. Various electrodes and a cannula were implanted into the animals at least one month before the experiments. Then monkeys were placed on monkey chairs with minimum restriction of body movement in an air-conditioned and sound proof room under an artificially controlled 12-hour light 12-hour dark cycle. The samples were dissolved in an artificial cerebrospinal fluid, which was then infused into the lateral or third ventricle through a cannula for 6 hours from 11:00 a.m. to 5:00

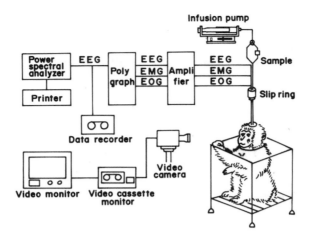

FIG. 4. BIOASSAY SYSTEM FOR SLEEP ANALYSES.

p.m. (Fig. 4). Sleep stages were monitored and determined by polygraphic recordings of EEG, EMG, and EOG (electrooculogram). The behavior of the monkey was monitored by a video recording system. All experiments were carried out with proper care and humane treatment of animals according to the NIH guideline for the care and use of laboratory animals.

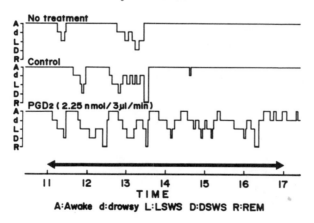

FIG. 5. SLEEP STAGE ALTERATION DURING INFUSION OF PGD_2 TO THE LATERAL VENTRICLE OF A CONSCIOUS MONKEY.

Fig. 5 shows the sleep diagrams of untreated, control, and PGD_2 infused monkeys. A,d,L,D,R stand for awake, drowsy, light and deep slow-wave sleep, and REM sleep, respectively. The sleep diagrams of untreated and artificial CSF-infused control monkeys were very similar, if not exactly identical. Like some human beings, this particular monkey takes a nap in the early afternoon. However, when about 2 nmoles/minute of PGD_2 were infused from 11 o'clock, drowsiness, light slow-wave sleep, and then deep slow-wave sleep were induced almost immediately, followed by occasional appearance of REM sleep, such a sleep pattern being almot identical to that of physiological sleep. The sleep-inducing activity is quite specific for PGD_2. Only D_3 is somewhat active, but PGE_2 is inhibitory and $F_{2\alpha}$, D_1, $9\beta-D_2$ and D_2 methylester are much less effective or inactive when 500 pmole/min of each PG were infused intraventricularly. This specificity coincides well with that of PGD_2 receptor in the monkey brain <u>in vitro</u>, suggesting that the process is probably receptor mediated.

In order to provide further evidence to show that PGD_2 induces physiological sleep, we compared power spectral data of EEG tracings of a Rhesus monkey infused with PGD_2 or artificial CSF. The spectral analysis permits dissection of an EEG signal into its frequency components and provides more qualitative and quantative information about the nature of sleep. The power spectral arrays of EEG obtained by infusion of PGD_2 during the day is essentially identical to those of the control animal and also to those of the experimental animal during the night, indicating that the sleep induced by PGD_2 during the day is indistinguishable from natural sleep during the night (Fig.6).

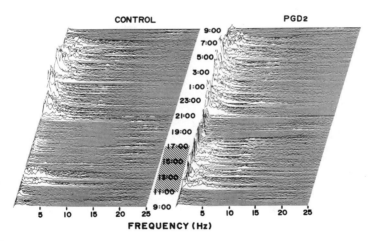

FIG. 6. POWER SPECTRAL ARRAYS DURING INFUSION OF PGD_2 IN RHESUS MONKEYS (2.5 NMOL/MIN).

Furthermore, after the termination of PGD_2 infusion, the circadian sleep pattern returned to normal and the nocturnal sleep was not affected, indicating that PGD_2 induces sleep without disturbing the sleep-awake rhythum. The infusion of PGD_2 caused a significant increase in power of the low frequency region with two sharp peaks in δ (delta) and θ (theta) wave regions (Fig. 7).

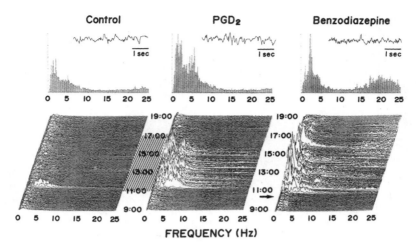

FIG. 7. POWER SPECTRAL ARRAYS OF EEG OF RHESUS MONKEY.

On the other hand, when bezodiazepine was administered per os shortly before 11 o'clock, the EEG tracing and power spectral arrays were clearly different in that there was a sharp peak in the δ wave region whereas the θ peak was almost nonexistent. Instead, the so-called benzodiazepine fast wave peak around 20 Hz was clearly evident. These data demonstrate that sleep induced by a sleep inducing drug is easily distinguishable from natural or PGD$_2$ induced sleep on the basis of EEG analysis.

In summary, 1. PGD$_2$ is the major PG in the CNS of the rat and other mammals including humans. 2. PGD$_2$ receptors are highly concentrated in the preoptic area, which is considered to be a center of sleep regulation. 3. Microinjection of PGD$_2$ into the preoptic area or intracerebroventricular infusion of as little as femtomole amounts of PGD$_2$ into rats and monkeys induces sleep which is indistinguishable from natural sleep on the basis of EEG, EMG, EOG, and behavior. 4. The effect is dose-dependent and specific for PGD$_2$. Other PG's are much less effective or totally inactive. On the other hand, PGE$_2$ inhibits sleep. 5. Inhibitors of PG synthesis decrease the amount of diurnal sleep of rats.

On the basis of these various lines of evidence, we conclude that prostaglandin D$_2$ induces sleep which is indistinguishable from physiological sleep and that PGD$_2$ and E$_2$ are the endogenous sleep-regulating substances which have been looked for by a number of investigators for so many years. What I have told you today is obviously not the final answer to solve the mystery of this complex phenomenon. However, it does provide clues that should lead to our ultimate understanding of the biological significance and biochemical mechanism of this interesting process.

Acknowledgement; This work has been carried out with the collaboration of the following coworkers: H. Onoe, H. Osama, K. Kin, H. Matsumura, R. Ueno, Research Development Corporation of Japan, Takatsuki, Y. Ishikawa, T. Nakayama, Osaka University, Osaka, K. Naitoh, K. Honda, S. Inoue, Tokyo Medical and Dental University, Tokyo, I. Fujita, H. Nishino, Y. Oomura, National Institute for Physiological Sciences, Okazaki.

REFERENCES

1. Yamashita A, Watanabe Y, Hayaishi O. Proc Natl Acad Sci USA 1980;80:6114-6118.

2. Nauta WJH. J Neurophysiol 1946;9:285-316.

3. Sterman MB, Clemente CD. Exp Neurol 1962;6:103-117.

4. Ueno R, Ishikawa Y, Nakayama T, Hayaishi O. Biochem Biophys Res Commun 1982;109(2):576-582.

5. Garcia-Arraras JE, Pappenheimer JR. J Neurophys 1983;49:528-533.

6. Krueger JM. In:Inoue S, Borbely AA, eds. Eighth Taniguchi International Symposium on Brain Sciences, Japan Scientific Societies Press, Tokyo, Japan.

7. Roberts II LJ, Sweetman BJ, Lewis RA, Austen KF, Oates JA, N Engl J Med 1980;303:1400.

8. Ueno R, Honda K, Inoue S, Hayaishi O. Proc Natl Acad Sci USA 1983;80:1735-1737.

9. Matsumura H, Honda K, Goh Y, Ueno T, Inoue S, Hayaishi O. Brain Res (in press).

10. Onoe H, Ueno R, Fujita I, Nishino H, Oomura Y, Hayaishi.O. Proc Natl Acad Sci USA (in press).

Advances in Prostaglandin, Thromboxane, and Leukotriene Research, Vol. 19, edited by B. Samuelsson, P. Y.-K. Wong, and F. F. Sun, Raven Press, Ltd., New York ©1989.

CYTOCHROME P450-DEPENDENT ARACHIDONATE METABOLITES:

BIOLOGICAL ACTIVITIES

J.C. McGiff and M.A. Carroll

Department of Pharmacology
New York Medical College
Valhalla, New York 10595 USA

Our studies of the past several years have addressed the biological importance of novel arachidonate metabolites formed via the cytochrome P450 monooxygenase system. We identified and characterized this pathway of arachidonic acid (AA) metabolism initially in epithelial cells isolated from the medullary thick ascending limb of Henle's loop (mTALH) of the rabbit kidney (1). This enzyme system is widely distributed, and the cytochrome P450-dependent oxygenated AA metabolites may, as prostanoids (2,3), make important contributions to the regulation of salt and water balance through renal tubular and hemodynamic actions as well as by effects on several transporting epithelia extrarenally.

Metabolism of AA via the cytochrome P450 monooxygenase system, the third pathway of AA metabolism, generates 1) epoxyeicosatrienoic acids (EETs): 5,6; 8,9; 11,12; 14,15 EETs, which can be enzymatically hydrolyzed by epoxide hydrolase to the corresponding dihydroxyeicosatrienoic acids (DHTs); 2) ω- and ω-1 hydroxylation products, 20- and 19-hydroxyeicosatetraenoic acids, and 3) monohydroxyeicosatetraenoic acids (HETEs). Cytochrome P450 exists in multiple forms which differ in substrate, and positional specificity and stereospecificity (4). Therefore, the predominance of one oxidation reaction over the other may be controlled by the isozyme composition of a given tissue or cell type.

The initial descriptions of the biological activities of AA metabolites arising from cytochrome P450 monooxygenases revealed similarities to prostanoids, i.e., they can act as secretagogues and local modulators of circulating hormones and their activity is usually circumscribed to the micro-environment of the cell of origin (5). Within segments of the nephron, cytochrome P450-dependent arachidonate metabolites, based on characterization of their principal biological activity, probably link renal tubular Na^+-K^+-ATPase activity to changes in local blood flow. They, thereby, couple a metabolic event to the regulation of zonal blood flow intrarenally. The evidence supporting this proposal will now be reviewed.

Incubation of mTALH cells with ^{14}C-labeled AA resulted in the formation of cytochrome P450-dependent oxygenated metabolites which were separated by reverse-phase chromatography into two major peaks designated P_1 and P_2 (6). The formation of these compounds was selectively stimulated by arginine vasopressin (AVP) and calcitonin at concentrations (10^{-10} to 10^{-8}M) shown to stimulate adenylate cyclase activity in the mTALH (7). As dibutyryl cAMP also stimulates cytochrome P450-AA metabolism by mTALH cells, these findings support the proposal of Morel (7) that segmentation of nephron responsiveness to hormones may be expressed through adenylate cyclase-sensitive receptors. For example, AVP stimulates two segments of the nephron, the cortical collecting tubules and the mTALH, via receptors coupled to adenylate cyclase. For each segment different metabolic pathways of AA metabolism are linked to AVP stimulation which is in accord with the findings that the natriuretic action of AVP is localized to mTALH (8) and can be dissociated from its effect on water reabsorption in the collecting system. For the latter site, prostanoids act to modulate the hydroosmotic action of AVP in contrast to the mTALH where cytochrome P450-dependent-AA metabolites either mediate or modulate the natriuretic action of AVP. A hormone-inducible modulator of Na^+-K^+-ATPase has long been sought (9), and our results indicate that this function may be invested in an AA metabolite arising from the cytochrome P450 system.

That the metabolites formed by a cytochrome P450 pathway in mTALH cells were capable of influencing cell function by altering ion transport was judged to be of paramount importance. We, therefore, examined the effects of P_1 and P_2 on Na^+-K^+-ATPase activity on a microsomal preparation of the canine heart (6). P_2 proved to be a potent inhibitor (IC_{50} ca 0.1 μM) of cardiac Na^+-K^+-ATPase, whereas P_1 was a weak inhibitor (IC_{50} ca 3 μM). Preliminary GC/MS identification indicated that P_2 contained a structure similar to that of 11,12 DHT (6) which presumably arises from transformation of 11,12 EET via an epoxide hydrolase. We have now confirmed the presence of 11,12 DHT in P_2. Thus, the cells of mTALH generate a compound that can affect the activity of the Na^+-K^+-ATPase pump. These findings suggest that a mechanism operating through AA metabolism in mTALH governs the reabsorption of sodium, potassium and chloride in this segment of the nephron.

The cytochrome P450-dependent AA metabolite(s) may, therefore, link hormonal stimulation to regulation of transport function of the mTALH. A corollary of this function is that the AA metabolite(s) can participate in the regulation of the countercurrent multiplication system for mediating water excretion. Persuant to this proposal, DHTs have been reported to inhibit osmotic water flow in the toad urinary bladder (10).

The vasomotor effect of the cytochrome P450-dependent AA metabolites generated by mTALH was examined using isolated blood vessels and perfused organs. P_1, but not P_2, relaxed rabbit pulmonary artery rings precontracted with phenylephrine: P_1 (ca 10^{-8}M) resulted in 40 to 60% relaxation, whereas 10^{-6}M P_2 did not affect vascular tone. Acetylcholine (10^{-7}M) relaxed vascular rings by 35 to 40%. We have reported that the mass spectrum of a component in P_1 possesses many of the structural features of the 5,6 EET (6) which has been shown to be a vasodilator (11). The 5,6 EET, unlike 8,9; 11,12 and 14,15 EETs, dilates the perfused rat-tail artery. It was the only cytochrome P450-dependent metabolite to decrease resistance of the tail artery, being equipotent to acetylcholine. The corresponding diol-5,6 DHT- as well as the γ-lactone of 5,6 EET - products arising from spontaneous decay of the 5,6 EET - were both inactive on the caudal artery. The 5,6 epoxide, in contrast to the 5,6 DHT and the other AA epoxides, may contribute to the regulation of blood flow to several vascular territories. Indeed, Proctor et al. have reported that 5,6 EET is a potent dilator of the intestinal microcirculation (12). It should be recalled that in the original description of AA metabolites formed by the cells of the mTALH (6) a substance with similar structural features and biological activity to the 5,6 epoxide was identified. The release of this substance into the renomedullary circulation has been suggested to link metabolic activity in this segment of the nephron to changes in local blood flow (13). It is possible with the use of pharmacological interventions to manipulate AA metabolism by the cytochrome P450 system either by inducers of the monooxygenases or depletors of cytochrome P450 (14). The flux of AA through the TALH and other renal cells containing this system can, thereby, be directed by changing the level of cytochrome P450.

The cytochrome P450-related metabolites generated by mTALH can be increased selectively by suprarenal renal aortic coarctation, a model of renal hypoperfusion associated with medullary hypoxemia and elevated blood pressure (13). After 8 days when hypertension was established, mTALH cell production of cytochrome P450-dependent AA metabolites was increased two-fold as compared to product formation by mTALH cells obtained from sham-operated normotensive rabbits. These AA metabolites were not increased in 2 rabbits that did not develop hypertension following aortic coarctation. A selective response to mTALH cells in this model of hypertension is suggested as AA metabolism was not elevated in other renomedullary cells obtained from the same hypertensive rabbits. The biological profile of AA metabolites was unchanged

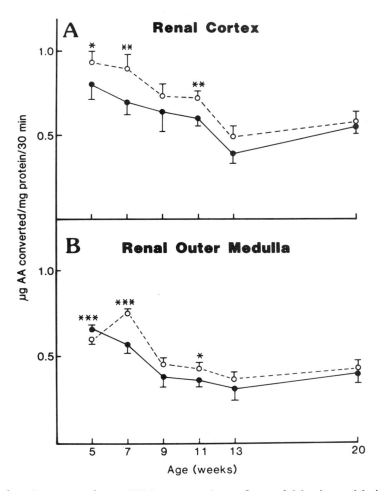

FIG. 1. Reverse-phase HPLC separation of arachidonic acid (AA) metabolites released by cells of the thick ascending limb of Henle's loop, obtained from sham-operated (upper panel) or hypertensive (lower panel) rabbits. The cytochrome P450-related AA metabolites, P_1 and P_2, had retention times of 18.8 min and 16.2 min respectively. No UV absorbance at 234 nm was detected, indicating the lack of conjugated diene structures.

in these hypertensive rabbits, i.e., vasodilator material and an inhibitor of Na^+-K^+-ATPase were associated with P_1 and $P_{2\downarrow}$ respectively. The latter may account for the reduced Na^+-K^+-ATPase activity reported in the renal outer medulla of hypertensive animals (15). The mTALH region of the nephron is extremely vulnerable to hypoxic injury, a susceptibility linked to the limited blood supply to this region and to the high rate of metabolism related to active reabsorption of sodium, potassium and chloride (16). Cytochrome P450-related AA metabolites may be released from mTALH cells, presumably, in response to both hypoxia and as an adaptation to hypoperfusion. These AA metabolites are able to reduce energy-dependent Na^+-K^+-ATPase activity and induce local vasodilation so as to maintain blood supply to the medulla, effects which could limit the degree of tissue injury.

Schwartzman and Abraham have conducted parallel studies on bovine corneal epithelium as this tissue has transport characteristics similar to those of mTALH; viz, active chloride transport, inhibitable by furosemide and coupled to Na^+-K^+-activated ATPase (17). The cotransport of NaCl in the corneal epithelium maintains stromal dehydration and, thus, corneal transparency. In this tissue AA is metabolized primarily by a cytochrome P450 monooxygenase to two biologically active products. One of these cytochrome P450-dependent AA metabolites inhibits Na^+-K^+-ATPase and has been identified as 12(R) HETE, previously shown to be the principal eicosanoid generated by the skin lesions of psoriasis (18). The other major AA product of the corneal epithelium probably arises from the 11,12 EET as does the 12(R) HETE. This second biologically active AA metabolite is a potent vasodilator, increases vascular permeability and supports angiogenesis (19). The biological effects produced by this substance mimic the inflammatory response of the cornea suggesting that this AA metabolite mediates the response of the eye to injury. The human cornea also possesses the enzymic machinery to produce these AA metabolites.

The most recent studies address the participation of cytochrome P450-dependent AA metabolites in the development of hypertension in the spontaneously hypertensive rat (SHR). Abnormalities of AA metabolism have been described in genetically hypertensive rats (20). Moreover, transient elevation of thromboxane formation occurs in the SHR coincident with the period of rapid blood pressure elevation, 5- to 13-weeks (21). It should be noted that thromboxane synthase is a cytochrome P450-containing enzyme (22). As elevation of blood pressure in the SHR can be ameliorated by renal transplant from a normotensive donor (23), abnormalities in renal function have been suggested to be responsible for the elevation of blood pressure in the SHR. Relative to this point, renal functional changes in salt and water excretion, renal blood flow and GFR are seen only in the young SHR, disappearing by the eighth week

(24). We examined whether some of the abnormalities of renal function in the young SHR are the functional expression of alterations in renal AA metabolism via the cytochrome P450-dependent pathway. The studies on the SHR were instigated by Abraham and Schwartzman and prosecuted by Sacerdoti and Escalante.

The initial study in testing this hypothesis by Sacerdoti et al. resulted in the demonstration that renal metabolism of AA by cytochrome P450-dependent monooxygenases was increased in the SHR only during the developmental phase of blood pressure elevation (5- to 13-weeks) when compared to the appropriate control normotensive rat, the WKY (25). To assess the contribution of enhanced metabolism of AA by the renal cytochrome P450 system to blood pressure elevation in the SHR, we studied the effects of suppression of renal cytochrome P450-AA metabolism (26). This was accomplished by inducing heme oxygenase which regulates the availability of heme for cytochrome P450. We treated the SHR with $SnCl_2$, a known inducer of renal heme oxygenase which spares that of liver and other tissues (27). Tin treatment resulted in depletion of renal cytochrome P450 and diminished AA metabolism by the heme-related monooxygenase, associated with prevention of hypertension in the SHR. This effect occurred only in the young SHR (7-weeks) not in the adult SHR. Blood pressure in the normotensive control WKY rat of either age was unaffected by tin treatment. This marked the first time that blood pressure in the most intensively studied animal model of human hypertension, the SHR, was maintained at normal levels by a therapeutic strategy targeted on a single enzyme. In the most optimistic reading of these studies, we suggest that they will reveal a "hypertension-specific gene product(s)" (28).

The studies reviewed above indicated that the novel metabolites of AA arising from the cytochrome P450 system contribute to the regulation of transport function and local blood flow in the eye, kidney and presumably other organs. Further, their biological properties suggest that they play a critical role in the regulation of the circulation.

REFERENCES

1. Ferreri NR, Schwartzman M, Ibraham NG, Chander PN, McGiff JC. J Pharmacol Exp Ther 1984;231:441-448.

2. McGiff JC. Ann Rev Pharmacol Toxicol 1981;21:479-509.

3. McGiff JC, Carroll MA. Am Rev Respir Dis 1987;136:488-491.

4. Schwartzman M, Carroll MA, Ibraham NG, Ferreri NR, Songu-Mize E, McGiff JC. Hypertension 1985;7(Suppl. I):I-136-I-144.

5. Capdevila J, Chacos N, Falck JR, Manna S, Negro-Vilar A, Ojeda SR. Endocrinology 1983;113:421-423.

6. Schwartzman M, Ferreri NR, Carroll MA, Songu-Mize E, McGiff JC. Nature (London) 1985;314:620-622.

7. Morel F Am J Physiol 1981;240:F159-F164.

8. Fejes-Toth G, Szenasi G. J Physiol (London) 1981;318:1-7.

9. Katz AI. Am J Physiol 1982;242:F207-F219.

10. Schlondorff D, Petty E, Oates J, Jacoby M, Levine SD. Am J Physiol 1987;253:F464-F470.

11. Carroll MA, Schwartzman M, Capdevila J, Falck JR, McGiff JC. Eur J Pharm 1987;138:281-283.

12. Protor KG, Falck JR, Capdevila J. Circ Res 1987;60:50-59.

13. Carroll MA, Schwartzman M, Baba M, Miller MJS, McGiff JC. Am J Physiol, in press.

14. Schwartzman ML, Abraham NG, Carroll MA, Levere RD, McGiff JC. Biochem J 1986;238:283-290.

15. Postnov YU, Reznikova M, Boriskina G. Pflugers Arch 1976;362:95-99.

16. Brezis M, Rosen S, Silva P, Epstein FH. J Clin Invest 1984;73:182-190.

17. Schwartzman ML, Abraham NG, Masferrer J, Dunn MW, McGiff JC. Biochem Biophys Res Commun 1985;132:343-351.

18. Schwartzman ML, Balazy M, Masferrer J, Abraham NG, McGiff JC, Murphy RC. Proc Natl Acad Sci USA 84:8125-8129.

19. Schwartzman ML, this volume.

20. Armstrong JM, Blackwell GJ, Flower RJ, McGiff JC, Mullane KM, Vane JR. Nature 1976;260:582-586.

21. Shibouta Y, Terashita Z, Inada Y, Nishikawa K, Kituchi S. Eur J Pharm 1981;70:247-256.

22. Haurand M, Ullrich V. J Biol Chem 1985;260:15059-15067.

23. Kawabe K, Watanabe TX, Shiono K, Sokabe K. Jpn Heart J 1978;19:87-89.

24. Beierwaltes WH, Arendshorst WJ, Klemmer PJ. Hypertension 1982;4:908-915.

25. Sacerdoti D, Abraham NG, McGiff JC, Schwartzman ML. Biochem Pharmacol 1987;37:521-527.

26. Escalante B, Sacerdoti D, Abraham NG, McGiff JC, Schwartzman ML. Hypertension 1987;10:359.

27. Kappas A, Maines MD. Science 1976;192:60-62.

28. Lovenberg WJ. Hypertension 1986;4(Suppl. 3):S3-S6.

ACKNOWLEDGMENTS

We thank Pam Blank for her secretarial help and Sallie McGiff for editing the manuscript. This work was supported by National Heart, Lung and Blood Institute Program Project Grant HL-34300 and Grant HL-25394, and by the American Heart Association Grant 86-112.

Advances in Prostaglandin, Thromboxane, and
Leukotriene Research, Vol. 19, edited by
B. Samuelsson, P. Y.-K. Wong, and F. F. Sun,
Raven Press, Ltd., New York ©1989.

COMPLEMENTARY DNA CLONE FOR SHEEP SEMINAL VESICLE

PROSTAGLANDIN ENDOPEROXIDE SYNTHASE (CYCLOOXYGENASE)

Diana Fagan, John Merlie, *Ned Siegel, Amiram Raz,
Jacqueline Mudd and Philip Needleman

Department of Pharmacology
Washington University School of Medicine
St. Louis, MO 63110

*Department of Biological Sciences
Monsanto Company
St. Louis, MO 63198

The important regulatory actions of prostaglandins and thromboxane in platelet activation, vascular tone and inflammatory reactions have been described; and the mechanism of action of cyclooxygenase, the rate-limiting enzyme in the formation of these arachidonic acid metabolites, has been extensively studied. Sheep seminal vesicle cyclooxygenase is a membrane associated homodimer of a 70 kDa glycoprotein (1-3) which catalyzes the bisoxygenation of arachidonic acid to the hydroperoxy prostaglandin G_2 as well as the peroxidative reduction of PGG_2 to the endoperoxide PGH_2 (4,5). These activities appear to be located on separate regions of the molecule as covalent acetylation and inactivation of the oxygenase by aspirin does not affect the peroxidase (3,6,7). Heme is required for both activities; however, only one heme moiety is bound per molecule (4,8,9). The heme binding-site and mechanism for the interaction of heme with both catalytic actions is not known. Many other questions relating to cyclooxygenase structure and membrane topography remain to be addressed.

An important step in these investigations has been the recent isolation and sequence analysis of complementary DNA clones encoding sheep seminal vesicle cyclooxygenase (10,11). The derived amino acid sequence for cyclooxygenase includes areas of identity with heme-binding proteins and myeloperoxidase and locates possible carbohydrate addition sites and hydrophobic areas of the molecule. These facts and discrepancies noted between the published sequences will be discussed.

RESULTS AND DISCUSSION

Clones encoding sheep seminal vesicle cyclooxygenase were isolated and the sequences published by our laboratory and by DeWitt and Smith (10). The clone described by DeWitt and Smith (10) is nearly identical to that reported by our laboratory (11); however, a few discrepancies are seen between the sequences.

Both clones contain nucleotides encoding an initiator methionine and 23 or 24 amino acids having all of the structural requirements for a leader peptide (12,13). As seen in Figure 1, the leader sequence published by DeWitt and Smith (10) differs from our clone by three amino acids. The arginine seen in position -22 of Dewitt and Smith's clone may be important as it places a charged residue closer to the N-terminus. We have no evidence to address these differences as only one clone of those isolated by our laboratory contained a complete leader sequence. Determination of the correct leader sequence will require isolation of additional clones containing a complete 5' end. Structural studies on cyclooxygenase may be continued in the absence of this information, as the leader peptide is cleaved from the protein and has no bearing on the activity of the mature hormone.

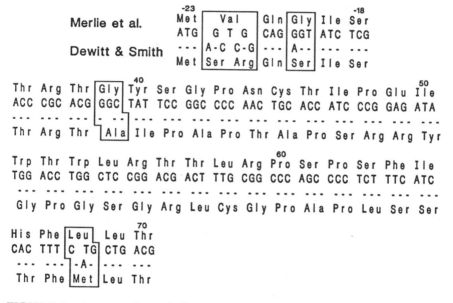

FIGURE 1. A comparison of disparate regions from the complementary DNA sequences published by Merlie et al. (11) and DeWitt and Smith (10). Nucleotide identity is indicated by a dash. Areas containing differences in the nucleotide sequence are enclosed in boxes.

A second area of disagreement exists (starting at position 39, Figure 1) with a 30 amino acid difference resulting from only two nucleotide changes. This discrepancy is significant as it includes a possible carbohydrate addition site, as seen in our sequence, and a possible hydrophobic segment, as seen in Dewitt and Smith's clone, which could act as a potential transmembrane region. We have chemically determined 43 residues from the N-terminus of purified sheep seminal vesicle cyclooxygenase (Figure 2) and the amino acid sequence supports the nucleic acid sequence published by our laboratory.

	...aa37	...aa38	...aa39	...aa40	...aa41	...aa42	...aa43
Observed signal	R	X	G	Y	S	X	P
Merlie et al.	R	T	G	Y	S	G	P
DeWitt & Smith	R	T	A	I	P	A	P

FIGURE 2. N-terminal amino acid sequence from purified sheep seminal vesicle cyclooxygenase. The amino acid sequence is compared to the sequence derived from the cDNA clone (11). Amino acid residue is indicated with numbering beginning at the N-terminal alanine of the mature protein

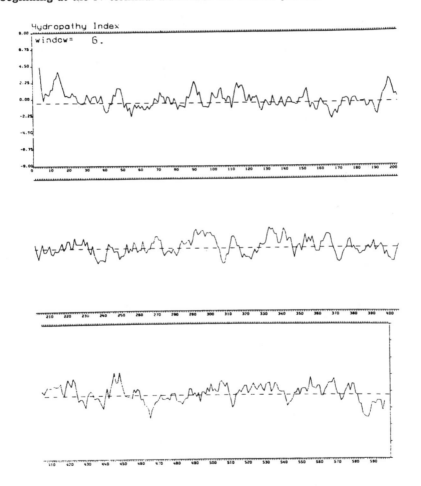

FIGURE 3. Hydropathy index was determined by the method of Kyte and Doolittle (14). Numbering begins at the initiator methionine.

The presence of a leader sequence and the demonstration of carbohydrate moieties associated with cyclooxygenase implies that at least a portion of the protein will be found in the lumen of the endoplasmic reticulum. An analysis of hydrophobicity (14) for the amino acids encoded by our cDNA clone is shown in Figure 3. The two hydrophobic regions beginning at positions 280 and 330, as indicated in Dewitt and Smith and as seen in Figure 3, have a hydropathy index of only 0.5 and -0.5 (14), suggesting that they are not functional transmembrane domains. The hydrophobic region beginning at position 280 is long enough to cross the endoplasmic reticulum membrane and has a hydropathy index (1.24) approaching that predicted for transmembrane domains (1.6, ref. 14). In addition, this sequence is preceded by two adjacent prolines and is followed by three charged amino acids (Figure 4). This sequence is similar to that seen in membrane-bound immunoglobulins, histocompatibility antigens, and in other integral membrane proteins containing a transmembrane domain (15,16). The prolines are likely an important component of a flexible peptide segment extending into the lumen of the endoplasmic reticulum. The cluster of charged amino acids may act as a signal for termination of protein transfer across the membrane. In our previous model (11), we suggested that this segment could act as a transmembrane region with the N-terminal portion of the molecule extending into the lumen of the endoplasmic reticulum.

```
                                         -23                        -1
                                         MVQGISLRFPLLLLLLSPSPVFS

                                30                                           60
ADPGAPAPVNPCCYYPCQHQGICVRFGLDRYQCDCTRTGYSGPNCTIPEIWTWLRTTLRP
                                          *

                                  90                                        120
SPSFIHFLLTHGRWLWDFVNATFIRDTLMRLVLTVRSNLIPSPPTYNIAHDYISWESFSN
   *                                                                           *

                              150                                         180
VSYYTRILPSVPRDCPTPMGTKGKKQLPDAEFLSRRFLLRRKFIPDPQGTNLMFAFFAQH

                           210                                          240
FTHQFFKTSGKMGPGFTKALGHGVDLGHIYGDNLERQYQLRLFKDGKLKYQMLNGEVYPP

                           270                                          300
SVEEAPVLMHYPRGIPPQSQMAVGQEVFGLLPGLMLYATIWLREHNRVCDLLKAEHPTWG

                           330                                          360
DEQLFQTARLILIGETIKIVIEEYVQQLSGYFLQLKFDPELLFGAQFQYRNRIAMEFNQL

                           390                                          420
YHWHPLMPDSFRVGPQDYSYEQFLFNTSMLVDYGVEALVDAFSRQPAGRIGGGRNIDHHI

                                  450                                        480
LHVAVDVIKESRVLRLQPFNEYRKRFGMKPYTSFQELTGEKEMAAELEELYGDIDALEFY

                           510                                          540
PGLLLEKCHPNSIFGESMIEMGAPFSLKGLLGNPICSPEYWKASTFGGEVGFNLVKTATL

                           570
KKLVCLNTKTCPYVSFHVPDPRQEDRPGVERPPTEL
```

FIGURE 4. Amino acid sequence derived from the cDNA clone (11). Amino acids are indicated by the single letter code. The first amino acid of the mature protein is indicated by position number 1. Symbols used in this figure are: ☒ S, site of acetylation by aspirin; *, possible carbohydrate addition site; ●, identity to heme-binding proteins; o, conservative change (23) from heme binding proteins; ■, identity to myeloperoxidase; □, conservative change from myeloperoxidase.

The sugar residues present on purified cyclooxygenase have been identified as being high mannose-linked sugars (2,17). An analysis of the predicted amino acid sequence for cyclooxygenase reveals four possible sites for N-linked glycosylation (18) (Figure 4). If our predicted location for the transmembrane portion of cyclooxygenase is correct, the three most N-terminal of these glycosylation sites would be exposed on the luminal side of the endoplasmic reticulum and, if present on the surface of the protein, accessible to glycosylating enzymes. If the remaining C-terminal carbohydrate addition site is found to be glycosylated, our model may need to be re-evaluated. Either a second transmembrane region is required for the C-terminal end of the molecule to be exposed to the lumen or cyclooxygenase may be located entirely in the lumen of the endoplasmic reticulum. However, both of these hypotheses contradict existing data suggesting the cyclooxygenase active site, identified by [^{3}H]aspirin labeling of intact microsomes, is present on the cytoplasmic face of the membrane (19). If all of the carbohydrate addition sites are utilized, this data may need to be re-examined.

A noncovalently-associated heme molecule is required for both the oxygenase and peroxidase activity of cyclooxygenase. Neither the heme-binding site, nor the location of the peroxidase has been identified. Areas of our clone contain sequence similarity to several heme-binding proteins (20,21) and to myeloperoxidase (22) (Figure 4). These regions are located on the C-terminal end of the molecule, between the hydrophobic segment and the aspirin-binding portion of the molecule. Thus, the cDNA sequence for cyclooxygenase suggests possible regions for heme-binding and peroxidase activity, sites for carbohydrate addition, and models for membrane topography which upon experimental examination may provide insight into the mechanism of action of cyclooxygenase.

ACKNOWLEDGEMENTS

This work was supported by National Institutes of Health Grants P01-DK38L1 and R01-HL2078.

1. Hemler M and Lands WEM. J Biol Chem 1976;251:5575-5579.

2. Van Der Ouderaa FJ, Buytenhek M, Nugteren DH and Van Dorp DA. Biochim Biophys Acta 1977;487:315-331.

3. Habenicht AJR, Goerig M, Grulich J, et al. J Clin Invest 1985;75:1381-1387.

4. Miyamoto T, Ogino N, Yamamoto S and Hayaishi O. J Biol Chem 1976;251:2629-2636.

5. Ohki S, Ogino N, Yamamoto S and Hayaishi O. J Biol Chem 1979;254:829-836.

6. Van Der Ouderaa FJ, Buytenhek M, Nugteren DH and Van Dorp DA. Eur J Biochem 1980;109:1-8.

7. Smith WL and Lands WEM. J Biol Chem 1971;246:6700-6704.

8. Ogino N, Ohki S, Yamamoto S and Hayaishi O. J Biol Chem 1978;253:5061-5068.

9. Roth GJ, Machuga ET and Strittmatter P. J Biol Chem 1981;256:10018-10022.

10. DeWitt DL and Smith WL. Proc Natl Acad Sci USA 1988;85:1412-1416.

11. Merlie JP, Fagan D, Mudd J and Needleman P. J Biol Chem 1988;263:3550-3553.

12. Austen BM. FEBS Letters 1979;103:308-313.

13. Strauss AW and Boime I. In: Fasman GD, ed. CRC Critical Reviews in Biochemistry, vol. 12, Boca Raton, FL, CRC Press, Inc, 1982;205-235.

14. Kyte J and Doolitle RF. J Mol Biol 1982;157:105-132.

15. Kimball ES and Coligan JM. In: Inman FP and Kindt TJ, eds. Contemporary Topics in Molecular Immunology, vol 9. New York: Plenum Press, 1983;1-63.

16. Von Heijne G. Eur J Biochem 1983;133:17-24.

17. Mutsaers JHGM, Van Halbeek H, Kamerling JP and Vliegenthart JFG. Eur J Biochem 1985;147:569-574.

18. Marshall RD. Biochem Soc Symp 1974;40:17-26.

19. DeWitt Dl, Rollins TE, Day JS, Gauger JA and Smith WL. J Biol Chem 1981; :10375-10382.

20. Leighton JK, DeBrunner-Vossbrinck BA and Kemper B. Biochemistry 1984;23:204-210.

21. Black SD and Coon MJ. In: Ortiz de Montellano PR, ed. Cytochrome P450: Structure, Mechanism, and Biochemistry. New York: Plenum Press, 1986;191-216.

22. Morishita K, Kubota N, Asano S, Kaziro Y and Nagata S. J Biol Chem 1987;262:3844-3851.

23. Dayhoff MO, Schwartz RM and Orcutt BC. In: Dayhoff MO, ed. Atlus of Protein Sequence and Structure, vol. 5. Washington: National Biomedical Research Foundation, 1979;345-362.

Advances in Prostaglandin, Thromboxane, and Leukotriene Research, Vol. 19, edited by B. Samuelsson, P. Y.-K. Wong, and F. F. Sun, Raven Press, Ltd., New York ©1989.

THE STRUCTURE AND FUNCTION OF MULTISPECIES OF PROTEIN KINASE C

K. Ogita, U. Kikkawa, M.S. Shearman, K. Ase, N. Berry, A. Kishimoto, and Y. Nishizuka

Department of Biochemistry, Kobe University School of Medicine, Kobe 650, Japan

Although once considered as a single entity (1), molecular cloning and enzymological analysis have revealed the existence of multiple subspecies of protein kinase C (PKC) in a number of mammalian species. These subspecies have a common structure closely related to, yet distinctly different from one another. The relative distribution of several PKC subspecies varies markedly with different areas of tissues and cell types examined. The structural heterogeneity, differential regional and cellular expression, and some prospectives of their physiological functions will be briefly summarized here. The integrated nomenclature used herein for several PKC subspecies and its correspondence to those to other workers are as given elsewhere (2-4).

THE HETEROGENEITY OF PROTEIN KINASE C FAMILY

Four cDNA clones which encode α-, βI-, βII-, and γ-subspecies were initially found in the bovine, rat, rabbit, and human brain, subsequently rabbit spleen cDNA libraries (see for a reviews, 5,6). The clone α, β(βI plus βII), γ are derived from genes located in different chromatosomes (7). Partial genomic analysis has clarified that βI- and βII-subspecies are derived from a single mRNA transcript by alternative splicing (2). These two subspecies differ from each other only in a short range of ~50 amino acid residues in their carboxyl terminal end region, yet possess in this region a high degree of sequence homology. Recently, another group of cDNA clones encoding additional three subspecies having δ-, ε-, and ζ-sequence have been isolated from rat brain library (4). These subspecies have a common structure closely related to, but clearly distinct from the four subspecies mentioned above. A cDNA clone corresponding to the rat brain ε-subspecies has also been isolated recently from a rabbit brain cDNA library (8).

The structures of PKC subspecies cloned to date are schematically shown in FIGURE 1. All subspecies are composed of a single polypeptide chain. The group of α-, βI-, βII-, and γ-subspecies each have four conserved (C_1-C_4) and five variable (V_1-V_5) regions, whereas the second group of δ- and ε-subspecies lack the C_2 region, yet the mass of the enzyme

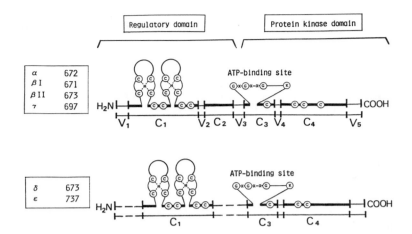

FIGURE 1. <u>Common</u> <u>structure</u> <u>of</u> <u>PKC</u> <u>subspecies</u>. C, G, K, X, and M represent cysteine, glycine, lysine, any amino acid, and metal, respectively. The numbers indicate amino acid residues of each subspecies. Other details are described in the text.

TABLE 1 <u>Regional</u> <u>distribution</u> <u>of</u> <u>PKC</u> <u>subspecies</u> <u>in</u> <u>rat</u> <u>brain</u>. The PKC subspecies were separated by chromatography on a hydroxyapatite column, which was connected to high performance liquid chromatography. Since βI- and βII-subspecies are not separated by conventional enzymological procedures, the relative ratio of these two subspecies was estimated by immunochemical procedures with subspecies-specific antibodies. The detailed procedures have been described previously (16). Specific activity is defined as pmoles of radioactive phosphate from [γ-^{32}P]ATP into calf thymus H1 histone per min per mg wet weight tissue under the standard conditions.

	Specific activity (units/mg protein)			
	α	βI	βII	γ
Whole brain	4.9	1.2	8.5	5.2
Cerebrum	2.8	0.3	10.3	3.2
Cerebellum	6.0	3.2	10.3	21.5
Hippocampus	10.8	0.3	12.9	8.3
Spinal cord	3.2	1.1	2.4	0.2

molecule is similar. The cDNA clone coding ζ-subspecies presently available does not contain a complete reading frame for the enzyme. In general, the enzyme is composed two, regulatory and catalytic, domains. The C_1 and C_2 regions appear to be regulatory domain. The conserved region C_1 contains a tandem repeat of a cysteine-rich sequence. This sequence matches the consensus sequence of "cysteine-zinc DNA-binding finger", which is found in many metalloproteins and DNA- binding proteins that are related to transcriptional regulation (9), but no obvious evidence is available indicating that PKC will bind to DNA.

On the other hand, the C_3 and C_4 regions appear to be the protein kinase domain, since this carboxyl-terminal half of the molecule shows large clusters of sequence homology to many other protein kinases. The conserved region C_3 has an ATP-binding sequence, GXGXXG----K, where G, K and X represent glycine, lysine, and any amino acid, respectively.

PKC was initially found as an undefined protein kinase which is present in many tissues and can be activated by limited proteolysis by Ca^{2+}-dependent neutral protease, calpain. The physiological significance of this proteolysis has not been established, but for reasons discussed later it may be related to down-regulation of PKC itself.

DIFFERENTIAL EXPRESSION AND TISSUE LOCALIZATION

Early studies using autoradiographic procedures with tritiated phorbol-12,13-dibutyrate have shown an uneven distribution of PKC in the brain (10,11). Northern blot analysis suggests tissue-specific expression of some PKC subspecies (7,12,13). In situ mRNA hybridization histochemistry has also shown a distinct distribution of the transcripts of some PKC subspecies in the rat brain and spleen (14). Immunohistochemical approach to identify PKC in the brain has shown different regional distribution of apparently distinct PKC subspecies (15). Using a combination of biochemical, immunological and cytochemical procedures with subspecies-specific antibodies, the relative activity and individual pattern of expression of multiple PKC subspecies have recently been examined extensively in this and other laboratories (16-24). TABLE 1 shows regional distribution of PKC subspecies in the rat brain.

PKC with γ-sequence is expressed only in the brain and spinal cord. This PKC subspecies develops post-natally and reaches maximum activity in the rat about three weeks after birth. The highest enzyme activity of γ-subspecies is found in the hippocampus (pyramidal cells), cerebral cortex, amygdaloid complex, and cerebellar cortex (Purkinje cell body, dendrites and axon, see FIGURE 2C). Immuno-electron microscopic analysis indicates that the γ-subspecies is associated with most membranous structures present throughout the cell.

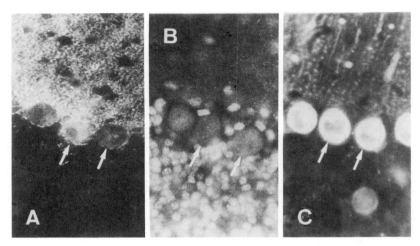

FIGURE 2. <u>Fluorescent micrographs of the rat cerebellar cortex</u>
<u>stained with subspecies-specific antibodies against PKC</u>. The
upper portion illustrates the molecular layer, and the lower
portion shows the granular layer. Arrows indicate the
Purkinje cell bodies. <u>A</u>. stained with antibodies against
ßII-subspecies. Under higher magnification, staining is
observed to be present in terminal-like structures in the
molecular layer and surrounding the Purkinje cell bodies. <u>B</u>.
stained with antibodies against ßI-subspecies. Granule cells
are specifically stained but no immuno-fluorescence is
detected in the molecular layer of Purkinje cells. <u>C</u>. stained
with antibodies against γ-subspecies. The detailed
experimental conditions are described elsewhere (24).

On the other hand, PKC's with βI- and βII-sequence are
expressed in the brain and many other tissues in different
ratios. These two subspecies differ from each other only in
the variable region V_5 as noted above. Normally, the activity
of βII-subspecies far exceeds that of the βI-subspecies.
Cytochemical analysis with the antibodies specific to each
subspecies indicates their clear distinct cellular expression.
FIGURE 2 illustrates the rat cerebellar cortex, where βI-
subspecies is localized mainly in the granular layer, whereas
βII-subspecies is found primarily in the molecular layer.

In contrast, α-subspecies appears to express commonly in
many tissues and cell types. Thus, one cell type does not
necessarily contain only one subspecies of PKC. In fact, most
tissues, such as liver, kidney, spleen, lung, testis, and heart,
contain α-, βI, and βII-subspecies in various ratios. Some
tissues such as heart and lung appear to possess additional
unidentified subspecies. Although the structure and genetic
identity of the group of δ-, ε-, and ζ-subspecies has not yet
been determined, preliminary studies have suggested that
multiple subspecies of PKC are co-expressed in a single cell

such as in T- and B-lymphocytes with apparently distinct intracellular location. The distinct regional expression and cellular localization of various PKC subspecies briefly mentioned above may be an important factor in determining a wide variety of responses of different tissues and cell types to external stimuli.

INDIVIDUAL ENZYMOLOGICAL PROPERTIES

PKC is more abundant in the brain than any other tissue. To date, three distinct fractions type I, II, and III, have been separated upon hydroxyapatite column chromatography (25). The structure and genetic identity of each fraction has been determined by comparison with the enzymes that were separately expressed in COS 7 cells after transfection with the respective cDNA-containing plasmids (2,3). Type I corresponds to the subspecies encoded by γ-sequence, type II is an unequal mixture of βI- and βII-subspecies, and type III has the structure having γ-sequence. Thus far, βI- and βII-subspecies can be distinguished from each other only by immunochemical methods, and show nearly identical kinetic properties (2,16). Type I, II, and III PKC exhibit a distinctly different mode of activation, kinetic properties, and most likely substrate specificity. It has been recently shown that the three fractions obtained from the rat and rabbit brain exhibit slightly different patterns of autophosphorylation, binding of phorbol ester, Ca^{2+}-sensitivity, and immunochemical reactivity (25,26). It has been further shown in this laboratory (27) that type I PKC is less sensitive to diacylglycerol but significantly activated by relatively low concentrations of free arachidonic acid. Type II PKC exhibits substantial activity without elevated Ca^{2+} levels, and responds well to diacylglycerol. Type III PKC is most sensitive to 1-stearoyl-2-arachidonylglycerol, which is the major species of diacylglycerol derived from inositol phospholipids.

It is a general problem in protein phosphorylation research that, following disruption of the cell, most protein kinases show an activity to phosphorylate many physiological and non-physiological substrate proteins. Although a number of proteins including cell surface receptors, enzymes, and many other proteins have been reported to serve as the phosphate acceptors of PKC in cell-free systems, it is difficult to assess the physiological significance of these proposed reactions (for a review, 28). Presumably, the PKC subspecies show different preference for substrate proteins which are located in specific intracellular compartments. In an in vitro experiment, the EGF receptor of cells of the A431 epidermoid carcinoma cell line was found to be phosphorylated most rapidly by the ubiquitous α-subspecies of PKC, whereas it is more slowly phosphorylated by the brain-specific γ-subspecies (29).

PROSPECTIVES OF PHYSIOLOGICAL FUNCTION

A synergistic interaction between Ca^{2+} and PKC proposed earlier (1) is now well recognized to underlie a variety of cellular responses to external stimuli. The biochemical basis of this synergistic action, however, still remains largely unexplored. Nevertheless, several important physiological functions have been assigned for PKC, including involvement in secretion and exocytosis, modulation of ion conductance, interaction and down-regulation of receptors, smooth muscle contraction, gene expression and cell proliferation (for a review, 28). PKC, however, appears to show a dual action, and exerts feedback control on the Ca^{2+}-signaling pathway. For instance, as illustrated in FIGURE 3, PKC may inhibit the receptor-mediated breakdown of inositol phospholipids. A number of reports have appeared to suggest that PKC also activates the Ca^{2+}-transport ATPase and Na^{+}/Ca^{2+} exchanger which remove Ca^{2+} from the cytosol (for a review, 28).

Such a negative feedback role of PKC is not confined to short-term responses such as the Ca^{2+}-transient, but may be extended to cell proliferation. The receptor for EGF has repeatedly been shown to be phosphorylated by PKC, resulting in a rapid decrease in high-affinity binding of EGF as well as inhibition of the ligand-induced tyrosine phosphorylation, termed down-regulation (for a review, 31). It is plausible

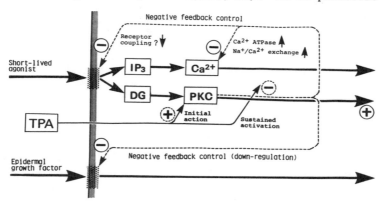

FIGURE 3. <u>Dual action of PKC and of TPA</u>. Unlike short-lived diacylglycerol, TPA appears to show a dual effect with a positive action to initially activate PKC, but with a negative action to degrade the enzyme during sustained activation. The detailed explanation is as given in the text. It does not exclude, however, a possible role for the proteolytically produced catalytically-active fragment of PKC (protein kinase M, see ref.30). DG represents diacylglycerol. IP_3 indicates inositol-1,4,5-trisphosphate.

that the treatment of cells with 12-O-tetradecanoylphorbol-13-acetate (TPA) causes disappearance of the PKC molecule itself, and thereby relieves the cell from down-regulation of the growth factor receptor, so that uncontrolled cell proliferation might occur. Indeed, a rapid, sometimes sustained, disappearance of PKC by treatment with TPA has been recognized for many cell types, including mouse epidermal cells (32). Presumably, under physiological conditions, the activation of PKC is transient, otherwise it would be degraded by proteolysis. Several subspecies co-expressed within a single cell disappear at different rates upon treatment with TPA.

In our earlier studies (30), it was shown that calpain I, which is activated at the micromolar range of Ca^{2+}, cleaves PKC in the presence of phosphatidylserine plus diacylglycerol or TPA, implying that the activated form of PKC is a target of calpain action. It is probable that this calpain-dependent proteolysis initiates the degradation of PKC molecules. No doubt, within the cell, TPA is more effective than diacylglycerol to initiate this enzyme degradation because of its stable properties. Thus, the tumor-promoter again provides a dual effect, furnishing a positive short-term activation of PKC, and then a negative action to initiate the degradation of the enzyme over a long time course (FIGURE 3).

Obviously, the negative feedback role of PKC emphasized above does not exclude the existence of a positive forward action of the enzyme. Plausible evidence seems to indicate a possible involvement of PKC in gene expression, such as some proto-oncogene activation. Several lines of evidence also suggest that PKC may have a crucial role in modulating many membrane functions including ion conductance and cross-talks of various receptors (for a review, 28). It is hoped that the heterogeneity of PKC briefly described here may open up another aspect for the research into signal transduction.

ACKNOWLEDGMENTS

This article is a part of the talk presented at the Taipei Conference on Prostaglandin and Leukotrience Research, and the authors(Y.N.) are grateful to the Organizing Committee for cordial invitation to the Conference. Some of the work presented herein was carried out in collaboration with the Biotechnology Laboratories of Takeda Chemical Industries and the Department of Pharmacology, Kobe University School of Medicine. The investigations reported from this laboratory were supported by research grants from the Research Fund of the Ministry of Education, Science and Culture, Japan; Muscle Dystrophy Association, U.S.; Yamanouchi Foundation for Research on Metabolic Disorders; Merck Sharp & Dohme Research Laboratories; Ajinomoto Central Research Laboratories; Meiji Institute Health Sciences; and New Lead Research Laboratories of Sankyo Company.

REFERENCES

1. Nishizuka Y, Nature 1984;308:693-697.
2. Ono Y, et al. Science 1987;236:1116-1120.
3. Kikkawa U, et al. FEBS Lett 1987;217:227-231.
4. Ono Y, et al. J Biol Chem 1988;263:in press.
5. Ono Y, Kikkawa U, Trends Biochem Sci 1987;12:421-423.
6. Nishizuka Y, BioFactors 1988;1:17-20.
7. Coussens L, et al. Science 1986;233:859-866.
8. Ohno S, Akita Y, Konno Y, Imajoh S, Suzuki K, Cell 1988;in press.
9. Berg J, Science 1986;232:485-487.
10. Nagle DS, Blumberg PM, Cancer Lett 1983;18:35-40.
11. Worley PF, Baraban JM, Snyder SH, J Neurosci 1986;6:199-207.
12. Knopf JL, Lee M-H, Sultzman LA, Kritz RW, Loomis CR, Hewick RM, Bell RM, Cell 1986;46:491-502.
13. Ohno S, et al. Nature 1987;325:161-166.
14. Brandt SJ, Niedel JE, Bell RM, Young III WS, Cell 1987;49:57-63.
15. Wood JG, Girard PR, Mazzei GJ, Kuo JF, J Neurosci 1986;6:2571-2577.
16. Shearman MS, Naor Z, Kikkawa U, Nishizuka Y, Biochem Biophys Res Commun 1987;147:911-919.
17. Mochly-Rosen D, Basbaum AJ, Koshland DE Jr, Proc Natl Acad Sci USA 1987;84:4660-4664.
18. Huang FL, Yoshida Y, Nakabayashi H, Knopf JL, Young III WS, Huang K-P, Biochem Biophy Res Commun 1987;149:946-952.
19. Girard PR, Stevens VL, Blackshear PJ, Merrill AH Jr, Wood JG, Kuo JF, Cancer Res 1987;47:2892-2898.
20. Kosaka Y, Ogita K, Ase K, Nomura H, Kikkawa U, Nishizuka Y, Biochem Biophy Res commun 1988;in press.
21. Kitano T, J Neurosci 1987;7:1520-1525.
22. Saito N, Kikkawa U, Nishizuka Y, Tanaka C, J Neurosci 1988;8:369-382.
23. Kose A, Saito N, Ito H, Kikkawa U, Nishizuka Y, Tanaka C, J Neurosci 1988;in press.
24. Ase K, et al. J Neurosci 1988;in press.
25. Huang K-P, Nakabayashi H, Huang FL, Proc Natl Acad Sci USA 1986;83:8535-8539.
26. Jaken S, Kiley SC, Proc Natl Acad Sci USA 1987;84:- 4418-4422.
27. Sekiguchi K, Tsukuda M, Ogita K, Kikkawa U, Nishizuka Y, Biochem Biophys Res Commun 1987;145:797-802.
28. Nishizuka Y, Science 1986;233:305-312.
29. Ido M, Sekiguchi S, Kikkawa U, Nishizuka Y, FEBS Lett 1987;219:215-218.
30. Kishimoto A, Kajikawa N, Shiota M, Nishizuka Y, J Biol Chem 1983;258:1156-1164.
31. Schlessinger J, J Cell Biol 1986;103:2067-2072.
32. Fournier A, Murray AW, Nature 1987;330:767-764.

Advances in Prostaglandin, Thromboxane, and Leukotriene Research, Vol. 19, edited by
B. Samuelsson, P. Y.-K. Wong, and F. F. Sun,
Raven Press, Ltd., New York ©1989.

ASPIRIN IN THE PREVENTION OF CATASTROPHES OF THE CORONARY CIRCULATION

John A. Oates, M.D.

The Vanderbilt University School of Medicine
Departments of Medicine and Pharmacology
Nashville, TN 37232

Aspirin is a potent inhibitor of the biosynthesis of thromboxane A_2 in platelets and thereby exerts a moderate inhibition of platelet aggregation. This anti-platelet action has led to evaluation of aspirin's ability to prevent morbidity and death from coronary disease in a number of large clinical trials. These studies have employed doses of aspirin that also block prostacyclin biosynthesis. This analysis examines the results of these aspirin trials from the perspective of the pathophysiology of the coronary ischemic syndromes, including the possible contribution of prostacyclin to the outcome of myocardial ischemia.

The catastrophic events of the coronary circulation, unstable angina, myocardial infarction and sudden cardiac death, are all initiated by a common pathophysiologic event, the rupture or fissuring of an atherosclerotic plaque with attendant thrombus formation (1). These mural thrombi are platelet rich and in their early stages may be very dynamic as exemplified by the transient reductions in flow in unstable angina. Although some patients with vasospastic angina may exhibit clinical features that are similar to the unstable angina syndrome, there are a number of lines of evidence supporting plaque rupture as the root cause of transient ischemia in unstable angina. This includes direct visualization of plaque fissures by angioscopy during coronary bypass grafting for patients with unstable angina (2), pathologic examination of the involved arteries (3, 4), arteriography (5, 6, 7) and several lines of evidence implicating platelet activation during this reversible ischemic syndrome. Studies demonstrating elevated levels of circulating platelet aggregates (8) and thromboxane B_2 levels in coronary sinus blood (9) are consistent with this conclusion, but are susceptible to the possible artifacts attendant to the activation of platelets and the release of thromboxane B_2 during withdrawal of blood. Measurement of the metabolites of thromboxane B_2, 2,3-dinor-thromboxane B_2 and 11-dehydro-thromboxane B_2, enable assessment of thromboxane B_2 biosynthesis without the artifact of its ex vivo formation. Studies in our medical center by FitzGerald et al., demonstrate striking increases in these circulating and urinary metabolites of thromboxane A_2 concurrent with unstable angina (10). This body of data supporting platelet thrombus formation as a key event in unstable angina strongly supports the use of anti-platelet therapy in this syndrome.

Again, with the exception of a few percent of myocardial infarctions that result from coronary vasospasm, it is axiomatic that plaque fissure with thrombus formation is the primary cause of the vascular occlusion in myocardial infarction, a concept further supported by the ability to reopen the vessels with thrombolytic therapy.

Although the pathophysiology of sudden cardiac death is multi-faceted, the data of Davies et al. (11) implicate fissuring of a lipid rich atheromatous plaque in most patients with cardiac sudden death. From this data, and the knowledge that ventricular fibrillation is the predominant terminal arrhythmia in such patients, it is assumed that the observed plaque ruptures and mural thrombi lead to ischemic ventricular fibrillation.

Based on the pathophysiologic inportance of platelet rich thrombi, it is not surprising that aspirin has been shown to reduce non-fatal myocardial infarction in all of the clinical trials (12). In addition, may of them show reduction of fatal myocardial infarction as well. Further, aspirin alone and together with streptokinase improves 5 week survival when used as treatment for myocardial infarctions (13). However, a major cause of death from coronary disease is sudden cardiac death. As this also stems from a mural thrombus, one would expect that aspirin would also reduce the prevalence of sudden cardiac death.

Data on sudden cardiac death have been reported in three large clinical trials during the past decade in which aspirin alone was used as the anti-platelet drug and in which beta blockers were used in only a minority of patients (14, 15, 16). Trials in which most patients were on beta blockers have been excluded from the examination of sudden cardiac death because of the powerful effect of beta blockers to prevent sudden cardiac death (17, 18). Two of these three trials have examined the secondary prevention of cardiac events and one was a primary prevention trial. In the two largest of the three trials, the Aspirin Myocardial Infarction Study and the U.S. Physicians Health Study, no reduction in cardiovascular mortality was seen despite significant reduction in myocardial infarction. In fact, there is a trend in all 3 studies for an increase in sudden cardiac death (Table 1). As plaque rupture is the common etiology of both myocardial infarction and sudden cardiac death, one would have expected that aspirin also would have reduced sudden cardiac death. Because aspirin did not decrease sudden cardiac death, it may be enhancing coupling between thrombus formation (occlusion) and ventricular fibrillation. As aspirin blocks prostacyclin biosynthesis in the doses employed in these trials, we have examined the effect of prostacyclin on the coupling of ischemia to ventricular fibrillation.

STUDIES OF ASPIRIN ALONE
THAT ADDRESS SUDDEN CARDIAC DEATH

SCD / 1000 ENTRANTS

	AMIS	PARIS I	USPHS
ASPIRIN	27	56	1.18
PLACEBO	20	44	0.82
INCREASE IN SCD WITH ASPIRIN	35%	27%	44%

TABLE 1. The occurrence of sudden cardiac death (SCD) within less than 1 hour in 3 large prospective, double-blind prevention trials conducted in the past decade evaluating aspirin as the only anti-platelet drug and in which the use of β-adrenoceptor blockers was infrequent. The trials are: the Aspirin Myocardial Infarction Study (AMIS), the Persantin/Aspirin Reinfarction Study (PARIS-I) and the U.S. Physician's Health Study (USPHS).

Ischemic ventricular fibrillation was induced in the unanesthetized dog by inflation of a balloon cuff on the circumflex coronary artery. In this model, ectopic ventricular beats were frequent for hours after ischemia whereas any ventricular fibrillation that ensued usually occurred within three minutes. To assess the effects of prostacyclin on ventricular fibrillation, a dose was selected that did not alter hemodynamics but did inhibit platelet aggregation. This dose of prostacyclin, 100 ng/kg/min, reduced the frequency of ventricular fibrillation from 53% in the control dog to 6% in the prostacyclin group (19). Further assessment of platelet-active eicosanoids on the coupling of ischemia to ventricular fibrillation was performed by examining effects of a thromboxane synthase inhibitor, RO-22-4679, a 1-substituted imidazole, on ischemic ventricular fibrillation. This inhibitor of thromboxane synthase reduced the frequency of ventricular fibrillation from 33.3% in the control animals to 6% in the RO-22-4679 treated group (20). Inhibition of thromboxane synthase has two potential biochemical consequences; it reduces the biosynthesis of thromboxane A_2 and at the same time causes accumulation of the prostaglandin endoperoxide, PGH_2, which under certain in vitro conditions as well as in normal humans leads to an increase of the biosynthesis of other prostaglandins, including prostacyclin and PGE_2 (21-23). To assess the possible contribution of prostaglandins formed from the accumulated endoperoxide to the beneficial effect of thromboxane synthase inhibition on ventricular fibrillation, a study was designed to compare the effects of the thromboxane synthase inhibitor alone and together with the inhibitor of endoperoxide biosynthesis, indomethacin (24). For this study, a structurally different thromboxane synthase inhibitor, U-63557A (5-[3' pyridinylmethyl] benzofuran-2-carboxylic acid) was employed, infused in a dose of 4 mg/kg. Ventricular fibrillation was completely abolished by U-63557A, in a contrast to a 38% occurrence in animals receiving vehicle. This beneficial effect of U-63557A, however, was completely abrogated by the concurrent administration of indomethacin 8 mg/kg; ventricular fibrillation occurred in 46% of the animals receiving inhibitors of the formation of both PGE_2 and thromboxane A_2.

From these experimental evaluations of ischemic ventricular fibrillation, it is concluded that exogenous prostacyclin inhibits ventricular fibrillation, and that generation of increased levels of prostaglandins, perhaps prostacyclin or PGE_2 (25), during thromboxane synthase inhibition also inhibits ventricular fibrillation.

Given the evidence that prostacyclin inhibits ischemic ventricular fibrillation, two important questions regarding the administration of aspirin to a patient at risk of sudden cardiac death are: (1) Do the doses of aspirin used in the clinical trials block prostacylin biosynthesis? and (2) Is prostacyclin released during myocardial infarction?

Evidence from several investigators has demonstrated that doses of aspirin greater than 80 mg daily will block the biosynthesis of prostacyclin in man. Studies in our laboratory demonstrated a reduction of the excretion of a urinary metabolite of prostacyclin, 2,3-dinor-6-keto-$PGF_{1\alpha}$ at aspirin doses of 80 mg or greater (26), and these doses reduce the biosynthesis of prostacyclin by arterial and venous tissue studied ex vivo following prior administration of aspirin (27-30). Accordingly, as the dose of aspirin employed in the large cardiovascular trials cited above was 325 mg every other day or greater, all of these studies examine the effects of inhibiting both thromboxane A_2 and prostacyclin.

The biosynthesis of prostacyclin during acute myocardial infarction has been evaluated by measuring the urinary excretion of 2,3-dinor-6-keto-$PGF_{1\alpha}$, a urinary metabolite of prostacyclin, in patients following acute myocardial infarction. The excretion of this prostacylin metabolite was found to be significantly and markedly elevated in patients with myocardial infarction, an elevation that correlated with peak plasma levels of creatine kinase (10). Thus, it is concluded that prostacyclin biosynthesis is markedly increased during the myocardial ischemia that leads to infarction.

The hypothesis that prostacyclin inhibits the coupling of ischemia to the ventricular fibrillation is therefore supported by several lines of evidence. Exogenous prostacylin inhibits ischemic ventricular fibrillation as does thromboxane synthase inhibition which acts by a prostaglandin dependent mechanism. Prostacylin biosynthesis is increased in myocardial infarction, and the doses of aspirin used in the large scale clinical trials on coronary disease were in the range that inhibit prostacyclin biosynthesis. Also consistent with the hypothesis is the observation that aspirin employed in trials in which beta blocker use is minimal does not prevent sudden cardiac death despite a clear reduction in the incidence in myocardial infarction.

The aspirin trials clearly demonstrate the potential of anti-platelet therapy in preventing myocardial infarction. Further research holds the promise of enabling inhibitors of platelet aggregation that also reduce sudden cardiac death and overall cardiovascular mortality. Such advances will be based on further research on the importance of prostacyclin in inhibiting the coupling of myocardial ischemia with fibrillation. Potential pharmacologic approaches to be considered include the administration of aspirin in lower doses and in different formulations, the use of thromboxane synthase inhibitors alone and in combination with thromboxane receptor antagonists, eicosapentaenoic acid, ticlopidine, inhibitors of the platelet glycoprotein receptors, and prostacyclin analogues. Given the fact that sudden cardiac death is the major cause of mortality in industrialized nations, elucidation and testing of anti-platelet therapy that will also reduce sudden cardiac death is a high scientific priority.

BIBLIOGRAPHY

1. Davies MJ, Thomas AC. Br Heart J 1985; 53: 363-73.

2. Sherman CT, Litvack F, Grundfest W, et al. N Engl J Med 1986; 315: 913-19.

3. Davies MJ, Thomas AC, Knapman PA, et al. Circulation 1986; 73: 418-27.

4. Falk E. Circulation 1985; 71: 699-708.

5. Vetrovec GW, Leinbach RC, Gold HK, et al. Am Heart J 1982; 104: 946.

6. Mandelkorn JB, Wolf NM, Singh S, et al. Am J Cardiol 1983; 52: 1-6.

7. Ambrose JA, Winters SL, Arora RR, et al. J Am Coll Cardiol 1986; 7: 472-8.

8. Schwartz MB, Hawiger J, Timmons S, et al. Thrombosis Hemostasis 1980; 43: 185-8.

9. Hirsh PD, Hillis LD, Campbell WB, et al. N Engl J Med 1981; 304: 685-91.

10. Fitzgerald DJ, Roy L, Catella F, et al. N Engl J Med 1986; 315: 983-9.

11. Davis MJ, Thomas A. N Engl J Med 1984; 310: 1137-40.

12. Anti Platelet Trialists' Collaboration. Br Med J 1988; 296: 320-31.

13. ISIS-2 (Second International Study Group of Infarct Survival) Collaborative Group. Lancet 1988; 2: 349-60.

14. Aspirin Myocardial Infarction Study Research Group. J Am Med Assoc 1980; 243: 661-9.

15. The Persantin-Aspirin Reinfarction Study Research Group. 1980; 62: 449-61.

16. The Steering Committee of the Physicians Health Study Group. N Engl J Med 1988; 318: 262-4.

17. The Norwegian Multicenter Study Group. N Engl J Med 1981; 304: 801-7.

18. β-Blocker Heart Attack Trial Research Group. J Am Med Assoc 1982; 247: 1707-14.

19. Starnes VA, Primm RK, Woosley RL, et al. J Cardiovasc Pharmacol 1982; 4: 765-9.

20. Huddleston CB, Lupinetti FM, Laws KH, et al. Circ Res 1983; 52: 608-13.

21. Marcus AJ, Weksler BB, Jaffe EA, et al. J Clin Invest 1980; 66: 979-86.

22. Needleman P, Wyche A, Raz A. J Clin Invest 1979; 63: 345-9.

23. FitzGerald GA, Brash AR, Oates JA, et al. J Clin Invest 1983; 72: 1336-43.

24. Catella F, Nowak J, FitzGerald GA. Am J Med 1986; 81: 23-9.

25. Hammon JW, Oates JA. Circulation 1986; 73: 224-6.

26. Au TLS, Collins GA, Harvey CJ, et al. Prostaglandins 1979; 18: 707-20.

27. FitzGerald GA, Oates JA, Hawiger J, et al. J Clin Invest 1983; 71: 676-88.

28. Preston FE, Whipps S, Jackson CA, et al. N Engl J Med 1981; 304: 76-9.

29. Hanley SP, Bevan J, Cockbill SR, et al. <u>Lancet</u> 1981; 1: 969-71.

30. Weksler BB, Pett SB, Alonso D, et al. <u>N Engl J Med</u> 1983; 308: 800-5.

31. Weksler BB, Goldman KT, Subramanian VA, et al. <u>Circulation</u> 1985; 71: 332-40.

Advances in Prostaglandin, Thromboxane, and Leukotriene Research, Vol. 19, edited by B. Samuelsson, P. Y.-K. Wong, and F. F. Sun, Raven Press, Ltd., New York ©1989.

BIOSYNTHESIS AND CONVERSIONS OF FATTY ACID ALLENE OXIDES

Mats Hamberg and Molly A. Hughes

Department of Physiological Chemistry,
Karolinska Institutet, S-104 01 Stockholm, Sweden

Conversion of an unsaturated fatty acid hydroperoxide into an α-ketol derivative was described by Zimmerman in 1966 (1). He found that preparations of flaxseed catalyzed the formation of 12-oxo-13-hydroxy-9($\underline{Z}$)-octadecenoic acid from 13($\underline{S}$)-hydroperoxy-9($\underline{Z}$),11($\underline{E}$)-octadecadienoic acid (13($\underline{S}$)-HPOD). The enzyme responsible for the conversion was called "hydroperoxide isomerase" and was subsequently identified in a number of other plants, $\underline{eg}$. corn (2). The mechanism of the transformation was recently clarified (3). Thus, two separate steps were involved, $\underline{i.e.}$ an enzymatic dehydration of 13($\underline{S}$)-HPOD into an unstable allene oxide, 12,13($\underline{S}$)-epoxy-9($\underline{Z}$),11-octadecadienoic acid, followed by spontaneous hydrolysis of the allene oxide into α-ketol. Because only the first step was an enzymatic reaction, a new name for the enzyme was proposed, $\underline{i.e.}$ "hydroperoxide dehydrase" (3).

The present chapter is a brief account of our studies on the formation and further conversions of allene oxides.

DETECTION OF FATTY ACID ALLENE OXIDES

Trapping Experiments. 13($\underline{S}$)-HPOD was added to a preparation of corn hydroperoxide dehydrase at 0^0. Aliquots were removed 10, 30, 60, 90 s and 5 min after addition of substrate and treated with 20 vol of methanol. Analysis by TLC revealed transient appearance of a trapping product, which was identified as 12-oxo-13-methoxy-9($\underline{Z}$)-octadecenoic acid (3). This finding suggested that 13($\underline{S}$)-HPOD when exposed to corn hydroperoxide dehydrase was converted into an unstable compound ($t_{1/2}$ at 0^0 about 33 s) that rapidly reacted with methanol to afford the trapping product or with water to afford α-ketol (FIG. 1).

Ultraviolet Spectrometry Experiments. 13($\underline{S}$)-HPOD was shaken at 0^0 with hydroperoxide dehydrase. Ice-cold acetonitrile (9 vol) was added, and the mixture was rapidly passed through a Sep-Pak silica cartridge into a spectrophotometric cuvette. Ultraviolet spectrometry demonstrated the presence in the eluate of an unstable compound exhibiting a strong absorption band with λ_{max} = 236 nm. That this material was identical to the unstable compound detected in the trapping experiments (see above) was supported by the finding that the half-lives (in 90% aqueous acetonitrile) of the unstable compounds detected by ultraviolet spectrometry and by the trapping technique were identical.

Isotope Experiments. 13($\underline{S}$)-[$^{18}O_2$]HPOD incubated with the enzyme preparation afforded 12-oxo-13-hydroxy-9($\underline{Z}$)-octadecenoic acid and 12-oxo-13-methoxy-9($\underline{Z}$)-octadecenoic acid both containing 1 atom of ^{18}O. The oxygen retained was located at C-12 (cf. ref. 4).

13($\underline{S}$)-[9,10,12,13-$^2H_4$]HPOD incubated with hydroperoxide dehydrase yielded 12-oxo-13-hydroxy-9($\underline{Z}$)-octadecenoic acid and 12-oxo-13-methoxy-9($\underline{Z}$)-octadecenoic acid containing 3 atoms of ^2H located at C-9, C-10, and C-13. The facts that the deuterium at C-12 of the precursor was lost and that the products were completely devoid of deuterium in the C-11 position argued against a mechanism previously proposed involving a hydride shift from C-12 to C-11 (5).

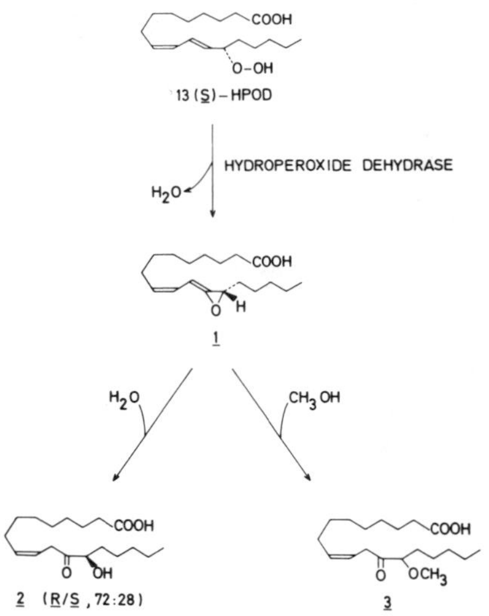

FIG 1. Mechanism of formation of α-ketol derivatives from fatty acid hydroperoxides. $\underline{1}$, 12,13($\underline{S}$)-epoxy-9($\underline{Z}$),11-octadecadienoic acid; $\underline{2}$, 12-oxo-13-hydroxy-9($\underline{Z}$)-octadecenoic acid; $\underline{3}$, 12-oxo-13-methoxy-9($\underline{Z}$)-octadecenoic acid.

The experiments described above showed that the unstable compound generated from 13($\underline{S}$)-HPOD in the presence of corn hydroperoxide dehydrase 1) retained one of the two hydroperoxide oxygens; 2) retained the hydrogens at C-9, C-10, and C-13 but not the hydrogen at C-12; 3) contained a chromophore absorbing at 236 nm (likely a conjugated diene); and 4) reacted with water to produce 12-oxo-13-hydroxy-9($\underline{Z}$)-octadecenoic acid and with methanol to produce 12-oxo-13-methoxy-9($\underline{Z}$)-octadecenoic acid. The structure established for the unstable compound on the basis of those results was 12,13($\underline{S}$)-epoxy-9($\underline{Z}$),11-octadecadienoic acid (12,13($\underline{S}$)-EOD)(3)(FIG. 1). Recent studies have shown that corn hydroperoxide dehydrase catalyzes a similar type of transformation of 9(S)-HPOD, i.e. into 9(S),10-epoxy-10,12(Z)-octadecadienoic acid (9(S),10-EOD)(Hughes M, Hamberg M, unpublished). The aqueous half-lives of 9(S),10-EOD and 12,13(S)-EOD were virtually identical (34 and 33 s, respectively).

CONVERSIONS OF FATTY ACID ALLENE OXIDES

Hydrolysis of Allene Oxides. As mentioned above, 12,13(S)-EOD and 9(S),10-EOD underwent rapid hydrolysis in aqueous medium to yield α-ketols. Steric analysis showed that the α-ketols had largely the R configuration (12-oxo-13-hydroxy-9(Z)-octadecenoic acid, 13(R)/13(S) = 72:28; 10-oxo-9-hydroxy-12(Z)-octadecenoic acid, 9(R)/9(S) = 74:26). Thus, formation of α-ketols from allene oxides apparently occurred by an $S_N 2$ type of displacement at the saturated epoxide carbon (resulting in inversion) as well as by an $S_N 1$ type of reaction involving the symmetrical oxyallyl zwitterion (resulting in racemization).

Reduction of Allene Oxides. Treatment of 12,13(S)-EOD with sodium borohydride in methanol yielded 12-hydroxy-9-octadecenoic acid. Identification was made by mass spectrometry and oxidative ozonolysis using the authentic compound (ricinoleic acid) as reference. When reduction was accomplished with sodium borodeuteride, 2 atoms of deuterium were incorporated into the 12-hydroxy-9-octadecenoic acid (at C-12 and C-13) whereas treatment of 12,13(S)-EOD generated from 13(S)-[9,10,12,13-^{2}H$_4$]HPOD with sodium borohydride led to the formation of 12-hydroxy-9-octadecenoic acid containing 3 atoms of deuterium (at C-9, C-10, and C-13). Thus, reduction of 12,13(S)-EOD by sodium borohydride occurred by addition of hydride at C-13, opening and ketonization of the allene oxide structure, and reduction of the 12-oxo group by addition of hydride at C-12.

Formation of Macrolactones. As described above, the fatty acid allene oxides 12,13(S)-EOD and 9(S),10-EOD were unstable in hydroxylic solvents such as water and methanol. As would be expected, stability was greatly enhanced in non-hydroxylic, water-miscible solvents such as acetonitrile and tetrahydrofuran. Thus, the half-life of 12,13(S)-EOD in acetonitrile/potassium phosphate buffer pH 7.4 (20:1, v/v) at 0⁰ was 7.4 min as compared to 33 s in buffer (6). Interestingly, in that case degradation of the allene oxide did not result in the formation of α-ketol but in two unique macrolactones, 12-oxo-9(Z)-octadecen-11-olide and 12-oxo-9(Z)-octadecen-13-olide (6). Experiments with 9(S),10-EOD showed a similar type of transformation, i.e. conversion into 10-oxo-12(Z)-octadecen-9-olide and 10-oxo-12(Z)-octadecen-11-olide (FIG. 2)(Hughes M, Hamberg M, unpublished).

Steric analysis showed that 10-oxo-12(Z)-octadecen-9-olide was essentially racemic (ratio between enantiomers, 52:48). It therefore seemed likely that macrolactone formation from 9(S),10-EOD (and 12,13(S)-EOD) occurred by way of the oxyallyl zwitterion in which there is no asymmetry (FIG. 2).

Formation of macrolactones required that the carboxyl group of the allene oxide exist in the form of the nucleophilic carboxylate anion. Thus, when 9(S),10-EOD was allowed to decompose in acidified acetonitrile solution, formation of macrolactones was inhibited. Instead, formation of 10-oxo-9-hydroxy-12(Z)-octadecenoic acid (α-ketol) and 10-oxo-13-hydroxy-11(E)-octadecenoic acid (γ-ketol), as well as a number of unidentified products was observed.

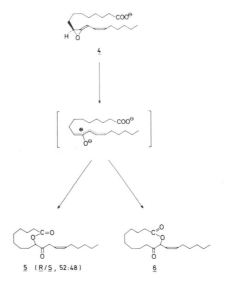

FIG. 2. Formation of macro-lactones from 9(S),10-EOD in acetonitrile/potassium phosphate buffer pH 7.4, 20:1 (v/v). 4, 9(S),10-epoxy-10,12(Z)-octadecadienoate; 5, 10-oxo-12(Z)-octadecen-9-olide; 6, 10-oxo-12(Z)-octadecen-11-olide.

<u>Formation of cyclopentenone derivatives</u>. The fatty acid allene oxides were stabilized in the presence of vertebrate serum albumins. Thus, the aqueous half-lives at 0° of 12,13(S)-EOD in the presence of 15 mg/ml of bovine, human, and equine serum albumins were 14.1 ± 1.8, 11.6 ± 1.2, and 4.8 ± 0.5 min, respectively, as compared to 33 s in the absence of albumin (7). Similarly, the half-life of 9(S),10-EOD in the presence of bovine serum albumin was 8.2 ± 1.0 min as compared to 34 s in the absence of albumin. Albumins have previously been found to stabilize thromboxane A_2 (8), prostaglandin I_2 (9), and leukotriene A_4 (10). Interestingly, with regard to the efficacy of the various albumins to stabilize 12,13(S)-EOD, the rank order was the same as that previously found for the stabilization of leukotriene A_4 (10), <u>i.e.</u> bovine > human > equine.

In the course of the studies on the stabilization of allene oxides by albumins, it was found that degradation of 12,13(S)-EOD in the presence of bovine serum albumin led to the formation of a novel cyclopentenone derivative, <u>i.e.</u> 3-oxo-2-pentyl-cyclopent-4-en-1-octanoic acid (FIG. 3)(7). Steric analysis demonstrated that the relative configuration between the side chains attached to the cyclopentenone ring was trans and that the compound was largely racemic (ratio between enantiomers, 58:42). Interestingly, degradation of 9(S),10-EOD in the presence of bovine serum albumin did not produce a cyclization product. It may be speculated that the lack of formation of a cyclopentenone derivative in that case could be attributed to the fact that the half-life of 9(S),10-EOD in the presence of bovine serum albumin (8.2 min) was significantly shorter than that found for 12,13(S)-EOD (14.1 min).

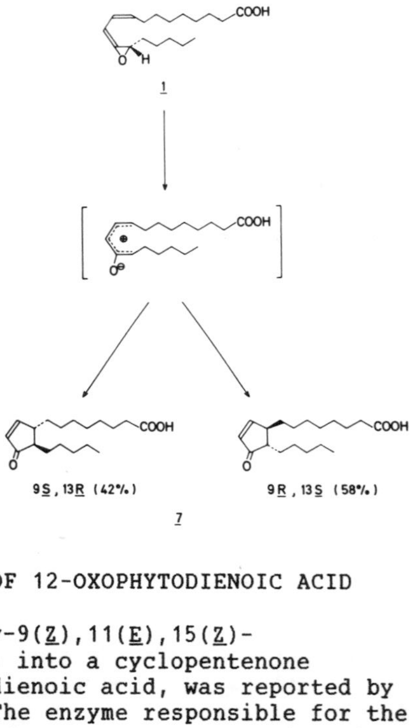

FIG. 3. Cyclization of 12,13(S)-EOD induced by bovine serum albumin (15 mg/ml). 1, 12,13(S)-epoxy-9(Z),11-octadecadienoic acid; 7, 3-oxo-2-pentyl-cyclo-pent-4-en-1-octanoic acid.

9S,13R (42%)   9R,13S (58%)

7

FORMATION AND CONFIGURATION OF 12-OXOPHYTODIENOIC ACID

Conversion of 13(S)-hydroperoxy-9(Z),11(E),15(Z)-octadecatrienoic acid (13(S)-HPOT) into a cyclopentenone derivative, 12-oxo-10,15(Z)-phytodienoic acid, was reported by Zimmerman and Feng in 1978 (11). The enzyme responsible for the conversion was called "hydroperoxide cyclase" and was identified in a number of plant tissues. Our finding that a cyclopentenone derivative can be formed from the allene oxide 12,13(S)-EOD in a non-enzymatic reaction (with bovine serum albumin) coupled with the fact that incubation of 13(S)-HPOT with corn hydroperoxide dehydrase afforded 12-oxophytodienoic acid (12) indicated that 12,13(S)-epoxy-9(Z),11,15(Z)-octadecatrienoic acid (the allene oxide generated from 13(S)-HPOT) may be converted into 12-oxophytodienoic acid via a non-enzymatic reaction. This proposal was further supported by experiments which have shown that, using conditions under which 12-oxophytodienoic acid is biosynthesized from 13(S)-HPOT, transient formation of 12,13(S)-epoxy-9(Z),11,15(Z)-octadecatrienoic acid can be detected by chemical and physical methods (Hamberg M, unpublished). Thus, only the hydroperoxide dehydrase activity would be required for the biosynthesis of 12-oxophytodienoic acid, although the existence in plant tissue of protein(s) influencing the cyclization of allene oxides into cyclopentenone derivatives cannot be excluded at this stage.

12-oxo-10,15($\underline{Z}$)-phytodienoic acid formed from 13($\underline{S}$)-HPOT in the presence of corn hydroperoxide dehydrase was found not to be optically pure but a mixture of enantiomers in a ratio of 82:18 (7). The absolute configurations of the enantiomers were recently determined using a derivative prepared from (+)-7-iso-jasmonic acid as reference (12). The major enantiomer of 12-oxophytodienoic acid was found to have the 9($\underline{S}$),13($\underline{S}$) configuration. Therefore, in the major enantiomer of 12-oxophytodienoic acid, the configurations of the side chain-bearing carbons are identical to the configurations of the corresponding carbons of (+)-7-iso-jasmonic acid, thus lending support to previous studies indicating that 12-oxophytodienoic acid serves as the precursor of (+)-7-iso-jasmonic acid in plant tissue (13). In this connection a recent study should be mentioned in which 12-oxophytodienoic acid generated by incubation of 13($\underline{S}$)-HPOT with an acetone powder of flaxseed was found to be completely racemic (14). Further studies are required in order to explain the different optical purities of 12-oxophytodienoic acid generated in the corn and flaxseed systems.

REFERENCES

1. Zimmerman DC, Biochem. Biophys. Res. Commun. 1966;23:398-402.
2. Gardner HW, J. Lipid Res. 1970;11:311-321.
3. Hamberg M, Biochim. Biophys. Acta 1987;920:76-84.
4. Gerritsen M, Veldink GA, Vliegenthart JFG, Boldingh, J, FEBS Lett. 1976;67:149-152.
5. Gardner HW, Lipids 1979;14:208-211.
6. Hamberg M, Chem. Phys. Lipids 1988;46:235-243.
7. Hamberg M, Hughes M, Lipids 1988, in press.
8. Folco GC, Granström E, Kindahl H, FEBS Lett. 1977;82:321-324.
9. Wynalda MA, Fitzpatrick, FA, Prostaglandins 1980;20:853-861.
10. Fitzpatrick FA, Morton DR, Wynalda MA, J. Biol. Chem. 1982;257:4680-4683.
11. Zimmerman DC, Feng P, Lipids 1978;13:313-316.
12. Hamberg M, Miersch O, Sembdner G, Lipids 1988, in press.
13. Vick BA, Zimmerman DC, Biochem. Biophys. Res. Commun. 1983;111:470-477.
14. Baertschi SW, Ingram CD, Harris TM, Brash AR, Biochemistry 1988;27:18-24.

Advances in Prostaglandin, Thromboxane, and Leukotriene Research, Vol. 19, edited by B. Samuelsson, P. Y.-K. Wong, and F. F. Sun, Raven Press, Ltd., New York ©1989.

ALLENE OXIDES AS INTERMEDIATES IN BIOSYNTHESIS

OF KETOLS AND CYCLOPENTENONES

Alan R. Brash[*], Steven W. Baertschi, Christiana D. Ingram[*], and Thomas M. Harris

Departments of Pharmacology[*] and Chemistry, Vanderbilt University, Nashville TN 37232

Recently, allene oxides have been implicated as intermediates in the conversion of hydroperoxy fatty acids to ketols and cyclopentenones in plants (1,2), and to prostaglandins and clavulones in certain corals (3,4). The natural allene oxides are formed from specific fatty acid hydroperoxides through catalysis by an allene oxide synthase or hydroperoxide dehydrase. Synthetic allene oxides have been more extensively studied, and the compounds are known to be prone to spontaneous cyclization and to hydrolysis (5).

RESULTS AND DISCUSSION

Allene oxide biosynthesis in flaxseed

Flaxseed, corn germ, and other plant tissues convert the 13(S)-hydroperoxide of α-linolenic acid to a 12-oxo,13-hydroxy α-ketol, and to a cyclopentenone named 12-oxophytodienoic acid (12-oxo-PDA) (6). Several lines of evidence point to an allene oxide, 12,13(S)-oxido-octadeca-9,11,15-trienoic acid as a common intermediate in these transformations (1,2). The allene oxide is extremely unstable. Using the methanol trapping method to intercept the intermediate, we estimated that the chemical half-life is about 16 seconds at 0°C and pH 7.4 (7); this is slightly less stable than the C18.2 analog of the compound (1).

Isolation of the allene oxides

We have now developed a procedure for the isolation and purification of the allene oxides derived from linoleic and α-linolenic acids (7). The method is based on a 5 second incubation of the hydroperoxide substrate with flaxseed enzymes at 0°C, followed by extraction with ice-cold hexane and formation of the methyl ester derivative using diazomethane. The methyl ester is stable in hexane, provided the temperature is kept at -10°C or below. Chromatographic purification was achieved by normal phase

HPLC on a short column operated at -15°C. Development of this method allowed isolation of the pure allene oxides in about 25% yield from the hydroperoxides. We characterized the structures of the C18.2 and C18.3 allene oxides by UV, CD, and NMR (7).

Allene oxide hydrolysis and cyclization

Strong circumstantial evidence suggested that the enzymic formation of the C18.3ω3 allene oxide is followed by the non-enzymatic breakdown to the α-ketol and the cyclopentenone 12-oxo-PDA (1,2). We were able to examine this question directly, using the pure allene oxide. When the methyl ester of the allene oxide was exposed to water, several polar products were detected, and the two most prominent derivatives were identified by UV, HPLC and GC-MS as the methyl esters of the 12-oxo,13-hydroxy α-ketol and 12-oxo-PDA. Analysis of the absolute configuration of the α-ketol revealed that the chirality of the 13-hydroxyl is very close that of the product formed in the presence of flaxseed enzymes. The 12-oxophytodienoic acid was found to be a racemic mixture with the side chains in the cis configuration. This is precisely the result obtained previously on 12-oxo-PDA formed in acetone powders of flaxseed (2). Thus, the two main products formed when isolated allene oxide is mixed with water are the same as those formed when hydroperoxide substrate is allowed to react with the enzymes in acetone powders. Clearly, biosynthesis of the allene oxide is enzymatic. Subsequent non-enzymic reactions can account for appearance of the α-ketol and 12-oxo-PDA.

Lipoxygenase pathway to the prostaglandins

An intriguing question regarding the natural allene oxides concerns the mechanism of transformation to chiral cyclopentanones such as the prostaglandins. The coral Plexaura homomalla contains about 1% of its wet weight as prostaglandins of the E and A series, with the main constituent being the methyl ester of PGA$_2$ acetate (8). These compounds have the same absolute configuration as prostaglandins of higher animals. In our studies of the metabolism of arachidonic acid in P.homomalla we detected an 8R-lipoxygenase pathway leading to formation of an α-ketol and a cyclopentenone with a PGA ring. In all respects, these in vitro reactions appear analogous to the transformations described in flaxseed. Most significantly, the prostaglandin-like cyclopentenone is racemic, with cis side chains. We have not detected the biosynthesis of a chiral prostanoid. How are the natural prostaglandins formed?

Detection of 11R-HETE in the phospholipids of P.homomalla

We questioned whether an isomer or derivative of arachidonic acid might be the natural substrate for conversion to the prostaglandins. In pursuit of this hypothesis, we examined the polar lipids of P.homomalla for the presence of unusual fatty acids. No isomers of arachidonate could be detected by reversed-phase HPLC and GC-MS analysis. However, we made an unexpected finding. Small amounts of a chiral HETE were detected in the phosphatidylcholine fraction.   The compound was identified by HPLC, UV, steric analysis and GC-MS as 11R-HETE.   Earlier we had found 11R-HETE as a very minor product formed in acetone powders of the coral (unpublished).   11R-H(P)ETE is a "frameshift" analog of 8R-H(P)ETE, and it might be formed by a minor 11R-lipoxygenase activity of the 8R-lipoxygenase.   However we were also led to question whether the 11R oxygenation might normally occur in the biosynthesis of the prostaglandins; (notably, the C-11 hydroxyl of PGE_2 is of the 11R configuration).   Consideration of this idea led to development of a new hypothesis to explain prostaglandin biosynthesis in the coral.

SCHEME   TWO POTENTIAL ROUTES TO PROSTAGLANDIN E_2

A proposal for PGE_2 biosynthesis in coral

The central concept of the hypothesis is that PGE_2 is the primary prostaglandin product of the pathway.   Two potential routes to PGE_2 are envisaged (Scheme); presently the evidence favors the left-hand route, via 11R-oxygenation of the allene oxide. The PGE_2 is then acetylated.   The 11-acetate of PGE is very unstable and (possibly non-enzymic) elimination of acetic acid will give PGA_2 15-acetate as the major end product stored in the coral.

An attractive aspect of the hypothesis is the concerted nature of the cyclization reaction. Also, the hypothesis does not require the existence of many new enzymes to explain the chiral trans configuration of the side chains, the appearance of hydroxyls on C-11 or C-15, or the PGE/PGA conversion. Several aspects of this hypothesis are open to straightforward experimental testing, and our current experiments are aimed at an assessment of these possibilities.

ACKNOWLEDGEMENTS

We thank the Department of Development & Natural Resources of the Cayman Islands for their cooperation in collection of samples of P. homomalla. This work is supported by NIH grants DK-35275 and ES-00267.

REFERENCES

1. Hamberg M. Biochim Biophys Acta, 1987;920:76-84.

2. Baertschi SW, Ingram CD, Harris TM, and Brash AR. Biochemistry, 1988;27:18-24.

3. Corey EJ, d'Alarcao M, Matsuda SPT, and Lansbury PT Jr. J Amer Chem Soc, 1987;109:289-290.

4. Brash AR, Baertschi SW, Ingram CD, and Harris TM. J Biol Chem, 1987;262:15829-15839.

5. Chan TH, and Ong BS. (1980) Tetrahedron 36, 2369-2289.

6. Vick BA, and Zimmerman DC, Plant Physiol, 1979;64:203-205.

7. Brash AR, Baertschi SW, Ingram CD, and Harris TM. Proc Nat Acad Sci USA, 1988; in press

8. Weinheimer AJ, and Spraggins RL. Tetrahedron Lett, 1969;59: 5185-5188.

Advances in Prostaglandin, Thromboxane, and
Leukotriene Research, Vol. 19, edited by
B. Samuelsson, P. Y.-K. Wong, and F. F. Sun,
Raven Press, Ltd., New York ©1989.

VERSATILE ARACHIDONATE 5-LIPOXYGENASE PURIFIED FROM PORCINE LEUKOCYTES —— 5S-OXYGENASE, LEUKOTRIENE A SYNTHASE AND 6R-OXYGENASE ACTIVITIES

Natsuo Ueda and Shozo Yamamoto

Department of Biochemistry, School of Medicine,
Tokushima University, Kuramoto-cho, Tokushima 770, Japan

Arachidonate 5-lipoxygenase catalyzes 5-oxygenation of arachidonic acid to produce 5-hydroperoxy-eicosatetraenoic acid (5-HPETE). The 5-hydroperoxy product is further converted to leukotriene (LT) A_4 by the catalysis of LTA synthase (1). It is now generally accepted that mammalian 5-lipoxygenase is a bifunctional enzyme and a single enzyme protein has both 5-oxygenase and LTA synthase activities (2). In this communication, we will report a novel 6R-oxygenase activity as a catalytic property of 5-lipoxygenase (3), and the lipoxin synthesis will be discussed in terms of these activities of 5-lipoxygenase (4).

5-Lipoxygenase which we purified from porcine leukocytes by immunoaffinity chromatography (1), was incubated with 5-HPETE at 24°C. Hydroperoxy product was reduced with borohydride, and analyzed by reverse-phase HPLC (FIG. 1A). As monitored at 270 nm for a conjugated triene, two major peaks A and B and several minor peaks were detected. The major peaks A and B comigrated with authentic 6-trans-LTB$_4$ and its 12-epimer. They are known to be degradation products of LTA$_4$ (5), which is produced from 5-HPETE by the LTA synthase activity of the purified enzyme (1). Previously, peaks E and F were tentatively identified as 5,6-dihydroxy-eicosatetraenoic acids (diHETEs), which were also thought to be hydrolytic products of LTA$_4$ (5). Upon our further investigations peak E was co-eluted with authentic 5S,6R-diHETE. It should be noted that the peak E was always bigger than peak F.

When the enzyme reaction with 5-HPETE was performed on ice, peak E corresponding to 5S,6R-diHETE was now a major product. The anaerobic condition markedly reduced the peak height. Furthermore, without pretreatment with borohydride the formation of 5S,6R-diHETE decreased. These results indicated that most of 5S,6R-diHETE was produced requiring molecular oxygen, and the primary product was presumably 5S,6R-dihydroperoxy acid.

In order to demonstrate the 6R-oxygenation without being affected by the LTA synthase activity, we incubated the purified enzyme with 5-HETE, which was an inactive substrate of LTA synthase. Upon HPLC one major peak appeared (FIG. 1B) and co-migrated with authentic 5S,6R-diHETE. Several minor peaks co-migrating with various 5,12-dihydroxy acids were also detected. Identity of the main product with 5S,6R-diHETE was confirmed as follows. UV spectrum of the major reaction product was indistinguishable from that of authentic 5S,6R-diHETE with a maximum at 273 nm and shoulders at 263 and 284 nm. Mass spectrum of the product was essentially identical with that of authentic 5S,6R-diHETE. Furthermore, by incubation with soybean lipoxygenase the reaction product was converted to lipoxin A as identified by its UV spectrum and HPLC profile. These results confirmed the identity of this product with 5S,6R-dihydroxy-7-trans-9-trans-11-cis-14-cis-eicosatetraenoic acid.

The 6R-oxygenation of 5-HETE was diminished in the absence of any of peroxide, calcium ion, and ATP. These compounds are required as activators for the 5-oxygenase and LTA synthase acti-

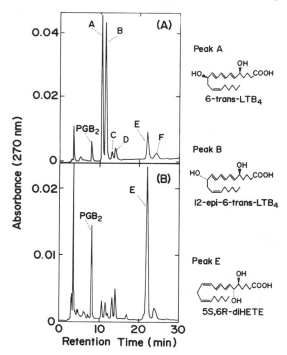

FIG. 1. 5-Lipoxygenase reactions with 5-HPETE and 5-HETE. The purified 5-lipoxygenase was incubated with 5-HPETE (A) or 5-HETE (B) at 24°C, and the borohydride-reduced products were analyzed by reverse-phase HPLC.

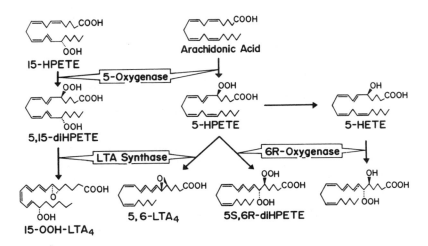

FIG. 2. Various reactions catalyzed by 5-lipoxygenase.

vities of 5-lipoxygenase (1,2). Furthermore, the 6R-oxygenase
activity was inhibited by two selective 5-lipoxygenase inhibitors, AA861 (6) and cirsiliol (7). These findings indicated
that the 6R-oxygenase activity was attributed to the catalysis
of 5-lipoxygenase.

FIG. 2 summarizes the reactions catalyzed by 5-lipoxygenase.
In addition to 5-oxygenation of arachidonic acid, the purified 5-
lipoxygenase catalyzed the conversion of 5-HPETE to LTA$_4$ and the
6R-oxygenation of 5-HPETE and 5-HETE. Since the 6R-oxygenation
of 5-HPETE proceeded at a rate lower than that of LTA$_4$ synthesis,
most of 5-HPETE endogeneously formed from arachidonic acid was
directed to the production of LTA$_4$. The 6R-oxygenation of 5-
HPETE by 5-lipoxygenase is equivalent to the 14R- and 8S-oxygen-
ation of 15-HPETE catalyzed by porcine leukocyte 12-lipoxygenase
(8) and rabbit reticulocyte 15-lipoxygenase (9).

We considered a possible lipoxin synthesis by these activities
of 5-lipoxygenase (4). 5,15-diHPETE was allowed to react with a
larger amount of the purified 5-lipoxygenase at 24°C for 5 min.
Reaction products were reduced with borohydride, and analyzed by
reverse-phase HPLC. When absorption at 301 nm was monitored for
a conjugated tetraene, several peaks were detected and compared
with authentic lipoxin isomers provided by Dr. Fitzsimmons and
Dr. Rokach of Merck Frosst Canada. The highest peak comigrated
with lipoxin A. The other peaks comigrated with 6-epimer of
lipoxin A, all-trans isomers of lipoxin A, and all-trans isomers
of lipoxin B, respectively. When the enzyme reaction was performed in the absence of air, the product profile was essentially
unchanged. The finding suggested that the lipoxin isomers were
produced by anaerobic conversion of 5S,15S-diHPETE to 15-hydro-
peroxy-5,6-epoxy compound by the LTA synthase activity followed

by non-enzymatic hydrolysis of the LTA_4-type product (FIG. 2), and there was a minor contribution of the 6R-oxygenase activity to aerobically produce trihydroperoxy derivative of lipoxin A.

REFERENCES

1. Ueda N, Kaneko S, Yoshimoto T, Yamamoto S. J Biol Chem 1986; 261:7982-7988

2. Samuelsson B, Dahlén S-E, Lindgren J, Rouzer C, Serhan CN. Science 1987;237:1171-1176

3. Ueda N, Yamamoto S. J Biol Chem 1988;263:1937-1941

4. Ueda N, Yamamoto S, Fitzsimmons BJ, Rokach J. Biochem Biophys Res Commun 1987;144:996-1002

5. Samuelsson B. Science 1983;220:568-575

6. Yoshimoto T, Yokoyama C, Ochi K, Yamamoto S, Maki Y, Ashida Y, Terao S, Shiraishi M. Biochim Biophys Acta 1982;713:470-473

7. Yoshimoto T, Furukawa M, Yamamoto S, Horie T, Watanabe-Kohno S. Biochem Biophys Res Commun 1983;116:612-618

8. Yokoyama C, Shinjo F, Yoshimoto T, Yamamoto S, Oates JA, Brash AR. J Biol Chem 1986;261:16714-16721

9. Bryant RW, Schewe T, Rapoport SM, Bailey JM. J Biol Chem 1985; 260:3548-3555

Advances in Prostaglandin, Thromboxane, and
Leukotriene Research, Vol. 19, edited by
B. Samuelsson, P. Y.-K. Wong, and F. F. Sun,
Raven Press, Ltd., New York ©1989.

UNUSUAL ROLE OF CALCIUM IN THE STIMULATION
OF THE 5-LIPOXYGENASE IN PT-18 CELLS

Jack Y. Vanderhoek, Becky M. Vonakis and Gary Fiskum

Department of Biochemistry, The George Washington University
School of Medicine, Washington, D.C. 20037

The biosynthetic sequence of events leading to the
formation of the biologically active leukotrienes starts with
the hydrolytic release of arachidonic acid from membrane lipids
and is followed by the oxygenation of arachidonic acid by the
5-lipoxygenase (5-LO) (1). However, many 5-LOs appear to exist
in a relatively inactive state even in the presence of
substrate and have to be stimulated before metabolites can be
produced (2). Various investigators have shown that formation
of 5-LO metabolites in intact human blood leukocytes and RBL-1
cells was markedly potentiated by the addition of the calcium
ionophore A23187 (3,4). We have previously reported that the
murine mast/basophil cell line PT-18 contains an inactive or
cryptic 5-LO and that this enzyme could be stimulated by
preincubation of the cells with the 15-LO product 15-
hydroxyeicosatetraenoic acid (15-HETE) (5). However, A23187
was much less effective in activating the 5-LO in PT-18 cells
whereas the isomeric 12-HETE was ineffective (5,6).
    Although various reports have confirmed that calcium was a
required cofactor for the (semi-)purified 5-LO enzyme from a
variety of sources (7,8), the results with PT-18 cells seem to
be anomalous. The purpose of this study was to elucidate the
role of cytosolic calcium in the activation of the 5-LO in
intact PT-18 cells.

MATERIALS AND METHODS

    PT-18 cells were grown as previously described (5) except
that a subline was used which did not require concanavalin A-
conditioned murine spleen cell supernatant. Fura-2-AM was
purchased from Calbiochem-Behring Diagnostics (San Diego, CA)
and 3,4,5-trimethoxybenzoic acid 8-(diethylamino)-octyl ester
(TMB-8) was obtained from Sigma Chemical Co. (St. Louis, MO).
PT-18 cells were harvested in the log phase of growth, washed
once and resuspended in RPMI-1640 (pH 7.4; without L-glutamine)
supplemented with 25 mM Hepes and 2 mg/ml dextrose at a
concentration of 7 X 10^6 cells/ml. The cells were kept on ice
prior to loading with Fura-2. For loading, 3.5 X 10^7 cells
were added to 5 ml of buffer kept at 37°C, followed by 5 μM
Fura-2 AM, and incubated at 37°C for 30 minutes. The cell
suspension was pelleted and the Fura-loaded cells were

resuspended in 5 ml of buffer without Fura-2 AM. The effect of various fatty acids on the cytosolic ionized calcium concentrations were monitored with a Perkin-Elmer LS-3 fluorescence spectrometer equipped with a 37° sample chamber. The samples were excited at 340 nm and fluorescent emission was monitored at 510 nm.

RESULTS AND DISCUSSION

Preincubating PT-18 cells with 17 μM 15-HETE prior to the addition of [^{14}C]-arachidonic acid (16 μM) stimulated the 5-LO activity (as measured by [^{14}C]-5-HETE formation) from 2.5 $\pm$ 1.4% dpm (control; n=10) to 15.5 $\pm$ 5.9% dpm (n=10). In the presence of 30 μM TMB-8, an intracellular calcium antagonist (9), the 15-HETE-induced stimulation was only 1.3 $\pm$ 0.6% dpm (n=4). This observation, coupled with the above mentioned calcium cofactor requirement of the 5-LO enzyme, could not explain the relative ineffectiveness of A23187 in enhancing the 5-LO in PT-18 cells and led us to examine the role of intracellular calcium ions in the activation of this cryptic LO.

The effects of various fatty acids on intracellular calcium levels were evaluated using PT-18 cells loaded with the calcium indicator dye Fura-2 (10) and monitoring the relative fluorescence intensity. At a fatty acid concentration of 15 μM, arachidonic acid was able to induce significant increases in fluorescence intensity, whereas 12-HETE or 15-HETE was relatively ineffective (Figure 1). None of these compounds exhibited significant fluorescence by themselves. On the other hand, when the fatty acid concentration was raised to 30 μM, both HETE isomers were more effective in increasing the intracellular calcium concentration but the order of potencies was arachidonic acid >>12-HETE>15-HETE. Ionomycin (5 μM), an ionophore known to translocate calcium across membranes thereby increasing cytosolic free calcium concentration (11), was 3-4 times more potent in enhancing fluorescence intensity than arachidonic acid (15 μM). Although previous reports have indicated that arachidonic acid and 12-HETE stimulated ^{45}Ca uptake in pancreatic islets (12) and neutrophils (13) respectively, the present study compares the potencies of these fatty acids in the same system.

To further examine whether intracellular calcium changes could be correlated with 5-LO stimulation, Fura-2 loaded PT-18 cells were pretreated with 15-HETE or ionomycin, followed by the addition of [^{14}C]-arachidonic acid. Although ionomycin and arachidonic acid induced large increases in cytosolic calcium levels, no corresponding increase in 5-LO activity (as measured by [^{14}C]-5-HETE formation) was observed. On the other hand, 15-HETE (15 μM) caused a very small increase in intracellular calcium, but a large increase in [^{14}C]-5-HETE formation. These

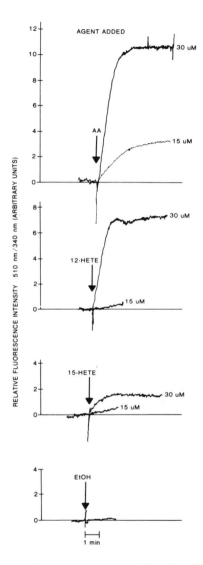

FIG 1. The effects of arachidonic acid, 12-HETE and 15-HETE on
the fluorescence of Fura-2 loaded PT-18 cells. PT-18 cells
(7×10^6 cells/ml) were loaded with 5 μM Fura-2, and incubated
with the indicated concentrations of arachidonic acid, 12-HETE,
15-HETE or ethanol (control vehicle). The intensities of the
signals reflect the amount of cytosolic calcium mobilization.
The results are representative of at least four different
experiments.

results indicate that the ability of arachidonic acid (and other fatty acids) to increase cytosolic calcium may not be important in the stimulation of this cryptic 5-LO but may be relevant in other cellular processes.

In conclusion, these studies suggest that the inability of 15-HETE to increase cytosolic calcium levels does not seem to interfere with its effectiveness in activating the cryptic 5-LO in PT-18 cells to its catalytically active state.

ACKNOWLEDGEMENTS

This work was supported by grants from the National Institutes of Health.

REFERENCES

1. Samuelsson B. *Science* 1983;220:568-575.
2. Vanderhoek JY, Bailey JM. In: Bailey JM, Ed. *Prostaglandins, Leukotrienes and Lipoxins*, New York: Plenum Publishing Corp., 1985;133-146.
3. Borgeat P, Samuelsson B. *Proc Natl Acad Sci USA* 1979;76:2148-2152.
4. Jakschik BA, Lee LH, Shuffer G, Parker CW. *Prostaglandins* 1978;16:733-748.
5. Vanderhoek JY, Tare NS, Bailey JM, Goldstein, AL, Pluznik DH. *J Biol Chem* 1982;257:12191-12195.
6. Vanderhoek JY, Pluznik DH. *Biochim Biophys Acta* 1985;837:119-122.
7. Jakschik BA, Sun FF, Lee LH, Steinhoff MM. *Biochem Biophys Res Comm* 1980;95:103-110.
8. Ueda N, Kaneko S, Yoshimoto T, Yamamoto S. *J Biol Chem* 1986;261:7982-7988.
9. Chiou CY, Malagodi MH. *Brit J Pharm* 1975;53:279-285.
10. Grynkiewicz G, Poenie M, Tsien T. *J Biol Chem* 1985;260:3440-3450.
11. Pollock WK, Rink TJ. *Biochem Biophys Res Comm* 1986;139:308-314.
12. Wolf BA, Turk J, Sherman WR, McDaniel ML. *J Biol Chem* 1986;261:3501-3511.
13. Naccache PH, Shaafi RI, Borgeat P, Goetzl EJ. *J Clin Invest* 1981;67:1584-1587.

*Advances in Prostaglandin, Thromboxane, and
Leukotriene Research*, Vol. 19, edited by
B. Samuelsson, P. Y.-K. Wong, and F. F. Sun,
Raven Press, Ltd., New York ©1989.

ENZYME IMMUNOASSAYS FOR CYCLOOXYGENASE

AND 12-LIPOXYGENASE OF HUMAN PLATELETS

T. Yoshimoto, H. Ehara, Y. Konishi, C. Yokoyama,
J. Murakami, S. Yamamoto, and *A. Hattori

Department of Biochemistry, Tokushima University
School of Medicine, Tokushima 770, Japan
*Department of Internal Medicine, Niigata University
School of Medicine, Niigata 951, Japan

In human platelets there are two pathways of arachidonic acid metabolism initiated by the reactions of cyclooxygenase and 12-lipoxygenase (1,2). The cyclooxygenase produces prostaglandin endoperoxides (PGG$_2$ and PGH$_2$) which are transformed into pro-aggregatory and vasoconstrictive thromboxane A$_2$. The 12-lipoxygenase oxygenates C-12 of arachidonic acid to give rise 12-HPETE which is then reduced to 12-HETE. The physiological role of 12-lipoxygenase has not yet been clarified. Recently we prepared monoclonal antibodies against these enzymes with partially purified enzyme preparations as antigens. By utilizing these antibodies, sensitive enzyme immunoassays of sandwich-type were developed for cyclooxygenase and 12-lipoxygenase of human platelets. The assays will allow a study on the pathophysiological dynamics of these enzymes.

ENZYME IMMUNOASSAY FOR CYCLOOXYGENASE

Using a partially purified cyclooxygenase of human platelet microsomes as an antigen, two species of monoclonal antibody (hPES-1 and hPES-2) were raised by the hybridoma technique (3). When cyclooxygenase was incubated with increasing amounts of antibody, the enzyme activity in the immunoprecipitate increased, and a maximum precipitation was attained with about 20 μg IgG of each antibody. Since these two antibodies seemed to recognize the same epitope of cyclooxygenase protein, an enzyme immunoassay of cyclooxygenase was developed by the use of hPES-1 and PES-5, the latter of which had been raised previously with bovine cyclooxygenase and cross-reacted with human enzyme (4). Peroxidase-labeled Fab' of PES-5 was prepared and incubated with cyclooxygenase, which was now labeled with peroxidase via the Fab' fragment. The immune complex was then precipitated with the aid of the other antibody (hPES-1). The peroxidase activity in the precipitate was determined by reaction with o-phenylenediamine and hydrogen peroxide following the increase of absorbance at 440 nm. The peroxidase activity was correlated with the amount of cyclooxygenase initially present in the assay mixture. When increasing amounts of the cyclooxygenase solubilized from human platelets were subjected to the standard enzyme immunoassay, the peroxidase activity in the immunoprecipitate increased in a linear fashion. The enzyme immunoassay thus established was over 100-times more sensitive than the cyclooxygenase activity assay measuring the conversion of ^{14}C-arachidonic acid to PGH_2.

A CASE OF CYCLOOXYGENASE ABNORMALITY

A female patient (47 years old) was investigated who showed a prolonged bleeding time and a reduced platelet aggregability (5). When a suspension of normal platelets was incubated with ^{14}C-arachidonic acid, four major product were observed upon thin layer chromatography; TXB_2, HHT, 12-HETE and 12-HPETE. In sharp contrast, patient's platelets produced only 12-HETE and 12-HPETE, and no cyclooxygenase products were detected in significant amounts. The solubilized cyclooxygenase of platelets from a normal subject or the patient was precipitated with an anti-cyclooxygenase antibody (hPES-1), and the immunoprecipitate was assayed for cyclooxygenase activity. The immunoprecipitate from normal platelets transformed arachidonic acid to PGH_2, whereas that from the patient's platelets showed no cyclooxygenase

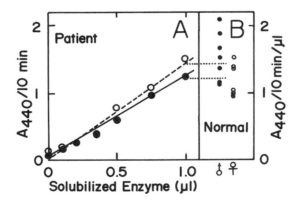

Fig. 1   Platelet cyclooxygenase content of a patient and normal subjects.   (A) Varing amounts of the solubilized enzyme from the patient were assayed in two occasions (o,●).   (B) The solubilized cyclooxygenase of normal platelets was subjected to standard enzyme immunoassay, and the cyclooxygenase content was expressed as A440 nm/10 min/2 x 10^6 platelets equivalent.

activity.   On the other hand, PGH$_2$ was converted to TXB$_2$ and HHT
at the same rate by platelets from both the normal subject and
the patient.   These results indicated that cyclooxygenase but not
thromboxane A synthase was impaired in patient's platelets.   The
solubilized preparation of the patient's platelets was subjected
to the standard enzyme immunoassay.   As shown in Fig. 1, the
patient's platelets in two separate determinations showed almost
the same enzyme level as normal platelets.   Furthermore, the
solubilized cyclooxygenase was precipitated by the antibody
(hPES-1) linked to Affi-Prep 10, and the immunoprecipitate was
analyzed by SDS-polyacrylamide gel electrophoresis followed by
staining with Coomassie Brilliant Blue.   Almost the same amount
of cyclooxygenase protein was detected in both normal platelets
and patient's platelets.   These lines of evidence indicated that
patient's platelets had an immunoreactive but catalytically
inactive cyclooxygenase protein.

ENZYME IMMUNOASSAY FOR 12-LIPOXYGENASE

12-Lipoxygenase was localized predominantly in the cytosol
fraction of human platelets (2).   The enzyme was partially
purified by ammonium sulfate fractionation (0-50% saturation)
followed by sequential chromatographies on DEAE-cellulose and
hydroxyapatite.   The enzyme thus purified by about 20 folds, was
used in the immunization of mice to prepare monoclonal anti-12-
lipoxygenase antibodies.   We obtained three species of antibody
(HPLO-1, HPLO-2 and HPLO-3).   When the 12-lipoxygenase of human
platelet cytosol was incubated with these antibodies the enzyme

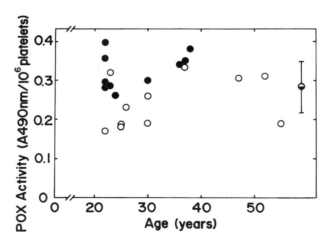

Fig. 2   Platelet 12-lipoxygenase content of normal subjects.
Platelets of male (o) and female (●) volunteers were subjected to
the standard enzyme immunoassay.   Mean and SD were also shown on
the right side.

activity in the immunoprecipitate increased depending upon the amount of each antibody. It should be noted that HPLO-2 did not cross-react with the 12-lipoxygenase purified from porcine leukocytes (6). HPLO-2 and HPLO-3 seemed to recognize different epitopes of 12-lipoxygenase protein. These two species of antibody were utilized to develop a peroxidase-linked immunoassay for 12-lipoxygenase of human platelets as discussed above for cyclooxygenase. The enzyme immunoassay was much more sensitive than the activity assay as assessed by the conversion of ^{14}C-arachidonic acid to 12-HPETE. The enzyme level in platelets of 22 normal subjects was screened by the enzyme immunoassay as shown in Fig. 2. Platelets from female subjects showed slightly higher enzyme content than those from male, but the difference was not statistically significant.

ACKNOWLEDGEMENTS

This work was supported by a grant-in-aid for scientific research from the Ministry of Education, Science and Culture of Japan, and grants from the Japanese Foundation of Metabolism and Diseases and Uehara Memorial Foundation.

REFERENCES

1. Hamberg M, Samuelsson B. Proc. Natl. Acad. Sci. USA 1974;71: 3400-3404

2. Nugteren DH. Biochim. Biophys. Acta 1975;380:299-307

3. Ehara H, Yoshimoto T, Yamamoto S, Hattori A. Biochim. Biophys. Acta 1988;960:35-42

4. Yoshimoto T, Magata K, Ehara H, Mizuno K, Yamamoto S. Biochim. Biophys. Acta 1986;877:141-150

5. Nakanishi K, Ikeda K, Hato T, Imai A, Kaneko H, Murakami A, Kumashima K, Kaido H, Kondo M, Hattori A, Fujita S, Kobayashi Y. Scand. J. Haematol. 1984;32:167-174

6. Yokoyama C, Shinjo F, Yoshimoto T, Yamamoto S, Oates JA, Brash AR. J. Biol. Chem. 1986;261:16714-16721

Advances in Prostaglandin, Thromboxane, and Leukotriene Research, Vol. 19, edited by B. Samuelsson, P. Y.-K. Wong, and F. F. Sun, Raven Press, Ltd., New York ©1989.

CHARACTERIZATION OF CGS 8515 AS A SELECTIVE

5-LIPOXYGENASE (5-LO) INHIBITOR

E.C. Ku, A. Raychaudhuri, G. Ghai, E.F. Kimble, W.H. Lee, C. Colombo, R. Dotson, D. White, T.D. Oglesby and J.W.F. Wasley

Research Dept., Pharmaceuticals Div., CIBA-GEIGY Corp., Summit, New Jersey 07901 U.S.A.

The pathophysiological importance of the 5-LO pathway has gained wide recognition since the discovery that leukotriene (LT) products are formed by this process (1). LTs are mediators of inflammation and host-response reactions (1).

Regulation of LT product formation in leukocytes and in target organs may be an important means of achieving therapeutic effects. Recent reports demonstrating the beneficial effects of 5-LO inhibitors in anaphylaxis (2), inflammatory responses (3) and antigen-induced bronchoconstriction in animals (4), and in the treatment of psoriasis in humans (5), have stimulated the search for therapeutic agents that inhibit LT biosynthesis.

This report profiles the pharmacological effects of a new 5-LO inhibitor, CGS 8515 {methyl 2-[(3,4-dihydro-3,4-dioxo-1-naphthalenyl)amino]-benzoate}, on arachidonic acid (AA) biotransformation and leukocyte function in <u>in vitro</u> and in animal models.

EFFECTS ON KEY ENZYMES OF AA METABOLISM

CGS 8515 inhibited the production of 5-LO products (5-HETE and LTB_4) in A23187-stimulated leukocytes (Table 1). The effect was concentration-dependent with an IC_{50} of 0.1 uM. With the exception of high concentrations (greater then 30 uM), CGS 8515 showed negligible effect on other key enzymes involved in AA metabolism (Table 1). The compound did not significantly affect leukocyte viability by the trypan blue test at a period up to 4 h.

The selective effect of CGS 8515 as a 5-LO inhibitor was shown to extend to a whole blood model based on LT formation stimulated by A23187. CGS 8515 preferentially inhibited the production of 5-LO (5-HETE, LTB_4 and LTC_4) over cyclooxygenase (CO) products (e.g. TxB_2) with a potency ratio of at least 20 in rat and 70 in human whole blood. CGS 8515 also affected 5-LO product formation at the tissue level. Over a concentration range of 0.3–1 uM, the compound significantly inhibited A23187–stimulated formation of peptido–LTs (LTC_4 and LTD_4) in rat lung (45–70%).

TABLE 1. Activity profiles in key enzymes of the
arachidonic acid cascade

Compound	5–LO	15–LO	IC_{50} Value (uM) 12–LO	CO	TxS
5,8,11,14–ETYA	13	0.2	0.7	6	N.D.
NDGA	2	6	4	5	N.D.
BW 755C	25	10	>30	10	N.D.
Indomethacin	150	>500	N.D.	15	N.D.
Propyl gallate	6	3	N.D.	170	N.D.
CGS 13080	4,000	>1,000	N.D.	3,600	0.003
AA 861	0.1	70	>30	>4,000	N.D.
CGS 8515	0.1	>500	>30	340	>50

N.D.= not determined. The assays were based on [^{14}C]AA conversion in guinea pig peritoneal leukocytes (5–LO), or with partially purified enzymes isolated from sheep seminal vesicles (CO), human platelets (12–LO and TxS) and human leukocytes (15–LO) as previously described (6,7). TxS = thromboxane synthase.

EFFECTS ON LT PRODUCTION IN ANIMAL SYSTEMS

The effect of CGS 8515 as a 5–LO inhibitor was confirmed in animal models. The compound dose–dependently inhibited the ex vivo production of 5–HETE and LTC_4 in rat blood over a dose range of 0.5–10 mg/kg, p.o. (Fig. 1). From these data, an approximate ED_{50} of 4 mg/kg can be derived for the inhibition of all three 5–LO metabolites (5–HETE, LTB_4 and LTC_4). AA 861 showed similar potency in this respect (data not shown). The effect of CGS 8515 persisted for at least 6 h after oral administration.

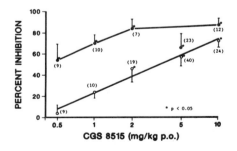

FIG. 1. Effects of CGS 8515 on ex vivo production of 5–LO products in rat blood. Blood samples were drawn 1 h after oral dosing and stimulated with A23187 (10 uM) and PAF (60 uM) for 15 min at 37°C (7). Plasma eicosanoid levels were assayed by RIA. Results shown are mean percent inhibition for the number of animals (n) indicated for 5–HETE (●) and LTC_4 (o).

Oral administration of CGS 8515 over the range of 5–50 mg/kg dose–dependently inhibited A23187–induced LTD_4 production from rat lung (data not shown).

PHARMACOLOGICAL EFFECTS IN ANIMAL MODELS

Compounds were tested in a rat model for effects on migration of leukocytes into the polyurethane sponge implants impregnated with carrageenan (7). CGS 8515, at oral doses of 2–5 mg/kg, significantly inhibited the accumulation of leukocytes in the sponge implants (Table 2). The degree of inhibition was comparable to that seen with the reference compounds AA 861 (5 mg/kg) and BW 755C (50 mg/kg).

TABLE 2.   Effects on carrageenan–induced leukocyte accumulation in the rat sponge model

Compound	Dose (3x per 24 h) mg/kg p.o.	Leukocyte Count (Cells/mm^3)	Percent Inhibition
BW 755C	Control	14,800 ± 700	–
	50	9,500 ± 540**	36%**
AA 861	Control	10,200 ± 790	–
	5	7,700 ± 710*	25%*
CGS 8515	Control	18,000 ± 1,900	–
	5	9,700 ± 1,400**	46%**
	Control	9,730 ± 790	–
	2	7,250 ± 690*	25%*
	5	6,700 ± 1,030*	29%*

* and ** designate $P < 0.05$ and $P < 0.01$, respectively. Animals (n = 10) were dosed with test compound 3 times (–1, 6 and 22 h after sponge implant). At 24 h, the sponges were removed for microscopic enumeration of leukocytes.

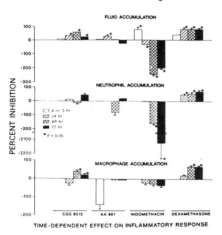

TIME-DEPENDENT EFFECT ON INFLAMMATORY RESPONSE

FIG. 2. Time–dependent effects of different agents on development of inflammatory response in the rat pleurisy model (8). Rats (n = 6–8) were dosed with test compound by the following schedules for determination of drug effects at different time points relative to carrageenan injection:
4–h at –1 h;
24–h at –1, 6 and 21 h;
48–h at –1, 6, 24 and 45 h;
72–h at –1, 6, 24, 48 and 69 h.
Exudate volume and differential leukocyte counts were determined as previously described (8).

The effects of CGS 8515 and reference compounds (indomethacin, AA 861 and dexamethasone) on leukocyte migration and exudate accumulation were studied in a rat pleurisy model (8). CGS 8515, at oral doses of 5–20 mg/kg, showed a distinct anti-inflammatory effect on exudate volume at time points as early as 24 h after carrageenan injection. This effect persisted through the 72 h time period. Although CGS 8515 failed to inhibit cell influx at the 24-h time point, it significantly suppressed the influx of mononuclear cells as the inflammation was allowed to become chronic at 48 and 72 h. Indomethacin, however, showed an enhancing effect on both fluid and neutrophil accumulation at these time points. Dexamethasone, on the other hand, inhibited fluid and leukocyte (neutrophil and macrophage) accumulation significantly throughout the entire 72-h study period.

Fig. 2 shows the differential effects of CGS 8515 (10 mg/kg), AA 861 (80 mg/kg), indomethacin (10 mg/kg) and dexamethasone (0.05 mg/kg) on fluid and leukocyte accumulation in the rat pleurisy model.

SUMMARY

1. CGS 8515 selectively inhibited 5-LO (IC_{50} = 0.1 uM) with negligible effect on CO, 12-LO, 15-LO and TxS at concentrations up to 100 uM.
2. CGS 8515 selectively inhibited A23187-induced formation of 5-LO products in rat and human whole blood with a 20–70 fold separation of effects over the formation of CO products.
3. Ex vivo and in vivo studies with rats showed that CGS 8515, at an oral dose of 2–50 mg/kg, significantly inhibited A23187-induced formation of LTs in whole blood and in the lung. The effect persisted for at least 6 h in the ex vivo blood model.
4. CGS 8515, at oral doses as low as 5 mg/kg, significantly suppressed exudate volume and leukocyte migration in the carrageenan-induced pleurisy and sponge models in the rat.

REFERENCES

1. Samuelsson B. Science 1983; 220:568–575.

2. Higgs GA. Prostaglandins Leukotrienes Med 1984; 13:89–92.

3. Creticos PS., Peters SP, Adkinson NF, et al. N Engl J Med 1984; 310:1626–1630.

4. Chustecka Z. In: The Scrip Leukotriene Report, Surrey (U.K.): PJB Publications, 1985.

5. Lassus A, Forsstrom S. Br J Dermatol 1985; 113:103–106.

6. Ku EC, McPherson SE, Signor C, Chertock H, Cash WD. Biochem Biophys Res Commun 1983; 112:899–906.

7. Kothari HV, Lee WH, Ku EC. Biochim Biophys Acta 1987; 921:502–511.

8. Almeida AP, Bayer BM, Horakova Z, Beaven MA. J Pharmacol Exp Ther 1980; 214:74–79.

Advances in Prostaglandin, Thromboxane, and Leukotriene Research, Vol. 19, edited by B. Samuelsson, P. Y.-K. Wong, and F. F. Sun, Raven Press, Ltd., New York ©1989.

PARTIAL PURIFICATION AND CHARACTERIZATION OF LEUKOTRIENE C_4 SYNTHASE FROM GUINEA PIG LUNG

T. Izumi, Z. Honda, N. Ohishi, S. Kitamura, Y. Seyama, and T. Shimizu

Department of Physiological Chemistry and Nutrition, Faculty of Medicine, University of Tokyo, Bunkyo-ku, Tokyo 113, Japan

Leukotriene (LT) C_4 synthase was solubilized from the microsomes of guinea pig lung by the treatment with a combination of CHAPS, digitonin, and KCl, and then it was partially purified by two steps of column chromatography which resulted in a complete resolution of the enzyme from glutathione $\underline{S}$-transferases (GSTs). The enzyme was extremely unstable. Glutathione protected the enzyme from inactivation, but other sulfhydryl group reducing reagents did not. The partially purified enzyme revealed high specificity towards 5,6-epoxide LTs.

INTRODUCTION

LTC_4 is synthesized by the enzymic conjugation of glutathione and LTA_4, and further metabolized to the additional cysteinyl-containing LTs that together constitute the slow reaction substance of anaphylaxis (1,2). This conversions of LTA_4 to LTC_4 have been observed in rat basophilic leukemia cells (3-5), rat liver (4), peritoneal macrophages of mice and rat (6), and human platelets (7). Solubilization of LTC_4 synthase from rat basophilic leukemia cells was reported in previous reports (4,5). However the properties of the enzyme and the relationship to other GSTs have not been fully elucidated.

MATERIALS AND METHODS

Enzyme assay.
LTC_4 synthase was assayed according to the method described in our previous paper (8). In brief, the standard reaction mixture contained 0.1 M Tris-HCl buffer, pH 8, 10 mM glutathione, 2 mg/ml of BSA, and enzyme. After preincubation at 37°C for 1 min, the reaction was started by the addition of 70 μM LTA_4 and carried out for 5 min at 37°C. The reaction was ter-

minated by the addition of the acidic organic solvent.   After
centrifugation, an aliquot of the supernatant was analyzed by
reversed-phase HPLC.   The product was identified by UV spectroscopy and the incorporation of (^{3}H) glutathione.
      GST activity was measured spectrometrically with 1 mM 1-
chloro-2,4-dinitrobenzene and 1 mM glutathione as substrates according to Habig <u>et al</u> (9).

      <u>Solubilization and purification of LTC$_4$ synthase from
microsomes of guinea pig lung</u>. (8)
      The microsomes (100,000 x g, pellet) from guinea pig lung
were treated with 1.5 % CHAPS, 0.75 % digitonin, 1 M KCl, 5 %
glycerol and centrifuged at 100,000 x g for 1 h.   The supernatant was applied onto a gel filtration column, Superose 12.
The collected active fractions were applied to an anion-
exchanger colunm, TSK DEAE-5PW.   After elution of proteins not
absorbing to the column, the concentration of KCl was raised to
1 M stepwisely.   The active fractions were combined, and
referred to as the partially purified LTC$_4$ synthase.

RESULTS

      <u>Solubilization and partial purification of LTC$_4$ synthase
from guinea pig lung</u>.
      By the combination of detergents (CHAPS and digitonin) and
KCl, the LTC$_4$ synthase activity was solubilized, and included in
a gelfiltration column.   While GST activities were eluted in two
major peaks, LTC$_4$ synthase activity was eluted in a single peak.
On the following anion-
exchange chromatography,
the remaining GST act-
ivity was recovered in
pass-through fractions,
while LTC$_4$ synthase activity was eluted with
0.2 M KCl (Fig. 1).
The partially purified
LTC$_4$ synthase showed a
specific activity of
39.3 nmol/mg·5 min and
no GST activity.   The
recoveries of protein
and the LTC$_4$ synthase
activity from the homo-
genates were 0.12 % and
2.5 %, respectively,
and this enzyme showed
a 21-fold enrichment
of the specific activity
from the homogenates.

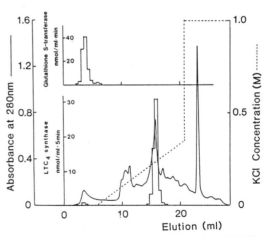

FIG. 1.   RESOLUTION OF LTC$_4$ SYNTHASE
AND GST BY ANION-EXCHANGE CHROMATO-
GRAPHY.   Active fractions from
Superose 12 were applied to a TSK
DEAE-5PW column.

Kinetic properties of LTC$_4$ synthase.

The K$_m$ values for LTA$_4$ and for glutathione were 36 μM and 1.6 mM, respectively, and the V$_{max}$ value of the partially purified LTC$_4$ synthase was 40 nmol/mg·min.

Stabilizing effect of glutathione on LTC$_4$ synthase.

The partially purified LTC$_4$ synthase was unstable (T$_{1/2}$ at 37°C = 3 min) (Fig. 2). When the enzyme was incubated with 2 mM glutathione, it was partially protected from inactivation, and no inactivation was observed with 10 mM glutathione. Neither dithiothreitol, 2-mercaptoethanol, cysteine, or oxidized form of glutathione had the protective effect.

Substrate specificity of LTC$_4$ synthase.

LTA$_4$ and four more epoxide LTs were evaluated as sub-strates for the partially purified LTC$_4$ synthase (Table 1). This enzyme had the similar K$_m$ and V$_{max}$ values towards LTA$_4$ as towards LTA$_4$ methyl ester. 14,15-LTA$_4$ and its methyl ester could not serve as good substrates, having higher K$_m$ and smaller V$_{max}$ values. 11,12-LTA$_4$ methyl ester was not converted. This enzyme did not have any GST activities when assayed with 1-chloro-2,4-dinitrobenzene, 1,2-dichloro-4-nitrobenzene, p-nitrophenethyl bromide, trans-4-phenyl-3-buten-2-one, 1,2-epoxy-3-(p-nitro phenoxy)propane, or ethacrynic acid.

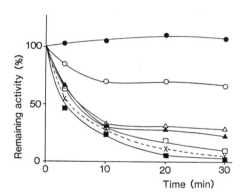

FIG. 2.   PROTECTIVE EFFECTS OF GLUTATHIUONE ON LTC$_4$ SYNTHASE.

The partially purified LTC$_4$ syn-thase was preincubated at 37°C.: without drug (X---X), with 10 mM glutathione (●), 2 mM glutathone (O), 1 mM dithiothreitol (△), 2 mM 2-mercaptoethanol (▲), 2 mM cysteine (□), and 5 mM oxidized form of glutathione (■).

TABLE 1.   Substrate speci-ficities of LTC$_4$ synthase

substrate	V$_{max}$ (nmol/mg·min)	K$_m$ (μM)
LTA$_4$	40	36
LTA$_4$ me*	32	20
14,15-LTA$_4$	13	130
14,15-LTA$_4$ me	13	70
11,12-LTA$_4$ me	not substrate	

*methyl ester

DISCUSSION

Solubilization and two subsequent steps of chromato-graphies resulted in complete resolution of LTC$_4$ synthase ac-tivity from GST activities. The partially purified LTC$_4$ syn-thase showed a 21-fold enrichment of the specific activity over the homogenates. Although more than 99 % of the protein was removed by those procedures, the specific activity was still rather low, possibly due to the instability of the enzyme. The partially purified enzyme from rat basophilic leukemia cells has also been reported as heat labile (5). While other sulfhydryl group reducing reagents did not stabilize LTC_4 synthase, glutathione had this effect. The apparent K_m value for glutathione was 1.6 mM. Thus, LTC_4 formation might be regulated by the glutathione concentrations.

LTA_4 and LTA_4 methyl ester served as substrates of the partially purified LTC_4 synthase, but 14,15-LTA_4 and its methyl ester were poor substrates and 11,12-LTA_4 methyl ester was not converted at all. Also, this enzyme did not act on other substrates of GSTs. On the other hand, rat cytosolic GSTs can convert all these epoxide LTs (8), and different types of human cytosolic GST were reported to conjugate glutathione to LTA_4 or LTA_4 methyl ester (10).

All these results indicate that LTC_4 synthase in guinea pig lung is a unique and specific enzyme.

REFERENCES

1. Lewis RA, Drazen JM, Corey EJ, and Austen, KF. In:Piper PJ ed. SRS-A and Leukotrienes Chichester:Reseach Studies Press, 1981;101-107.

2. Hammarström S. Ann Rev Biochem 1983;52:355-377.

3. Jakschik BA, Harper T, and Murphy RC. J Biol Chem 1982;257: 5346-5349.

4. Bach MK, Brashler JR, and Morton DR Jr. Arch Biochem Biophys 1984;230:455-465.

5. Yoshimoto T, Soberman RJ, Lewis RA, and Austin, KF. Proc Natl Acad Sci USA 1985;82:8399-8403.

6. Abe M, Kawazoe Y, Tunematsu H, and Shigematsu N. Biochem Biophys Res Commun 1985;127:15-23.

7. Pace-Asciak CR, Klein J, and Spielberg SP. Biochim Biophys Acta 1986;877:68-74.

8. Izumi T, Honda Z, Oishi N, Tsuchida S, Sato K, Kitamura S, Shimizu T, and Seyama Y. Biochim Biophys Acta 1988;(in press)

9. Habig WH, Pabst MJ, and Jakoby WB. J Biol Chem 1974;249: 7130-7139.

10. Soderström M, Mannervik B, Oring L, and Hammarström S. Biochem Biophys Res Commun 1985;128:265-270.

Advances in Prostaglandin, Thromboxane, and
Leukotriene Research, Vol. 19, edited by
B. Samuelsson, P. Y.-K. Wong, and F. F. Sun,
Raven Press, Ltd., New York ©1989.

Properties of leukotriene A$_4$-hydrolase from guinea pig liver

Haeggström, J., T., Bergman, T., Jörnvall, H.,
and Rådmark, O.

Department of Physiological Chemistry
Karolinska Institutet
S-104 01 Stockholm, Sweden

Leukotriene A$_4$-hydrolase converts the allylic epoxide leukotriene A$_4$ (LTA$_4$) into the chemotactic agent leukotriene B$_4$ (LTB$_4$). This enzyme has been purified from different blood cells (1-3) and from lung tissue (4). LTA$_4$-hydrolase was also present in plasma from several species (5) as well as in liver from guinea pig and man (6). Also another epoxide hydrolase, i.e. cytosolic epoxide hydrolase (cEH) was demonstrated to convert LTA$_4$. In this case the product was 5(S),6(R)-di-hydroxy-7,9-trans-11,14-cis-eicosatetraenoic acid (5,6-DHETE)-(7). This paper describes some characteristics of LTA$_4$-hydrolase purified from guinea pig liver.

Methods

The purification procedure is outlined in table 1. For more details, and additional methodology it is referred to the original paper (8).

Results and Discussion

LTA$_4$-hydrolase from guinea pig liver was purified 1200-fold, to about 85% homogeneity in good yield (close to 20%). The enzyme was similar to its human counterpart in many respects, but also it displayed some special features, primarily a higher catalytic activity.

The starting material for the enzyme purification (100.000 x g supernatant from liver homogenate) contained cEH as well as LTA$_4$-hydrolase. However alredy after the first anion exchange chromatography (DEAE cellulose) these two enzyme activities were separated. This shows that also in liver tissue, LTA$_4$-hydrolase and cEH are two different enzymes which convert the same substrate (LTA$_4$) to different products (LTB$_4$ and 5,6-DHETE respectively).

PURIFICATION OF LTA$_4$ HYDROLASE FROM GUINEA-PIG LIVER

Aliquots of the enzyme from each step of purification were incubated with LTA$_4$ (100 µM) at 37°C for 1 min. Analysis and quantitation of LTB$_4$ was performed with reverse-phase HPLC. Enzymatic activity is expressed as nmol LTB$_4$ formed per min.

Fraction	Volume	Total protein	Total activity	Specific activity	Yield	Purifi-cation
	(ml)	(mg)	(nmol/min)	(nmol/mg/min)	(%)	-fold
Cytosol	102	1835	730	0.4	-	-
Precipitations	40	975	1420	1.5	100	1
AcA-44	265	500	1450	2.9	102	2
DEAE-cellulose	80	62	860	14	61	9
Mono-Q	21	18	800	44	56	29
Hydroxyapatite	13.5	2.6	445	171	31	114
Mono-P	1.1	0.15	270	1800	19	1200

The kinetics of the hydrolysis of LTA$_4$ by the guinea pig liver enzyme were studied. The optimal pH was around 8 and the time course was characterized by the previously observed quick initial burst of product formation, in combination with selfinactivation of the enzyme. However LTA$_4$-hydrolase from guinea pig liver was considerably more active than the human enzyme. This became evident when purified enzyme was incubated at 37°C (see table 1). Mainly due to the instability of LTA$_4$ however, activity assays of LTA$_4$-hydrolase at 37°C are somewhat uncertain. Therefore the activity of guinea pig liver LTA$_4$-hydrolase was elucidated at lower temperatures, and the values at 37°C were determined by extrapolation. Incubation series with different amounts of substrate were performed at -10°C, +0°C and +10°C. Glycerol (30% v/v) was added to prevent freezing. The resulting three graphs describing the relationships between initial velocity and substrate concentration are shown in Fig 1A, and three sets of K_m and v_{max} were obtained, which were used in the respective Arrhenius plots.

Fig 1B thus illustrates how the apparent v_{max} at 37°C could be deduced as 68 µmol/mg/min. This number is substantially higher than previously published data for the human enzyme (below 3 µmol/mg/min). We believe this is not only due to methodological discrepancies, since determination of v_{max} for the guinea pig liver enzyme performed at 37°C also gave a higher number (10 µmol/mg/min). A similar plot of pK_m against 1/T yielded an apparent K_m at 37°C of 27µM. This is in the same range as for the human enzyme.

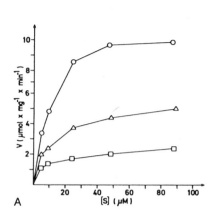

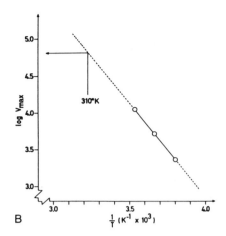

Fig. 1A. Dependency of intitial velocity of substrate concentration at +10°C(o), 0°C (Δ) and -10°C ( ). Aliquots of purified enzyme (0.33 μg dissolved in 100 μl 50 mM Tris-HCl, pH 8.0, with 30% glycerol) were incubated with LTA₄ (5-90 μM) for 5 s. Reactions were stopped with 5 vols. of methanol. Internal standard PGB₁ (150 ng/sample) was added prior to acidic ether extraction and analysis by reverse-phase HPLC.

Fig. 1B. Plot of log V_{max} vs. 1/T (Arrhenius plot). Dashed line indicates extrapolation.

The apparent second order rate constant (k_{cat}/K_m) for guinea pig liver LTA₄-hydrolase was calculated from these data as $3 \times 10^6 \, M^{-1} \times s^{-1}$. The same constant for the conversion of LTA₄ to 5,6-DHETE by cEH was lower (1.3×10^5) (9), indicating the higher efficiency of the enzymatic hydrolysis leading to LTB₄.

		(Ile)								
1	2	3	4	5	6	7	8	9	10	
Pro -	Glu -	Val -	Val -	Asp -	Thr -	Cys -	Ser -	Leu -	Ala	-
706	475	430	461	413	149	286	199	360	377	

		(Ser)							
11	12	13	14	15	16	17	18	19	20
Ser -	Pro -	Ala -	Thr -	Val -	Cys -	Arg -	Thr -	Lys -	His
180	259	348	96	300	117	130	82	240	48

Fig. 2. N-terminal amino acid sequence. Gas-phase sequencer analysis combined with reverse-phase HPLC phenylthiohydantoin identification were performed with ~ 1 nmol of enzyme. Values given are pmoles recovered. Differing residues in human leukocyte LTA₄ hydrolase are given within parentheses.

The guinea pig liver LTA_4-hydrolase was also studied regarding physical properties[4]. The MW (70.000) and Stokes radius (3.0 nm) were similar to the human enzyme, however in the N-terminal sequence two out of twenty amino acids were different (fig 2). Possibly, additional stuctural features could explain the high catalytic activity of LTA_4-hydrolase in guinea pig liver.

Acknowledgements

We thank Dr. Tapio Puustinen for presenting this paper at the Taipei Conference. This project was supported by grants from the Swedish Medical Research Council (03X-217, 03X-07467, 03X-3532), from O.E. & Edla Johanssons Stiftelse, and from Petrus & Augusta Hedlunds Stiftelse.

References

1. Rådmark, O., Shimizu, T., Jörnvall, A. and Samuelsson, B.: (1984) J. Biol. Chem., 259, 12339-12345.

2. McGee, J and Fitzpatrick, F.: (1985) J. Biol. Chem., 260, 12832-12837.

3. Evans, J.F., Nathaniel, D.J., Zamboni, R.J. and Ford-Hutchinson, A.W.: (1985) J. Biol. Chem., 260, 10966-10970.

4. Ohishi, N., Izumi, T., Minami, M., Kitamura, S., Seyama, Y., Ohkawa, S., Terao, S., Yotsumoto, H., Takaku, F. and Shimizu, T.: (1987) J. Biol. Chem., 262, 10200-10205.

5. Fitzpatrick, F., Haeggström, J., Granström, E. and Samuelsson, B.: (1983) Proc. Natl. Acad. Sci. USA, 80, 5425-5429.

6. Haeggström, J., Rådmark, O. and Fitzpatrick, F.A.: (1985) Biochem. Biophys. Acta, 835, 378-384.

7. Haeggström, J., Meijer, J. and Rådmark, O.: (1986) J. Biol. Chem., 261, 6332-6327.

8. Haeggström, J., Bergman, T., Jörnvall, H. and Rådmark, O.: (1988) Eur. J. Biochem., accepted for publication.

9. Haeggström, J., Wetterholm, A., Hamberg, M., Meijer, J., Zipkin, R. and Rådmark, O.: (1988) Biochim. Biophys. Acta, 985, 469-476.

Advances in Prostaglandin, Thromboxane, and Leukotriene Research, Vol. 19, edited by
B. Samuelsson, P. Y.-K. Wong, and F. F. Sun,
Raven Press, Ltd., New York ©1989.

11,12-LEUKOTRIENE A_4: SYNTHESIS AND METABOLISM

Ichiro Miki[1], Shigeto Kitamura[2], Takao Shimizu and Yousuke Seyama

Department of Physiological Chemistry and Nutrition,
Faculty of Medicine, University of Tokyo, Tokyo 113, Japan

SUMMARY

11(S),12(S)-oxido-5Z,7E,9E,14Z-eicosatetraenoic acid (11,12-LTA_4) was chemically synthesized from 12-hydroperoxy-eicosatetra-enoic acid (12-HPETE). 11,12-LTA_4 methyl ester was nonenzymical-ly hydrolyzed to at least four products. These products were identified to be epimers of 5,12(S)-dihydroxy-eicosatetraenoic acid methyl ester (5,12(S)-diHETE-Me) and epimers of 11,12-diHETE-Me. In addition to the above nonenzymic products, 11,12-LTA_4 was converted to 11,12-LTC_4 by the rat liver glutathione S-transferase, and to an isomer of 11,12-diHETE by homogenates of the guinea pig adrenal gland and liver.

12(S)-HPETE was synthesized from arachidonic acid in various tissues of mammals (1-3). The physiological significance of 12-lipoxygenase has not yet been clarified. To examine further conversion of 12-HPETE and its biological significance, we chemi-cally synthesized 11,12-LTA_4 methyl ester (4). In this study, we report the metabolism of this compound.

MATERIALS AND METHODS

Materials
Commercial sources of reagents, and the detailed conditions of synthesis of 11,12-LTA_4 methyl ester are described in Ref. 4.

---

[1] On leave from Pharmaceutical Research Laboratories, Kyowa Hakko Kogyo Co., Ltd., Nagaizumi, Sunto, Shizuoka 411, Japan
[2] On leave from Tokyo Research Laboratories, Kyowa Hakko Kogyo Co., Ltd., Machida, Tokyo 194, Japan

HPLC conditions

A column (TSK ODS-80TM, 0.46 x 15 cm, Tosoh, Japan) was eluted with solvent I (acetonitrile/methanol/water/acetic acid, 300/100/300/0.6, v/v/v/v, containing 0.05 % EDTA Na_2, adjusted pH to 5.6 with ammonia water), at a flow rate of 1 ml/min (5).

Enzymic conversion of 11,12-LTA₄

11,12-LTA₄ methyl ester (0.5 µg) was incubated with rat liver glutathione S-transferase in a reaction mixture consisting of 0.1 M Tris-HCl buffer, pH 8.0, 20 mM glutathione, and 10 mg/ml bovine serum albumin (BSA).

Alternatively, 11,12-LTA₄ (0.5 µg) was incubated with tissue homogenates of guinea pig in a reaction mixture consisting of 0.1 M Tris-HCl buffer, pH 7.3, and 10 mg/ml BSA. These reactions were terminated by the addition of solution A (acetonitrile/methanol/acetic acid, 150:50:3, v/v/v, containing 1 µg/ml prostaglandin B_2 as an internal standard). The mixture was kept standing at -20°C for at least 30 min, followed by centrifugation (10,000 x g, 10 min). To the supernatant, one-sixth volume of 0.35 % EDTA Na_2 was added, and the aliquot (50 µl) was analyzed by HPLC.

RESULTS

Nonenzymic Hydrolysis of Methyl Ester of 11,12-LTA₄

Methyl ester of 11,12-LTA₄ was nonenzymically hydrolyzed to at least four compounds (FIG. 1A). Peaks 1 and 2 were determined as epimers of 5,12(S)-diHETE-Me. Peak 3 was separated into two

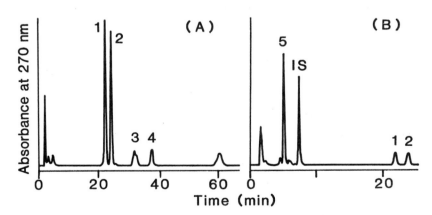

FIG. 1. HPLC analysis of the products from 11,12-LTA₄ methyl ester. (A); Acid-hydrolyzed products of 11,12-LTA₄-Me were analyzed by HPLC. Absorbance at 270 nm was monitored. (B); 11,12-LTA₄-Me was incubated with rat liver glutathione S-transferase. Prostaglandin B_2 was added as an internal standard (IS).

peaks with different C values (23.6 and 24.4) by gas chromatography-mass spectrometry. Both showed same mass spectra of
11,12-diHETE-Me.

Enzymic Products of 11,12-LTA$_4$

Glutathione conjugate of methyl ester of 11,12-LTA$_4$

11,12-LTA$_4$ methyl ester was metabolized to a glutathione conjugate (11,12-LTC$_4$ methyl ester) by the glutathione S-transferase
(FIG. 1B). An incorporation of the radioactivity to the peak 5
was observed when incubated with [^{3}H]glutathione (5). Formation
of 11,12-LTC$_4$ depended on the enzyme amount, and heat treatment
of the enzyme abolished the formation of peak 5.

Incubation with guinea pig homogenates

11,12-LTA$_4$ was incubated with cytosols and microsomes from
various tissues (TABLE I). Cytosols had higher specific activity
than microsomes in every tissues. The adrenal gland and liver
had the highest specific activitiy. The product was identified
as 11,12-diHETE by UV spectra and GC-MS analysis.

DISCUSSION

The methyl ester of 11,12-LTA$_4$ was hydrolyzed to at least four
compounds. Peaks 1 and 2 were identified to be epimers of
5,12(S)-diHETE-Me. Peak 3 had mass spectra of 11,12-diHETEs. The
structure of peak 4 could not be determined. 11,12-LTA$_4$ was
metabolized to 11,12-LTC$_4$ and 11,12-diHETE with rat liver glutathione S-transferase and guinea pig tissue homogenate, respectively (FIG. 2). LTA$_4$ is metabolized to 5,6-diHETE by the

TABLE I. Tissue distribution of 11,12-LTA$_4$ hydrolysis activity

Tissues	Specific activity (nmol/min/mg protein)	
	Cytosol	Microsome
Adrenal gland	1.25	0.31
Liver	0.74	0.23
Small intestine	0.29	0.05
Brain	0.25	0.01
Kidney	0.18	0.05

Tissues of female guinea pigs (Hartley, 250 g body weight)
were homogenized using a Potter-Elvehjem homogenizer in 3 volumes
(v/w) of 0.1 M Tris-HCl buffer, pH 7.8, containing 0.1 M NaCl, 2
mM EDTA Na$_2$ and 0.5 mM dithiothreitol, and centrifuged at 10,000
x g for 10 min. The supernatant was further centrifuged at
105,000 x g for 1 hour (cytosol). The precipitate was washed and
resuspended in the homogenizing buffer (microsome).

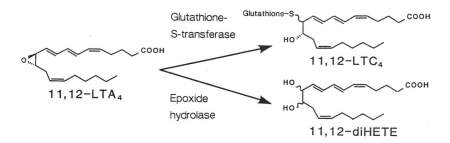

FIG. 2. Enzymic conversions of 11,12-LTA₄

cytosolic epoxide hydrolase (6). The enzyme which produces
11,12-diHETE is a kind of cytosolic epoxide hydrolases. Although
the enzymic formation of 11,12-LTA₄ has not so far been demonstrated, the natural occurrence of 11,12-diHETE was reported
(2,7). The biological activity of the enzymic products of 11,12-
LTA₄ is unclear. However, the acquisition of chemically synthesized 11,12-LTA₄ makes it possible to determine the physiological
significance of 12-lipoxygenase pathway.

REFERENCES

1. Nugteren DH. Biochim Biophys Acta 1975;380:299-307.

2. Samuelsson B. Science 1983;220:568-575.

3. Shimizu T, Takusagawa Y, Izumi T, Ohishi N, Seyama Y.

   J Neurochem 1987;48:1541-1546.

4. Kitamura S, Shimizu T, Izumi T, Seyama Y. FEBS Lett 1987;213:

   169-173.

5. Izumi T, Honda Z, Ohishi N, Kitamura S, Tsuchida S, Sato K,

   Shimizu T, Seyama Y. Biochim Biophys Acta 1988 (in press).

6. Haeggstrom J, Meijer J, Radmark O. J Biol Chem 1986;261:

   6332-6337.

7. Westlund P. in: Samuelsson B, Paoletti R, Ramwell PW, eds.

   Advances in Prostaglandin, Thromboxane and Leukotriene

   Research, vol 17A. New York: Raven Press, 1987;99-104.

Advances in Prostaglandin, Thromboxane, and
Leukotriene Research, Vol. 19, edited by
B. Samuelsson, P. Y.-K. Wong, and F. F. Sun,
Raven Press, Ltd., New York ©1989.

METABOLISM OF PEPTIDE LEUKOTRIENES IN THE RAT

J. Rokach, A. Foster, D. Delorme and Y. Girard

Merck Frosst Canada Inc., P.O. Box 1005,
Pointe Claire-Dorval, Québec, H9R 4P8

Recently, a major focus in leukotriene research has been
centered on the metabolism of the carbon backbone, not only to
further understand its regulatory role, but also to identify and
quantify the major eliminated metabolites in animal models and
man (1-6). Using a line of inbred rats (7) having a non
specific bronchial hyperreactivity as an asthma model (8), our
goals were to first observe the distribution and elimination of
the peptide leukotrienes in these rats and secondly to elucidate
the metabolic pathway that these mediators follow before
elimination. After evaluation of these processes our next aim
was to measure leukotriene levels upon antigen challenge in the
above rats.

RESULTS AND DISCUSSION

The distribution and elimination processes of the peptide
leukotrienes were investigated by intravenous administration of
tritiated leukotrienes. Administration of [^{3}H]LTC$_4$ (1)
resulted in a rapid systemic clearance of radioactivity (5 min)
from the blood (Fig. 1, left panel). Although the peptide
leukotrienes have very short systemic half-lives, it was of
interest to obtain information on their metabolic fate in
blood. Incubation of [^{3}H]LTC$_4$ in rat whole blood (38°C)
resulted in a 30% conversion (5 min) to LTD$_4$ and LTE$_4$ (Fig.
1, right panel). 80% conversion was achieved after 30 min but,
as this time point is physiologically not relevant in vivo, it
can be concluded that only minor metabolism of LTC$_4$ occurs in
rat blood during the systemic partition.

Intravenous administration of [^{3}H]LTC$_4$ also resulted in a
significant time-related biliary excretion of 69 ± 4.1% (n=6
over 60 min, Fig. 2, left panel) of administered radioactivity
with a urinary recovery of only 0.9 ± 0.3% (n=3 over 60 min).
Similar results were obtained with tritiated LTD$_4$ and LTE$_4$
recovering 62 ± 7.5% and 52 ± 1.5% of administered
radioactivity respectively from the bile. These data suggest
that the leukotrienes are eliminated from the systemic
circulation by an efficient uptake mechanism in the liver
resulting in biliary excretion as the major route of elimination.

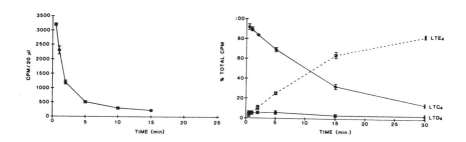

FIG. 1:   Left panel: Clearance of total radioactivity from the
circulation of the anesthetized rat following the
intravenous administration of [^{3}H]LTC$_4$. Right
panel: time course of the metabolism of [^{3}H]LTC$_4$
in rat whole blood <u>in vitro</u>.

The metabolic composition of radioactivity in the bile vs time
is illustrated in Fig. 2 (right panel).

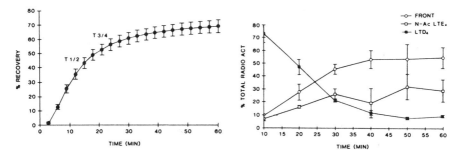

FIG. 2:   Left panel: Recovery of total radioactivity from the
bile after [^{3}H]LTC$_4$ administration. Right panel:
composition of radioactivity recovered from the bile
vs time following intravenous [^{3}H]LTC$_4$
administration.

The initial HPLC profile of radioactivity in the bile after
[^{3}H]LTC$_4$ administration showed (Fig. 3, top panel) in
addition to LTD$_4$ and N-acetyl LTE$_4$ (4,5) a large amount of
radioactivity at the solvent front. Further fractionation of
this peak (middle and bottom panels) revealed the presence of
three major polar metabolites which were isolated.
Identification of these metabolites was performed by UV and HPLC
correlation with synthetic standards, including derivatization.
These metabolites were identified as 20-carboxy-N-acetyl LTE$_4$
(2), 18-carboxy-N-acetyl LTE$_4$ (dinor) and 16-carboxy-14,15-
dihydro-N-acetyl LTE$_4$ (tetranor). Further proof of the

saturation at the position 14,15 in the latter was derived by oxidative ozonolysis. These metabolites have been reported recently to be generated <u>in vitro</u> by incubation of [^{3}H]LTE$_4$ with isolated rat hepatocytes (9).

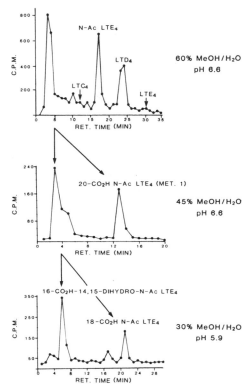

FIG. 3:   HPLC separation of polar metabolites.

Characterization of these metabolites has allowed us to clearly demonstrate that peptide leukotrienes undergo N-acetylation followed by ω and subsequent β-oxidation in the rat (Fig. 4).

Synthesis of the above-mentioned synthetic standards was accomplished using a general process involving initial condensation of a common epoxy diene aldehyde with the appropriate phosphonium salt (Fig. 5).

To demonstrate the production of leukotrienes in an asthma model, ovalbumin was administered via tracheal instillation to sensitized inbred rats (7) this resulted in an elevation of airways pressure consistent with an anaphylactic response. Bile was collected before and after antigen challenge (30 min samples) in order to characterize and quantify peptide leukotriene levels using a combination of reverse phase HPLC and LTC radioimmunoassay techniques. Significant elevations of

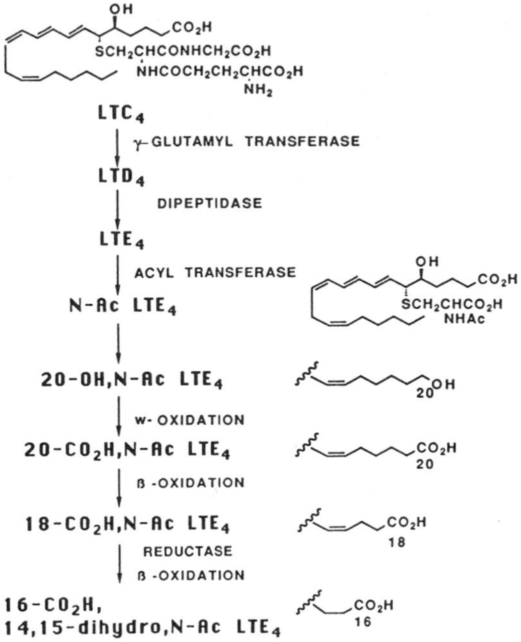

FIG. 4: Leukotriene metabolic pathway.

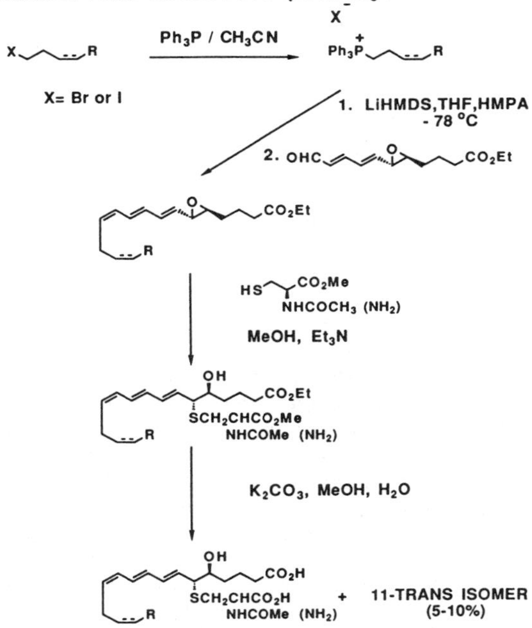

FIG. 5: General synthesis.

LTC_4, LTD_4 and N-Ac LTE_4 were observed under these
conditions. The polar metabolites described above do not
crossreact with this antibody. An intriguing aspect of the
metabolic profile obtained upon antigen challenge was the
presence of a significant immunoreactive component having the
same retention time as LTC_4. This product was further
identified to be LTC_4 by UV spectroscopy and by its enzymatic
conversion by γ-glutamyl transpeptidase to LTD_4.

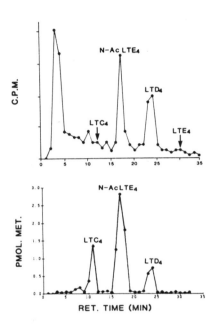

FIG. 6:   In vivo Leukotriene Production

CONCLUSION

   In summary, we have shown that the major route of elimination
of peptide leukotrienes is via the bile duct in the rat. Also,
identification of biliary metabolites demonstrates that
leukotrienes undergo N-acetylation, followed by ω and
subsequent β-oxidation. Furthermore, significant biliary
levels of peptide leukotrienes were obtained following pulmonary
anaphylaxis in sensitized hyperreactive rats. Thus, this model
would be suitable for testing the efficacy of leukotriene
inhibitors on leukotriene production in vivo. In order to
accurately monitor leukotriene biosynthesis in vivo, it will be
necessary to consider these polar metabolites either alone or in
combination with the previously known mediators.

REFERENCES

1. Foster A., Fitzsimmons B., Rokach J. and Letts G. (1987) Biochim Biophys Acta 921, 486-93.

2. Foster, A., Fitzsimmons, B., Rokach, J. and Letts, G. (1987) Biochem. Biophys. Res. Comm. 148 (3), 1237-45.

3. Ezra, D., Foster, A., Cirino, M., Rokach, J. and Letts, L.G. (1987) Prostaglandins 33 (5), 717-725.

4. Hagmann W., Denzlinger C., Rapp S., Weckbecker G. and Keppler D. (1986) Prostaglandins 31, 239-52.

5. Orning L., Norin E., Gustatsson B. and Hammarström S. (1980) J Biol Chem 261(2) 766-71.

6. Keppler, D., Huber, M., Hagman, W., Ball, H.A., Guhlmann, A. and Kastner, S. (1987) Annals of the New York Academy of Sciences (in press).

7. Holme G. and Piechuta H. (1981) Immunology 42, 19-24.

8. Brunet G., Piechuta H., Hamel R., Holme G. and Ford-Hutchinson A.W. (1983) J. Immunol 131 434-38.

9. Stene, D.O., Murphy, R.C. (1988) J. Biol. Chem. 263(6) 2773.

Advances in Prostaglandin, Thromboxane, and Leukotriene Research, Vol. 19, edited by B. Samuelsson, P. Y.-K. Wong, and F. F. Sun, Raven Press, Ltd., New York ©1989.

SEQUENTIAL FORMATION OF LEUKOTRIENE E_4 METABOLITES BY ISOLATED RAT HEPATOCYTES

Danny O. Stene and Robert C. Murphy

Department of Pharmacology, University of Colorado Health Sciences Center, Colorado, 80262, USA.

An understanding of the role that sulfidopeptide leukotrienes play in mediating physiological and pathophysiological events *in vivo* is complicated by the fact that these substances are potent effectors of biological responses such as smooth muscle contraction and enhanced capillary permeability (1). Investigation of the production of leukotrienes *in vivo* is further hampered by the inaccessibility of the site of synthesis and a convenient means of collecting an appropriate physiological fluid in which the sulfidopeptide leukotrienes might be found. An alternative approach to study of the *in vivo* production of leukotrienes would be to measure the quantity of sulfidopeptide leukotrienes present in a collecting, integrating fluid such as urine. This approach is complicated by the fact that due to rapid uptake and metabolism of the sulfidopeptide leukotrienes by the liver, hepatic metabolism prior to subsequent elimination into the urine may occur. Thus, it is necessary to understand the metabolic fate of such leukotrienes in order to assess whether or not a metabolite would appear in urine which might adequately reflect leukotriene production *in vivo*.

The liver is known to have an efficient uptake system for the sulfidopeptide leukotrienes (2,3). In the rat, a major hepatic metabolite has been identified as N-acetyl-LTE_4 (4) as well as omega-oxidized N-acetyl-LTE_4 (5). Several novel beta-oxidation products of sulfidopeptide leukotrienes from the isolated rat hepatocyte have been reported (6). These metabolites included N-acetyl-LTE_4 (A), 20-carboxy-N-acetyl-LTE_4 (B), 18-carboxy-dinor-N-acetyl-LTE_4 (C), and a major metabolite identified as 16-carboxy-tetranor-dihydro-N-acetyl-LTE_4 (D). The time course for the production of these metabolites by the isolated hepatocyte is presented in this report as well as the effect of substrate concentration on the distribution of these novel metabolites.

MATERIALS AND METHODS

Hepatocytes from Sprague-Dawley rats were isolated by the collagenase perfusion method previously described (6). Cells were suspended in 10 mM Tris buffer, containing 1 mM Ca^{++} at 3×10^6 cells/ml. Cells (either 5 or 10 ml) were kept under an atmosphere of 95% O_2, 5% CO_2 with gentle shaking at 37°C. Synthetic LTE_4 and $[14,15-^3H_2]-LTE_4$ was added to the incubation after 10 min preincubation. Cell viability was measured by trypan blue exclusion and was greater than 85% for all experiments reported.

Following the incubation period, chilled ethanol was added (80% ethanol final concentration) to stop metabolism and precipitate proteins. This was stored at -70°C over night. After centrifugation, the ethanolic supernatant was evaporated under vacuum to dryness and the residue resuspended in water. Loss of tritium counts at this stage indicated conversion of LTE_4 tritium label to volatile components. The solution was partially purified by solid phase extraction (6) and then subjected to reverse phase HPLC using a linear gradient from 80% solvent A to 100% of solvent B. Solvent A was 16.6 mM ammonium acetate, pH 4.5, 132 uM EDTA; solvent B was 90% methanol, 10% solvent A, 0.1% acetic acid, 132 uM EDTA. The effluent from the HPLC was monitored by a photodiode array detector and an on-line scintillation detector after mixing the effluent with scintillation cocktail. Metabolites were quantitated by UV spectroscopy and radioactivity content.

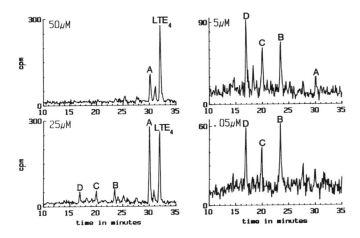

Figure 1. RP-HPLC radiochromatograms of tritium labeled LTE_4 metabolites from isolated hepatocytes (3 x 10^6 cells/ml, 30 min) at the concentrations indicated (50 uM - 0.05 uM). The identity of the metabolites was determined by co-migration with biologically derived and synthetic standards. A. N_{AC}-LTE_4; B. 20-COOH-N_{AC}-LTE_4; C. 18-COOH-N_{AC}-LTE_4; D. 16-COOH-DH-N_{AC}-LTE_4.

RESULTS AND DISCUSSION

As can be seen in Figure 1 the metabolism of LTE_4 was dependent upon the concentration of LTE_4 exposed to the isolated rat hepatocytes. When 50 uM LTE_4 was incubated with cells (3 x 10^6 cells/ml) for 30 min, the only metabolite observed was N-acetyl-LTE_4 in addition to unreacted LTE_4. However, at intermediate substrate concentration (5-10 uM) the 30 min incubation period resulted in almost complete metabolism of LTE_4 to the previously identified beta-oxidation products. At very low substrate concentrations, loss of tritium label was up to 45% of the total indicating metabolism of LTE_4 beyond the 16-COOH-dihydro metabolite. The formation of each of the metabolites of LTE_4 as a function of LTE_4 substrate concentration is presented in Figure 2.

O Total w/β-oxidized Metabolites
◇ Metabolite A (N_{ac}-LTE_4)
□ LTE_4

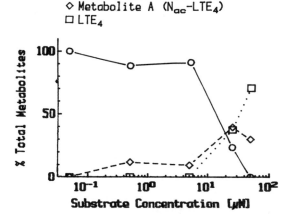

Figure 2. Effect of LTE_4 concentration on the extent of metabolisms by rat hepatocytes in the formation of metabolites at 30 min.

The time course for the appearance of metabolites in the hepatocyte incubation is presented in Figure 3. At early time points N-acetyl-LTE_4 predominated while after 40 min the major metabolites were the 18-carboxy-dinor-N-acetyl-LTE_4 and 16-carboxy-dihydro-tetranor-N-acetyl-LTE_4. The further conversion of these metabolites to 16-carboxy-tetranor-tetraene-N-acetyl-LTE_4 and 14-carboxy-hexano-N-acetyl-LTE_4 was extensive at these later times. These metabolites were not quantitated since they lost the tritium label and have an altered UV absorbance spectrum (6).

Since the observed major metabolites all involved an acetylation of the amino group of the cysteine residue of LTE_4 as well as the fact that the N-acetyl-LTE_4 metabolite itself was maximally produced prior to any of the beta-oxidized metabolites, the potential precursor role of N-acetyl-LTE_4 for the omega-oxidation and subsequent beta-oxidation reactions was considered. This is opposed to the possibility that the formation of omega-oxidized and beta-oxidized products preceded the N-acetylation step (5). The observed relative metabolite concentrations at 0, 2, 10, 20, and 40 min was compared to theoretical values obtained using a sequential model of LTE_4 metabolism to N-acetyl-LTE_4, then to 20-carboxy-N-acetyl-LTE_4 and subsequent steps of beta-oxidation (Figure 3). Assuming first order kinetics, the sequential rate constants were empirically chosen for the best fit. The close-agreement between observed and calculated metabolite concentrations support the hypothesis that the beta-oxidized metabolites of LTE_4 are preceded by N-acetylation of LTE_4 in the isolated rat hepatocyte.

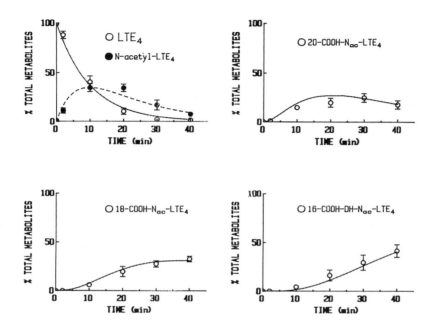

Figure 3. Time course of LTE_4 metabolism by isolated rat hepatocytes, (5 uM LTE_4, 3×10^6 cell/ml, n=3). The curves were generated by an empirical fitting of a sequential first order kinetic model $[LTE_4 \rightarrow N_{AC}\text{-}LTE_4 \rightarrow 20\text{-}COOH\text{-}N_{AC}\text{-}LTE_4 \rightarrow 18\text{-}COOH\text{-}N_{AC}\text{-}LTE_4 \rightarrow 16\text{-}COOH\text{-}DH\text{-}N_{AC}\text{-}LTE_4]$ to the observed metabolite levels.

ACKNOWLEDGEMENTS

This work was supported, in part, by a grant from the National Institutes of Health (HL25785).

REFERENCES

1. Lewis RA and Austen KF, <u>J. Clin. Invest.</u> 1984; 73:889-897.
2. Hagman W, Denglinger C, and Keppler D, <u>Circ. Shock</u> 1984; 14:223-235.
3. Armstad K, Vehara N, Orranius S, Orning L, and Hammarstrom S, <u>Biochem. Biophys. Res. Commun.</u> 1982; 104:1434-1440.
4. Keppler D, Hagman W., Rapp S, Denglinger C, and Koch HK, <u>Hepatology</u> 1985; 7:224-228.
5. Orning L, <u>Eur. J. Biochem.</u> 1987; 170:77-85.
6. Stene DO and Murphy RC, <u>J. Biol. Chem.</u> 1988; 263:2773-2778.

Advances in Prostaglandin, Thromboxane, and Leukotriene Research, Vol. 19, edited by B. Samuelsson, P. Y.-K. Wong, and F. F. Sun, Raven Press, Ltd., New York ©1989.

METABOLISM OF LEUKOTRIENE B4 AND RELATED SUBSTANCES

BY POLYMORPHONUCLEAR LEUKOCYTES

William S. Powell, Sandra Wainwright, and Francine Gravelle

Endocrine Laboratory, Royal Victoria Hospital, 687 Pine Avenue West, Montreal, Quebec, Canada, H3A 1A1, and Department of Medicine, McGill University, Montreal, Quebec, Canada

The major pathway for the metabolism of arachidonic acid in neutrophils is the formation of 5-hydroxy-6,8,11,14-eicosatetraenoic acid (5-HETE) and LTB4. LTB4 is a potent chemotactic agent for polymorphonuclear leukocytes (PMNL), and stimulates aggregation and degranulation of these cells (1). The biological action of LTB4 is limited by its metabolism to omega-oxidation products by LTB4 20-hydroxylase. Although this enzyme metabolizes other substrates related in structure to LTB4, the latter compound is the preferred substrate (2). The products of this reaction, 20-hydroxy-LTB4 and omega-carboxy-LTB4, generally have considerably less biological activity than LTB4 (3).

We recently found that LTB4 and its 6-trans isomers are metabolized by an additional pathway in PMNL, in which one of the three conjugated double bonds is reduced to give a conjugated diene. The "reductase" pathway in human PMNL is the major route of metabolism of 12-epi-6-trans-LTB4, which is not a good substrate for LTB4 20-hydroxylase (4). In rat PMNL, which possess much less LTB4 20-hydroxylase activity than human PMNL, LTB4 is also metabolized primarily by the reductase pathway (5).

RESULTS AND DISCUSSION

Incubation of porcine leukocytes with LTB4 resulted in the formation of two major products, both of which had longer HPLC retention times (87 and 98 min) than that of the substrate (85 min). These metabolites did not have the characteristic UV absorption spectra of leukotrienes, but rather had absorption maxima at about 230 nm, suggesting that one of the three conjugated double bonds of the substrate had been reduced.

The mass spectrum of the methyl ester, trimethylsilyl ether derivative of the metabolite with the shorter retention time, which has a C-value of 23.4, exhibited fragment ions at m/z 496 (M), 481 (M-15), 465 (M-31), 406 (M-90), 395 (C_5 to C_{20}), 391 (M-15-90), 385 (C_1 to C_{12}), 375 (M-31-90), 316 (M-2x90), 305 (395-90), 295 (385-90), 269 (C_1 to C_{10}), 255 (C_1 to C_9), 229 (C_1

to C7), 213 (C12 to C20), 205 (385-2x90), 203 (C1 to C5), 181, 131, 129, 119, and 105. This mass spectrum indicates that this product is a dihydro metabolite of LTB4, in which one of the 3 conjugated double bonds has been reduced. The mass spectrum of dihydroLTB4 is clearly different from that of the corresponding derivative of dihydro-12-epi-6-trans-LTB4 (5,12-dihydroxy-7,9,14-eicosatrienoic acid), which we identified after incubation of 12-epi-6-trans-LTB4 with human PMNL (4). Since the mass spectra of LTB4 and 12-epi-6-trans-LTB4 are virtually identical, this suggests that the two double bonds between carbons 5 and 12 may be in different positions in these two metabolites. The ion at m/z 229 (231 in the deuterium-labeled compound; see below) would suggest that a double bond is present between carbons 6 and 7, and therefore that this dihydro metabolite is identical to 5,12-dihydroxy-6,8,14-eicosatrienoic acid (i.e. 10,11-dihydroLTB4). The positions of the double bonds forming the conjugated diene were confirmed by oxidative ozonolysis of dihydro[1-14C]LTB4, which gave rise to 5-hydroxy[1-14C]adipate, indicating that these double bonds are in the 6 and 8 positions.

DihydroLTB4 could have been formed by one of two mechanisms. One possibility is that one of the double bonds of LTB4 could have been directly reduced. However, in most cases, reduction of a double bond is preceded by oxidation of an associated hydroxyl group. This is true in the formation of dihydro prostaglandins, which are not formed by the direct reduction of prostaglandins, but rather via 15-oxo intermediates (6) as shown below:

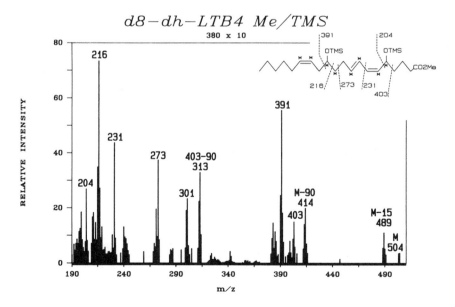

FIG. 1. Mass spectrum of deuterium-labeled dihydroLTB4

PG ⟶ 15-oxoPG ⟶ 13,14-dihydro-15-oxoPG ⟶ 13,14-dihydroPG

To determine which mechanism is correct, porcine PMNL were incubated with $[5,6,8,9,11,12,14,15^{-2}H]LTB_4$ and the products were analyzed by GC-MS. The mass spectrum of the methyl ester, trimethylsilyl ether derivative of deuterium-labeled dihydroLTB₄ (Fig. 1) exhibited fragment ions at m/z 504 (M; 8d), 489 (M-15; 8d), 414 (M-90; 8d), 403 (C_5 to C_{20}; 8d), 399 (M-15-90; 8d), 391 (C_1 to C_{12}; 6d), 383 (M-31-90; 8d), 324 (M-2x90; 8d), 313 (403-90; 8d), 301 (391-90; 6d), 273 (C_1 to C_{10}; 4d), 259 (C_1 to C_9; 4d), 231 (C_1 to C_7; 2d), 216 (C_{12} to C_{20}; 3d), 211 (391-2x90; 6d), 204 (C_1 to C_5; 1d), 186, 159, 131, 123, and 109. This mass spectrum is in agreement with the fragmentation pattern assigned for the mass spectrum of the corresponding derivative of unlabeled dihydroLTB₄ as described above. The ions at m/z 204 and 216 indicate that deuterium atoms are present in the 5- and 12-positions of deuterium-labeled dihydroLTB₄. This clearly demonstrates that one of the double bonds of LTB₄ can be directly reduced by porcine PMNL, without the requirement for an oxo intermediate. However, there was an ion at m/z 215 in the mass spectrum of the deuterium-labeled compound, suggesting that partial loss of the hydrogen at C_{12} does occur, presumably due to the formation of a 12-oxo compound (Fig. 2).

The presence of the 12-oxo metabolite referred to above was confirmed by the mass spectra of various derivatives of the second metabolite of LTB₄ (retention time, 98 min) formed by porcine PMNL. This product could could be converted to an O-methyloxime derivative, indicating that an oxo group was present. The mass spectrum of the methyl ester, trimethylsilyl ether derivative of the hydrogenated metabolite clearly indicated that the oxo group is in the 12-position and the hydroxyl group in the 5-position. This product would therefore be identical to 5-hydroxy-12-oxo-6,8,14-eicosatrienoic acid (i.e. 10,11-dihydro-12-oxoLTB₄). Experiments in which dihydro-oxoLTB₄ and dihydroLTB₄ were incubated with porcine PMNL

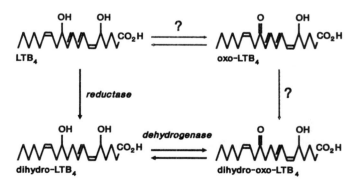

FIG. 2. Scheme for the metabolism of LTB₄ by porcine PMNL

indicated that these two products were interconverted. This could explain the partial loss of deuterium from the 12-position during the formation of dihydroLTB4. It is possible that dihydro-oxoLTB4 could be formed exclusively from dihydroLTB4. However, preliminary evidence suggests that the dihydro-oxo metabolite may also be formed from 12-oxoLTB4, which could be an intermediate in this reaction (Fig. 2).

TABLE 1. Specificity of reductase pathway in porcine PMNL.

Substrate	% Remaining	% Dihydro	% Dihydro-oxo
LTB4	16	30	44
12e-6t-8c-LTB4 [a]	11	32	21
12-HETE	1	22	34
15-HETE	54	5	11
13h-18:2	34	15	32
PGE2	100	0	0

[a] 12-epi-6-trans-8-cis-LTB4

The reductase/dehydrogenase pathway appears to be fairly specific for LTB4 and related substances containing a 12-hydroxyl group preceded by two double bonds (Table 1). 13-Hydroxy-9,11-octadecadienoic acid, is also metabolized, but not as rapidly as LTB4, whereas 15-HETE is a relatively poor substrate, and prostaglandins are not metabolized at all. In addition to the products shown in Table 1, 6-trans-LTB4 is a good substrate, whereas 12-epi-6-trans-LTB4 is metabolized more slowly. The latter two products are also substrates for a second reductase/dehydrogenase pathway in porcine PMNL, which appears to be similar to the pathway of metabolism of these compounds in human PMNL. The latter pathway involves oxidation of the 5-hydroxyl group, rather than that in the 12-position (4). Consequently, these two 6-trans isomers of LTB4 are metabolized to tetrahydro and tetrahydro-oxo products by these cells.

REFERENCES

1. Ford-Hutchinson AW. Federation Proc 1985;44:25-29.

2. Powell WS. J Biol Chem 1984;259:3082-3089.

3. Ford-Hutchinson AW, Rackham A, Zamboni R, Rokach J, Roy S. Prostaglandins 1983; 25-37.

4. Powell WS, Gravelle F. J Biol Chem 1988;263:2170-2177.

5. Powell WS. Biochem Biophys Res Commun 1987;145:991-998.

6. Hamberg M, Samuelsson B. J Biol Chem 1971;246:1073-1077.

Advances in Prostaglandin, Thromboxane, and Leukotriene Research, Vol. 19, edited by
B. Samuelsson, P. Y.-K. Wong, and F. F. Sun,
Raven Press, Ltd., New York ©1989.

ON THE GENERATION OF LIPOXINS AND NOVEL RELATED COMPOUNDS

BY HUMAN NEUTROPHILS: RELATIONSHIP TO LEUKOTRIENE PRODUCTION

Charles N. Serhan

Hematology Division, Department of Medicine
Brigham and Women's Hospital and Harvard Medical School
75 Francis Street, Boston, MA   02115

While the 5-lipoxygenase (LO) is key in the formation of
leukotrienes (LT), another major route of arachidonate metabolism
is initiated by the 15-LO which is widely distributed throughout
mammalian tissues (1).   Interactions between LO pathways lead to
the formation of lipoxins (LX) which display a spectrum of
activities distinguishable from those of leukotrienes and
prostaglandins (1).   Activated human leukocytes can generate both
LXA_4 and LXB_4 from 15-HETE, an event which can lead to their
formation during cell-cell interactions (2).   In addition,
lipoxins can be generated from arachidonic acid by human
eosinophils (3), porcine leukocytes (4) and mastocytoma cells
(5).   Here, utilizing an improved detection system which employed
a gradient-HPLC and photodiode array detector, the production of
LT, LX and related compounds was examined in human neutrophils.
Evidence is presented for (a) the generation of lipoxins from
endogenous sources; (b) identification of three novel compounds;
(c) the different metabolic fates of mono-HETE's and (d)
inhibition of superoxide anion generation and LT biosynthesis by
15-HETE with human neutrophils.

METHODS

Neutrophils (PMN) were prepared from fresh blood obtained from
healthy volunteers by dextran sedimentation and Ficoll-Hypaque
gradient.   These suspensions contained 98 $\pm$ 1% PMN and their
integrity was monitored both before and during incubations by
exclusion of trypan blue (6,7).   Products were extracted and
isolated with an RP-HPLC system equipped with an Altex
Ultrasphere-ODS column and a photodiode array spectral detector
linked to an AT&T PC6300.   Post-run analyses were performed with
a Nelson Analytical 3000 series chromatography data system
(Paramus, NJ) and Wavescan 2140-202 (Bromma, Sweden) software

(6,7). Synthetic eicosanoids were from Biomol Research Laboratories, Inc. (Philadelphia, PA). Products were identified according to published criteria including analysis by GC-MS (2,6,7).

RESULTS AND DISCUSSION

Production of Lipoxins by PMN: Since the balance between LO products may be of importance in both pathophysiological and physiological circumstances, new methodologies were sought which could resolve the products (7). Here, neutrophils were prepared and incubated with A23187 (5 μM, 20 min) within 2.5 h post-venipuncture. Following extraction, materials were injected into a RP-HPLC equipped with a rapid spectral detector and analytical software. A representative post-HPLC analysis of the products is given in Figure 1 (n=7). Profiles obtained at both 270 and 300 nm were recalled from stored UV spectral data obtained from an individual injection (material from 30×10^6 cells). In addition to LT (monitored at 270 nm), tetraene containing products (300 nm) were generated by activated PMN from endogenous sources. They were LXA_4, LXB_4 and their all-trans isomers. In this system, 8-trans-LXB_4 and 14S-8-trans-LXB_4 coeluted as did 11-trans-LXA_4 and 6S-11-trans-LXA_4 (RP-HPLC was performed with free acid, cf. ref. 2).

These cells generated three novel tetraene-containing products, two eluted before LXB_4 and the other before the trans-isomers of LXA_4. For purposes of comparison, the chromatographic profile of a mixture of authentic materials resolved by this system is given in Figure 1 (lower panel). The amounts of triene-containing products were greater than those of tetraene-containing compounds and the amounts of both LX and LT formed by neutrophils were dependent upon the dose of A23187 (7).

Identification of Novel Compounds: Addition of 15-HETE to A23187-stimulated PMN led to a dose dependent increase in the formation of tetraene products (n=23). The new compounds were examined to determine their stereochemistry. The properties of the neutrophil-derived products were compared to those of synthetic materials by HPLC, GC-MS and bioassay (6). These studies showed that one of the new compounds is 5S,6R,15S-trihydroxy-9,11,13-trans-7-cis-eicosatetraenoic acid or the 7-cis-11-trans-isomer of LXA_4 (7-cis-11-trans-LXA_4). The material beneath I proved to be a 5,14,15-trihydroxy-6,8,10,12-eicosatetraenoic acid (C 24.2 –24.3) while the material beneath II proved to be a 5,6,15-trihydroxy-7,9,11,13-eicosatetraenoic acid (C 24.1 –24.2) (Figure 2). The properties of these two compounds did not match those of synthetic materials (6,7).

Metabolic Fates of HETEs: Studies were performed to determine if exogenous 5-HETE is also a substrate for LX formation (7).

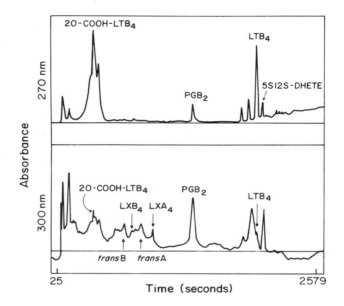

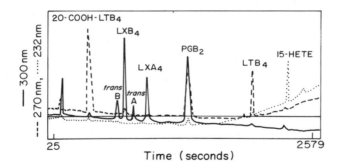

FIG. 1. <u>Lipoxygenase products generated by human neutrophils from endogenous sources.</u>
<u>Upper panel:</u> Profiles obtained from incubation of human PMN (30 x 10^6 cells/1 ml) stimulated with A23187 (5 μM) for 20 min, 37°C. Following extraction, samples were injected into a RP–HPLC equipped with a rapid spectral detector. Post–HPLC analyses were performed with a Wavescan 2140–202 program and a Nelson Analytical 3000 series chromatography data system (9). <u>Lower panel:</u> Profile of authentic materials chromatographed from a mixture by this system following a single injection.

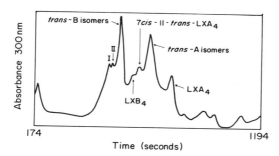

FIG. 2. <u>RP-HPLC profile of lipoxins and related compounds from</u>
<u>human neutrophils.</u> PMN (30 x 10^6/10 ml) were incubated with
15-HETE (35 μM) and A23187 (2.5 μM) for 20 min, 37°C. Products
were analyzed as in Fig. 1. The lipoxin region of the profile
(cf. Fig. 1) was expanded from 174-1194 seconds; products were
collected and characterized (8,9).

———

5-HETE was transformed by activated neutrophils to 5,15-DHETE
(7.7%), 5,20-HETE (11.3%) and low levels of 5S,12S-DHETE (1.4%)
while 64% remained as 5-HETE (Figure 3). In the absence of
A23187, 5-HETE was converted to 5,20-HETE (12.6%) alone
indicating that ω-oxidation is a major route of metabolism of
HETE in the unstimulated neutrophil (7). In addition, these
findings indicate that unlike 15-HETE, 5-HETE is not a precursor
for the formation of LX and suggest that the 14(15)-epoxytetraene
is not generated from 5-HETE by neutrophils.

Inhibition of Neutrophil Responses: Exposure of A23187-
stimulated PMN to 15-HETE led to a dose-dependent generation of
LX while blocking LT production (Figure 4). In contrast, LTB_4
formation was not altered in the presence of exogenous 5-HETE.
15-HETE also inhibited $O_2^{\overline{\cdot}}$ generation both in response to A23187
(2.5 μM) and f-met-leu-phe (10^{-7} M). With both stimuli, the
action of 15-HETE on $O_2^{\overline{\cdot}}$ generation was dose-dependent (7).

In summary, results indicate that human neutrophils can
generate lipoxins and three novel compounds from endogenous
sources (7). The complete stereochemistry of one of the
products, 7-cis-11-trans-LXA_4, and its biological activity was
established (6). In contrast to the utilization of 15-HETE,
activated neutrophils did not generate either lipoxins or related
products from exogenous 5-HETE. During the time course and dose
response of conversion of 15-HETE to lipoxins by neutrophils,
both leukotriene B_4 and superoxide anion generation is inhibited
(7). Together, these findings suggest that activation of the
15-LO may play an important role in modulating cellular responses
of interest in inflammation.

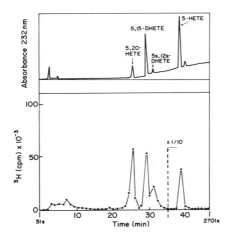

FIG. 3. <u>HPLC profile of products obtained from A23187-stimulated neutrophils incubated with 5-HETE/^{3}H-5-HETE.</u>
   Neutrophils (30 x 10^6) were incubated with 5-HETE (50 μM), ^{3}H-5-HETE and A23187 (2.5 μM) for 15 min at 37°C.
   <u>Upper panel</u>: Chromatogram plotted at absorbance 232 nm from spectral data recorded at 220-360 nm. <u>Lower panel</u>: Radioactivity plot of materials collected following RP-HPLC (n=3).

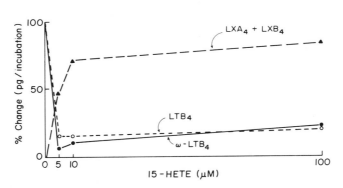

FIG. 4. <u>Relationship between LT and LX production.</u>
   PMN (30 x 10^6) with incubation with A23187 (2.5 μM) in the presence and absence of varying amounts of exogenous 15-HETE for 20 min at 37°C. Data are presented as the percent change in products following addition of 15-HETE (n=3).

Acknowledgments

The author thanks Eileen Reardon for technical assistance and Mary Halm Small for skillful preparation of the manuscript. This work was supported by NIH #1-R29-GM38765-01 and aided by grant 13-506-867 from the American Heart Association, Massachusetts Affiliate, Inc. C.N.S. is a recipient of the J.V. Satterfield Arthritis Investigator Award from the National Arthritis Foundation and a Fellow of the Medical Foundation, Inc. (Boston, Mass.).

REFERENCES

1. Samuelsson B, Dahlén S-E, Lindgren JA, Rouzer CA, Serhan CN. Science 1987; 237:1171-1176.

2. Serhan CN, Nicolaou CK, Webber SE, et al. J Biol Chem 1986; 261:16340-16345.

3. Serhan CN, Hirsch U, Palmblad J, Samuelsson B. FEBS Lett 1987; 217:242-246.

4. Lam BK, Serhan CN, Samuelsson B, Wong PY-K. Biochem Biophys Res Commun 1987; 144:123-131.

5. Lazarus SC, Zocca E. FASEB Journal 1988; 2:A409 (Abstract 656).

6. Nicolaou KC, Marron B, Veale CA, et al. (submitted).

7. Serhan CN (submitted).

Advances in Prostaglandin, Thromboxane, and
Leukotriene Research, Vol. 19, edited by
B. Samuelsson, P. Y.-K. Wong, and F. F. Sun,
Raven Press, Ltd., New York ©1989.

PHARMACOLOGICAL ACTIVITIES OF LIPOXINS
AND RELATED COMPOUNDS.

Sven-Erik Dahlén

Department of Physiology, and Institute of Environmental Medicine,
Karolinska Institutet, S-104 01 Stockholm, Sweden.

Several biological activities have been reported for the
lipoxins (LX)(Fig.1). For example, LXA4 (5S,6R,15S-trihydroxy-
7,9,13-trans-11-cis-eicosatetraenoic acid) is a potent activator of
Protein Kinase C (1) and may affect leukocyte function in vitro (2).
In vivo, LXA4 induces arteriolar dilation in the hamster cheek
pouch (3) and rat preglomerular circulation (4), whereas it constricts
the rat tail artery (5). Furthermore, both LXA4 and
LXB4 (5S,14R,15S-trihydroxy-6,10,12-trans-8-cis-eicosatetraenoic
acid) inhibit cytotoxicity induced by natural killer cells (6). This
chapter will elaborate on the actions of lipoxins and related
compounds in smooth muscle preparations.

ACTIONS OF LIPOXINS IN SMOOTH MUSCLE PREPARATIONS.

When examined in spasmogenic assays, LXA4 displayed a rather
specific profile of activity (3). Thus, it constricted strips of guinea
pig lung but had no direct effect on the ileum and trachea of the
same species. More recently, it was observed that LXA4 contracts
human bronchi (7), and that both LXA4 and LXB4 can relax the
guinea pig aorta (8). The pharmacodynamics of the lipoxins in each
model are discussed henceforth.

Contractile effect.

Lipoxin A4 (0.03-10 µM) induced dose-dependent and very long-
lasting contractions of the guinea-pig lung strip (3,7,9). The effect of
LXA4 resembled the "slow reacting response" elicited with cysteinyl-
leukotrienes (cysLTs:LTC4, LTD4 and LTE4). At the highest dose,
the response to LXA4 approached maximal tissue contractility, thus
indicating that LXA4 was a complete agonist.

The contractile effect of LXA4 in the lung strip was associated
with release of thromboxane(TX) A2 (7,10). The generation of TXA2
was however not a consequence of the contraction response per se
(10). Nevertheless, similar to what has been found for cysLTs under

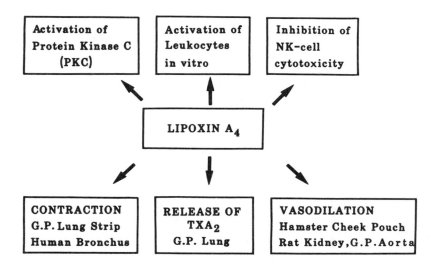

FIG. 1. Biological activities of lipoxin A_4(LXA$_4$).

the present experimental conditions (11), indomethacin blocked release of TXA$_2$ from the lung strip without affecting the peak amplitude of the contraction response to LXA$_4$ (3,7).

In contrast, several structurally unrelated antagonists for cysLTs (FPL 55712, LY-171883, L-648,051, ICI 198,615) inhibited the contraction response to LXA$_4$ in a competitive manner (7,9,unpublished)(Fig.2). Since lipoxygenase inhibitors failed to alter the contraction induced by LXA$_4$ (7), it was concluded that LXA$_4$, rather than causing release of leukotrienes, directly activated the smooth muscle at a site with similar characteristics as the receptor(s) for cysLTs. This conclusion was substantiated by the finding that specific cross-desensitization could be induced between LXA$_4$ and the cysLTs (7).

With the aid of stereochemically defined compounds (reviewed in 12), it has been possible to outline structure-activity relations (SAR) for LXA$_4$ in the lung strip (7,13). Evidently, the presence of alcohol groups at both carbon atoms 5(C-5) and 6(C-6) in LXA$_4$ are essential for spasmogenic activity. For example, 5(S)-HETE, 5(S),15(S)-DHETE, 14(R),15(S)-DHETE and 15(S)-HETE are considerably less active than LXA$_4$. Likewise, LXB$_4$, which has its hydroxyls positioned at C-5, C-14 and C-15, causes but relaxation of the lung strip. In addition, the orientation of the two hydroxyls at C-5 and C-6 appears crucial, because 6S-LXA$_4$ is nearly inactive (14). On the other hand, changes in the tetraene sequence appears to have comparatively minor influence on the contractile activity, because octahydro-LXA$_4$, which has the same geometry of the alcohol groups

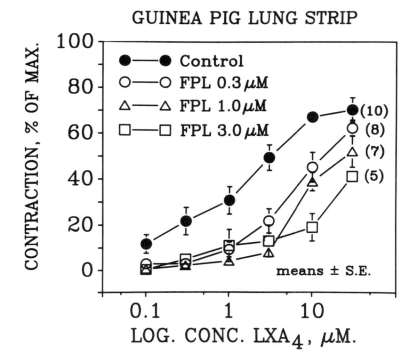

FIG. 2. The antagonist of cysteinyl-leukotrienes, FPL 55712, causes dose-dependent inhibition of the cumulative dose-response relation for lipoxin A4(LXA4) in the guinea pig lung strip.

as LXA4, but lacks double bonds altogether, lost only one log order of magnitude in potency.

The structure-activity studies, therefore, seem to provide the stereochemical explanation for the observed interaction between LXA4 and the cysLTs. Thus, LXA4 and the cysLTs have several structural features in common, for example a system of conjugated double bonds at the same positions (-7,9-trans-11-cis). In particular, both LXA4 and the cysLTs have polar groups at C-5 and C-6 with the relative orientation 5S,6R. Moreover, it is known that the 5S,6R-orientation of the hydroxyl and cysteinyl-substituent, respectively, is one very important determinant of the contractile activity of cysLTs (15). Likewise, the 5S,6R-hydroxyls were crucial for the spasmogenic activity of LXA4 (13,14).

In this context, it is of interest that LXA4 contracts human bronchi in a manner which is almost identical to that observed in the lung strip, including sensitivity to antagonists for cysLTs (7). It

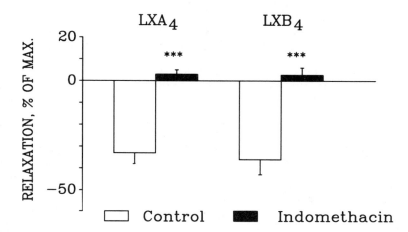

FIG. 3. Indomethacin (10 μM, 30 min pretreatment) blocks the relaxations induced in the precontracted guinea pig aorta by lipoxins A(LXA4) and B(LXB4). Mean responses ± S.E. in indicated number of experiments.

is noteworthy that, eventhough the guinea pig lung strip contains several types of contractile elements, its responsiveness to many mediators appear to correlate with the reactivity of human airways.

Leukotriene Antagonism.

In spite of the observed interaction between LXA4 and cysLTs in the lung strip, LXA4 failed to contract the guinea pig ileum (3). Therefore, although both the lung strip and the ileum are sensitive to cysLTs, the receptors in the two tissues obviously differ with respect to sensitivity for LXA4. In fact, it was observed that LXA4 causes a dose-dependent inhibition of the contraction response to LTC4 in the ileum (7). Similar observations have been made in the guinea-pig trachea (7). Thus, in the ileum, LXA4 behaves as an antagonist, whereas it is a full agonist for contraction in the lung strip. The observations with LXA4 enforce other indications that there are multiple and tissue-specific receptors for cysteinyl-LTs(15).

Cyclooxygenase-Dependent Relaxation.

In contrast to their differential activity in the lung strip, LXA4 and LXB4 both relaxed the guinea pig aorta (Fig.3)(8). The responses were predominantly, if not exclusively, endothelium-dependent. The potency of LXA4 and LXB4 was identical, and both compounds caused dose-dependent relaxations in concentrations which were similar to that of acetylcholine (0.1-10 μM). Moreover, pretreatment with indomethacin effectively annulled the relaxations induced by the lipoxins (Fig.3), but left the response to acetylcholine unaffected. Since, TXA_2, as well as prostaglandin(PG) $F_{2\alpha}$ or D_2, is contractile in this preparation, and PGE_2 causes a biphasic response (contraction followed by relaxation), it is only PGI_2 that mimics the indomethacin-sensitive response to the lipoxins. Therefore, it is concluded that the lipoxins induced a functionally important release of PGI_2 in the guinea pig aorta.

Somewhat surprisingly, the methyl-ester of LXA_4 was inactive on aortic strips from guinea pigs, rats or rabbits (7,8). This is different from the situation in the guinea pig lung strip, where the free acid and methyl ester consistently produce qualitatively similar responses. The difference may indicate that a free carboxyl group at C-1 is required for the vascular relaxation induced by lipoxins. Considered together, it is apparent that the SARs for the relaxant property of lipoxins differ from those required for the spasmogenic action in the lung strip. Since 15-HETE also may cause cyclooxygenase-dependent relaxations of the guinea pig aorta (16), it is suggested that the polar group at C-15 is important for the relaxation of vascular smooth muscle induced by lipoxins. In line with this proposal, 15-HPETE caused a vasodilation of the hamster cheek pouch which was similar to that induced by LXA_4 (3).

CONCLUSIONS

The pharmacology of the lipoxins has so far mostly been characterized for LXA_4 (Fig.1). As discussed in this chapter, LXA_4 may stereoselectively interact with certain smooth muscles at a "5S,6R-site" shared with the cysteinyl-leukotrienes. This site may also be involved in the evoked release of TXA_2 from the guinea pig lung. On the other hand, the vasodilation observed in vivo and in the guinea pig aorta may relate to the presence of a hydroxyl group at C-15, because LXA_4, LXB_4 and 15-HETE are equally active in these respects. At least in vitro, the relaxant property of the lipoxins can be explained in terms of generation of a cyclooxygenase product, presumably PGI_2.

Finally, although potentially important interactions may thus occur between lipoxins and other eicosanoids, it should be recognized that lipoxins, in most systems, have profiles of activity which are distinct from those of other arachidonic acid metabolites (discussed in ref. 7). Moreover, it is evident that the exploration of the biology of the lipoxins and related lipoxygenase products will continue to be an exciting area of research.

ACKNOWLEDGEMENTS

Supported by grants from the Swedish Medical Research Council (project 14X-4342), the Swedish Association Against Chest and Heart Diseases, the Swedish Association Against Asthma and Allergy (RmA), the Institute of Environmental Medicine, the Swedish Environment Protection Board (5324067-7), and Karolinska Institutet.

REFERENCES

1. Hansson A, Serhan CN, Haeggström J, Ingelman-Sundberg M, Samuelsson B, Morris J. Biochem Biophys Res Commun. 1986;134:1215-1222.

2. Serhan CN, Hamberg M, Samuelsson B. Proc Natl Acad Sci USA 1984;81:5335-5339.

3. Dahlén S-E, Raud J, Serhan CN, Björk J, Samuelsson B. Acta Physiol Scand 1987;130:643-648.

4. Badr KF, Serhan CN, Nicolaou KC, Samuelsson B. Biochem Biophys Res Commun 1987;145:408-414.

5. Lam BK, Wong PY-K. In Wong PY-K, Serhan CN, eds. Lipoxins: Biosynthesis, Chemistry and Biological Activities, New York, Plenum Press, 1988;51-60.

6. Ramstedt U, Ng J, Wigzell H, Serhan CN, Samuelsson B. J Immunol 1985;135:3434-3438.

7. Dahlén S-E, Franzén L, Raud J, et al. In Wong PY-K, Serhan CN, eds. Lipoxins: Biosynthesis, Chemistry and Biological Activities, New York, Plenum Press, 1988; 107-130.

8. Matsuda H, Dahlén S-E, Haeggström J, Nicolaou KC, Hedqvist P. (submitted).

9. Spur, BW, Jacques C, Crea AE, Lee TH. In Wong PY-K, Serhan CN, eds. Lipoxins: Biosynthesis, Chemistry and Biological Activities, New York, Plenum Press, 1988; 147-154.

10. Wikström E, Westlund P, Nicolaou KC, Dahlén S-E. Ag Actions (in press).

11. Dahlén S-E, Hedqvist P, Westlund P, Granström E, Hammarström S, Lindgren JÅ, Rådmark O. Acta Physiol Scand 1983;118: 393-403.

12. Webber SE, Veale CA, Nicolaou KC. In Wong PY-K, Serhan CN, eds. Lipoxins: Biosynthesis, Chemistry and Biological Activities, New York, Plenum Press, 1988;61-78.

13. Dahlén S-E, Veale CA, Webber SE, Marron BA, Nicolaou KC, Serhan CN. Ag Actions (in press).

14. Serhan CN, Nicolaou KC, Webber SE, Veale CA, Dahlén SE, Puustinen TJ, Samuelsson B. J Biol Chem 1986;261:16340-16345.

15. Krell RD,Brown FJ,Willard AK,Giles RE. In Chakrin LW,Bailey DM, eds. The Leukotrienes,Chemistry and Biology. Orlando,Academic Press 1984;271-299.

16. Matsuda H, Dahlén S-E, Puustinen T, Hedqvist P. (submitted).

Advances in Prostaglandin, Thromboxane, and Leukotriene Research, Vol. 19, edited by B. Samuelsson, P. Y.-K. Wong, and F. F. Sun, Raven Press, Ltd., New York ©1989.

FORMATION OF LIPOXINS BY RAT BASOPHILIC LEUKEMIA CELLS

Carol F. Ng, Bing K. Lam[*], Kirkwood A. Pritchard, Jr.[+], Michael B. Stemerman[+], Pat Hejny and Patrick Y-K Wong

Departments of Pharmacology and [+]Medicine, New York Medical College, Valhalla, New York 10595 and [*]Department of Rheumatology and Immunology, Harvard Medical School, Boston, Massachusetts, U.S.A.

INTRODUCTION

A new class of conjugated trihydroxy tetraenes derived from oxygenation of arachidonic acid (AA) and eicosapentaenoic acid (EPA) via interactions between the 5- and 15-lipoxygenase pathways have been reported by Serhan et al. (1) and Wong et al. (2). This group of new compounds referred to as Lipoxin A_4/B_4 and A_5/B_5, respectively, exhibits interesting biological functions (1,3). It has been suggested that these conjugated tetraene compounds can be formed by cell-cell interactions, utilizing 15-HPETE or 15-HETE (15-hydroxyeicosatetraenoic acid) from lung alveolar macrophages, endothelial cells, eosinophils and neutrophils (4). Rat basophilic leukemic cells (RBL-1), which contain 5-lipoxygenase have been shown to produce slow reacting substances of anaphylaxis when stimulated by calcium ionophore A23187. In this report we examined the formation of lipoxin from RBL-1 cells when stimulated by various agents.

MATERIALS AND METHODS

Calcium ionophore A23187, fMLP (formyl-methionyl-leucyl-phenylalanine and PMA (phorbol myristate acetate) were purchased from Sigma Co. (St. Louis, Mo.). 15-HPETE was prepared by incubating $[1-^{14}C]$-arachidonic acid with soybean lipoxygenase as described (5). Lipoxin A_4 and B_4 standards were generously supplied by Dr. J. Rokach of Merck Frosst Canada. RBL-1 cells (American Type Tissue Culture) were grown in suspension cultures in MEM supplemented with 20% fetal bovine serum (Sigma). After harvest, the cells were washed and suspended in Dulbecco's phosphate-buffered saline, pH 7.4. The cell suspension ($2-3 \times 10^8$) was added to an incubation vessel containing 15-HPETE ($16\mu M$) dissolved in a minimum volume of ethanol. Either calcium ionophore A23187 ($5\mu M$), fMLP ($22\mu M$) or PMA ($2\mu M$) was then added to the suspension and incubated for 30 min at $37^{\circ}C$ and stopped by the addition of two volumes of ethanol. After extraction, the sample was

analyzed by RP-HPLC as described (1). Lipoxin-like substances
were collected, methylated with diazomethane and reinjected onto
the same column and eluted with methanol/water (65:35) (1). The
identity of lipoxins were determined by the criteria of their
ultra-violet spectrum (UV), co-elution with synthetic standards
and by GC/MS (2,6).

RESULTS AND DISCUSSION

Incubation of RBL-1 cells with 15-HPETE and either A23187,
fMLP or PMA generated products with a UV spectrum indicative
of conjugated tetraene compounds. Following incubation and
extraction, the lipid soluble materials were purified by RP-
HPLC, which revealed 3 major and 1 minor peaks (Fig. 1) showing
typical UV spectrum of lipoxin (1). These fractions were collected and processed as described above. Four peaks showing the
same lipoxin UV spectra were obtained. The major peak (R.T. 22
min) which co-eluted with LXB_4ME standard was converted to
trimethylsilyl derivative and analyzed by GC/MS. The C-value
was 24.0 and the mass spectrum showed ions of high intensity at
m/z: 173 (base peak), 203. Ions of lower intensities were
observed at 582(M), 409, 394 and 379. These ions are similar to
those reported for LXB_4 (1). Other components having similar
UV data were tentatively assigned as isomers of LXB_4. Peaks
II and III (Fig. 1) were collected, methylated and reinjected
onto second RP-HPLC. Five peaks displaying the same UV spectra
was obtained. The major fraction (R.T. 25 min), which co-eluted
with LXA_4ME standard was converted to the trimethylsilyl derivative and further analyzed by GC/MS. The C-value was 24.1 and
the prominent ions were at m/z 203 (base peak), 171, 173. Ions
of lower intensity were observed at m/z 582(M), 482 and 379.
These ions and C-value were identical to those reported for
LXA_4 (1).

In comparing the three agonists used to stimulate the
production of lipoxins, particularly LXA_4, the greatest amount
was generated with A23187 (4.8$\pm$1.0 μg). This was followed
by the chemotactic peptide fMLP (2.0$\pm$0.74 μg), which is
58% less than that produced with A23187. The smallest amount
was generated with the addition of PMA (0.65$\pm$0.25 μg),
showing 86% less than A23187 (Fig. 2). In addition, both A23187
and fMLP stimulated the formation of LXB_4 (1.2$\pm$0.57 μg
and 0.55$\pm$0.07 μg, respectively). However, LXB_4 production
was not detected with the addition of PMA. Interestingly, the
addition of either purified PLA_2 (10μg) (6) or AA
(50μM) to RBL-1 cells did not produce any detectable
lipoxin-like substances.

Biological activity of LXA_4 generated from RBL-1 cells was
examined in an isolated preparation of rat tail artery. The
preparation was suspended in a 6 ml organ bath filled with
oxygenated Krebs solution and kept at 37°C. The tissue was
precontracted with 0.125μM phenylephrine (PE). Following
relaxation of the tissue, administration of 3nM LXA_4 from

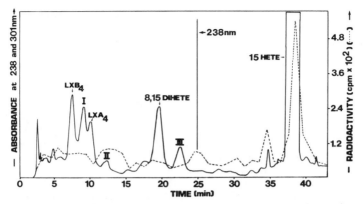

Fig. 1: RP-HPLC chromatogram of 15-HPETE metabolites isolated after incubation of RBL-1 cells with 15-[1-^{14}C]-HPETE.

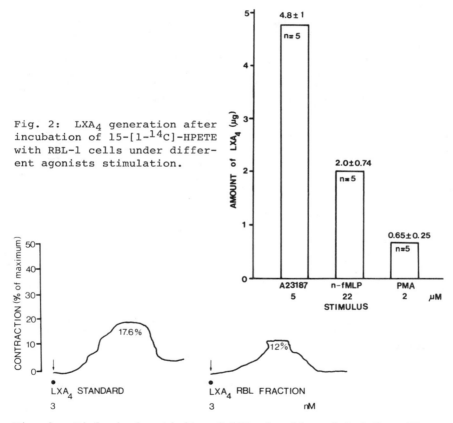

Fig. 2: LXA$_4$ generation after incubation of 15-[1-^{14}C]-HPETE with RBL-1 cells under different agonists stimulation.

Fig. 3: Biological activity of LXA$_4$ fraction eluted from RP-HPLC (Ref Fig. 1) as compared with LXA$_4$ synthetic standard on perfused rat tail arteries.

RBL-1 fractions display 12% of the maximum contraction induced
by PE, whereas a known LXA_4 standard (3nM) elicited 17.6% of
the maximum contraction. Since some isomers of LXA_4 do not
possess biological activity (3), this would account for the
difference in the musculotropic response observed with the
standard as compared to the biological sample containing isomers
of LXA_4. The existence of several LXA_4 isomers was further
confirmed by the second RP-HPLC chromatography analysis. These
results suggest that RBL-1 cells can utilize exogenous 15-HPETE
to generate lipoxins. Agonists such as A23187 and fMLP may
mobilize calcium to activate the 5-lipoxygenase pathway for the
consumption of exogenous 15-HPETE. This then leads to the
generation of 5,15-diHPETE, epoxytetraene intermediates, and
finally the formation of lipoxins. The addition of exogenous AA
or the release of endogenous AA by either PLA_2 or PLC
stimulated by PMA, did not produce any detectable amounts of
products. These results suggest that 5-lipoxygenase in RBL-1
cells may be compartmentalized and coupled to different pools of
phospholipids. This compartmentalization may not allow the liberated AA to gain access to the lipoxin generating system. Thus,
we can conclude that RBL-1 cells can use 15-HPETE or 15-HETE donated by neighboring cells to make lipoxins when concurrently
the 5-lipoxygenase pathway is activated by stimuli that induce
an influx of calcium. The fact that the amount of lipoxins
generated varies with different agonists suggests the involvment
of different receptors mediating cellular events and possibly
the induction of different cellular sites for the oxidative
burst metabolism. Once the cell has generated and released
these biologically active products, such as lipoxin, they can
further attenuate or amplified the physiological response of
neighboring cells.

REFERENCES

1. Serhan C.N., Hamberg, M. and Samuelsson, B. (1984). Proc.
   Natl. Acad. Sci. 81:5335-5339.
2. Wong, P.Y-K, Hughes, R. and Lam, B. (1985). Biochem.
   Biophys. Res. Commun. 126:763-772.
3. Dahlen, S.E., Franzen, L., Raud, J., Serhan, C.N., Westlund,
   P., Wikstrom, E., Bjorck, T., Matsuda, H., Webber, S.E.,
   Veale, C.A., Puustinen, T., Haeggstrom, J., Nicolaou, K.C.
   and Samuelsson, B. (1988). in Lipoxins, Biosynthesis,
   Chemistry and Biological Activities, ed. by Wong, P.Y-K and
   Serhan, C.N., Plenum Press, New York, pp. 107-130.
4. Serhan, C.N. and Samuelsson, B. (1988). in Lipoxins,
   Biosynthesis, Chemistry and Biological Activities, ed. by
   Wong, P.Y-K and Serhan, C.N., Plenum Press, New York, pp.
   1-14.
5. Hamberg, M. and Samuelsson, B. (1967). J. Biol. Chem.
   24:5329-5333.
6. Lam, B.K., Serhan, C.N., Samuelsson, B. and Wong, P.Y-K
   (1987). Biochem. Biophys. Res. Commun. 144(1):123-131.

Advances in Prostaglandin, Thromboxane, and Leukotriene Research, Vol. 19, edited by B. Samuelsson, P. Y.-K. Wong, and F. F. Sun, Raven Press, Ltd., New York ©1989.

MECHANISM OF FORMATION OF LEUKOTRIENES AND LIPOXINS FROM

ARACHIDONIC ACID CATALYZED BY HOMOGENOUS LIPOXYGENASE FROM

POTATO TUBERS

C. C. Reddy, J. Whelan[*], M. K. Rao, and P. Reddanna

Department of Veterinary Science and Department of Nutrition[*], The Pennsylvania State University, University Park, PA 16802

Lipoxygenases (LOXs) are a group of closely related enzymes responsible for the dioxygenation of various polyenoic fatty acids containing all-cis-methylene interrupted double bonds such as linolenic acid, arachidonic acid (AA), and eicosapentaenoic acid (EPA). Hydroperoxyeicosatetraenoic acids (HPETEs) are the immediate oxygenation products of AA during LOX catalyzed reaction, and these semistable intermediates are enzymatically transformed into a spectrum of compounds, including leukotrienes (LTs) and lipoxins (LXs), which exhibit much higher biological potency. In these studies, we have demonstrated that an electrophoretically pure LOX from potato tubers exhibits not only the 5- and 8-LOX activities reported previously (1) but also 9-, 11-, 12- and 15-LOX activities, thus generating all six possible HPETEs from AA. Also, we have obtained evidence to suggest that the nonregiospecificity of the enzyme is responsible for the synthesis of various LTs and LXs from AA.

METHODS

Purification of LOX From Potato Tubers

Lipoxygenase from red potato tubers was partially purified initially by procedures involving conventional protein purification steps such as ammonium sulfate fractionation and ion-exchange chromatography. An electrophoretically pure LOX preparation was then obtained by high pressure liquid chromatography (HPLC) steps employing hydrophobic interaction and anion-exchange columns. The details are published elsewhere (2).

Isolation and Characterization of Single- and Dual-Site Oxygenation Products of AA Catalyzed by the Purified Potato LOX

The large scale reactions were carried out in an oxygenated buffer system containing 0.15 M potassium phosphate with an excess of potato LOX. The reaction was initiated by the addition of AA (0.133 mM) and incubated at 30°C for 2 min for the generation of single-site oxygenation products (i.e. HPETEs) and 15 min for the generation of dual-site oxygenation products (i.e., diHPETEs and diHETEs). The reaction was terminated by acidification to pH 3.0 with 6N HCl and the products extracted twice with hexane:ether (1:1, v/v). The organic extracts were pooled, dried with anhydrous sulfate, and evaporated to dryness. The residues were reconstituted in an appropriate HPLC solvent system. The individual HPETEs were converted to their respective HETEs by reduction with either sodium borohydride or the selenium-dependent glutathione peroxidase system. Both HPETEs on HETEs were analyzed by HPLC on SP-column (Altech preparative μ-porasil, 10 mm x 50 cm) using hexane:2-propanol:acetic acid (984:15:1, v/v/v). DiHPETEs and diHETEs were analyzed initially by a reverse-phase (C-18) column using methanol:acetic acid:water and the individual peaks were further separated on a preparative SP-HPLC column. The enzymatic oxidation products of AA were characterized by different analytical criteria which included: 1) cochromatography with the standards, 2) proton NMR, and 3) absorption and mass spectral analyses. The diHETE standards were prepared by a combination of different LOX activities involving soybean LOX and the purified potato LOX with appropriate precursors, or by the nonenzymatic hydrolysis of LTA$_4$s which were synthesized by a biomimetic method (3).

Formation of Lipoxins

Synthesis of LXs catalyzed by potato LOX was demonstrated with 5(OH),15(OOH)-eicosatetraenoic acid (ETE) and 5(OOH),15(OH)-ETE as substrates. The latter compounds were prepared by the action of soybean LOX and potato 5-LOX on 5-HETE and 15-HETE respectively. For the generation of LXs, the reaction was carried out in an oxygenated 0.15 M potassium phosphate buffer, pH 6.3 using either 5(OH),15(OOH)- or 5(OOH),15(OH)-ETE as substrate. The reactions were monitored spectrophotometrically using a Beckman DU-7 scanning spectrophotometer.

RESULTS AND DISCUSSION

When AA was incubated with the purified potato LOX, six major peaks with an UV absorption maximum at 235 nm, characteristic of a diene conjugation system, were resolved on SP-HPLC. The individual peaks were characterized by mass spectral analyses of the respective hydroxy compounds and found to be 12-, 15-, 11-, 9-, 8-, and 5-HPETEs in the increasing order of elution time. 5-HPETE accounted for ~60% of the total HPETEs formed. The relative concentrations of the other HPETEs were determined to be approximately 8-(12%), 9-(10%), 11-(7%), 15-(5%), and 12(5%). Interestingly the product profile (HPETE pattern) of crude potato LOX was identical to that of the pure enzyme, thus indicating that there appears to be only one type of LOX in potato tubers. The pH of the reaction had a profound effect on the enzyme activity as well as the profile of the oxygenation products of AA. Maximal LOX activity was obtained around pH 6.5; and it markedly decreased with increasing pH. The relative quantities of individual HPETEs changed dramatically with an increase in pH. As the pH of the reaction increased to 8.0 and above, positional specificity of the enzyme became more selective. For example, at pH 9.0 the formation of 8-HPETE was more than 5-HPETE while other HPETEs were not detectable.

When the reaction time of AA with the potato LOX was prolonged, the 236/268 nm ratio was significantly decreased, indicating the loss of conjugated diene system in favor of the conjugated trienes. If the potato LOX can act at all possible positions in the dioxygenation of AA then six diHPETEs would be expected to be formed as a result of dual LOX activities (Fig. 1a). Indeed, all six diHPETEs (i.e., 5,12- 8,15-, 9,15-, 5,11-, 9,11-, and 5,15-diHPETEs) were detected in the potato LOX reaction with AA as substrate. Furthermore, it is now believed that the biosynthesis of 5,6- and 14,15-LTA$_4$s is also the result of dual lipoxygenase activity (1, 4, 5); however, as opposed to the diHPETE production, the formation of a given LTA$_4$ is dependent on the sequential action of two specific LOXs. Therefore, it is conceivable that the potato LOX, as a result of its nonregiospecificity, can catalyze the formation of all possible LTA$_4$s from AA (Fig. 1b). Since the allylic epoxides are not stable under aqueous conditions, one expects to observe different diHETEs in the reaction mixture as a result of nonenzymatic hydrolysis of LTA$_4$s (Fig. 1b). All possible diHETEs were indeed isolated and characterized by several analytical criteria, including their characteristic UV absorption spectra. Not only does our data confirm that 5,6-LTA$_4$ synthase activity is associated with the potato LOX but it also suggests that all possible LTA$_4$s can be formed from AA as a result of the nonregiospecificity of the purified potato LOX. Furthermore, our studies using 5(OOH),15(OH)-ETE and 5(OH),15(OOH)-ETE as substrates with the purified potato LOX resulted in the generation of different compounds identified as the all-_trans_-isomers of LXA$_4$ and LXB$_4$. It is also reasonable to expect that LXA$_4$ and LXB$_4$ could be formed via the potato LOX-catalyzed reactions. For example, when 5(S),15(S)-diHETE(EZZE) is acted upon by the 8- and 12-LOX activities associated with the potato enzyme followed by the reduction, it

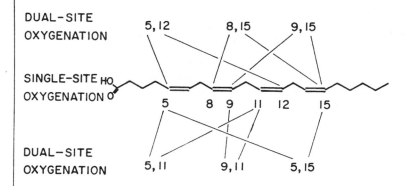

SINGLE AND DUAL-SITE OXYGENATION PRODUCTS OF
POTATO LIPOXYGENASE WITH ARACHIDONIC ACID

DUAL-SITE OXYGENATION

SINGLE-SITE OXYGENATION

DUAL-SITE OXYGENATION

Ia

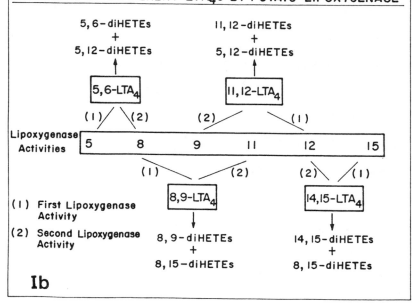

SYNTHESIS OF DIFFERENT LTA$_4$'s BY POTATO LIPOXYGENASE

5,6-diHETEs + 5,12-diHETEs

11,12-diHETEs + 5,12-diHETEs

5,6-LTA$_4$

11,12-LTA$_4$

(1) (2)   (2)   (1)

Lipoxygenase Activities   5   8   9   11   12   15

(1)   (2)   (2)   (1)

(1) First Lipoxygenase Activity

(2) Second Lipoxygenase Activity

8,9-LTA$_4$

14,15-LTA$_4$

8,9-diHETEs + 8,15-diHETEs

14,15-diHETEs + 8,15-diHETEs

Ib

should yield 5(S),6(R),15(S)-triHETE(EEZE) or LXA_4, and 5(S),14(R),15(S)-triHETE(EZEE) or LXB_4 respectively. Based on this information, we propose that the potato enzyme can catalyze the synthesis of LXs by the sequential action of three specific LOX activities associated with this enzyme. Also, we have demonstrated further that the potato LOX can act at all possible positions of EPA and docosahexaenoic acid.

In summary, we have shown that the potato LOX, by virtue of its nonregiospecificity towards the site of insertion of O_2 in polyenoic acids, exhibits unique characteristics in the formation of all possible HPETEs, diHETEs, LTs and LXs. Also, it is conceivable that the mechanism of biosynthesis of LTs and LXs catalyzed by mammalian LOXs might be analogous to the plant enzymes.

REFERENCES

1.   Shimizu T, Radmark O, Samuelsson B. Proc Natl Acad Sci (USA) 1984;81:689-693.

2.   Whelan J, Reddanna P, Prasad G, Reddy CC. In: Lands WEM, ed. Polyunsaturated Fatty Acids and Eicosanoids, Proc AOCS Short Course, AOCS Press, Champaign, Illinois, 1988;468-473.

3.   Chang M, Rao MK, Reddanna P, Li CH, Tu C-PD, Corey EJ, Reddy CC. Arch Biochem Biophys 1987;259:536-547.

4.   Maas RL, Brash AR. Proc Natl Acad Sci (USA) 1983;80:2884-2888.

5.   Wong PY-K, Westlund P, Hamberg M, Granstrom E, Chao PH-W, Samuelsson B. J Biol Chem 1985;260:9162-9165.

*Advances in Prostaglandin, Thromboxane, and
Leukotriene Research*, Vol. 19, edited by
B. Samuelsson, P. Y.-K. Wong, and F. F. Sun,
Raven Press, Ltd., New York ©1989.

THE FORMATION OF LIPOXINS AND 6,7-DIHYDROLIPOXINS BY 5-LIPOXYGENASE AND REDUCTASE PARTIALLY PURIFIED FROM POTATO TUBERS

Hsiao-Yung Ho[+] and Patrick Y-K Wong

Department of Pharmacology, New York Medical College,
Valhalla, N.Y. and [+]Institute of Biomedical Science,
Academic Sinica, Nankang, Taiwan, R.O.C.

INTRODUCTION

Lipoxygenase products, in general, plays an important role in inflammatory responses, immunity, and other physiological and pathophysiological processes (1). A new class of conjugated trihydroxy tetraenes derived from oxygenation of arachidonic acid (AA) and eicosapentaenoic acid (EPA) by multiple lipoxygenation between the 5- and 15-lipoxygenase pathways has been reported by Serhan et al. (2) and Wong et al. (3). These two groups of new compounds were referred to as Lipoxins (LX)A_4, LXB$_4$, LXA$_5$ and LXB$_5$, respectively (4). The initial oxygenation of C-15 position of AA (EPA) leading to the formation of 15-HPETE (15-HPEPE) is the first step in the formation of lipoxins. Ueda et al. (5) reported that LXA$_4$ and LXB$_4$ can also be synthesized by 12-lipoxygenase from 15-HPETE. Lipoxins exhibit interesting biological activities (6) which stimulates the release of superoxide anion without stimulating aggregation of human neutrophils. Lipoxin A$_4$ has been shown to cause contractions of parenchymal strips of guinea pig lung, and dilates arterioles in the hamster cheek pouch (4). Other activities of LXA$_4$ includes activation of protein kinase C (6) and as with LXB$_4$ inhibits the activity of natural killer cells (7). In this report, 5-lipoxygenase, which is enriched in the potato tubers was partially purified and used to study the mechanism and generation of lipoxins. During this study we also observed the existence of 6,7-dihydro-reductase activity in partially purified potato enzyme which generates the 6,7-dihydro-lipoxin B$_4$ from the incubation with 15-HPETE.

MATERIALS AND METHODS

The potato homogenate was obtained by brief homogenization of potato tubers (Russet Burbank) in pH 4.5 acetate buffer, filtration through gauze and precipitation with ammonium sulfate (50% saturation after a prior precipitation at 25% saturation), dissolution in pH 6.8 phosphate buffer, and dialysis as described by Sekiya et al. (8). The partially purified potato enzyme (15 mg of protein) was added to an incubation vessel containing 15-HPETE in ethanol (the amount of ethanol was less than 1%) and 1.0 ml of 50mM phosphate buffer (pH 6.8). The suspension was incubated for 30 min in a shaking water bath at 37° C and reaction was stopped by the addition of two to three volumes of ethanol. The incubation precipitate was filtered and the ethanolic filtrate was evaporated to dryness. The residue was dissolved in 2 ml of distilled water and sodium borohydride was added, followed by incubation on ice for 10 min. The mixture was acidified to pH 3 with 1M citric acid and extracted with diethyl ether. The solvent was evaporated, and the dry residue was dissolved in small amount of methanol. RP-HPLC on a dual pump system equipped with a Vercopak C18 column (3.9mm x 30cm, 10u), a Rheodyne Model 7125 sample injector and a 700 max variable wavelength detector (Shimadzu SPD-6AV). The products were eluted with a linear gradient of methanol/water/acetic acid (50:50:0.01 v/v) (solvent A) to methanol (solvent B) for 40 min at a flow rate of 1 ml/min. UV detector was set at 301 nm for detection of LXs.

The methyl ester of the LXs and dihydro LXs was converted to trimethylsilyl ester as described by Wong et al. (3). The sample was dissolved in hexane ($25\mu l$) and injected into the gas chromatography-mass spectrometer (Hewlett-packard 5988 A) equipped with a cross methyl silicone capillary column (0.3mm x 12m). Helium flow was set at 16 ml/min and oven temperature was programmed from 130°C to 300°C at 5°C/min, injector temperature at 250°C, ion source at 200°C. Electron energy was set at 70 ev.

RESULTS AND DISCUSSION

Incubation of potato enzyme, partially purified from potato tubers, with 15-HPETE generated products with a UV spectrum indicative of both conjugated tetraene (λmax at 301 nm and shoulders at 287 nm and 315 nm) and conjugated triene (λmax at 268 and shoulders at 258 nm and 279 nm) compounds (Figs. 1A and 2A). Following incubation and extraction of the lipid materials were further purified by RP-HPLC, the conjugated triene compounds co-eluted with the tetraene compounds, were collected, methylated and converted to trimethylsilyl derivatives for GC/MS analysis. The mass spectra with base peak at m/z 173 and ions of high intensity at m/z 203 and 275 were monitored. Ions of low intensity were observed at m/z 582, 492 and 409 with M of 582. There were eight isomers with C-value of 24.0, 24.2, 24.25, 24.3, 24.35, 24.4, 24.55 and 24.6, which all contained m/z 582. Their mass-spectra were similar to those reported for LXB_4 and its isomers (9) (Fig. 1A).

A new conjugated triene component was observed on GC which

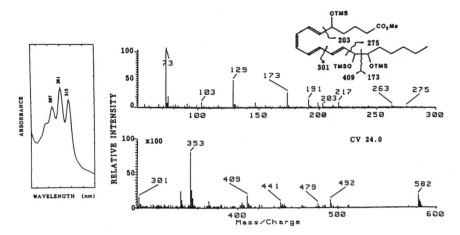

Fig. 1: U.V. spectrum of Lipoxin fractions after incubation of partially purified potato 5-lipoxygenase with 15-HPETE (A). Mass spectrum of the methylester trimethylsilyl derivative of LXB$_4$ isolated and purified from RP-HPLC (B).

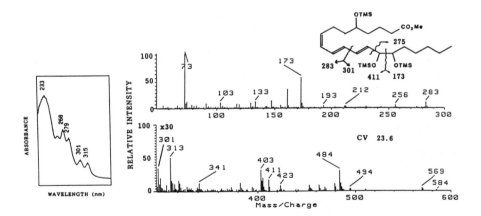

Fig. 2: U.V. Spectrum of a dihydro-lipoxin fraction after incubation of partially purified potato reductase with 15-HPETE (A). Mass spectrum of the methylester trimethylsilyl derivative of 6,7-dihydro-LXB$_4$ isolated and purified from RP-HPLC (B).

gives a C-Value of 23.5 and the mass spectrum showed ions at m/z
584(M), 569(M-15), 494(M-90), 484(M-100), 411(M-173), 303, 203
and 173 (Fig. 1B). Molecular ion of this new compound was found
to be 584 with two mass units higher than that of LXB_4.
Together with the U.V., C-value and the mass-spectrum of this
compound suggested that this is a dihydro metabolite of
LXB_4, in which the $C_{6,7}$ double bonds has been reduced.
The assignment of 6,7-dihydro — LXB_4 is in agreement with its
UV absorption which indicates the presence of a conjugated
triene rather than a tetraene system.

In this report, 5-lipoxygenase partially purified from
potato tubers was used to synthesize lipoxins and various
isomers with the LXB_4 as the major product. A reductase
activity was also present in the potato enzyme because of the
dihydro product was detected in the incubation mixture and
identified by GC/MS.

REFERENCES

1. Samuelsson B, Dahlen SE, Lindgren J, Rouzer CA, Serhan CN.
    Science, 1987;237:1171-1176

2. Serhan CN, Hamberg M, Samuelsson B. Proc Natl Acad Sci USA,
    1984;81:5335-5339

3. Wong PYK, Hughes R, Lam B. Biochem Biophys Res. Commun,
    1985;126:765-772

4. Dahlen SE, Raud J, Serhan CN, Bjork J, Samuelsson B. Acta
    Physiol Scand, 1987;130:643-647

5. Ueda, N., Yokoyama, C., Yamamoto, S., Fitzsimmons, B.J.,
    Rokach, J., Oates, J. and Brash, A.R. Biochem. Biophys.
    Res. Commun., 1987;1063-1069.

6. Hansson A, Serhan CN, Haeggstron J, Ingelman-Sundberg M,
    Samuelsson B. Biochem Biophys Res. Commun,
    1986;134:1215-1222

7. Ramstedt U, Ng J, Wigzell H, Serhan CN, Samuelsson B. J
    Immunol 1985;135:3434-3436

8. Sekiya J, Aoshima H, Kajiwara T, Togo T, Hatanaka A, Agric
    Biol Chem, 1977;41:827

9. Serhan, C.N., Hamberg, M., Samuelsson, B., Morris, J. and
    Wishka, D.G. Proc. Natl. Acad. Sci. USA, 1986;83:1983-1987.

Advances in Prostaglandin, Thromboxane, and
Leukotriene Research, Vol. 19, edited by
B. Samuelsson, P. Y.-K. Wong, and F. F. Sun,
Raven Press, Ltd., New York ©1989.

BRAIN HEPOXILINS: FORMATION AND ACTION

C. R. Pace-Asciak[1]*, S. Asotra*, L. Pellerin**, L.S. Wolfe**,
E. J. Corey***, P. Wu****, N. Gurevich****, and P. L. Carlen****

*The Research Institute, The Hospital for Sick Children, Toronto M5G 1X8,
**The Montreal Neurological Institute, Montreal H3A 2B4, Canada
***Department of Chemistry, Harvard University, Cambridge, USA
****Addiction Research Foundation and The Playfair Neurosciences Unit,
Departrments of Medicine (Neurology), Physiology and Pharmacology, University
of Toronto M5S 1A8, Canada

Hepoxilins (HxA$_3$ and HxB$_3$) are hydroxy epoxide derivatives of arachidonic acid derived from 12-HPETE (1-3). ^{18}Oxygen studies have shown that both oxygen atoms of the hydroperoxide group of 12-HPETE are retained during its isomerisation into the hepoxilins (4). This isomerisation has been shown to occur in platelets (5,6), lung (1,4,7) as well as in the absence of enzymes, e.g. with hemoglobin and hemin (3,4). The hepoxilins are formed by isolated perifused pancreatic islets (2,8) where they act to stimulate the glucose dependent release of insulin, and are capable of transporting calcium across fetal membranes (8), although they are mostly devoid of biological activity in a variety of other test systems we have used. These include smooth muscle, arterial blood pressure and Na/K ATPase (unpublished). The hepoxilins are inactivated through an epoxide hydrolase into the corresponding trihydroxy derivatives termed trioxilins, TrX (1,10). We have recently shown that the hepoxilins are formed by homogenates of the cerebral cortex, pons, median eminence and pituitary of the rat (11), and that the hepoxilins are found in the circulation of the rat after intravenous bolus injection of arachidonic acid (12). Previous studies have shown that glutamate and norepinephrine induce 12-HETE formation by intact pieces of the rat cerebral cortex (13). Because of the recent findings with Aplysia sensory neurons showing that 12-HPETE is capable of exhibiting changes in membrane potential and an increase in hyperpolarization (14), we felt that the actions of 12-HPETE are probably mediated via its transformation into the hepoxilins, since we had previously shown that 12-HPETE is rapidly transformed into the hepoxilins (1-4, 8). The present paper describes the formation of hepoxilin A$_3$ by intact pieces of the cerebral cortex and the effect of various neurotransmitters and other compounds on the formation of both 12-HETE and hepoxilin A$_3$; we further provide for the first time preliminary electrophysiological evidence that hepoxilin A$_3$ acts in the mammalian CNS (hippocampal CA1 neurons) with a persistent membrane hyperpolarization, prolongation of the post-spike train afterhyperpolarization (AHP) and an enhancement of both the early and late phases of the orthodromic inhibitory postsynaptic potential (IPSP).

MATERIALS AND METHODS

Materials: Deuterium-labelled (D4) methyl ester of HxA$_3$ (deuterium atoms at positions 5,6,14,15) was saponified to the free acid by reaction with ethanol/1N

---

[1] To whom correspondence should be addressed

sodium hydroxide (1/1, v/v) at room temperature and was subsequently hydrolysed to TrXA3 by acidification with 1N HCl and extracted with ethyl acetate (12). 9-HOTE was prepared from linolenic acid through photochemical oxygenation using methylene blue as initiator and purified by HPLC (unpublished).

Biochemical experiments: Adult male Wistar rats (approx. 250 g) were purchased from Charles River Labs. Inc.(Montreal, Canada). Rats were sacrificed by decapitation, the brain was dissected, and the cerebral cortex was removed, washed with buffer (2.68 mM KCl, 1.47 mM KH$_2$PO$_4$, 136.9 mM NaCl, 15.2 mM NaH$_2$PO$_4$) and chopped into fine pieces with a sharp scalpel blade. The brain pieces were incubated in 3 ml of the same buffer containing 4 mM CaCl$_2$ in open vessels for 20 min at 37°C. The incubations were terminated by cooling on ice, addition of 1N HCl to bring the medium to pH 3 and the mixture was left on ice for 30 min. Deuterium labelled TrXA3 (50 ng) was added followed by 3 ml methanol. The mixture was brought to 10% methanol by the addition of water, and it was separated on a C18-SEPPAK cartridge (Waters) previously saturated with methanol and water. After the sample had been loaded, the cartridge was eluted with water, followed by increasing amounts of methanol in water/acetic acid. The hepoxilins were eluted from the SEPPAK with methanol/water/acetic acid (65/35/0.4) and the HETEs were eluted with methanol/water/acetic acid (90/10/0.4).

Derivatisation for GCMS: Samples from the SEPPAK were converted to the methyl ester tBDMSi ether derivatives for EI-GCMS through procedures published previously (11).

EI-GCMS: A Hewlett-Packard 5970 GCMS (MSD) was used for the assay of the hepoxilins on a 60 meter DB-1 capillary column (J&W Scientific) directed into the source. Helium was employed as carrier gas at a linear velocity of 30 cm/sec. The mass spectrometer was operated in the EI mode (70eV) with a source pressure at 8.10^{-5} Torr. Sample was injected on column in 1 µl hexane at an oven temperature of 50°C. The oven temperature was raised at 20°/min to a final temperature of 300°C. Data was acquired in the SIM mode with TrXA3 detected using two groups of ions, i.e. m/z 255/257 and 285/287, the former ion in each group detecting the endogenous (Do) product, the latter fragment detecting the D4 carrier.

Electrophysiological experiments: Male Wistar rats (150 - 170 g) were anaesthetised with halothane and decapitated. The brain was dissected and coronal hemisphere (400 µm) sections were cut with a vibratome in ice-cold medium. The slices were stored in oxygenated (95% O$_2$- 5% CO$_2$) artificial cerebrospinal fluid (ACSF) for at least 1 h at room temperature of the following composition in mM: Na$^+$ 154; K$^+$ 4.25; Ca^{2+} 2; Mg^{2+} 2; Cl$^-$ 131.5; HCO$_3^-$ 26; HPO$_4^-$ 1.25; SO$_4^{-2}$ 2; dextrose 10. The pH was maintained at 7.4. For recording, a slice was transferred to a modified interface-type Haas electrophysiological recording chamber at 34°C. Standard electrophysiological recording techniques were employed (15,16). Glass micropipettes filled with 3M KCl or 3M potassium acetate and having resistances from 60 to 150 Meg Ohm were used for the intracellular recordings done with an Axoclamp II microelectrode amplifier. Data was recorded on chart paper and stored on tape. Appropriate amounts of hepoxilin

A3 methyl ester were dissolved in 50 μl DMSO and diluted with 50 ml of ACSF to give final concentrations of 0.5, 5 and 10 μM. Hepoxilin A3 at a concentration of 100 μM was also focally drop-applied onto the stratum radiatum or stratum oriens inside the slice tissue. Stratum radiatum afferents were stimulated orthodromically by monopolar or concentric bipolar tungsten electrodes using 5 to 40 μA.

RESULTS

Biochemical experiments: Rat brain is capable of releasing a variety of HETEs. However, only 12-HETE appears to be increased upon incubation or upon stimulation. Figure 1 shows an HPLC profile of HETEs released from the control (unstimulated) brain incubated for 20 min, and brain incubated with the calcium ionophore, A23187, for the same time period. A marked stimulation of 12-HETE was seen with A23187, but also with neurotransmitters such as norepinephrine, L-glutamate, and other compounds such as n-methyl D-aspartate (NMDA) and carbachol. Since the hepoxilins are formed through activation of the 12-lipoxygenase pathway, we chose to investigate whether their release also follows the release of 12-HETE. Figure 2 shows the GCMS/SIM-profiles demonstrating the formation of HxA3 (as TrXA3) in brain samples stimulated by the ionophore, A23187. Table 1 compares the relative appearance of 12-HETE and HxA3 under various conditions of stimulation.

TABLE 1. <u>Formation of 12-HETE and HxA3 by rat cerebral cortex pieces</u>

Condition	Product (ng/0.5g tissue)*	
	12-HETE**	HxA3***
Control 5 min	6.2 ± 1.4^a	10.7 ± 0.3^c
Control 20 min	$12.7 \pm 1.1^{a,b}$	$13.9 \pm 0.9^{c,d}$
" + A23187 (10μM)	51.7 ± 7.2^b	14.8 ± 0.8^d
" + L-glutamate (100μM)	17.0 ± 0.6^b	14.1 ± 0.8^d
" + NMDA (100μM)	17.7 ± 7.3^d	13.7 ± 0.9^d
" + Norepinephrine (100μM)	28.1 ± 5.3^b	12.5 ± 1.0^d
" + Carbachol (100μM)	31.8 ± 2.4^b	14.7 ± 0.6^d

*Values represent the mean ± SEM of triplicate determinations. Students t-test: letters denote groups compared, a,b) $p<0.025$, c) $p<0.005$, d) NS.
**Analysis by HPLC
***Analysis by EI-GCMS

Electrophysiological experiments: At all doses employed (Table 2), HxA3 consistently hyperpolarized the resting membrane potential by 1 to 4 mV, but this effect was not associated with any significant changes in the neuronal input

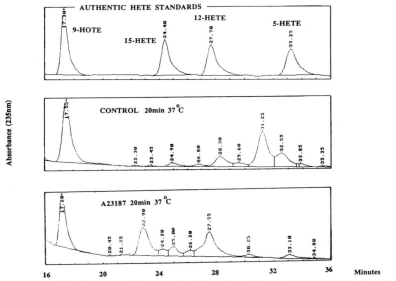

FIG. 1. HPLC profile (reversed phase) showing the release of HETEs by incubated pieces of the rat cerebral cortex. Top profile represents authentic standards, middle profile represents brain pieces incubated for 20 min without additions, and lower profile shows the stimulation by the ionophore, A23187 (10μM).

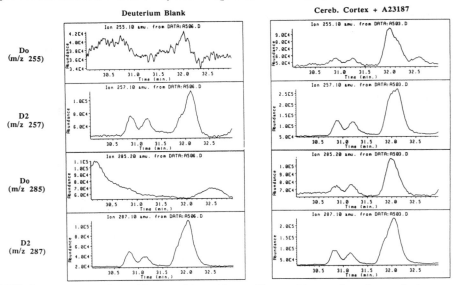

FIG. 2. EI-GCMS selected ion profiles of hepoxilin A3 (detected as the methyl ester t-BDMSi ether derivative of TrXA3) using D4 TrXA3 as internal standard. The profiles show the composition of the deuterium blank (left panels) and that of an extract obtained from incubation of rat cerebral cortex pieces with the ionophore, A23187 (right panels).

TABLE 2. <u>Electrophysiological responses* of CA1 hippocampal neurons to hepoxilin A$_3$</u>

Dose	RMP (hyperpolarization)	AHP (prolongation)	EPSP (no change)	IPSP (enhancement)
1. Perfusion				
0.5 µM	2/2	2/2	N/A	N/A
5 µM	4/4	4/4	3/3	3/3
10 µM	2/2	2/2	2/2	2/2
2. Drop-application				
100 µM	3/3	3/3	N/A	N/A

* = number of responding cells / number of cells tested. RMP = resting membrane potential; AHP = afterhyperpolarization; EPSP = excitatory postsynaptic potential; IPSP = inhibitory postsynaptic potential; N/A = not assessed.

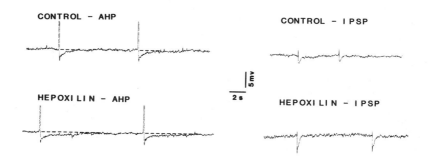

FIG. 3. Electrophysiological recordings showing the effects of HxA$_3$ on the AHP and IPSP in the rat hippocampal CA1 neurons. AHPs followed a train of 6 spikes before (control) and 9 min after beginning of HxA$_3$ perfusion (10 µM). RMP = -74 mV. IPSPs were recorded before (control) and 25 min after HxA$_3$ perfusion (5 µM). RMP = -63 mV.

resistance. With perfusion, the hyperpolarization gradually developed over a 7 min period. Drop application caused a small (< 2 mV) hyperpolarization within 10 to 20 sec which lasted up to 40 sec.

The AHP, which is thought to be due to a Ca^{2+}-mediated potassium conductance, was prolonged up to 2-fold by perfusion (Fig. 3) and up to 1.5-fold by drop application (not shown). The prolongation following drop application lasted 1 - 4 min.

EPSPs were not affected. However, a marked enhancement of the IPSP was observed (up to 2-fold). This increase included both the early chloride-dependent and the later potassium-dependent phases of the IPSP (Fig. 3).

In two cells that were perfused with 10 µM HxA$_3$ for 30 min, the effects were partially reversed after 20 min washout.

DISCUSSION

The present results indicate that the hepoxilins are formed by tissues other than the platelets (5,6), and the lung (1,4,7). It has previously been shown that pancreatic islet cells in vitro have the capacity to form 12-HPETE (17-19); we have shown that this product is avidly transformed in the absence of hemoglobin into both hepoxilins A$_3$ and B$_3$ (2). The present results add further evidence that HxA$_3$ is formed by intact pieces of the rat cerebral cortex. It is not clear from the data presented (Table 1) why hepoxilin formation was not stimulated by the various neurotransmitters in parallel to 12-HETE synthesis as both products have already been shown to be derived through the same pathway (1, 3, 4). We further provide in this paper preliminary electrophysiological evidence that one of the hepoxilins (HxA$_3$) is capable of inducing neuronal responses at doses that lie within the amounts that can be formed in brain tissue. The mechanism of the RMP hyperpolarization by HxA$_3$ is unclear, especially since there was no associated conductance increase. The prolongation of the AHP is a postsynaptic phenomenon related to increased K^+ conductance possibly due to an increased Ca^{2+} entry or increased sensitivity of the K^+ channel to ambient intracellular Ca^{2+} ions. The increase by HxA$_3$ of both the early and late phases of the IPSP suggest a presynaptic effect, which also could be related to intracellular Ca^{2+} mobilization. To our knowledge, this is the first demonstration of hepoxilin actions on central mammalian neurons suggesting that in addition to their demonstrated insulin-secretory effects on islet β-cells, these products may play important neuromodulatory roles in the brain and other tissues.

ACKNOWLEDGEMENTS

The present study was supported by grants to CRP-A (MRC #MT-4181), to LSW (MRC #MT-1345), and to PLC (MRC #MT-7980; OMH #971-87-89).

REFERENCES

1. Pace-Asciak CR, Granstrom E and Samuelsson B, J Biol Chem 1983;258:6835-6840.

2. Pace-Asciak CR and Martin JM, Prostaglandins Leukotrienes Med 1984;16:173-180.

3. Pace-Asciak CR, Biochim Biophys Acta 1984;793:485-488.

4. Pace-Asciak CR, J Biol Chem 1984;259:8332-8337.

5. Jones RL, Kerry PJ, Poyser NL et al. Prostaglandins 1978;16:583-589.

6. Bryant RW and Bailey JM, Prostaglandins 1979;17:9-18.

7. Pace-Asciak CR, Mizuno K and Yamamoto S, Biochim Biophys Acta 1982;712:142-145.

8. Pace-Asciak CR, Martin JM, Corey EJ and Su WG, Biochem Biophys Res Commun 1985;128:942-946.

9. Derewlany LO, Pace-Asciak CR and Radde I, Can J Physiol Pharmacol 1984;62:1466-1469.

10. Pace-Asciak CR, Klein J and Speilberg SP, Biochim Biophys Acta 1986;875:406-409.

11. Pace-Asciak CR, Biochim Biophys Res Commun 1988;151:493-498.

12. Pace-Asciak CR, Lee SP and Martin JM Biochim Biophys Res Commun 1987;147:881-884.

13. Pellerin L and Wolfe LS, Trans Amer Soc Neurochem 1988;19:76 (Abstract).

14. Piomelli D, Volterra A, Dale N, et al Nature 1987;328:38-43.

15. Carlen PL, Gurevich N and Durand D, Science 1982;215:306-309.

16. Blaxter TJ, Carlen PL, Davies MF and Kutjan PW, J Physiol 1986;373:181-194.

17. Metz S, vanRollins M, Strife R, et al. J Clin Invest 1983;71:1191-1205.

18. Walsh M and Pek SB, Life Sci 1984;34:1699-1706.

19. Turk J, Colca JR and McDaniel ML, Biochim Biophys Acta, 1985;834:23-36.

Advances in Prostaglandin, Thromboxane, and Leukotriene Research, Vol. 19, edited by B. Samuelsson, P. Y.-K. Wong, and F. F. Sun, Raven Press, Ltd., New York ©1989.

REDUCED 12-LIPOXYGENASE

ACTIVITY IN PLATELETS OF PATIENTS

WITH MYELOPROLIFERATIVE DISORDERS

M. Okuma, K. Kanaji, F. Ushikubi, H. Uchino, *J. Murakami, *T. Yoshimoto, and *S. Yamamoto

The First Division, Department of Internal Medicine, Faculty of Medicine, Kyoto University, Kyoto 606, Japan and *Department of Biochemistry, School of Medicine, Tokushima University, Tokushima 770, Japan

In human platelets, a greater portion of arachidonic acid is oxygenated via the 12-lipoxygenase pathway rather than the cyclooxygenase pathway. A deficiency of platelet 12-lipoxygenase activity was found in some patients with myeloproliferative disorders (MPD) (1,2). However, this abnormality of the enzyme has not yet been well characterized.

REDUCED ACTIVITY OF 12-LIPOXYGENASE

Blood from 9 normal volunteers and 7 MPD patients with reduced or undetectable activity of platelet 12-lipoxygenase was collected in 0.1 volume of 3.8% trisodium citrate, and washed platelets were suspended in 300 mM sucrose (2×10^6 platelets/μl) (3). An aliquot of the washed platelets was disrupted by sonication, and the homogenate was centrifuged for 12 min at 12,000g and 4°C (4). The supernatant (F1) was collected and its aliquot was further centrifuged for 60 min at 105,000g and 4°C. After removal of the supernatant (F2), the pellet was rinsed and suspended in the same volume of the sucrose solution (F3) as that of F2. Intact platelets and their subcellular fractions were incubated with arachidonic acid for 5 min at 37°C in the absence or presence of $CaCl_2$ (3). Arachidonate metabolites extracted in ethyl acetate were analyzed and quantitated by reversed phase high performance liquid chromatography (3). 12-HETE production by intact 10^8 platelets of normal subjects and the patients was 1162 ± 203 ng (M ± SD, n = 9) and 68 ± 107 ng (n = 7), respectively. One of the 7 patients showed essentially no production of 12-HETE by intact platelets as well as by any subcellular fraction. All the

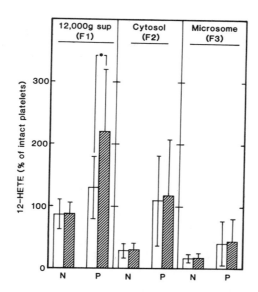

Fig. 1. 12-HETE production by subcellular fractions of normal
subjects (N) and MPD patients (P) in the absence (open columns)
or presence (hatched columns) of 2.5 mM $CaCl_2$. M ± SD (n = 9 for
N; n = 6 for P); *, p < 0.01

other patients showed reduced production of 12-HETE. These 6 patients were used in the following studies. In normal platelets,
the amounts of 12-HETE produced by F1, F2 and F3 were about 87%,
31% and 17%, respectively, of that by intact platelets, and were
not significantly affected by the addition of $CaCl_2$ (Fig. 1). On
the other hand, the 12-HETE production by F1, F2 and F3 of the 6
patients was 131%, 112% and 42%, respectively, and the addition
of $CaCl_2$ to the reaction mixture significantly increased the synthesis of 12-HETE by F1 (p < 0.01 by Student's paired t-test),
although such an effect of Ca^{2+} was not observed with the other
subcellular fractions (Fig. 1). The requirement of the mammalian
5-lipoxygenase for Ca^{2+} was earlier reported (5). Furthermore,
12-lipoxygenase from rat basophilic leukemia cells was stimulated
by Ca^{2+} (6). On the other hand, human platelet 12-lipoxygenase
was unaffected by Ca^{2+} (7,8). This was confirmed by our data on
normal platelets. However, the lipoxygenase activity of F1 prepared from platelets of the patients was significantly enhanced
by Ca^{2+}. The reason for this stimulating effect of Ca^{2+} on F1
(not on F2 and F3) from the patients' platelets is unclear at the
moment.

In normal subjects, 12-HETE production by any subcellular
fraction of platelets was not more than that by intact platelets.
In most patients, however, the lipoxygenase activity was higher
in F1 and F2 than in intact platelets, suggesting a possibility

that there was an endogenous inhibitor of 12-lipoxygenase. Intact platelets from one of the patients were mixed with various
numbers of normal platelets, and the mixtures were incubated with
arachidonic acid. 12-HETE production increased as the percentage
of normal platelets was increased, and reached a plateau when
normal platelets accounted for 60% of the total platelets. Furthermore, the addition of the 12,000g pellet of the patient's
platelets did not reduce the 12-HETE synthesis by Fl of normal
platelets and of the patient. Thus, a possible involvement of an
inhibitory factor could be ruled out.

QUANTIFICATION OF 12-LIPOXYGENASE BY ENZYME IMMUNOASSAY

As described by Yoshimoto et al. in a separate chapter of this
volume, a peroxidase-linked immunoassay of sandwich type was developed utilizing monoclonal anti-human 12-lipoxygenase antibodies. Two separate species of antibody which recognized different sites of the enzyme protein were utilized to develop a
method to determine the amount of 12-lipoxygenase protein rather
than the activity of enzyme. The precipitate of the whole immune
complex was subjected to the assay of peroxidase activity, and
the result was correlated with the 12-lipoxygenase content. This
method was applied to determine the 12-lipoxygenase content in F2
from the patients' platelets in which the 12-lipoxygenase activity was abnormally reduced. As shown in Fig. 2, when the increasing amounts of the platelet cytosol from three patients were examined by the enzyme immunoassay, the peroxidase activity in the
immunoprecipitate leveled off with more than 3×10^6 platelets.
In contrast, the activity of peroxidase immunoprecipitated from
the platelet cytosol of normal subjects increased linearly as the
amount of the cytosol was raised in the same range. As far as

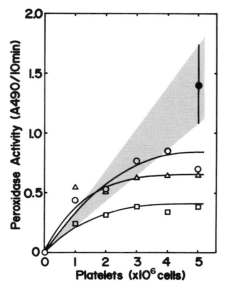

Fig. 2. 12-lipoxygenase contents
in the platelets of three MPD pa-
tients ($\bigcirc$, $\triangle$, $\square$). Mean and
SD of 22 normal subjects are
shown by the closed circle and
the shaded area.

the enzyme levels were compared with smaller amounts of the platelet cytosol, there was no significant difference in the 12-lip-
oxygenase content between the MPD patients and normal subjects.
Since the partially purified 12-lipoxygenase added to the platelet cytosol of patients was recovered in the yield of almost 100
%, the loss of linearity may not be attributed to the presence of
certain substances in the patient's platelets which interfered
with the immunoassay. The mechanism for the loss of linearity
in the peroxidase activity of the patients' platelets remains to
be eluciated.

REFERENCES

1. Okuma M, Uchino H. Blood 1979; 54:1258-1271.

2. Schafer A I. N Engl J Med 1982; 306:381-386.

3. Kanaji K, Okuma M, Ushikubi F, Uchino H. Prostaglandins
   Leukotrienes Essent Fatty Acids 1988; 31:155-161.

4. Okuma M, Yamashita S, Numa S. Blood 1973; 41:379-389.

5. Jakschik B A, Sun F F, Lee L -H, Steinhoff M M. Biochem
   Biophys Res Commun 1980; 95:103-110.

6. Hamasaki Y, Tai H -H. Biochim Biophys Acta 1984; 793:393-398.

7. Lagarde M, Croset M, Authi K S, Crawford N. Biochem J 1984;
   222:495-500.

8. Wallach D P, Brown V R. Biochim Biophys Acta 1981; 663:361-
   372.

*Advances in Prostaglandin, Thromboxane, and
Leukotriene Research*, Vol. 19, edited by
B. Samuelsson, P. Y.-K. Wong, and F. F. Sun,
Raven Press, Ltd., New York ©1989.

ON THE ORIGIN OF 12-HYDROXYEICOSATETRAENOIC ACID
IN PSORIATIC SCALE

John L. Humes and Evan E. Opas

Department of Inflammation Research
Merck Sharp and Dohme Research Laboratories
Rahway, N.J. 07065, USA

A characteristic of psoriasis is the elevated levels of
certain free fatty acids and their metabolites in affected
skin. Hammerstrom and colleagues in 1975 demonstrated large
increased amounts of 12-HETE in psoriatic epidermis as
compared to uninvolved tissue (1). The pathology of this
disease is characterized at least in part by polymorphonuclear
leukocytes (PMNs) infiltration and the abnormal proliferation
of epidermis. Recent data have suggested that 12-HETE can be
a mediator of these events. Goetzl and Sun showed that
12-HETE was chemotactic for PMNs (2). Chan and colleagues
demonstrated epidermal cell proliferation in response to
intradermal administration of this agent (3).

Recently Woollard found that the 12-HETE extracted from
psoriatic scale was in fact the 12-R enantiomer and not 12-S-
HETE that is synthesized by platelets (4). Of potential
importance are the in vitro findings that 12-R-HETE is more
potent than 12-S-HETE to promote PMN chemotaxis (5). Evans
and colleagues have shown that the 12-R enantiomer is more
active than the 12-S-HETE to induce rat PMN aggregation (6).
In addition, these workers have shown that 12-R-HETE
competitively displaced the binding of [^{3}H]-LTB$_4$ to human
leukocyte membranes (6). In this system 12-R-HETE was 10-fold
more potent than 12-S-HETE. Thus the finding that 12-R-HETE
is present in elevated levels in psoriatic scale has
stimulated speculation that this eicosanoid may at least in
part be responsible for the inflammation and cellular
proliferation associated with this disease.

We have recently confirmed by a new and different method
(7) the work of Woollard that psoriatic scale contained
predominantly 12-R-HETE. In this procedure, 12-R or 12-S
isomers were incubated with a potato preparation of
5-lipoxygenase. The synthesized substrate-specific diHETEs,
5-S,12-R and 5-S,12-S were readily separated on reverse phase
high performance chromatography. However in contrast to the
fact that psoriatic scale contained 12-R, our studies showed
that homogenates of human epidermis synthesized predominantly
12-S-HETE (7).

These combined observations present a question — "What are the origins of 12-R-HETE found in psoriatic scale?" At least five explanations are proposed.

1. Different 12-lipoxygenases
2. P_{450} catalyzed oxygenations
3. Coupled oxidation and reduction
4. Isomerization
5. Auto/Photo oxidation of arachidonic acid (AA)

Our recent studies clearly demonstrated that epidermal homogenates synthesize 12-S-HETE as determined by the 5-lipoxygenase enzyme method to determine the stereoconfiguration (7). However the 12-lipoxygenase found in human skin differs pharmacologically from the 12-lipoxygenase found in human platelets (8). These studies evaluated several key compounds, which were all developed as 5-lipoxygenase inhibitors, for their effect on epidermal and platelet lipoxygenase. Takeda's AA861 and the "active metabolite" of Syntex's Lonapalene were inactive when evaluated as platelet 12-lipoxygenase inhibitors (8) but were inhibitors of human epidermal 12-lipoxygenase (7). Merck's L-651,896 was more potent as a epidermal 12-lipoxygenase inhibitor than as an inhibitor of the platelet enzyme, with IC_{50} values of 1.4 versus 5.9 uM respectively (7,9).

Capdevila and colleagues reported that 12-R-HETE was the principle 12-HETE synthesized by rat liver P_{450} preparations (10). However our studies showing that epidermal homogenates synthesize 12-S-HETE suggested that P_{450} oxygenases are not responsible for the 12-R isomer found in psoriatic scale. In addition, Nakadate et al. showed that carbon monoxide, an inhibitor of P_{450} oxygenations, did not inhibit 12-HETE synthesis in mouse skin homogenates (11). Similarly we have shown that 12-HETE synthesis by human epidermal homogenates was not stimulated by NADPH or inhibited by SKF525A (7). Thus the data when evaluated in concert tends to exclude the P_{450} system as the source of 12-R-HETE.

The direct enzymatic or chemical isomerization of 12-R to 12-S-HETE has not been reported. The possibility that 12-S-HETE could be oxidized to 12-ketoeicosatetraenoic acid which would be then subsequently reduced to 12-R-HETE has similarly not been documented.

Lesional psoriatic skin may provide an attractive environment for the photo and autooxidation of AA as large amounts of AA are present in areas exposed to molecular oxygen and ultraviolet radiation as well as potentially other environmental oxidation catalysts. In this scenario equimolar amounts of both 12-S- and 12-R-isomers would be formed. Subsequently the S-isomer but not the R-isomer would be preferentially esterified into cellular phospholipids and triglycerides thus leaving 12-R-HETE as the product found in psoriatic scale. Thus psoriatic scale would be analogous to a fossilized record of biochemical events that previously occurred in the inflammation of the lesional epidermis and dermis.

Studies employing 12-lipoxygenase preparations derived from psoriatic epidermis and dermis to determine which isomer is synthesized will be necessary to establish the origin of 12-R-HETE found associated with psoriatic scale. The understanding of the mechanism would thus permit the design of therapeutic agents to control the formation and evaluate the contribution of 12-R-HETE to this disease.

REFERENCES

1. Hammarstrom S, Hamberg M, Samuelsson B, Duell EA, Stawiski M and Voorhees JJ, Proc Natl Acad Sci 1975;72:5130-5134.

2. Goetzl EJ and Sun FF, J Exp Med 1979;150:406-411.

3. Chan CC, Duhamel L and Ford-Hutchinson AW, J Invest Dermatol 1985;85: 333-334.

4. Woollard PM, Biochem Biophys Res Commun 1986;136:169-176.

5. Cunningham FM, Greaves MW and Woollard PM, Br J Dermatol 1986;87:107a.

6. Evans JF, Leblanc Y, Fitzsimmons BJ, Charleson S, Nataniel D and Leveille C, Biochimica et Biophysica Acta 1987;917:406-410.

7. Opas EE, Argenbright LW and Humes JL, Brit J Dermatol In press.

8. Opas EE, Argenbright LW, Pacholok SG, Weinstein MJ and Humes JL, Clin Res 1987;35(5):795a.

9. Bonney RJ, Davies P, Dougherty H, et al. Biochem Pharmacol 1987;35:3885-3891.

10. Capdevila J, Yadagiri P, Manna S and Falck Jr. Biochem Biophys Res Commun 1986;141:1007-1011.

11. Nakadate T, Aizu E, Yamamoto S and Kato R, Prostaglandin Leukotrienes and Medicine 1986;21:305-319.

Advances in Prostaglandin, Thromboxane, and Leukotriene Research, Vol. 19, edited by B. Samuelsson, P. Y.-K. Wong, and F. F. Sun, Raven Press, Ltd., New York ©1989.

ARACHIDONATE 15-LIPOXYGENASE FROM HUMAN LEUKOCYTES: Purification and structural homology to other mammalian lipoxygenases

Elliott Sigal, Dorit Grunberger, Charles S. Craik*, George H. Caughey, Jay A. Nadel
Cardiovascular Research Institute, Departments of Medicine, *Pharmaceutical Chemistry, *Biochemistry and Biophysics
San Francisco, California 94143

The enzyme 15-lipoxygenase catalyzes the hydroperoxidation of arachidonic acid to form 15-hydroperoxyeicosatetraenoic acid. This is the first step in the formation of the mono-hydroxy acid 15-hydroxyeicosatetraenoic acid (15-HETE), the dihydroxy acids 8,15 diHETE and 14,15 diHETE and the trihydroxy acids, lipoxin A and B(1). The biological functions of these 15-lipoxygenase metabolites may include the stimulation of mucus release from cultured human airway(2), chemotaxis of human neutrophils(3), inhibition of natural killer cell activity(1) and contraction of guinea pig lung strips(1). The 15-lipoxygenase pathway is the predominant pathway for arachidonic acid metabolism in human lung homogenates(4), isolated human airway epithelial cells(5), human eosinophils(6), and human keratinocytes(7). We have recently described a method for purifying human 15-lipoxygenase to homogeneity from eosinophil-enriched leukocytes (8). In this paper, we summarize the results of the purification procedure and report the N-terminal amino acid sequence of the human 15-lipoxygenase. Sequence similarity with other mammalian lipoxygenases suggests that the enzymes of the lipoxygenase family are related structurally.

Cells were obtained from the peripheral blood of subjects with hypereosinophilia. Arachidonate 15-lipoxygenase was purified from the 100,000 x g supernatant of these leukocytes using ammonium sulfate precipitation, hydrophobic-interaction chromatography, and high pressure liquid chromatography on hydroxyapatite and cation exchange columns. The details of these procedures and the enzyme assays are described elsewhere(10). One unit of enzyme activity is defined as the amount of enzyme required to generate one nmol of 13-OH linoleic acid under standard assay conditions.

Enzyme activity was localized to the 100,000 x g supernatant, suggesting a cytosolic origin. The 15-lipoxygenase in the 30-60% ammonium sulfate fraction was very hydrophobic as indicated by its elution from phenyl-Sepharose at approximately 0% ammonium sulfate. The

protein's elution from the Mono S column at pH 7 suggests
that the enzyme is cationic at neutral pH. The results of a
purification experiment combining differential
centrifugation, ammonium sulfate precipitation,
hydrophobic-interaction, hydroxyapatite and cation-exchange
chromatography are shown in **Table 1**. A single protein
peak, co-eluting precisely with a peak of lipoxygenase
activity, was obtained in the final chromatographic step.
This purification began with 3×10^9 leukocytes (25%
eosinophils and 75% neutrophils) and approximately 1800-
fold purification of 15-lipoxygenase was achieved.

TABLE 1. Purification of 15-lipoxygenase from human leukocytes

Fraction	Vol (ml)	Total protein (mg)	Total activity (units)	Specific Activity (units/mg)	Yield (%)	Purification (fold)
Supernatant (100,000 x g)	60	152	16,419	108	100	--
Precipitate (30-60%)	15	52.5	10,946	208	67	1.9
Phenyl-Sepharose	10	0.891	6,055	6,796	37	62.9
Hydroxyapatite	9	0.066	1,187	17,985	7.2	160
Mono S	2	0.001	198	198,000	1.2	1800

The activity of the purified enzyme was unchanged in the
presence or absence of calcium. In contrast, calcium
enhanced the acitivty of the crude enzyme(9), suggesting
that either calcium stabilizes the crude enzyme, or the
purification procedure removes a calcium dependent
stimulatory factor.

The major products produced from linoleic acid and
arachidonic acid by the action of the purified lipoxygenase
were identical to that of synthetic 13-OH linoleic acid and
15-HETE, respectively, as determined by ultraviolet
spectroscopy, normal phase- and reverse phase-HPLC, and
mass spectrometry.

The results from SDS/polyacrylamide gel electrophoresis of
samples obtained from each purification step are shown in
Fig 1. In the purified preparation, one major protein band
(apparent M_r, 70,000) was observed (lane 4). In addition,
one major amino acid sequence was obtained from the
purified protein. Comparison of the amino-terminal sequence
of the human 15-lipoxygenase with known sequences of other
lipoxygenases (**Fig 2**) reveals 71% sequence identity with
the rabbit reticulocyte lipoxygenase(10) and 36% sequence
identity with the human 5-lipoxygenase(11,12). Furthermore,
when one considers the sequence similarity at positions
5,8,11,13 and 14, there is 60% sequence similarity among
all three mammalian lipoxygenases. In contrast, a search
of the entire sequence of the soybean lipoxygenase
isoenzyme 1(13) failed to locate any sequence identity to

the N-terminal sequence of the human 15-lipoxygenase. These
results suggest that the mammalian lipoxygenases are
members of an homologous family of proteins.

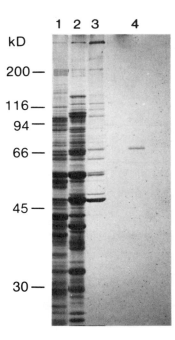

Fig. 1. Polyacrylamide
gel electrophoresis of
fractions obtained during
the purification of human
15-lipoxygenase. The samples
are 30-60% precipitate (lane
1), phenyl-Sepharose (lane
2), hydroxyapatite (lane 3),
and Mono S cation exchange
(lane 4). (Reproduced with
permission from [8])

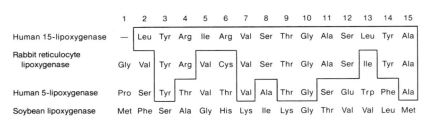

	1	2	3	4	5	6	7	8	9	10	11	12	13	14	15
Human 15-lipoxygenase	—	Leu	Tyr	Arg	Ile	Arg	Val	Ser	Thr	Gly	Ala	Ser	Leu	Tyr	Ala
Rabbit reticulocyte lipoxygenase	Gly	Val	Tyr	Arg	Val	Cys	Val	Ser	Thr	Gly	Ala	Ser	Ile	Tyr	Ala
Human 5-lipoxygenase	Pro	Ser	Tyr	Thr	Val	Thr	Val	Ala	Thr	Gly	Ser	Glu	Trp	Phe	Ala
Soybean lipoxygenase	Met	Phe	Ser	Ala	Gly	His	Lys	Ile	Lys	Gly	Thr	Val	Val	Leu	Met

Fig. 2. N-terminal amino acid sequences for human
leukocyte 15-lipoxygenase, rabbit reticulocyte
lipoxygenase, human 5-lipoxygenase and soybean 15-
lipoxygenase. Sequence identity is indicated by the bold
lines. (Reproduced with permission from [8])

The complete structural relationship between the rabbit
reticulocyte lipoxygenase and the human 15-lipoxygenase

remains unknown. Despite the fact that others have presented functional and immunological data(14) suggesting that the reticulocyte lipoxygenase is unique to reticulocytes, we speculate, based on the strong sequence identity shown here, that these two lipoxygenases, from different species and different tissues, are closely related in their structure. In view of this, the human 15-lipoxygenase of eosinophils, airway epithelial cells and keratinocytes should be evaluated for the degradative functions of the reticulocyte lipoxygenase such as the ability to degrade mitochondrial membranes selectively and to inhibit cellular respiration by decreasing the synthesis of ATP. Such degradative properties may be important in the pathophysiology of inflammatory and allergic responses.

In summary, we have purified the human 15-lipoxygenase to homogeneity and obtained N-terminal amino acid sequence which suggests that the mammalian lipoxygenases are structurally related. The availability of homogeneous 15-lipoxygenase is expected to play a key role in elucidating other relationships among the various lipoxygenases as well as permitting the study of 15-lipoxygenation of arachidonic acid at the molecular level.

1. Samuelsson B, Dahlen SE, Lindgren JA, Rouzer CA, Serhan CN. *Science* 1987;220:568-575.
2. Marom Z, Shelhamer JH, Sun F, Kaliner M. *J. Clin. Invest.* 1983;72:122-127.
3. Shak S, Perez D, Goldstein IM. *J. Biol. Chem.* 1983;258:14948- 14953.
4. Hamburg M, Hedquist P, Radegran K. *Acta. Physiol. Scand.* 1980;110:219-221.
5. Hunter JA, Finkbeiner WE, Nadel JA, Goetzl EJ, Holtzman MJ. *Proc. Natl. Acad. Sci.* 1980;82:4633-4637.
6. Turk J, Mass RL, Brash AR, Roberts LJ,II, Oates JA. *J. Biol. Chem.* 1982;257:7068-7076.
7. Burrall BA, Wintroub BU, Goetzl EJ. *Biochem. and Biophys. Res. Com.* 1985;133:208-213.
8. Sigal E, Grunberger D, Craik CS, Caughey GH, Nadel JA. *J. Biol. Chem., in press.*
9. Sigal E, Grunberger D, Cashman JR, Craik CS, Caughey GH, Nadel JA. *Biochem. and Biophys. Res. Com.* 1988;150:376-383.
10. Thiele BJ, E Black, J Fleming, B Nack, SM Rapoport, PR Harrison *Biomed. Biochim. Acta* 1987;46:S120-123.
11. Dixon RAF, Jones RE, Diehl RE, Bennett CD, Kargman S, Rouzer CA, *Proc. Natl. Acad. Sci.* 1988;85:416-420.
12. Matsumoto T, Funk CD, Radmark O, Hoog JO, Jornvall H, Samuelsson B.*Proc. Natl. Acad. Sci.* 1988;85:26-30.
13. Shibata D, J Streczko, JE Dixon, M Hermodson, R. Yazdanparast, B Axelrod *J. Biol. Chem.* 1987;262:10080-10085.
14. Rapoport SM, Schewe T, Wiesner R, et. al. *Eur. J. Biochem.* 1979;96:545-561.

Advances in Prostaglandin, Thromboxane, and Leukotriene Research, Vol. 19, edited by
B. Samuelsson, P. Y.-K. Wong, and F. F. Sun,
Raven Press, Ltd., New York ©1989.

TRANSFORMATION OF 15-HYDROPEROXYEICOSATETRAENOIC ACID TO
15-KETO-PENTADECA-5,8,11,13-TETRAENOIC ACID BY HYDROPEROXIDE
LYASE IN RABBIT LEUKOCYTES

Yuh-Ling Lin[+] and Patrick Y-K Wong

[+]Institute of Biomedical Science, Academia Sinica,
Nankang, Taiwan, R.O.C. and Department of Pharmacology,
New York Medical College, Valhalla, N.Y. 10595, U.S.A.

Oxygenation of polyunsaturated fatty acid leads to the
formation of various fatty acid hydroperoxides such as 5-HPETE,
12-HPETE and 15-HPETE and 15-HPETE (1). These fatty acid
hydroperoxides are unstable and spontaneously as well as
enzymically transformed to the coresponding hydroxyl
derivatives. Recently, hydroperoxides of arachidonic acid (AA)
were found in lipid extracts of the clastogenic mixture derived
from lymphocyte culture medium (2). Thus, during cell-cell
interaction hydroperoxides of AA such as 15-HPETE, released from
leukocytes, lymphocytes, and platelets can exert their effects
on neighbouring cells. Intact polymophonuclear leukocytes
(PMNL) was found to produce mainly the 5-lipoxygenase product of
AA and small amount of 15-lipoxygenase products. However,
sonicated PMNL or activated PMNL showed higher 15-lipoxygenase
activity on the formation of various 15-series of leukotrienes.
We reported here the presence of hydroperoxide lyase activity in
rabbit leukocytes which may represent a new mechanism for the
metabolism of 15-hydroperoxides of AA. Furthermore, the
hydroperoxie lyase activity in leukocytes can prevent certain
toxic effects on other hydroxyperoxides that may disturb the
cellular hemostasis in the target cells.

MATERIALS AND METHODS

[1-^{14}C] 15-HPETE was prepared by incubation of of
[1-^{14}C]-arachidonic acid (AA) mixed with pure non-label
arachidonic acid (Nuchek, Mn) and soybean lipoxygenase I as
described by Hamberg and Samuelsson (3). Fresh rabbit leukocyte
was obtained from ten rabbits venous blood by heart puncture and
prepared by Dextran sedimentation as perveiouly described (4).
The cell preparations were contaminated with platelets and
mononuclear leukocytes (5). The leukocytes were suspended in
dalbecco's phosphate buffered salne (PBS), pH 7.4 an adjusted to
50 x 10^6 cell/ml. The viability of the cells as measured by

the trypan blue exclusion test was found to be greater than 95%. The cell suspension in 10 ml of PBS was incubated for 10 min at 37°C with [1-^{14}C] 15-HPETE (30μM final concentration) under a normal atmosphere. The reactions were terminated by addition of 3 volumes of ethanol. The incubation precipitate was filtered and the ethanolic filtrate was evaporated to dryness. The residue was acidified and extracted with ethylacetate. The ethylacetate fraction was evaporated to dryness and the residue was redissolved in 200 μl of solvent (A) and injected into a Waters associate dual pump HPLC system equipped with a U-6K injector and a 481 λmax variable wavelength U.V. detector and a RP-ultrasphere ODS column (C18-ODS, 5U, 10 mm x 25 cm, Beckman, Palo Alto, CA). The products were eluted with a linear gradient of methanol/water/ acetic acid (60:40:0.05, V/V) (solvent A) to methanol (solvent B) for 40 mins at a flow rate of 1 ml/min. Fractions are collected with on-line fractions collector and a portion of each fraction was removed for estimation of recovery of radioactivity. The methylester of the polar metabolite (Fig. 1A) (10μg) was converted to trimethylsilyl esters as described by Wong et al. (5). The dried sample was dissolved in hexane (25 μl) and injected into the gas chromatograph-mass spectrometer (Hewlett-Packard 5899-B) equipped with a cross methyl silicone capillary column (0.3 mm x 12 m). Helium flow were set at 16 ml/min and oven temperature was programmed from 180°C to 300°C at 5°/min. Electron energy was set at 70 ev.

RESULTS AND DISCUSSION

Incubation of [1-^{14}C] 15-HPETE with rabbit peripheral blood leukocytes resulted in the formation of a new polar metabolite (retention time of 9.5 min) having strong single band ultra-violet absorption at 280 nm (Fig. 1A). This compound accounted for about 7% of total radioactivity recovered. The strong U.V. max at 280 nm suggested the presence of a conjugated dienone structure which will shift from U.V. max from 280 nm to 233 after the reduction by NaBH$_4$ (Fig. 1B). After reduction to its alcohol forms, the sample was methylated for further purification by RP-HPLC and was subsequently converts to trymethylsilylester derivative as described (5). The methylester trimethylsilylester of the reduced polar metabolite was then subjected to gas chromatograph-mass spectrometric analysis. This compound gives a C-value of 18.5 and the electron impact mass spectrum (EI) (Fig. 2B) showed ions at M/Z: 336(M$^+$), 321(M-15), 321(M-15), 305(M-31), 246(M-90), 181(M-155), 155([CH]$_4$-CH$_2$-OTMS), and 103(CH$_2$-OTMS). Molecular ion of 336 suggest that the metabolite contains 15 carbons instead of 20 carbons. Ions at 155 and 103 strongly suggested the cleavage between C$_{10-11}$ and between C$_{14-15}$, respectively. Taken together the mass spectra data and the U.V. spectra the reduced polar metabolite was identified as the methylester trimethylsilylester of 15-hydroxypentadeca-

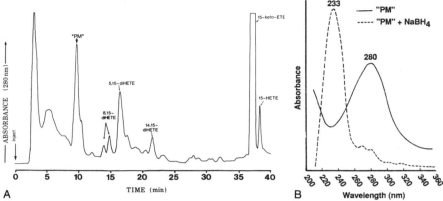

A

B

Fig 1:   RP-HPLC chromatography of ethyl acetate extract obtained
from incubations of 15-HPETE and rabbit peripheral leukocytes
(A), and U.V. spectra of "PM" before and after sodium
bonohydride reduction (B).

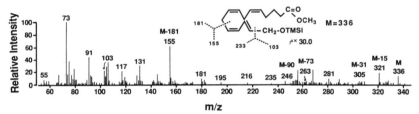

Fig. 2:   Mass spectrum of the methylester trimethylsilylester
derivative of "PM" after NaBH$_4$ reduction.

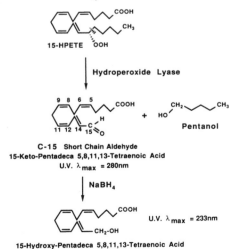

Fig. 3:   Proposed schematic pathways for the transformation of
15-HPETE to 15-keto-pentadeca-5,8,11,13-tetraenoic acid.

5,8,11,13-tetraenoic acid. Thus, the polar metabolite was
identified as 15-keto-pentadeca-5,8,11,13-tetraenoic acid, a new
de novo, previously unknown metabolite of 15-HPETE derived from
rabbit leukocyte (Fig. 3). Control experiments with heated and
ethanol-treated leukocytes fail to produce this metabolite.

Lipoxygeanse catalyzes the incorporation of molecular O_2
into certain polyunsaturated fatty acids. The enzyme is present
in a variety of cell types as well as in plants and fungus. In
1966, Zimmerman (6) reported the presence of hydroperoxide
isomerase in flax seed, which converted linoleic acid
hydroperoxides to an α-keto fatty acid. Galliard et al. (7)
reported that 12-lipoxygenase contain hydroperoxide lyase
activity.

In this report we described the presence of the
hydroperoxide lyase-like enzyme in rabbit leukocytes can cleave
the 15-HPETE or orther hydroperoxides to form the corresponding
short-chain aldehydes. Thus, the presence of an active enzyme
such as "hydroperoxide lyase" in leukocytes may provide a de
novo protective mechanism by controlling the intracellular lipid
hydroperoxide level and prevent the clastogenic action and
cellular damage (8). Recently, Glasgow et al. (9) reported that
porcine leukocytes convert exogenous AA to
12-oxo-dodeca-5,8,10-trienoic acid. They proposed that this
12-carbon short-chain aldehyde is formed from 12-HPETE by a
cleavage reaction catalyzed by the leukocyte 12-lipoxygenase
that this aldehyde product has significant biological actiity in
the activation of leukocytes. Whether the C-15 short-chain
aldehyde has similar biological activity as C-12 aldehyde and
its cellular localization in leukocyte remain to be established.

REFERENCES

1. Samuelsson, B. (1983) Science, 220:568-575.
2. Carutti, P. (1985) Science 227:375-381.
3. Hamberg, M. and Samuelsson, B. (1967) J. Biol. Chem.
    242:5329-5335.
4. Lam, B.K., Hirai, A., Yoshida, S., Tamura, Y. and Wong,
    P.Y-K (1987) Biochem. Biophys. Acta 917:398-405.
5. Wong, P.Y-K., Westlund, P., Hamberg, M., Granstrom, E.,
    Chao, P.H-W and Samuelsson, B. (1987) J. Biol. Chem.
    259:2683-2686.
6. Zimmerman, D.C. (1966) Biochem. Biophys. Res. Commun.
    23:398-402.
7. Galliard, T., Phillips, D.R. and Frost, D.J. (1973) Chem.
    Phys. Lipid 11, 173-180.
8. Ochi, T. and Carutti, P.A. (1987) Proc. Natl. Acad. Sci.
    U.S.A. 84:990-994.
9. Glasgow, W.C., Harris, T.M. and Brash, A.R. (1986) J. Biol.
    Chem. 261:200-204.

Advances in Prostaglandin, Thromboxane, and Leukotriene Research, Vol. 19, edited by B. Samuelsson, P. Y.-K. Wong, and F. F. Sun, Raven Press, Ltd., New York ©1989.

LEUKOCYTES BIOSYNTHESIZE LEUKOTOXIN

(9,10-EPOXY-12-OCTADECENOATE)

-- A NOVEL CYTOTOXIC LINOLEATE EPOXIDE --

Takayuki Ozawa, Satoru Sugiyama, Mika Hayakawa

Department of Biomedical Chemistry,
Faculty of Medicine, University of Nagoya,
Tsuruma, Showa-ku, Nagoya 466, Japan

Many patients with deep and extensive burns die after recovering from primary shock (late death). Why do burn patients die in this phase ? To resolve the answer is the aim and motive of our study, because it provides us with new maneuvers to treat burn patients resulting in increases in the eventual survival rate. It is postulated that toxic substances synthesized in burned skin are transferred into general circulation and cause multiple organ damage. However, the responsible substance remains unknown. We reported (1) that toxic substances exist in human burned skin by using high performance liquid chromatography. Recently, we succeeded in clarifying the chemical structure of a toxic substance using gas chromatography/mass spectrometry, nuclear magnetic resonance, and ozonolysis (2). It is a linoleate epoxide, 9, 10-epoxy-12-octadecenoate, the chemical structure of which is shown in Fig. 1. We demonstrated that the linoleate epoxide is biosynthesized by neutrophils from linoleate as a substrate (2). The biosynthesis is sensitive to carbon monooxide, and not to lipoxygenase inhibitor (3). Accordingly, it is concluded that neutrophil microsomal cytochrome P-450 dependent monooxygenase is responsible for the synthesis. The linoleate epoxide shows a highly toxic effect on mitochondria, a key organelle in the energy metabolism. Thus, it was given the name leukotoxin. The same substance is synthesized by the rice plant as a self defensive substance toward a fungus, *Pyricularia oryzae*' infection (4). We also confirmed (5) that leukotoxin shows anti-fungal and anti-bacterial activities. Moreover, leukotoxin exhibited a dominant cytotoxic activity toward human tumor cells as well as normal cells (6). Hence, it is considered that leukotoxin is like a double edged sword; namely, a self defence substance and a cytotoxic one with its over production. In the present paper, we introduce the effect of leukotoxin on lung and heart, though leukotoxin has various pathophysiological roles.

HEMODYNAMIC EFFECT OF LEUKOTOXIN

To test the hemodynamic effect of leukotoxin, various dosis of leukotoxin were administered to anesthetized dogs. Table 1 summarizes the results of leukotoxin injections for aortic flow, left ventricular dP/dt, and aortic blood pressure. Administration of leukotoxin, 30 μmol/kg, showed severe cardiac dysfunction. Furthermore, all dogs given leukotoxin 150 μmol/ kg were dead within 45 min. Although we confirmed (7) that administration of the same dosis of linoleic acid showed a slight decrease in these hemodynamic parameters, leukotoxin showed a prominent cardio-depressive effect.

LEUKOTOXIN AND PULMONARY INJURY

Because adult respiratory distress syndrome (ARDS) shows a high mortality rate, its genesis has attracted much interest. Recent advances emphasized the role of neutrophils. Clinical features of ARDS are ascribed to the increase in the permeability of pulmonary artery and endothelial cell damage. We examined (8) bronchoalveolar lavage fluid (BALF) in patients with ARDS and normal volunteers. As summarized in Table 2, neutrophil recruitment was observed. Increases in albumin concentration and in angiotensin converting enzyme (ACE) activities, which are presumptive markers of permeability and endothelial cell damage, were demonstrated. Furthermore, we detected a considerable amount of leukotoxin in patients with ARDS. In animal experiments, administration of leukotoxin to rats causes pulmonary edema, which was evidenced by increases in lung wet weight/body weight ratios and dry weight/wet weight ratios (9). Albumin concentration and ACE activities were also increased in BALF of rats administered with leukotoxin. Moreover, structural findings such as edematous changes of the lung, swelling of the alveolar epithelium, and endothelial cell were observed. These morphological findings are similar to those observed in patients with ARDS (10). These results suggest that leukotoxin synthesized from accumulated neutrophils in the lung is closely linked with the development of ARDS.

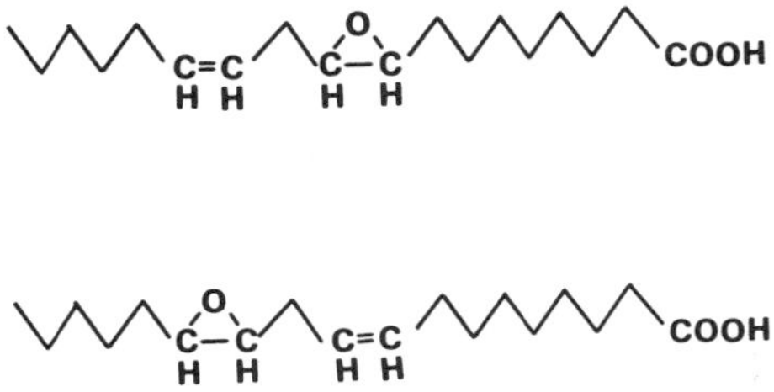

Fig. 1.
Chemical structures of leukotoxin (upper panel) and its isomer (12,13-epoxy-9-octadecenoate).

Table 1. Hemodynamic effect of leukotoxin

	0	5	30 (min)
Aortic flow (1/min)			
Control	0.74 ± 0.07	0.69 ± 0.05	0.71 ± 0.06
Leukotoxin	0.74 ± 0.04	0.40 ± 0.07*	0.30 ± 0.04*
LV dP/dt (mmHg/sec)			
Control	2250 ± 99	2183 ± 135	2200 ± 141
Leukotoxin	2040 ± 205	1140 ± 217*	1220 ± 213*
Systolic pressure (mmHg)			
Control	107 ± 2.5	105 ± 2.6	99 ± 4.9
Leukotoxin	106 ± 7.1	75 ± 9.2*	78 ± 5.9*
Diastolic pressure (mmHg)			
Control	69 ± 1.5	69 ± 2.0	68 ± 4.6
Leukotoxin	67 ± 6.3	48 ± 6.5*	48 ± 10.6*

mean ± SE   * P < 0.01 vs. Control

Table 2. Changes in various makers in lung lavages in patients with ARDS

	Control	ARDS
Contents of Leukotoxin (nmol/lung lavage)	< 3.0	38.5 ± 21.9
Number of Neutrophil (X10[5])	0.80 ± 0.12	12.0 ± 3.4*
Albumin Concentrations (mg/dl)	31.8 ± 11.2	168 ± 70.7*
ACE Activities (units/ml)	0.34 ± 0.08	0.99 ± 0.11*

mean ± SE.   * P < 0.01 vs. Control

CONCLUSION

We emphasized here that leukotoxin, an epoxygenase product, is closely related to the development of various pathological conditions including burn. The aim of this study is not completely resolved, the responsible factor for burn toxin has been clarified, but prevention of late death in patients with burn remains unsettled. The elucidation of linoleate cascade reaction, illustrated in Fig. 2, will contribute to not only the treatment of burns but also to the understanding of the genesis of the inflammatory process.

Linoleate Cascade Reaction

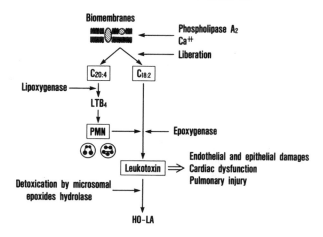

Fig. 2. Schematic presentation of linoleate cascade reaction. $C_{20:4}$: Arachidonic acid, $C_{18:2}$: Linoleic acid, HO–LA: 9-hydroxy-octadecenoate, PMN: Polymorphonuclear leukocyte

REFERENCES

1. Yokoo K, Hayakawa M, Sugiyama S, et al. J. Clin. Biochem. Nutr. 1980; 1: 121–127.
2. Ozawa T, Hayakawa M, Takamura T, et al. Biochem. Biophys. Res. Commun. 1980; 134: 1071–1078.
3. Ozawa T, Sugiyama S, Hayakawa M, Taki F, Hanaki Y, Biochem. Biophys. Res. Commun. (in press)
4. Kato T, Yamaguchi Y, Uyehara T, Yokoyama T, Namai T, Yamanaka S. Tetrahedron Lett. 1983; 24: 4715–4718.
5. Hayakawa M, Sugiyama S, Takamura T, et al. Biochem. Biophys. Res. Commun. 1980; 137: 424–430.
6. Ozawa T, Nishikimi M, Sugiyama S, Taki F, Hayakawa M, Shionoya H. Biochem. Int. 1988; 16: 369–373.
7. Fukushima A, Hayakawa M, Sugiyama S, Ajioka M, Ito T, Satake T, Ozawa T. Cardiovasc. Res. 1988; 22: 213–218.
8. Ozawa T, Sugiyama S, Hayakawa M, et al. Am. Rev. Respir. Dis. 1988; 137: 535–540.
9. Hu J-N, Taki F, Sugiyama S, Asai J, Izawa Y, Satake T, Ozawa T. Lung (in press)
10. Jones R, Langleben D, Reid LM. In: The pulmonary circulation and acute lung injuey (Said SI ed) pp137–188, 1985, Futura Publishing Co. Inc. New York

Advances in Prostaglandin, Thromboxane, and Leukotriene Research, Vol. 19, edited by B. Samuelsson, P. Y.-K. Wong, and F. F. Sun, Raven Press, Ltd., New York ©1989.

PHOTOAFFINITY LABELLING AND ISOELECTRIC FOCUSING OF THE

HUMAN PLATELET THROMBOXANE A_2/PROSTAGLANDIN H_2

(TXA_2/PGH_2) RECEPTOR

D.E. Mais and P.V. Halushka

Departments of Cell and Molecular Pharmacology and
Experimental Therapeutics and Medicine
Medical University of South Carolina
Charleston, SC 29425

INTRODUCTION

Photoaffinity ligands have been utilized in a variety of ways to characterize a broad spectrum of membrane bound receptors. Coupled to such techniques as SDS-PAGE and/or isoelectric focusing, physical characteristics of the receptor can be determined, such as molecular weights, the presence of subunits and isoelectric points. There have been two previous reports of photoaffinity ligands for the human platelet TXA_2/PGH_2 receptor (1-2), however neither of these studies used the radiolabelled probes to characterize the receptor.

The purpose of the present study was to determine the isoelectric point via isoelectric focusing of the human platelet TXA_2/PGH_2 receptor that was photoaffinity labeled with [^{125}I]PTA-Azido, a TXA_2/PGH_2 receptor antagonist.

MATERIALS AND METHODS

The chemical structure of [^{125}I]PTA-Azido is shown in Figure 1. The synthesis and characterization of this compound have been described elsewhere (3-4). Photoaffinity labelling was carried out using washed human platelets prepared by previously described methods and resuspended in a Tris-NaCl-dextrose buffer (5). The washed platelets (0.5 ml, 5 x 10^8 plts/ml) were incubated with approximately 2-4 µCi of [^{125}I]PTA-Azido in both

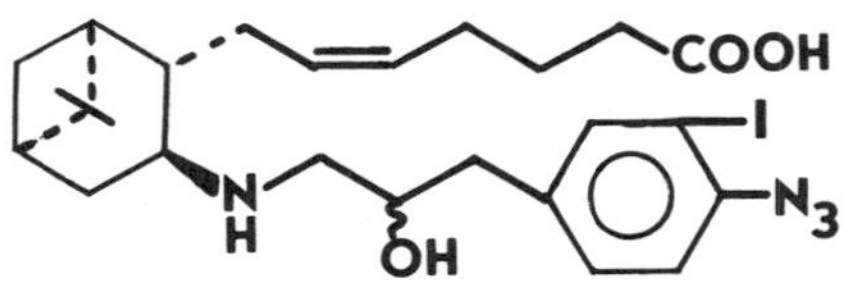

FIG. 1. CHEMICAL STRUCTURE OF [^{125}I]PTA-AZIDO.

the absence of a competing ligand and presence of the thromboxane receptor antagonist L657925 (250 nM) (5). Incubations of
10 min at 37°C were followed by a 1.5-2 min photolysis with a
hand held ultraviolet lamp (Ultra-violet Products, Inc., San
Gabriel, CA) at a distance of 5 cm. The platelets were pelleted
and dissolved in the sample buffer (urea-triton X-100-dithio-
threitol) containing ampholytes (LKB, Piscataway, NJ) with a pH
range of 4.0-6.5. Isoelectric focusing was conducted in a
vertical slab gel of 4% acrylamide. Approximately 100 μg of
protein (100 μl) were applied to the lanes 1 and 2 and twice
that amount was applied to lanes 3 and 4 and focusing was
carried out at room temperature at 4800 volt-hrs. The gel was
stained for protein by Coomassie blue, destained and dried onto
filter paper. Prior to staining, adjacent non-protein
containing lanes were cut into 0.5 cm bands and placed in 1 ml
distilled water to determine the pH which was used to determine
the pH gradient. Autoradiography was performed at -70°C using
Kodak X-omat film and Dupont Camera cassettes with intensfying
screens for 2-5 days.

RESULTS AND DISCUSSION

Figure 2 shows the results of photoaffinity labelling of platelets with [¹²⁵I]PTA-Azido followed by isoelectric focusing and
autoradiography. Lane 1 represents the control lane in which
platelets were incubated with [¹²⁵I]PTA-Azido in the absence of
competing ligand. Lane 2 is similar to lane 1 except incubation
of the platelets with [¹²⁵I]PTA-Azido was conducted with L657925
(250nM) present. Lanes 3 and 4 are the same as 1 and 2 but
twice as much protein was applied. As can be seen, there are
several bands labelled in lane 1 which are absent in lane 2.
Presumably representing protein which was specifically labelled
with [¹²⁵I]PTA-Azido. The isoelectric points of these proteins
correspond to 5.6, 5.3, 5.1, and 4.9. One or more of these
bands may represent the binding portion of the human platelet
TXA_2/PGH_2 receptor. Since multiple specifically labelled
proteins are observed, the possibility exists that variable
degrees of phosphorylation and/or glycosylation of the receptor
may occur. In preliminary studies utilizing 2-dimensional gel
electrophoresis, the protein band possessing a pI value of 5.6
corresponds to a protein of 43kDa and the proteins with the pI
value of 5.3, 5.1 and 4.9 corresponded to a molecular weight of
27 kDa. Alternatively, the multiple labelled bands may represent proteolysis or photolysis fragments.

   The ligand [¹²⁵I]PTA-Azido represents a significant improvement over previously published photoaffinity ligands for the
human platelet TXA_2/PGH_2 receptor. The ligands used in the
previous studies, either possessed low affinity or could not be
radiolabelled (1,2). The affinity of [¹²⁵I]PTA-Azido for the
TXA_2/PGH_2 receptor was measured kinetically and found to be 11
nM (5). Thus, while this represents a significant improvement
over previous ligands, an affinity of 11 nM remains loose enough

that during the photolysis reaction a variety of platelet proteins are labelled. One or more of the specifically labelled proteins may represent the TXA_2/PGH_2 receptor or a nearest neighbor protein to the TXA_2/PGH_2 receptor.

Isoelectric focusing of membrane bound proteins have been utilized for a variety of receptors for both purificiation and characterization. It has been observed that many receptors possess pI values in the range of 4.0 to 6.0 (6). Thus, it appears that this receptor may have a pI in a range previously reported for other receptors.

[^{125}I]PTA-Azido should prove useful in probing alterations in the structure of the TXA_2/PGH_2 receptor under conditions which alter its function. In addition, its availability should help in the purification of the receptor.

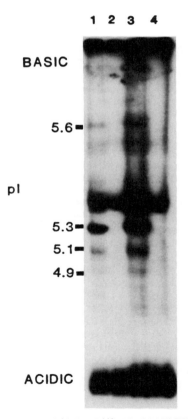

FIG. 2. AUTORADIOGRAM OF ISOELECTRIC FOCUSED WASHED HUMAN PLATELETS WHICH HAVE BEEN PHOTOAFFINITY LABELLED WITH [^{125}I]PTA-AZIDO.

ACKNOWLEDGEMENTS

Supported in part by HL36838 and HL29566.   Dr. Halushka is a
Burroughs-Wellcome Scholar in Clinical Pharmacology.   The
authors wish to thank Ms. Nita Pike for her secretarial assistance.

REFERENCES

1.   Mais DE, Burch R, Oatis J, Knapp D and Halushka PV. Biochem
      Biophys Res Comm 1986; 140:128-133.

2.   Arora S, Kattelman E, Lim C, LeBreton G and Venton P. J
      Med Chem 1987;30:918-924.

3.   Mais DE, DeHoll D, Sightler H and Halushka PV. Eur J
      Pharmacol 1988; In press.

4.   Mais DE and Halushka PV. J Labelled Compds and
      Radiopharmaceut 1988; In press.

5.   Mais DE, Yoakim C, Guindon Y, Gillard J, Rokach J and
      Halushka PV. Submitted.

6.   Lilly L, Eddy B, Schaber J, Fraser C, and Venter J. In
      Venter J. and Harrison L. eds. Receptor purification
      procedures, New York: Alan R. Liss, Inc. 1984; 77-96.

Advances in Prostaglandin, Thromboxane, and Leukotriene Research, Vol. 19, edited by B. Samuelsson, P. Y.-K. Wong, and F. F. Sun, Raven Press, Ltd., New York ©1989.

FURTHER STUDIES WITH 5E AND 5Z ANALOGUES OF PGI$_2$ IN PLATELETS AND VASCULATURE

D. Oliva, S. Giovanazzi, M. Lograno, N. Mongelli[+], A. Corsini, R. Fumagalli and S. Nicosia

Institute of Pharmacological Sciences, 20133 Milan - Italy
[+]Farmitalia-Carlo Erba Research Institute - 20100 Milan - Italy

Since the discovery of PGI$_2$, a great effort has been devoted to establish whether PGI$_2$-receptors on platelets differ from those present at vascular level. In fact, the concomitant occurrence of antiplatelet and smooth muscle relaxing activities (cAMP-mediated processes) has so far hindered wider clinical applications of PGI$_2$. In this respect, only a clearcut difference between platelet and vascular receptors could allow the development of a stable PGI$_2$-analogue with a high degree of selectivity toward either one of the target cells. Although the first suggestion of some intrinsic differences between the platelet and vascular PGI$_2$-receptors has been put forward by Whittle et al. (1), the first direct evidence of such a difference at the receptor/binding site level has been obtained in our laboratory (2-4).

In fact, by assaying the effect of a number of PGI$_2$-analogues in human platelets and in rabbit mesenteric artery, we found that the 5Z epimer of carbacyclin (5Z-carbacyclin) behaved as a full agonist on human platelets, displaying the same efficacy as PGI$_2$ both as activator of adenylate cyclase (AC) and as inhibitor of aggregation. On the contrary, 5Z-carbacyclin was a partial agonist on rabbit vascular myocytes, because not only it failed to attain the maximal effect reached by PGI$_2$ and PGE$_1$, but also it counteracted their effect both in AC stimulation and vascular muscle relaxation.

However, it must be pointed out that data obtained in different species (rabbit vascular myocytes vs human platelets)

had been compared. Therefore, aim of our work was to establish if 5Z-carbacyclin behaves as a full agonist of PGI_2-receptors in rabbit platelets as well, ruling out the problems of species specificity. In addition, by the use of two other PGI_2-analogues, namely the epimers FCE 22177 (5E-FCE) and FCE 22176 (5Z-FCE) from Farmitalia Carlo Erba, Italy, we addressed the problem of whether the moiety comprising carbon 5 might play a key role in the interaction with PGI_2-receptors at vascular or platelet levels.

METHODS

Adenylate cyclase activity was measured according to Salomon et al. (5) in a crude membrane preparation from either rabbit platelets or myocytes cultured from rabbit mesenteric artery (6). Membrane preparation and incubation conditions were as previously described (7,8). Inhibition of collagen-induced platelet aggregation was evaluated in platelet rich plasma by the turbidimetric technique of Born (9).

RESULTS AND DISCUSSION

Fig. 1 shows the dose-response curves of 5Z-carbacyclin and PGE_1, for the inhibition of rabbit platelet aggregation induced by 1 $\mu g/\mu l$ collagen. 5Z-carbacyclin is able to induce the same maximal response as PGE_1 (100% inhibition), displaying, however, a lower potency than the reference compound (IC_{50} = 4.07×10^{-9} and 9.12×10^{-7} M for PGE_1 and 5Z-carbacyclin, respectively). The finding that even in rabbit platelets 5Z-carbacyclin shows the same efficacy of PGE_1 as an antiaggregating agent, rules out the

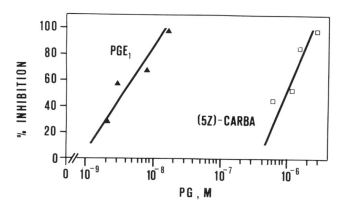

Fig. 1: Dose-response curves for the inhibition of rabbit platelet aggregation by PGE_1 (▲) and 5Z-carbacyclin (□). Aggregation was induced by 1 $\mu g/\mu l$ collagen.

possibility that the partial agonist properties reveald by the compound in rabbit mesenteric artery, but not in human platelets (2-4), could be due simply to species differences.

Concerning the other issue we addressed, i.e. whether the agonist/antagonist properties of 5Z-carbacyclin are a peculiarity of this compound or are linked to the configuration at carbon 5, we evaluated the effect ot two other PGI_2-analogues, 5E-FCE (isosteric with PGI_2) and 5Z-FCE (isosteric with 5Z-carbacyclin) on AC activity in membranes of rabbit platelets and myocytes cultured from rabbit mesenteric artery. PGE_1 has been used as a reference compound instead of PGI_2, since it is more easily handled and, as already demonstrated (2,7), it interacts with the same receptors as PGI_2. Table I shows that all the three

TABLE 1

Effect of FCE 22176 (5Z), FCE 22177 (5E) and PGE_1 on adenylate cyclase activity in membranes from rabbit platelets and mesenteric artery myocytes.

Additions	Concentration M	cAMP (pmol/mg prot. x min)	
		Platelets	Mesenteric artery
------	------	39.58± 1.62	8.21±0.72
5Z-FCE	3×10^{-6}	82.41± 4.21	10.40±0.35
	10^{-5}	171.57± 8.98	10.56±1.37
	2×10^{-5}	---	10.67±0.23
	3×10^{-5}	311.20±17.08	---
	5×10^{-5}	---	11.88±0.25
	10^{-4}	454.35± 8.10	11.85±0.38
	3×10^{-4}	---	11.96±0.33
	5×10^{-4}	388.15±22.36	---
5E-FCE	10^{-6}	102.92±17.69	8.95±0.20
	3×10^{-6}	168.47+ 2.22	9.55±0.56
	10^{-5}	308.66±28.84	12.35±0.14
	3×10^{-5}	402.45±19.86	13.92±0.27
	10^{-4}	488.70±34.21	16.83±0.46
	3×10^{-4}	413.43±21.02	17.66±0.24
	10^{-3}	---	15.10±0.81
PGE_1	10^{-5}	136.30± 6.34	---
	5×10^{-5}	287.92± 9.17	---
	10^{-4}	350.37±16.48	---
	5×10^{-4}	451.62±23.19	---
	10^{-3}	406.76±12.13	---

prostaglandins are able to stimulate AC activity dose-dependent-ly, reaching the same maximal effect ($\leq$ 12 fold stimulation) in membranes from rabbit platelets. The pattern appeared completely different when the activation of AC was evaluated in membranes of rabbit myocytes. In fact, 5Z-FCE failes to reach the same maximal response elicited by its 5E-epimer, confirming that the configuration at carbon 5 in the structure of a PGI_2-analogue influences the mode of interaction of the compound with PGI_2-receptors. The present findings, along with the results of previous studies with the two epimers of carbacyclin (2,3), strengthen the hypothesis that the receptors for PGI_2 at platelet level differ from those present at vascular level.

REFERENCES

1. Whittle BJR, Moncada S. In: Ellis GP, West GB, eds. Progress in Medicinal Chemistry, vol 21. Amsterdam, New York and Oxford: Elsevier, 1984; 238-279.

2. Nicosia S, Oliva D, Noè MA, Corsini A, Folco GC, Fumagalli R. In: Samuelsson B, Paoletti R, Ramwell PW eds. Advances in Prostaglandin, Thromboxane and Leukotriene Research, vol. 17. New York: Raven Press, 1987; 474-478.

3. Corsini A, Folco GC, Fumagalli R, Nicosia S, Noè MA, Oliva D. Br J Pharmac 1987; 90:255-261.

4. Oliva D, Nicosia S. Pharm Res Comm 1987; 19:735-765.

5. Salomon Y, Londos C, Rodbell M. Anal Biochem 1974; 58:541-548.

6. Ross R. J Cell Biol 1971; 50:172-186.

7. Lombroso M, Nicosia S, Paoletti R, Whittle BJR, Moncada S, Vane JR. Prostaglandins 1984; 27:321-333.

8. Oliva D, Noè MA, Nicosia S, et al. Eur J Pharmacol 1984; 105:207-213.

9. Born GVR. Nature 1962; 194:927-929.

Advances in Prostaglandin, Thromboxane, and
Leukotriene Research, Vol. 19, edited by
B. Samuelsson, P. Y.-K. Wong, and F. F. Sun,
Raven Press, Ltd., New York ©1989.

ENHANCEMENT OF CATECHOLAMINE RELEASE MAY BE
MEDIATED BY PROSTAGLANDIN E RECEPTOR-STIMULATED
PHOSPHOINOSITIDE METABOLISM

*S. Ito, *M. Negishi, *H. Yokohama, *T. Tanaka,
*H. Hayashi, **T. Katada, †M. Ui, and *O. Hayaishi

*Hayaishi Bioinformation Transfer Project, Research
Development Corporation of Japan, Minami-ku, Kyoto
601; **Department of Life Science, Faculty of
Science, Tokyo Institute of Technology, Midori-ku,
Yokohama 227; and †Department of Physiological
Chemistry, Faculty of Pharmaceutical Sciences,
University of Tokyo, Bunkyo-ku, Tokyo 113, Japan

Prostaglandins of the E series (PGE) produce a
broad range of biological actions in diverse tissues.
The initial step in these cellular mechanisms of action may modulate adenylate cyclase activity through
specific receptors, the existence of which was first
demonstrated in 1972 using membranes from rat fat
cells (1). Since then, PGE_2 binding to membranes has
been reported in various mammalian tissues. However,
attempts to further analyze the structural properties
of functional PGE receptors have accomplished little.
We have recently demonstrated that PGE_2 can induce a
drastic increase in catecholamine release from cultured bovine adrenal chromaffin cells in the presence of
ouabain, an inhibitor of Na^+,K^+-ATPase (2). This
chapter describes the characterization of PGE receptor
in bovine adrenal medulla and its signal transduction
system in relation to catecholamine release.

RESULTS

Characterization of PGE Receptor

As reported previously (3), cell membranes isolated from bovine adrenal medulla bind PGE_2 with high
affinity and specificity. Specific binding of PGE_2
was more than 90%. The rate and magnitude of the
total binding of PGE_2 were dependent on temperature,
while nonspecific binding of PGE_2 was relatively

independent of temperature. The dissociation of bound [^{3}H]PGE$_2$ was accelerated by GTP in a dose-dependent manner, and half-maximal stimulation was observed at 10 μM GTP. These results suggest the formation of high-affinity complex of hormone, receptor and a GTP-binding protein (HRG complex). The interaction of PGE receptor and a GTP-binding protein was confirmed by the reconstitution experiment in phospholipid vesicles (4). Cross-linking of [^{3}H]PGE$_2$-prelabeled membrane fraction with the bifunctional cross-linker dithiobis (succinimidyl propionate), DSP, resulted in a complete loss of the ability of GTP to promote the dissociation of HRG complex. This cross-linking makes the complex stable in the detergent and molecular properties of the solubilized PGE receptor can be characterized by virtue of [^{3}H]PGE$_2$ already bound to it.

To characterize PGE receptor in bovine adrenal medulla, [^{3}H]PGE$_2$-prelabeled membrane fraction was cross-linked by 1 mM DSP for 5 min, solubilized with 20 mM CHAPS, and the solubilized proteins were analyzed by a series of column chromatographies. Among lectins tested, only wheat germ agglutinin (WGA) had the ability to adsorb the solubilized [^{3}H]PGE$_2$-receptor complex, which was specifically eluted from the WGA column with N-acetylglucosamine. The eluate from the WGA column was adsorbed to GTP-Sepharose, indicative of the association of a GTP-binding protein. Such a PGE receptor complex was further analyzed by gel filtration. A symmetrical peak of radioactivity was eluted at the position of Mr=200,000. By subtracting the Mr of a GTP-binding protein (about 90,000) from that of HRG complex, an apparent Mr of PGE receptor was estimated to be 110,000 (5).

Signal Transduction Mechanism of PGE$_2$ in Bovine Chromaffin Cells

In the presence of ouabain, PGE$_2$ stimulated a slow and longlasting catecholamine release from chromaffin cells. The effect was specific for PGE$_1$ and PGE$_2$. PGF$_2$α and PGD$_2$ were two to three orders of magnitude less effective. The specificity was very similar to that of potency of inhibition of [^{3}H]PGE$_2$ binding to chromaffin cells by these PGs, indicating that this process is probably mediated through a specific receptor. Although the signaling systems used by cells often display extensive heterogeneity from tissue to tissue, most tissues seem to have at least two major signal transduction systems across the cell membrane: the adenylate cyclase system and phosphoinositide metabolism. Until now, PGE$_2$ has been known to elicit its biological actions by modulating the cAMP levels in diverse tissues. In the plasma membrane from adrenal medulla and chromaffin cells, forskolin and NaF plus $AlCl_3$ enhanced the basal adenylate cyclase activity, suggesting the participation of a stimulatory GTP-binding protein in the activation of adenylate cyclase. However, PGE_2 did not stimulate the cAMP level at concentrations up to 10 µM. The cAMP analogue dibutyryl cAMP did not cause catecholamine release from ouabain-treated cells. On the other hand, we found that PGE_2, like muscarine, induced a concentration-dependent formation of inositol phosphates (IPs): rapid rises in IP_3 and IP_2 followed by a slower accumulation of IP_1. This effect of phosphoinositide metabolism was accompanied by an increase in cytosolic free Ca^{2+}. Then we compared the effects of various PGs on IP formation and increment of intracellular free Ca^{2+} ($[Ca^{2+}]i$) and catecholamine release from chromaffin cells.

Fig. 1 clearly demonstrates that the effect of PGs and muscarine on catecholamine release was parallel to those on the accumulation of IPs and the increment of $[Ca^{2+}]i$. All three parameters examined were well correlated with the ability of each PG to displace [^{3}H]PGE_2 from membranes. These results indicate that the effect of PGE_2 on catecholamine release is mediated by its specific receptor linked to phosphoinositide metabolism in adrenal medulla.

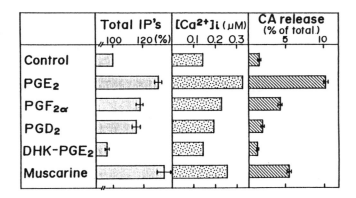

FIG. 1. Comparison of the effects of various PGs and muscarine on IP formation, increment of $[Ca^{2+}]i$ and catecholamine release in chromaffin cells. [^{3}H]IP formation over a 2-min incubation, $[Ca^{2+}]i$ at the peak, and catecholamine release for 15 min in the presence of ouabain were compared among stimulants.

DISCUSSION

TABLE 1. Signal transduction mechanisms of PGE

Signal transduction mechanism	Tissue
1. Adenylate cyclase: Stimulation	Brain
	Liver
	Many other tissues
2. Adenylate cyclase: Inhibition	Adipose tissue
	Kidney medulla
3. Ca^{2+} mobilization	Swiss 3T3 cell
4. Phosphoinositide metabolism	Adrenal medulla

Table 1 summarizes the signal transduction mechanisms of PGE. Although PGE have been shown to increase the cAMP level in many tissues and cell types via stimulation of adenylate cyclase, PGE can also attenuate hormone-stimulated synthesis of cAMP in some other tissues. Recently a rather high concentration of PGE_1 was reported to mobilize Ca^{2+} in Swiss 3T3 cells. The present study is the first demonstration that PGE_2 can stimulate phosphoinositide metabolism, which in turn induces catecholamine release in the presence of ouabain. Subdivision of PGE receptors has been proposed by Coleman and his coworkers (6) based on the difference in agonist and antagonist sensitivity among tissues. The difference in signal transduction mechanisms of PGE also strongly suggests the existence of subtypes in PGE receptors, in analogy with adrenergic receptors. Therefore, PGE receptor in bovine adrenal medulla may be a new type of PGE receptor which is coupled to phosphoinositide metabolism.

REFERENCES

1. Kuehl FA Jr, and Humes JL. Proc Natl Acad Sci USA 1972;69:480-484.
2. Yokohama H, Tanaka T, Ito S, Negishi M, Hayashi H, and Hayaishi O. J Biol Chem 1988;263: 1119-1122.
3. Karaplis AC, and Powell WS. J Biol Chem 1981; 256:2414-2419.
4. Negishi M, Ito S, Yokohama H, et al. J Biol Chem 1988;263:(in press).
5. Negishi M, Ito S, Tanaka T, et al. J. Biol Chem 1987;262:12077-12084.
6. Coleman RA, Kennedy I, and Sheldrick RLG Advances in PG TX and LT Research 1987;17:467-470.

*Advances in Prostaglandin, Thromboxane, and
Leukotriene Research*, Vol. 19, edited by
B. Samuelsson, P. Y.-K. Wong, and F. F. Sun,
Raven Press, Ltd., New York ©1989.

CO-EXPRESSION OF LEUKOTRIENE B$_4$ AND LEUKOTRIENE D$_4$ RECEPTORS ON HUMAN MONOCYTIC LEUKEMIA U-937 CELLS

Henry M. Sarau and Seymour Mong*

Department of Molecular Pharmacology and Immunology*
Smith Kline & French Laboratories, P.O. Box 7929
King of Prussia, PA   19406

INTRODUCTION

LTB$_4$ and LTD$_4$ are important metabolites of arachidonoyl-5-lipoxyenase pathway that have potent, yet diverse biological activities. LTD$_4$ induces vascular and airway smooth muscle contraction, increases vascular permeability, induces the synthesis of prostanoids and is a myocardial depressant. LTB$_4$ is a potent inflammatory mediator that induces chemo-taxis, aggregation, chemokinesis, enzyme secretion and super-oxide generation in inflammatory cells (for review see 1 & 2). Results published from a number of laboratories clearly demonstrated that the biological effects of LTB$_4$ and LTD$_4$ are mediated through distinct membrane bound receptors. LTD$_4$ receptors from guinea pig lung, human lung, rat basophilic leukemia (RBL-1) cells and a primary culture of sheep tracheal smooth muscle (STSM) cells have been identified and characterized (7-11).

In the current study, we discovered that LTB$_4$ and LTD$_4$ receptors are co-expressed on differentiated human monocytic leukemia (U-937) cells, thus this offers a unique opportunity for a direct quantitative comparison of these two receptors. The specificity profiles, the regulatory components and factors, the transducer proteins, the PI metabolism and the $[Ca^{2+}]_i$ mobilization responses were therefore characterized in detail.

RESULT

Equilibrium Saturation Binding of Radioligands to Receptors

Saturation binding of [^{3}H]LTB$_4$ and [^{3}H]LTD$_4$ to DMSO differentiated U-937 cell membranes was performed to determine the dissociation constant (K$_d$) and the density of binding sites (B$_{max}$). Under standard conditions, the nonspecific binding of [^{3}H]LTB$_4$ to U-937 cell membranes was linearly dependent upon the concentration of [^{3}H]LTB$_4$. Specific binding of [^{3}H]LTB$_4$ to the receptor component increased with increasing concentrations of [^{3}H]LTB$_4$ (0.02 to 0.2 nM) and then reached a plateau level at 1 to 2 nM of [^{3}H]LTB$_4$ (Fig. 1A). These results suggested that [^{3}H]LTB$_4$ bound to a low-capacity, saturable and high affinity site in the U-937 cell membranes. The specific binding data were transformed by the method of Scatchard (13) and yielded a linear plot (Fig. 1B). These results suggested that [^{3}H]LTB$_4$ bound to a single class of high-affinity receptor sites in U-937 cell membranes. The K_d determined from six saturation studies was .15 $\pm$ .06 nM and the B_{max} was 300 $\pm$ 86 fmol/mg protein.

Binding of [^{3}H]LTD$_4$ to the nonspecific sites of U-937 cell membranes was linearly dependent upon the concentration of [^{3}H]LTD$_4$. Specific binding of [^{3}H]LTD$_4$ to the membranes was dependent upon the concentration of [^{3}H]LTD$_4$ (0.02 to 1.0 nM) and then reached a plateau level (Fig. 1C). Using a non-linear least square best-fit computer analysis program, the saturation binding data was best-described by the model for a single class of specific binding sites. Transformation of the data by the Scatchard method yielded a linear plot (Fig. 1D). The K_d and B_{max} for six saturation studies were 0.35 $\pm$ 0.12 nM and 440 $\pm$ 96 fmol/mg, respectively. These results suggested that [^{3}H]LTD$_4$ bound to a single single class of high affinity, low-capacity and saturable receptors in U-937 cell membranes.

When the undifferentiated U-937 cell membranes were used for radioligand saturation binding studies, the K_d and B_{max} for [^{3}H]LTD$_4$ binding were 0.42 $\pm$ 0.12 nM and 170 $\pm$ 56 fmol/mg protein respectively. The K_d and B_{max} for [^{3}H]LTB$_4$ could not be accurately determined because the specific binding was barely detectable (<10 fmol/mg). These results demonstrated that when U-937 cells were differentiated with DMSO, both types of receptors, i.e., [^{3}H]LTB$_4$ and [^{3}H]-LTD$_4$, were induced and co-expressed in membrane preparations. Table 1 summarizes these results.

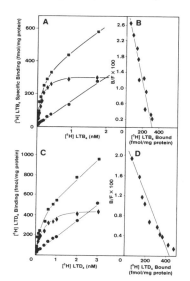

Figure 1. Saturation binding of leukotrienes to membrane receptors. Binding of [^{3}H]LTB$_4$ (A) or [^{3}H]LTD$_4$ (C) to U-937 cell membranes indicated as specific (♦), non-specific binding (•) and total binding (■). Scatchard plots of the specific binding for [^{3}H]LTB$_4$ (B) and [^{3}H]LTD$_4$ (D) are also shown.

Pharmacological Specificity of LTD₄ and LTB₄ Receptors

Radioligand competition studies were used to determine the rank order potency and the binding affinity of several LTB$_4$ agonist analogs for the [^{3}H]LTB$_4$ receptor site. All LTB$_4$ analogs tested competed in a dose-dependent fashion with [^{3}H]LTB$_4$ for binding to receptor sites. The K_i for LTB$_4$, 2-nor-

LTB$_4$, 20-OH-LTB$_4$ and 6-trans-LTB$_4$ were 0.24 nM, 0.92 nM, 0.8 nM, and 114 nM, respectively (Table 2). These results indicate a rigid binding requirement for the LTB$_4$ receptor. A series of agonist and antagonist analogs was used to characterize the [^{3}H]LTD$_4$ specific binding sites. The K$_i$ for LTD$_4$, LTE$_4$ 5R,6S-LTD$_4$ and LTB$_4$ were 0.65 nM, 42 nM, 61 nM and 100 µM respectively. The rank order potency of the agonists was equivalent to that determined using guinea pig lung or RBL-1 cell membrane receptors or in the guinea pig tracheal smooth muscle contraction assay. 5-HETE, 20-OH LTB$_4$ and 20-COOH LTB$_4$ showed no significant inhibition of [^{3}H]-LTD$_4$ binding at 10 µM (Table 2).

TABLE 1 Comparative Characteristics of LTB$_4$ and LTD$_4$ Receptors in U-937 Cell Membranes

	[^{3}H]-LTB$_4$	[^{3}H]-LTD$_4$
Binding Affinity[a] (nM)	0.15±0.06	0.35±0.12
Density (fmol/mg)	300±86	440±96
Regulation by:		
(a) G Protein	[b]G$_i$	[c]G$_i$ and G$_p$
(b) Monovalent cation (Na$^+$)	inhibition	inhibition
(c) Divalent cations (Ca^{2+} & Mg^{2+})	enhancement	enhancement

[a]Binding affinity expressed as K$_d$. [b] G$_i$ inhibitory or islet activating protein sensitive guanine nucleotide binding protein. [c]G$_p$, phosphoinositide phospholipase C selective guanine nucleotide binding protein.

LTB$_4$ and LTD$_4$ Induced [Ca^{2+}]$_i$ Mobilization

The [Ca^{2+}]$_i$ mobilization in differentiated U-937 cells induced by LTB$_4$ and LTD$_4$ was demonstrated and characterized. When fura-2 loaded differentiated U-937 cells were treated with 100 nM LTB$_4$, rapid transient increases in [Ca^{2+}]$_i$ were monitored as changes in the fura-2/Ca^{2+} fluorescence signal. The characteristics of the LTB$_4$ induced changes in [Ca^{2+}]$_i$ in the presence of 1 mM extracellular Ca^{2+} ([Ca^{2+}]$_o$), included a rapid rise (maximum signal within 5-10 sec) followed by a slow

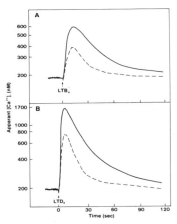

Figure 2. [Ca^{2+}]$_i$ mobilization induced by LTB$_4$ and LTD$_4$. Differentiated U-937 cells were loaded with fura-2 and challenged with 100 nM LTB$_4$ (A) or LTD$_4$ (B). The fura-2/Ca^{2+} fluorescence change was recorded either in the presence (___) of or absence (---) of 1 mM [Ca^{2+}]$_o$ in the KRH buffer.

decline over 2 min to a new steady state level, significantly higher than the initial baseline (Fig. 2A). The peak $[Ca^{2+}]_i$ levels calculated were 634 ± 68 nM which represents a greater than 200% increase of $[Ca^{2+}]_i$ over basal levels (186 ± 22 nM).

LTD₄ (100 nM) also induced mobilization of $[Ca^{2+}]_i$ in differentiated U-937 cells (Fig. 2B). In the presence of 1 mM $[Ca^{2+}]_o$, the maximal response was reached in 5-10 sec and slowly returned toward baseline but remained significantly higher than baseline after 5 min. The maximal response was 3-5 fold higher than the LTB₄ response in the same cells. The peak $[Ca^{2+}]_i$ level was 1760 ± 130 nM which is 8-10 fold higher than the basal $[Ca^{2+}]_i$ level of 186 ± 22 nM. Similar to the LTB₄ receptor-mediated $[Ca^{2+}]_i$ mobilization, >50% of the $[Ca^{2+}]_i$ mobilization was dependent on $[Ca^{2+}]_o$. Similar to the observations for LTB₄, the response was more transient in the presence of low levels of $[Ca^{2+}]_o$ (Fig. 7B). The calcium channel blockers, nifedipine, diltiazem and verapamil (10 to 20 µM) did not affect LTB₄ or LTD₄-induced $[Ca^{2+}]_i$ mobilization (data not shown).

TABLE 2   Binding Affinity of Leukotriene Analogs to [³H]-LTB₄ and [³H]-LTD₄ Receptors in U-937 Cell Membranes

Compounds	[³H]-LTB₄ (nM)	[³H]-LTD₄ (nM)
LTB₄	0.24	> 10 µM
20-OH-LTB₄	0.8	> 10 µM
20-COOH-LTB₄	11	> 10 µM
6-trans-LTB₄	114	NT[a]
2-nor-LTB₄	0.9	NT
5-HETE	2200	> 10 µM
12-HETE	260	NT
LTD₄	> 10 µM	0.65
LTE₄	> 10 µM	42
5R,6S-LTD₄	> 10 µM	61

[a]NT: not tested.

Polyphosphoinositide Metabolism Induced by LTB₄ and LTD₄

[³H]Inositol labeled differentiated U-937 cells were pre-incubated at 37°C for 10 min and then stimulated with 1 µM LTB₄ or 1 µM LTD₄ for 10 sec. Typical profiles of the inositol phosphates are shown in Fig. 3. In the absence of a stimulus there were very low IP₃ levels (Fig. 3A) but after stimulation with maximally effective concentrations of either LTB₄ (Fig. 3B) or LTD₄ (Fig. 3C) there was a rapid hydrolysis of PIP₂ to Ins (1,4,5)P₃ and increases in IP₄ and Ins (1,3,4)P₃. The LTB₄ and LTD₄-induced changes in PI metabolism were time- and concentration-dependent (data not shown). The concentration required to produce 50% of the maximal effect on IP₃ synthesis after 20 sec of stimulation was 6-12 nM for both LTB₄ and LTD₄, which was in good agreement with the $[Ca^{2+}]_i$ mobilization results (data not shown). The maximal increase in Ins (1,4,5)P₃ after LTD₄ stimulation was at 2 sec the earliest possible time point, while the LTB₄ maximum was reached at 5 sec (data not shown). It is apparent from Fig. 3 that increased synthesis of IP₃ isomers and IP₄ was substantially higher with maximally effective concentrations of LTD₄ relative to LTB₄. These changes in PI metabolism correlate with the observed changes in $[Ca^{2+}]_i$ mobilization by the leukotrienes.

DISCUSSION

The criteria for the establishment of leukotriene receptors in U-937 cells were based on the specificity of the radioligand binding characteristics and the correlations of the accompanying signal transduction responses. Binding of [³H]LTB₄ to to differentiated U-937 cell membranes was saturable, of high-affinity and regulated by divalent cations, Na⁺ and guanine nucleotides. Most important, the rank order potencies of the LTB₄ analogs in binding to the membrane receptors directly correlated with that of the $[Ca^{2+}]_i$ mobilization activities in U-937 cells. These observations clearly demonstrate that LTB₄ receptors in U-937 cells represent physiologically and pharmacologically important receptors. Such receptors have been associated with chemotaxis, chemokinesis and other pro-inflammatory activities in PMN, macrophage and monocyte.

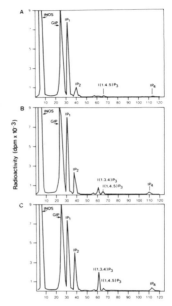

Figure 3. Phosphatidylinositide metabolism by LTB₄ and LTD₄. [³H]-inositol prelabeled differentiated U-937 cells were stimulated with maximally effective concentrations (1 μM) of LTB₄ and LTD₄ for 10 sec. The typical HPLC profile of PI metabolites for no agonist (top), LTB₄ (middle) and LTD₄ (bottom) are presented.

Binding of [³H]LTD₄ to the U-937 cell membranes was saturable, specific and of high-affinity. LTD₄ and LTE₄ type agonists specifically competed with [³H]LTD₄ binding to the receptors. Most importantly, the rank order potency, for these agonists and antagonists, in binding to the U-937 cell membrane receptors was equivalent to those reported for guinea pig lung PIP₂ hydrolysis (11), thromboxane and prostacyclin synthesis (12) and tracheal smooth muscle contraction (8). These observations clearly indicate that the LTD₄ receptors in U-937 cells represent physiologically and pharmacologically important receptors. Such receptors have been associated with the pharmacological activities of peptidoleukotrienes in a variety of cells, tissues and species.

The early phases of the signal transduction mechanism(s)

induced by these receptors appear to be similar. Both types of receptors e.g. the LTB_4 receptors in rabbit, rat and human PMNs and the LTD_4 receptors in guinea pig lung, rat basophilic leukemia cells and primary culture of sheep tracheal smooth muscle cells were coupled to a G protein regulated phospholipase C. Binding of the agonist ligands to the respective receptors promoted a high-affinity ligand-receptor-G protein ternary complex formation. In cells and tissues, binding of the agonist ligands resulted in the activation of PLC, hydrolysis of phosphoinositides with the formation of intracellular messengers; i.e. IP_3 and DAG. IP_3 and DAG mobilized $[Ca^{2+}]_i$ and activated protein kinase C, respectively, and resulted in a variety of biochemical, cellular and pharmacological responses in vitro and in vivo.

In agreement with the mobilization data we have shown that stimulation of differentiated U-937 cells by LTB_4 and LTD_4 results in the rapid hydrolysis of PIP_2 by phospholipase C. The inositol phosphates formed by maximally effective concentrations of the leukotrienes were resolved by HPLC. The two IP_3 isomers (Ins $(1,4,5)P_3$ and Ins $(1,3,4)P_3$, IP_2 and IP_4 all increased rapidly in a time- and concentration-dependent manner after leukotriene stimulation. The magnitude of the PI response correlated with the $[Ca^{2+}]_i$ mobilization response, in that the LTB_4 response was much smaller than LTD_4.

A major distinction of receptor-G protein-PIP_2-PLC coupling for LTB_4 and LTD_4 receptors in U-937 cells is in the "efficiency" of coupling between the receptor and the catalyst, PLC. As demonstrated in the current study, in membrane preparations isolated from differentiated U-937 cells, the density of LTB_4 receptors (B_{max} = 300 $\pm$ 86 fmol/mg) appeared to be similar to that of the LTD_4 receptor (B_{max} = 440 $\pm$ 96 fmol/mg). Yet, the LTD_4 receptor induced maximal $[Ca^{2+}]_i$ mobilization (1760 $\pm$ 130 nM) was approximately 2.5 to 3-fold higher than that induced by the LTB_4 receptor suggesting that the coupling efficiency of LTD_4 receptor induced $[Ca^{2+}]$ mobilization was substantially higher.

In summary, the results showed that LTB_4 and LTD_4 receptors are co-expressed in differentiated U-937 cells. Both types of receptors are coupled to phosphoinositide hydrolysis and $[Ca^{2+}]_i$ mobilization. U-937 cells offer an excellent model for the studies of leukotriene receptor biology, signal transduction mechanism and receptor-effector coupling.

REFERENCES

1. Piper, P.J. *Physiol. Rev.* 1984; 64: 744.
2. Samuelson, B. *Science* 1983; 220: 568.
3. Goldman, D.W. and E.J. Goetzl. *J. Exp. Med.* 1984; 159: 1027.
4. Showell, H.J., P.H. Naccache, P. Borgeat, S. Picard, P. Vallerand, E.L. Becker, and R.I. Sha'afi. *J. Immunol.*

128: 811-816 (1982).
5. Mong, S., G. Chi-Rosso, J. Miller, K. Hoffman, K.A. Razgaitis, P.E. Bender, and S.T. Crooke. <u>Mol. Pharmacol.</u> 1986; 30: 235.
6. Benjamin, C.W., P.L. Rupple, and R.R. Gorman. <u>J. Biol. Chem.</u> 1985; 260: 14208.
7. Pong, S.S. and R.N. DeHaven. <u>Proc. Natl. Acad. Sci USA,</u> 1983; 80: 7415.
8. Mong, S., H-L. Wu, M.O. Scott, M.A. Lewis, M.A. Clark, B.M. Weichman, C.M. Kinzig, J.G. Gleason, and S.T. Crooke. <u>J. Pharmacol. Exp. Ther.</u> 1985; 234: 316.
9. Lewis, M.A., S. Mong, R.L. Vesgella, and S.T. Crooke. <u>Biochem. Pharmacol.</u> 1985; 34: 4311.
10. Sarau, H.M., S. Mong, J.J. Foley, H-L. Wu, and S.T. Crooke. <u>J. Biol. Chem.</u> 1987; 262: 4034.
11. Mong, S., K. Hoffman, H-L. Wu, and S.T. Crooke. <u>Mol. Pharmacol.</u> 1987; 31: 35.
12. Mong, S., H-L. Wu, M.A. Clark, J.G. Gleason and S.T. Crooke, J. Pharmacol. Exp. Ther. 1986; 239-63.

Advances in Prostaglandin, Thromboxane, and
Leukotriene Research, Vol. 19, edited by
B. Samuelsson, P. Y.-K. Wong, and F. F. Sun,
Raven Press, Ltd., New York ©1989.

INVOLVEMENT OF PEPTIDOLEUKOTRIENES IN ANTIGEN-DEPENDENT THROMBOXANE (TX) SYNTHESIS IN IgG1-SENSITIZED GUINEA PIG LUNGS

John B. Cheng, Joann Pillar, Maryrose Conklyn, Robbin Breslow,
John Shirley and Henry J. Showell

Department of Immunology and Infectious Diseases
Central Research Division, Pfizer Inc., Groton, CT 06340. U.S.A.

ABSTRACT

Lungs from IgG1-sensitized guinea pigs synthesize both leukotrienes (LTs) and thromboxane (Tx) upon *ex vivo* antigen challenge. This study was undertaken to investigate whether antigen-dependent Tx synthesis could result from prior formation of LTD_4. In IgG1-sensitized lungs, LTD_4 effectively induced Tx formation ($ED_{50} = 2$-4 nM). In these lungs, the levels of antigen-dependent formaion of LTD_4 (8-26 nM formed by 0.01-10 $\mu g/ml$ antigen challenge) were 2-7 X greater than the ED_{50} value of LTD_4-stimulated Tx synthesis. In addition, incubation of the sensitized lungs with ICI-198,615, a LTD_4 antagonist, prior to antigen-challenge prevented Tx formation ($IC_{50} = 0.01$ μM). Our results indicate that LTD_4 generated from IgG1-sensitized lungs could play a prominent role in stimulating Tx synthesis. LTC_4 may also be involved because of rapid formation of LTC_4 upon antigen-stimulation and its capacity to induce Tx synthesis.

INTRODUCTION

Despite direct bronchoconstricting activity, LTC_4 and LTD_4 have been shown to stimulate Tx synthesis in normal guinea pig lungs (1,2). Formation of Tx can be demonstrated as early as 0.5 min post LTD_4 challenge and by as little as 0.1 nM of LTC_4 (3,4). Since lungs taken from IgG1-sensitized guinea pigs produce a significant amount of both LTD_4 and TxB_2 upon *ex vivo* antigen challenge (5,6), the sensitized tissue should be an excellent system for testing the hypothesis that increased TxB_2 production could result from prior formation of LTD_4. Specifically, we set out to investigate (I) whether LTD_4 could cause Tx production from IgG1-sensitized lung fragments, (II) whether the level of LTD_4 generated from the lung could be sufficient to induce Tx synthesis, and (III) whether treatment of the lungs with ICI-198,615 (6), a potent LTD_4 antagonist, could suppress antigen-dependent Tx synthesis.

METHODS

Isolation and purification of anti-ovalbumin (anti-OA) IgG1 antibody:

Male Hartley guinea pigs were immunized with ovalbumin (OA) precipitated onto alum as described previously (4). The pooled hyperimmune serum was the source for the isolation of anti-OA IgG1. Purification procedures of anti-OA IgG1 were according to previous described methods (7,8).

Guinea pig passive sensitization and chopped lung preparation:

The sensitization protocol and the chopped lung assay were performed according to the methods indicated previously (5,8). The antibody dose of 0.5 mg/Kg was used for sensitization (8).

Measurements of LTC_4, LTD_4, LTB_4, TxB_2 and histamine:

TxB_2, a stable metabolite of TxA_2, was measured by a radioimmunoassay (NEN, Boston, MA) and histamine levels were determined by a double-isotopic enzymatic assay (9). LTC_4, LTD_4 and LTB_4 were measured using reverse phase HPLC and UV detection (5).

[³H]LTD₄ receptor binding assay:

This assay was reported previously (10). The data obtained from competition studies for [³H]LTD_4 binding sites were analyzed by a non-linear least square curve fitting program developed by Lundon Software, Inc. (Cleveland, OH).

RESULTS AND DISCUSSION

Incubation of 0.6 g of lung tissues from IgG1-sensitized guinea pig with 10 μg/ml of OA for 20 min resulted in the formation of significant amounts of LTB_4 ($\sim$20 ng/g lung), LTD_4 ($\sim$50 ng/g), TxB_2 ($\sim$2.5 μg/g) and histamine ($\sim$4 μg/g).

As shown in FIG. 1, the amount of LTB_4, LTD_4 or TxB_2 produced after OA challenge increased with incubation time, reaching equilibrium in about 16 min, and was constant for up to 64 min. A time course study indicated that LTD_4 and LTB_4 were the stable metabolites of the 5-lipoxygenase pathway of arachidonic acid metabolism in the lung preparation, and that the kinetics of LTB_4 and LTD_4 synthesis was similar to that for TxB_2.

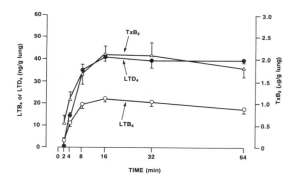

FIG. 1. Time Course of Antigen-Induced LT and Tx Synthesis in IgG1-Sensitized Lung Fragments.

Similar to its effect on unsensitized tissue (1-3), LTD_4 stimulated dose-dependent formation of TxB_2 from IgG1 sensitized lung fragments (FIG. 2A). The ED_{50} value of the LTD_4 effect was 4.1 $\pm$ 1.9 nM (n = 3). In addition, the response of sensitized tissue fragments to LTD_4 was rapid (t½ = 2 min) and reached a maximum at 10 min. Incubation of sensitized lung fragments with 0.1 μM LTB_4 or 0.2 μM PAF for 20 min caused an increase in TxB_2 production; however, the TxB_2 level produced was significantly less than that seen with LTD_4.

To determine if the LTD$_4$ formed by OA challenge is sufficient to induce Tx synthesis, lung fragments were incubated with OA (0.01-10 μg/ml) and the amount of LTD$_4$ synthesized at 20 min was quantified. As shown in FIG. 2B, the levels of LTD$_4$ formed were in the range of 8 to 26 nM. These levels are 2-7 fold greater than the ED$_{50}$ as determined using exogenous LTD$_4$, indicating that the amount of LTD$_4$ formed by antigen-challenged lung fragments is more than sufficient to induce Tx synthesis.

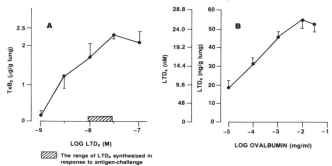

FIG. 2. A. LTD$_4$-Dependent Tx Synthesis from IgG1-Sensitized Lung Fragments.
B. Antigen-Dependent LTD$_4$ Production from IgG1-Sensitized Lung Fragments.

To examine the possibility of endogenously-generated LTD$_4$ being a prerequisite for Tx formation, we determined the ability of ICI-198,615 to inhibit antigen-induced Tx production. As shown in FIG. 3, pretreatment of sensitized lungs with ICI-198,615 inhibited the response in a dose-dependent manner. In addition, approximately 90% of the TxB$_2$ formed was inhibited by the high concentration (1 μM) of ICI-198,615, suggesting that the majority of the Tx synthesized is mediated via the formation of LTD$_4$. This suggestion was further strengthened by the ability of ICI-198,615 to directly inhibit the response due to LTD$_4$ (FIG. 3). Since neither WEB-2086, a PAF antagonist, nor pyrilamine prevented antigen- or LTD$_4$-induced TxB$_2$ production (IC$_{50}$ >30 μM), PAF or histamine are unlikely to be involved in Tx synthesis. Non-linear least square analysis of LTD$_4$/[³H]LTD$_4$ and ICI-198,615/[³H]LTD$_4$ competition curves revealed that LTD$_4$ interacted with a single homogenous population of [³H] LTD$_4$ receptor binding sites in lung membranes (Ki = 0.4 nM), and that ICI-198,615 competed effectively with [³H]LTD$_4$ for the receptor site (Ki = 8.7 nM). The Ki value of ICI-198,615 obtained from the competition curve is close to the Kb value (3 nM) determined for the inhibition of TxB$_2$ release, suggesting that the effect of ICI-198,615 on LTD$_4$- or antigen-dependent response is mediated through the LTD$_4$ receptor site.

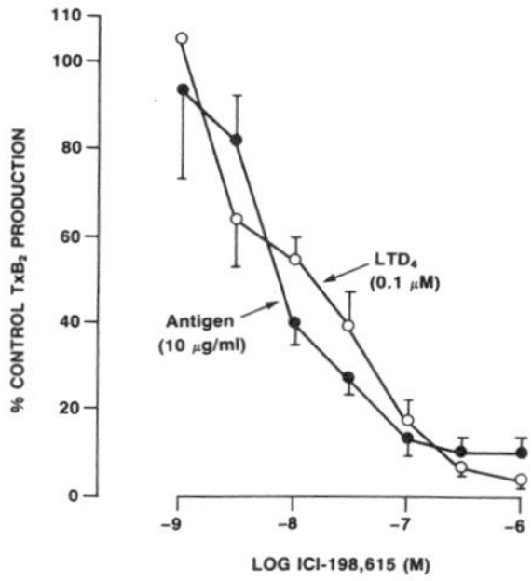

FIG. 3. Effect of ICI-198,615 on Antigen- and LTD$_4$-Induced
Tx Synthesis from IgG1-Sensitized Lung Fragments.

Besides LTD_4, LTC_4 produced by the IgG1 sensitized lungs may also be involved. Previous experiments with lungs taken from actively-sensitized (IgG1-dependent) guinea pigs (5) demonstrated that following antigen challenge LTC_4 was rapidly synthesized (LTC_4 levels peaked at 3 min post challenged). In addition, LTC_4 stimulated Tx synthesis with an ED_{50} value of 10 ± 0.6 nM (n = 3) under conditions where >90% conversion of LTC_4 to LTD_4 was blocked by AT-125 (11), an irreversible inhibitor of γ-glutamyl transpeptidase. In the presence of AT-125, ICI-198,615 prevented both antigen- and LTC_4-dependent Tx synthesis ($IC_{50} = 0.018$ and 0.025 μM, respectively).

These experiments provide evidence that in antigen-challenged lung fragments of IgG1-sensitized guinea pigs, the formation of Tx occurs secondary to the synthesis of LTD_4/LTC_4 and this is most likely mediated through a LTD_4 receptor type. While the cells responsible for LTD_4/LTC_4-dependent Tx synthesis in the lung fragments remain unclear, cell culture studies indicate that they can stimulate the formation of TxB_2 and 6-keto-$PGF_{1\alpha}$ from both smooth muscle cells and vascular endothelial cells (12,13). It is therefore possible that these cells are, at least partly, responsible for Tx synthesis in this guinea pig chopped lung preparation.

REFERENCES

1. Piper PJ. *Physiol. Rev.* 1984; 64:744-761.

2. Dahlen S-E. *Acta Physiol. Scand.* 1983; Suppl.5 12:1-51.

3. Mong S, Wu H-L, Clark MA, *et al. J. Pharmacol. Exp. Therap.* 1987; 239: 63-70.

4. Regal JF. *Immunopharmacol.* 1984; 8:111-119.

5. Cheng JB, Eskra JD, Pillar J. *Pharmacol. Exp. Therap.* 1987; 241:786-792.

6. Synder DW, Giles RE, Keith RA, *et al. J. Pharmacol. Exp. Therap.* 1987; 243:548-556.

7. Conklyn MJ, Showell HJ. 1987; New England Pharmacologists 6th Annual Meeting. Abstract #25.

8. Cheng JB, Conklyn MJ, Pillar J, *et al. Fed. Proc.* 1987; 46:931.

9. Shaff RE, Beaven MA. *Anal. Biochem.* 1979; 94:425-430.

10. Cheng JB, Lang D, Bewtra A, *et al. J. Pharmacol. Exp. Therap.* 1987; 232:80-87.

11. Allen L, Meck R, Yunis A. *Res. Commun. Chem. Pharmacol.* 1980; 27:175-182.

12. Clark MA, Cok M, Mong S, *et al. Europ. J. Pharmacol.* 1985; 116:207-220.

13. Cramer EB, Pologe L, Pawlowski, *et al. Proc. Natl. Acad. Sci. (U.S.A.)* 1983; 80:4109-4113.

Advances in Prostaglandin, Thromboxane, and Leukotriene Research, Vol. 19, edited by B. Samuelsson, P. Y.-K. Wong, and F. F. Sun, Raven Press, Ltd., New York ©1989.

MOLECULAR DIVERSITY OF HUMAN LEUKOCYTE RECEPTORS

FOR LEUKOTRIENES

Catherine H. Koo, Jeffrey W. Sherman,
Laurent Baud and Edward Goetzl

Howard Hughes Medical Institute and Departments
of Medicine and Microbiology-Immunology,
University of California Medical Center,
San Francisco, California 94143-0724

The chemotactic emigration, tissue accumulation and activation of polymorphonuclear leukocytes (PMNLs) are central elements of inflammation that are regulated by a variety of mediators, of which the products of complement pathways and the leukotrienes are the most potent. PMNLs express distinct subsets of receptors for LTB4, LTC4 and LTD_4 that transduce unique profiles of functional effects of each leukotriene. While LTB_4 induces chemotaxis, lysosomal enzyme secretion and generation of superoxide, and enhances adherence to surfaces (1,2), LTD_4 selectively increases adherence without other detectable effects (2,3). The presence of a population of PMNL receptors specific for each type of leukotriene has been demonstrated by binding studies of radiolabeled leukotrienes. Specific cell surface receptors for LTB_4 have been described by several groups of investigators (4-7), whereas the existence of specific receptors for LTC_4 and LTD_4 on PMNLs has only recently been described (8).

RECEPTORS FOR LTB4

The receptors for LTB_4 on PMNL exist in two affinity states (4,6) that appear to be coupled to separate functions of PMNLs. A high affinity state with a mean Kd of 0.3nM constitutes approximately 2-9% of the total receptors, whereas the remaining receptors are in a subset that displays a mean Kd of 61nM. Chemotactically deactivated PMNLs that can still degranulate in response to LTB_4 display a selective loss of the high affinity receptors without alteration of the low affinity receptors (4). This finding suggests that occupancy of high affinity receptors mediates adherence and chemotaxis, while the low affinity receptors are coupled to the lysosomal secretory and oxidative metabolic responses (4).

191

The addition of guanosine di- and triphosphates and their
analogs to membrane preparations reversibly converts a portion
of the high affinity receptors to a low affinity state (9).
That this conversion of affinity states reflects involvement
of a guanine nucleotide binding protein (G-protein) is
supported by the observation that the addition of LTB_4 to
PMNL membranes greatly enhances the binding of the
radiolabeled non-hydrolyzable guanosine triphosphate analog,
GMP-PNP, to a pertussis toxin sensitive G-protein (9). The
possible existence of receptor-G-protein complexes is
supported by size fractionation chromatography of solubilized
PMNL membrane proteins (Fig. 1). Gel filtration of PMNL
membrane proteins solubilized in the detergent
3-[(3cholamidopropyl)-dimethylammonio]-1-propanesulfonate
(CHAPS) (10) revealed the presence of two peaks of $[^3H]LTB_4$-
binding activities with apparent molecular weights of 66kD
and 144 kD. The smaller LTB_4-binding is presumably the
receptor-micelle complex whereas the higher molecular weight
moiety may consist of a complex of the receptor protein and
G-protein. Further characterization of the two LTB_4-binding
activities will be necessary in order to determine which
complex contains the high affinity LTB_4 receptors.

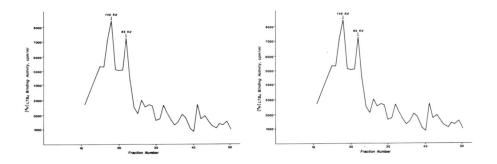

FIG. 1. Gel filtration on Sephacryl S-200 of CHAPS-
solubilized PMNL membranes. To determine the $[^3H]LTB_4$-binding
activity of each fraction, bound $[^3H]LTB_4$ was separated from
unbound ligand by rapid filtration through polyethyleneimine-
treated glass fiber filters.

RECEPTORS FOR SULFIDOPEPTIDE-LEUKOTRIENES

The leukocyte receptors for LTC_4 and LTD_4 differ from LTB_4 receptors in both binding characteristics and cellular distribution. Whereas LTB_4 receptors are located primarily on plasma membranes (7,11), one-third of the total cellular LTC_4 binding sites are associated with membranes and the remaining two-thirds are localized in the lysosomal granules (8). The receptors on both membranes and granules display homogeneous $[^3H]LTC_4$-binding properties, consistent with the presence of a single population of binding sites, with mean densities of 15.9 pmol/mg of protein and 3 pmol/mg of protein, respectively. The Kd value calculated for membrane receptors of 38.3 nM was the same as that detected of receptors in intact PMNL, which was significantly higher than that for granule receptors (13.4nM). The stereoselectivity of the receptors was the same in both cellular fractions and intact cells. The possibility of glutathione S-transferase contributing to the binding activity of the preparations was excluded since LTC_4-binding was insensitive to the addition of bilirubin and hematin (8).

The biochemical transductional events elicited by occupancy of receptors with sulfidopeptide leukotrienes was investigated in HL-60 cell derived myelocytes. Both LTC_4 and LTD_4 evoked increases in the cytosolic intracellular calcium concentration $([Ca^{+2}]_i)$ which attained a peak more rapidly for LTD_4 than LTC_4 and was transient for both. The finding that inhibition of LTC_4 conversion to LTD_4 by serine-borate suppressed both the LTC_4-induced rise in $[Ca^{+2}]_i$ and the concurrent increase in adherence of HL-60 myelocytes to Sephadex G-25 suggested that the slower response and lower EC_{50} of LTC_4 were due to a requisite conversion of inactive LTC_4 to the active LTD_4. The biochemical response appeared to be LTD_4 receptor mediated, since the specific LTD_4 receptor antagonist SKF 102922 inhibited the LTD_4-induced increase in $[Ca^{+2}]_i$. The source of Ca^{+2} appeared to be extracellular and the rise in $[Ca^{+2}]_i$ was suppressed by lanthanum, but was not affected by nifedipine nor accompanied by any changes in membrane potential. That pertussis toxin treatment of HL-60 myelocytes eliminated the LTD_4-induced elevation of $[Ca^{+2}]_i$ suggests that LTD_4 receptors may be linked to a G-protein mediated transductional mechanism similar to that characteristic of LTB_4 receptors (12).

Another similarity between LTB_4 and LTD_4 receptor mediated biochemical pathways is the alteration in intracellular pH (pH_i) induced by ligand binding to the cell surface (13-14). Unlike the peptide chemotactic factors and LTB_4 which initiates first a transient acidification and then a prolonged alkalinization of the cytoplasm, LTD_4 evokes only an increase in pH_i with a half maximal response at 1-2nM LTD_4. As for $[Ca^{+2}]_i$ changes, LTC_4 has no effect on pH_i (15). As the alkalinization response was sensitive to inhibition by $1\mu M$ ethylisopropylamiloride, the increase in pH_i elicited by LTD_4 thus appears to be associated with activation of the NA^+/H^+ antiport. The cytoplasmic alkalinization, however, was not coupled to the more rapid increase in $[Ca^{+2}]_i$ evoked by LTD_4, since an increase in pH_i was observed in the absence of any extracellular source of Ca^{+2} (15). Thus the increase in intracellular cytosolic calcium levels and the intracellular alkalinization response are separate and not sequential events induced by LTD_4.

The distinct profiles of PMNL responses to each leukotriene are mediated by a separate subset of receptors, each of which exhibits a unique specificity, affinity and cellular distribution. Although the separate subsets of receptors may share some cellular pathways in the activation of PMNLs, different types of leukotriene receptors exhibit distinctive transductional biochemistry and functional effects.

REFERENCES

1. Goetzl EJ, Pickett WC. J Immunol 1980;125:1789-1791.

2. Goetzl EJ, Brindley LL, Goldman DW. Immunology 1983;50:35-41.

3. Dahlen S-E, Bjork J, Hedqvist P, et al. Proc Natl Acad Sci USA 1981;78:3887-3891.

4. Goldman DW, Goetzl EJ. J Exp Med 1984;159:1027-1041.

5. Lin AH, Ruppel PL, Gorman RR. Prostaglandins 1984;28:837-849.

6. Kreisle RA, Parker CW. J Exp Med 1983;157:628-641.

7. Bomalaski JS and Mong S. Prostaglandins 1987;33:855-867.

8. Baud L, Koo CH, Goetzl EJ. Immunology 1987;62:53-59.

9. Sherman JW, Goetzl EJ, Koo CH. J Immunol 1988 (in press).

10. Koo CH, Healy A, Goetzl EJ. Fed Proc 1988;2:A668.

11. Goldman DW, Gifford LA, Marotti T, Koo CH, Goetzl EJ. Fed Proc 1987;46:200-203.

12. Baud L, Goetzl EJ, Koo CH. J. Clin Invest 1987;80:983-991,

13. Faucher N, Naccache PH. J Cell Physiol 1987;132:483-491.

14. Grinstein S. Furuya W. Biochem Biophys Res Commun 1984; 122:755-762.

15. Baud L, Goetzl EJ, Koo CH. J Cell Physiol 1988 (in press).

Advances in Prostaglandin, Thromboxane, and Leukotriene Research, Vol. 19, edited by B. Samuelsson, P. Y.-K. Wong, and F. F. Sun, Raven Press, Ltd., New York ©1989.

INHIBITION OF IN VITRO GUINEA PIG EOSINOPHIL
CHEMOTAXIS BY LEUKOTRIENE B_4 ANTAGONIST U-75,302

Bruce M. Taylor, Christine I. Czuk, Marshall N. Brunden*,
Donn G. Wishka[+], Joel Morris[+], and Frank F. Sun

Department of Hypersensitivty Diseases Research, *Biostatistics
[+]Metabolic Diseases Research, The Upjohn Company
Kalamazoo, MI 49001 USA

There is increasing evidence to suggest that eosinophils are prominent effector cells associated with the chronic airway inflammation in asthma. Eosinophil secreted inflammatory mediators such as sulfidopeptide leukotrienes (LT) or platelet activating factor (PAF) have been implicated in the development of late phase bronchoconstriction and hyperresponsiveness in atopic patients after antigen provocation (1). Dunn and coworkers (2) observed massive infiltration of eosinophils into bronchoalveolar tissue and epithelial lining fluid in the antigen challenged sensitized guinea pigs during the period 18-54 hours after antigen challenge. A novel leukotriene B_4 antagonist U-75,302 (3,4) was shown to partially block this late phase cellular response (I.M. Richards, personal communication, 1988), suggesting that LTB_4 may be a mediator of this cell influx. While LTB_4 is an active chemoattractant for eosinophils from guinea pig and man (5,6), the mode of action of U-75,302 as an inhibitor of eosinophil chemotaxis has not been examined. This report describes the effect of chemoattractants on in vitro migration of guinea pig eosinophils and its inhibition by U-75,302.

Guinea pigs were injected intraperitoneally with 0.5 ml of horse serum twice a week for two weeks and peritoneal cells were collected by lavage with Hanks buffer without calcium or magnesium (HBSS). The cells were washed once and red blood cells were removed by hypotonic lysis. Eosinophils were separated by centrifugation on discontinuous Percoll density gradients. Eosinophils (85-95%) were collected in two bands at density 1.09 and 1.10. The majority of contaminating cells were mononuclear and could be removed by adherence during a differential plating in RPMI medium with 10% fetal calf serum for 90 minutes. The two bands of eosinophils had slightly different density, but identical morphology under optical microscopy. They behaved identically in several biochemical and functional tests. Therefore, the two bands were mixed and used in subsequent experiments.

The purified eosinophils were suspended in HBSS at 1×10^7 cells/ml and incubated with 20 µCi/ml of $Na_2^{51}CrO_4$ for 30 minutes at room temperature. After two washes the cells were suspended in complete HBSS (1.2 mM of $CaCl_2$) containing 3 mg/ml guinea pig serum albumin and added to the top compartment of a blind Boyden chamber. The bottom compartment was filled with complete HBSS without albumin. Chemoattractants were added to the bottom compartment only and inhibitors were added to both compartments in equal concentration. The two compartments were separated by a 8 µ Nucleopore polycarbonate membrane on the cell side and a 3 µ Millipore nitrocellulose membrane on the chemoattractant side. Total radioactivity for the chamber was adjusted to 10,000 cpms and the counts associated with cells that penetrated into the 3 µ membrane were normalized and used as measure of cell migration. Chemokinesis was assessed by adding chemoattractants to both chambers at the same concentration. Each experiment was performed in duplicate to quadruplicate in order to achieve statistical significance.

Guinea pig eosinophils exhibited marked migration responses toward LTB_4, formyl-Met-Leu-Phe (fMLP) and zymosan activated guinea pig plasma (ZAP). Dose response studies showed that LTB_4 was maximally active at 10 nM and ZAP reached maximal level at 1:10 dilution. FMLP was active at 1 nM but the maximal response it induced was somewhat smaller than that elicited by optimal concentrations of LTB_4 and ZAP. The two ECF-A tetrapeptides val-gly-ser--glu and ala-gly-ser-glu were active at 2 uM. PAF, bacterial endotoxin or interleukin-1 were ineffective at relevant concentrations.

The contribution of elevated random movement (chemokinesis) to the total response was measured for both LTB_4 and ZAP. For LTB_4, chemokinesis accounted for 60-70% of the total response. ZAP induced almost exclusive (> 90%) directional chemotaxis with very little random movement. This result is similar to that obtained for human eosinophils by Czarnetzki and Rosenbach (6).

When the inhibitor U-75,302 (10 µM and 1 µM) was added to both compartments of the Boyden chamber with 20 nM of LTB_4 as chemoattractants added to the lower compartment, in three experiments the average total migratory responses was reduced by 33% (67.44±3.35% of control) and 14% (85.72±4.25% of control) respectively. U-75,302 at 1 µM also reduced the ZAP (1:10) induced eosinophils migration by an average of 28% (72% of control) in two experiments. At 10 µM, U-75,302 possesses significant directional chemotaxis when added as a chemoattractant to the lower compartment. If U-75,302 was added along with LTB_4 to the lower compartment but not to the upper compartment, the agonist activity prevailed and the inhibitory effect would not be observed. However, U-75,302 apparently lacks chemokinetic activity. When it was present in both upper and lower compartments at identical concentration (from 0.1 to 10 uM) in the absence of a chemoattractant, there was no detectable cell migration. Therefore, the inhibition effect of U-75,302 could only be seen when the inhibitor was present in both compartments. These experimental conditions seem to simulate the in vivo situation when circulating eosinophils encounter the administered inhibitor in the blood before they come into contact with a chemoattractant diffused in from a distant site.

In this study, we found LTB_4, fMLP and zymosan activated plasma are the most effective chemoattractants for the directional migration of ^{51}Cr labelled guinea pig eosinophils. The results are similar to those obtained by previous investigators using different techniques (5-7). The guinea pig eosinophil migration responses are quite different from that of human cells. Human eosinophils are very responsive to PAF, (8-10) while guinea pig cells are not responsive to PAF. LTB_4 has been considered as a weak (10) or inactive (9) chemoattractant for human eosinophils, but as shown in the present study, it is among the most potent chemotactic agonists for guinea pig cells. There is also a considerable species difference in the pattern of arachidonic acid metabolites produced by these eosinophils. After activation by calcium ionophore, guinea pig eosinophils synthesize thromboxane B_2 and leukotriene B_4 as their major products, while human cells synthesize leukotriene C_4 and 15-HETE. The differences in both the biochemistry and the functions of lipid mediators cast the doubt whether guinea pig airway eosinophilia is a suitable model for the study of human diseases.

However, the data clearly demonstrates that the putative LTB_4 antagonist U-75,302 inhibits LTB_4 and complement component induced guinea pig eosinophil migration in vitro. The inhibitory effect is weak (33% at 10 uM) but highly reproducible. Because of the poor aqueous solubility of U-75,302, we were not able to block the cell migration response greater than 50% in order to calculate the potency in a more quantitative term. The inhibition of complement component stimulated eosinophil chemotaxis indicates that the inhibitor lacks agonist specificity. But, Clancy et al (11) had shown that human polymorphonuclear leukocytes could be activated by complement component C5a to express a functional 5-lipoxygenase that formed LTB_4. Perhaps secondary synthesis of LTB_4 by the responding cell is a required step for the chemotactic action of zymosan activated plasma and that step is inhibited by U-75,302.

We conclude that the inhibition of antigen induced late phase airway eosinophilia in guinea pigs by U-75,302 can be partially attributed to the antagonism of LTB_4 induced cell migration in vivo.

1) de Monchy, J.G.R., Kauffman, H.F., Venge, P., Koeter, G.H., Jansen, H.M., Sluiter, H.J., and deVries, K., Am. Rev. Respir. Dis., 131:373-376, (1985).

2) Dunn, C.J., Elliott, G.A., Oostveen, J.A., and Richards, I.M., Am. Rev. Resp. Dis., 137:541-547, 1988.

3) Lin, A.H., Morris, J.L, Wishka, D.G. and Gorman, R.R., Ann. N.Y. Acad. Sci., 524:196-200, 1988.

4) Morris, J.L. and Wishka, D.G., Tetrahedron Letters, 29:(2), 143-146, 1988.

5) Czarnetzki, B.M. and Mertensmerier, R., Prostaglandins 30:5-11, (1985).

6) Czarnetzki, B.M. and Rosenbach, T., Prostaglandins 31:851-858, (1986).

7) Ogawa, H., Kunkel, S.L., Fantone, J.C., and Ward, P.A., Am. J. Pathol., 105:149-155, 1981.

8) Sigal, C.E., Valone, F.H., Holtzman, M.J., and Goetzl, E.J., J. Clin. Immunol., 7179:184, 1987.

9) Tamura, N., Agrawal, D.K., Suliaman, F.A., and Townley, R.G., Biochem. Biophys. Res. Communs., 142:638-644, 1987.

10) Wardlaw, A.J., Moqbel, R., Cromwell, O., and Kay, A.B., J. Clin. Invest., 78:1701-1706, 1986.

11) Clancy, R.M., Dahinden, C.A., and Hugli, T.E., Proc. Nat. Acad. Sci. USA, 80:7200-7204, 1983.

Advances in Prostaglandin, Thromboxane, and Leukotriene Research, Vol. 19, edited by
B. Samuelsson, P. Y.-K. Wong, and F. F. Sun,
Raven Press, Ltd., New York ©1989.

THE ROLE OF THROMBOXANE A_2 IN EXPERIMENTAL AND HUMAN MODELS OF CHRONIC GLOMERULAR DAMAGE

C. Patrono, *A. Pierucci and **P. Salvati

Dept. of Pharmacology, Catholic University School of Medicine,
00168 Rome; *Division of Nephrology, University of Rome
"La Sapienza", 00100 Rome and **Farmitalia Carlo Erba
Research Laboratories, 20159 Milan, Italy.

Thromboxane $(TX)A_2$ is a labile derivative of prostaglandin (PG) endoperoxide metabolism that amplifies platelet response to a variety of aggregating agents (1). In addition, TXA_2 contracts vascular smooth muscle and glomerular mesangium through receptor-mediated actions resulting in changes in intracellular calcium (2). Platelets represent a major source of TXA_2 production, though the presence of a TX-synthase has been reported in other cell types, including macrophages and glomerular epithelial and mesangial cells (3).

Qualitative as well as quantitative changes in glomerular PG-endoperoxide metabolism have been described or postulated in both clinical and experimental models of chronic glomerular disease (4). Enhanced intrarenal production of TXA_2 has been characterized as a common metabolic feature of many such models, although the cellular source(s) and mechanism(s) responsible for this biochemical abnormality have remained largely hypothetical. Some insight into the pathophysiologic significance of increased glomerular TXA_2 synthesis was provided by the use of TX-synthase inhibitors and receptor antagonists, i.e. drugs blocking the synthesis or contractile actions of TXA_2.

ASSESSMENT OF GLOMERULAR TXA_2 BIOSYNTHESIS

Largely indirect evidence supports the notion that the urinary excretion of primary unmetabolized eicosanoids including TXB_2, may represent a fraction of intrarenal eicosanoid production (5). The evidence concerning urinary TXB_2, as obtained in humans, derives from infusion studies of exogenous TXB_2 in healthy subjects (6), from the investigation of patients with lupus nephritis (7) and from pharmacologic studies of selective and non-selective cyclooxygenase inhibitors in health and disease (5). These human studies have measured the urinary excretion of TXB_2 and 2,3-dinor-TXB_2, a major derivative of the ß-oxidation pathway of systemic TXB_2 metabolism, and have demonstrated a dissociation of their excretory pattern possibly suggestive of a renal vs extra-renal origin. No information of similar nature is available in animal studies, even though measurements of urinary TXB_2 have been used extensively in rat and murine models of glomerular disease. Thus, the inference made in the latter studies that urinary TXB_2 may reflect intrarenal TXA_2 production is largely speculative and not supported by the appropriate experimental evidence.

Measurement of ex vivo glomerular TXB_2 production in response to added substrate or other stimuli, represents a capacity-related index conceptually similar to the measurement of serum TXB_2 i.e. platelet TXB_2 production in response to endogenously formed thrombin. These measurements have been used extensively to monitor disease-associated changes in glomerular PG-endoperoxide metabolism. The relationship of enhanced glomerular TXB_2 production, as detected ex vivo, to the actual rate of TXA_2 biosynthesis in vivo remains, however, to be defined. Perhaps more importantly than a quantitative assessment, measurement of eicosanoid production in isolated glomeruli may provide useful information on qualitative differences in disease-related expression of PG-endoperoxide metabolism, possibly reflecting changes in the cellular source(s) of a particular eicosanoid (e.g. TXA_2) or the biochemical cooperation between resident and infiltrating cells.

ANIMAL MODELS OF PROGRESSIVE GLOMERULAR SCLEROSIS

Proteinuria, hypertension and glomerular sclerosis in the viable portion of the remnant kidney occur in rats after ablation of more than 70% of renal mass. Pharmacologic intervention studies performed by S. Klahr and his associates over the past 12 years have suggested that at least two mechanisms may be responsible for the development of progressive glomerular sclerosis in this model (8): a) increased transmission of systemic blood pressure to glomerular capillaries, resulting in intraglomerular hypertension and b) other factors involving platelet aggregation and intraglomerular coagulation.

Rats with a remnant kidney showed a higher TXB_2 excretion rate than control animals (9). Moreover, long-term administration of OKY-1581, a selective TX-synthase inhibitor, increased renal blood flow (RBF) and glomerular filtration rate (GFR), decreased proteinuria, lowered blood pressure and markedly improved renal histology (9). It is of interest that in the studies of Purkerson et al. (8,9), most of the maneuvers designed to decrease the progressive glomerulosclerosis also resulted in marked decreases in arterial blood pressure. These included OKY-1581, aspirin when given alone in low doses (5 mg/kg body weight) or in combination with dipyridamole (50 and 10 mg/kg, respectively), heparin, coumadin and a combination of antihypertensive drugs. The following sequence of events has been suggested by these Investigators (8): reduced renal mass causing vasodilation of arterioles in residual glomeruli would lead to hyperperfusion and intraglomerular hypertension. The latter will result in mechanical damage of the endothelium of glomerular capillaries followed by platelet aggregation, intraglomerular thrombosis and release of factors which may produce hyperplasia and hypertrophy of medium and small arterioles and subseguent sclerosis of the tissue.

Conflicting results have been obtained by Zoja et al. (submitted), showing that selective inhibition of platelet TXB_2 generation by low-dose aspirin (a loading dose of 100 mg/kg followed by 15 mg/kg daily) failed to protect rats with reduced renal mass from the development of progressive glomerular sclerosis. These Investigators have argued that the beneficial results obtained by Purkerson et al. (9) with a selective TX-synthase inhibitor might be attributed to an effect on TXA_2 synthesis by resident glomerular cells (not inhibited by low-dose aspirin) or to lowering of systemic blood pressure.

The Milan normotensive rat strain (MNS) is characterized by a genetically determined, age-related glomerular sclerosis accompanied by heavy proteinuria and deterioration of renal function (10). Increased glomerular production of TXB_2 has been described in this model of spontaneous glomerular damage not associated with systemic hypertension. Long-term administration of FCE 22178, a selective TX-synthase inhibitor, reduced proteinuria, preserved renal function and improved renal hystology with no significant change in systemic blood pressure (submitted). These results would support the contention that selective inhibition of intraglomerular TXA_2 production per se is responsible for the prevention of progressive glomerular damage irrespective of changes in arterial blood pressure.

Whether intraglomerular platelet activation and/or enhanced TXA_2 production by glomerular mesangial and epithelial cells is the primary target of FCE 22178 remains to be determined. This drug inhibits TXB_2 production in isolated MNS glomeruli at significanty lower concentrations than in whole blood from the same animals (unpublished observations), a finding at variance with previous results obtained with dazoxiben and other imidazole-analogue TX-synthase inhibitors.

Thus, "tissue-selective" inhibitors, such as FCE 22178, may help to clarify the relative contribution of glomerular vis-a-vis platelet TX-synthase in the progression of glomerulosclerosis.

ROLE OF TXA_2 IN LUPUS NEPHRITIS

A complex alteration in renal arachidonate metabolism has been described in patients with lupus nephritis, the most consistent and specific features of which are reflected by enhanced urinary excretion of TXB_2 and decreased excretion of 6-keto-$PGF_{1\alpha}$ (7). The severity of such biochemical alterations correlates with the activity of renal lesions and with deteriorating renal function (7). In these patients, PGI_2 represents an important determinant of glomerular haemodynamics and its suppression by cyclooxygenase inhibitors accounts for the reduction in renal function associated with these drugs (7).

More recently, the functional significance of enhanced intrarenal TXA_2 production has been explored by means of a TXA_2-receptor antagonist and low-dose aspirin (submitted). BM 13,177 caused a statistically significant increase in RBF and GFR when infused iv for 48 h in patients with diffuse proliferative lupus nephritis. In contrast, the daily administration of aspirin (20 mg bid) was not associated with any statistically significant change in urinary TXB_2 excretion or renal function, despite virtually complete suppression of platelet cyclooxygenase activity. Thus, enhanced intrarenal synthesis of TXA_2 by cells other than platelets has pathophysiological effects on glomerular haemodynamics. Long-term studies of TXA_2-receptor antagonists and/or tissue-selective TX-synthase inhibitors will help to define the role of this biochemical alteration in the progression of lupus nephropathy.

We thank M.L. Bonanomi for expert editorial assistance.

REFERENCES

1. Hamberg M, Svensson J, Samuelsson B. Proc Natl Acad Sci USA 1975;72:2994-2998.

2. Mené P, Simonson MS, Dunn MJ. In: Dunn MJ, Cinotti GA, Patrono C, eds. Renal eicosanoids, New York: Plenum Press, 1988 (in press).

3. Schlondorff D. Am J Med 1986;81(2B):1-11.

4. Patrono C, Pierucci A. Am J Med 1986;81(2B):71-83.

5. Patrono C, Dunn MJ. Kidney Int 1987;32:1-12.

6. Patrono C, Ciabattoni G, Pugliese F, Pierucci A, Blair IA, FitzGerald GA. J Clin Invest 1986;77:590-594.

7. Patrono C, Ciabattoni G, Remuzzi G, et al. J Clin Invest 1985;76:1011-1018.

8. Purkerson ML, Joist JH, Yates J, Klahr S. Mineral Electrolyte Metab 1987;13:370-376.

9. Purkerson ML, Joist JH, Yates J, Valdes A, Morrison A, Klahr S. Proc Natl Acad Sci USA 1985;82:193-197.

10. Brandis A, Bianchi G, Reale E, Helmechen U, Kunn K. J Lab Invest 1986;55:234-243.

Advances in Prostaglandin, Thromboxane, and
Leukotriene Research, Vol. 19, edited by
B. Samuelsson, P. Y.-K. Wong, and F. F. Sun,
Raven Press, Ltd., New York ©1989.

PROSTACYCLIN SYNTHESIS IS INCREASED DURING PROPRANOLOL

THERAPY FOR ESSENTIAL HYPERTENSION

M. L. Beckmann, A. S. Nies, and J. G. Gerber

University of Colorado School of Medicine
Division of Clinical Pharmacology, Depts. of Medicine and Pharmacology
4200 E. Ninth Avenue, Denver, CO 80262, U.S.A.
(Supported by USPHS Grants HL21308, GM07063, RR00051, and RR01152;
Dr. Gerber is a Burroughs Wellcome Scholar in Clincal Pharmacology)

Because of their various effects on vascular tone, sympathetic nervous system function, renal function and renin release, prostaglandins have been considered potentially important in blood pressure control (1). A role for prostaglandins in the etiology of hypertension has never been established, but the non-steroidal antiinflammatory drugs (NSAIDs) that inhibit prostaglandin production have been shown to interfere with the efficacy of several types of antihypertensive drugs (1-3). In addition some investigators have reported that NSAIDs can raise arterial pressure in patients with essential hypertension.

When propranolol is first administered to patients with hypertension, cardiac output falls, peripheral vascular resistance rises and arterial pressure is little changed. However, with continued propranolol treatment some patients (the propranolol responders) have a fall in arterial pressure associated with a reduction of vascular resistance to baseline (4). The mechanism of this delayed antihypertensive effect in the responders is unknown. Our study was designed to test the hypothesis that vascular prostacyclin synthesis is increased by propranolol associated with its antihypertensive effect. We also wished to quantify the hypertensive effect of the NSAID, indomethacin, and determine whether this effect was sufficient to explain the ability of the NSAID to inhibit the antihypertensive efficacy of propranolol.

METHODS

Five male and five female caucasian patients with essential hypertension (135-165/95-105 mmHg) were studied in a randomized, double-blind, crossover trial. All patients were free of medications for two weeks. They then received either placebo or indomethacin (50 mg bid) for one week followed by propranolol (100 mg bid) for two weeks. Drugs were then discontinued for a two week washout period. Patients then received the alternate regimen (placebo or indomethacin) and repeated the first half of the study. Patients were seen weekly during washout and indomethacin/placebo periods and twice weekly during propranolol therapy. At each visit arterial pressure was determined in the supine and sitting positions, and urine was obtained for measurement of the major urinary metabolite of prostacyclin, 2,3 dinor-6-keto-$PGF_{1\alpha}$ (PGIM).

203

PGIM was measured by a gas-chromatographic-negative ion, chemical ionization technique using deuterated PGIM (kindly provided by Dr. John Pike, Upjohn) as the internal standard (5,6). The urinary excretion of PGIM has been shown to reflect the total body synthesis of PGI_2 (7,8).

Data were analyzed by analysis of variance or Student's t-test as appropriate and presented as means ± standard error of the mean. Statistical significance was defined as $p \leq 0.05$.

RESULTS

Propranolol reduced mean arterial pressure (MAP) in 7 of 10 patients (Table 1); three were termed non-responders due to failure of propranolol to reduce MAP by at least 5 mmHg in the supine and standing positions. Indomethacin alone increased MAP significantly in the sitting position. The subsequent addition of propranolol to indomethacin resulted in a fall of MAP, but the reduction of MAP was significantly greater when propranolol was administered alone (-17.5±1.7 mmHg supine; -12.4±1.5 mmHg sitting) than when it was added to indomethacin (-8.0±2.9 mmHg supine; -8.5±2.2 mmHg sitting). A significant weight gain was seen with the combination of propranolol and indomethacin (1.6±0.6 kg).

TABLE 1. Effects of propranolol and/or indomethacin in responders

	Control	Placebo	Propranolol	Control	Indo	Prop/Indo
MAP mmHg (supine)	115.8 ±2.5	117.8 ±1.6	100.3[a,b] ±2.0	115.7 ±1.1	119.6 ±2.9	111.6[c] ±2.5
MAP mmHg (sitting)	120.6 ±2.4	120.1 ±2.0	107.7[a,b] ±1.6	120.5 ±1.3	126.0[a] ±1.4	117.5[c] ±2.5
PGIM ng/g creatinine	59.9 ±21.6	63.2 ±12.7	135.6[a,b] ±17.6	67.0 ±12.3	42.7[a] ±10.6	52.3 ±8.8
Weight kg	88.9 ±5.4	88.2 ±5.5	89.1 ±5.4	89.2 ±5.5	90.1 ±5.9	90.8[a] ±5.8

[a]Different from Control (p<0.05)
[b]Different from Placebo (p<0.05)
[c]Different from Indo (p<0.05)

Propranolol therapy was associated with a significant increase in the excretion rate of PGIM in the responders whereas indomethacin reduced PGIM excretion (Table 1). A group of age and sex matched normotensive controls had a significantly higher PGIM excretion rate (185.0±33.5 ng/g creatinine) than did the untreated hypertensive patients. However, during propranolol therapy the PGIM excretion rate in the responders was not significantly different from that in the untreated normotensive group. The non-responders had an increase in PGIM excretion with propranolol therapy that was significantly smaller than that seen in the responders (+28.7±10.7 ng/g creatinine in non-responders vs +72.4±13.3 ng/g in the responders), and the PGIM excretion rate in the non-responders always remained significantly lower than in the normotensive controls.

DISCUSSION

We found that the antihypertensive effect of propranolol was associated with an increase in the excretion rate of PGIM that is thought to reflect the total body synthesis of PGI_2. Since the major source of PGI_2 is vascular endothelium, our finding implies an increase in vascular PGI_2 synthesis. During treatment with the cyclooxygenase inhibitor, indomethacin, PGIM excretion rate was reduced associated with an increase in MAP. Subsequent administration of propranolol did not increase PGIM excretion or reduce MAP below control values. The ability of indomethacin to abolish the antihypertensive effect of propranolol was a combination of two factors. Indomethacin increased MAP when given alone, and it attenuated the reduction of arterial pressure produced by propranolol. These data suggest that propranolol may have prostaglandin-dependent and prostaglandin-independent antihypertensive mechanisms.

The increase in PGIM excretion rate during propranolol treatment was only to the range exhibited by the normotensive controls. Thus, the increase was not of a magnitude to suggest that PGI_2 could act as a circulating substance (7). Rather, the increase in vascular PGI_2 synthesis may contribute to a reduced MAP only to the extent that such levels contribute to blood pressure homeostasis in normals. In the non-responders there was a small rise in PGIM excretion during propranolol therapy but not to the level seen in the responders, implying that elevation of PGI_2 synthesis to the range of our normotensive controls may be contributing to the antihypertensive response to propranolol. Alternatively, the relative hypotension during propranolol therapy in the responders may have caused the increased PGI_2 synthesis.

No previous clinical studies have attempted to assess the ability of propranolol to increase PGI_2 production. Studies in vitro indicate that propranolol may have the ability to increase PGI_2 production in some circumstances (9,10). The most relevant animal experiment indicated that the PGI_2 synthetic capacity of aortic tissue obtained from spontaneously hypertensive rats was increased in those animals that had been treated with the active l-isomer but not the d-isomer of propranolol (11).

During the combination of indomethacin and propranolol the patients' weight increased significantly, suggesting that sodium retention could also be an important variable in this study. Sodium retention has been associated with elevated arterial pressure and a reduced response to diuretics and adrenergic blockers, and may have contributed to the attenuated response to propranolol in the presence of indomethacin (12-14). With indomethacin alone the increase in weight was not significant although there was a rise in arterial pressure. This hypertensive effect has been suggested to be related to a rise in vascular resistance secondary to an increased sensitivity to endogenous vasoconstrictors as a result of cyclo-oxygenase inhibition (1,12).

In conclusion, we have demonstrated that successful therapy of essential hypertension with propranolol is associated with an increase in PGI_2 synthesis as reflected by the urinary excretion of the major metabolite, PGIM. Indomethacin reduced the basal PGIM excretion rate and increased arterial pressure. Indomethacin also blocked the increase in PGIM associated with propranolol therapy and blunted the hypotensive effect of propranolol. As a result of indomethacin's hypertensive effect and its ability to blunt the antihypertensive effect of propranolol, the combination of indomethacin and propranolol did not reduce arterial pressure below the baseline value.

REFERENCES

1. Stoff J. Am J Med 1986;80(Suppl 1A):56-61.

2. Watkins J, Abbott EC, Hensby CN, Webster J, Dollery CT. Br Med J 1980; 281:702-705.

3. Radack KL, Deck CC, Bloomfield SS. Annals Int Med 1987;107:628-635.

4. Tarazi RC, Dustan HP. Am J Cardiol 1972;29:633-640.

5. Falardeau P, Oates JA, Brash AR. Analyt Biochem 1981;115:359-367.

6. FitzGerald GA, Lawson J, Blair IA, Brash AR. Adv Prostagland Thrombox Leukotri Res 1985;15:87-90.

7. Brash AR, Jackson EK, Saggese CA, Lawson JA, Oates JA, FitzGerald GA. J Pharmacol Exp Ther 1983;226:78-87.

8. FitzGerald GA, Brash AR, Falardeau P, Oates JA. J Clin Invest 1981;68:1272-1276.

9. Mostaghim R, Maddox Y, Ramwell PW. J Pharmacol Exp Ther 1986;239:792-801.

10. Gotoh S, Ogihara T, Ohsu H, Nakamaru M, Masao K, Saeki S, Kumahara Y. Prostagland Leukotri Med 1984;8:537-544.

11. Nishimiya T, Webb JG, Daniell HB, Oatis J, Walle T, Gaffney TE, Halushka P. Clin Res 1987;35:579A.

12. Brown J, Dollery C, Valdes G. Am J Med 1986;81(Suppl 2B):43-55.

13. Freis E. Circulation 1976;53:589-595.

14. Dustan H, Tarazi R, Bravo E. N Engl J Med 1972;286:861-866.

Advances in Prostaglandin, Thromboxane, and Leukotriene Research, Vol. 19, edited by B. Samuelsson, P. Y.-K. Wong, and F. F. Sun, Raven Press, Ltd., New York ©1989.

ROLE OF TXA$_2$ IN THE PATHOGENESIS OF SEVERE

ANGIOTENSIN II-SALT HYPERTENSION

Mahesh Mistry and Alberto Nasjletti[*]

Department of Pharmacology, University of Tennessee, Memphis, TN 38163 and [*]Department of Pharmacology, New York Medical College, Valhalla, NY 10595

Increased urinary excretion of TXB$_2$ and/or elevated production of TXB$_2$ by vascular and renal structures accompany the development of hypertension in spontaneously hypertensive rats (1,2), rats with renal ablation hypertension (3), Dahl salt-sensitive hypertensive rats (4), and 2-kidney 1-clip hypertensive rats (5). Since TXA$_2$, the precursor of TXB$_2$, produces vasoconstriction, the possibility arises that TXA$_2$ contributes to the pathogenesis of hypertension and associated vascular and renal disturbances in models of hypertension featuring augmentation of TXA$_2$ synthesis. In agreement with this notion, it has been reported that inhibitors of thromboxane synthetase lower blood pressure in spontaneously hypertensive rats (1) and in rats with renal ablation hypertension (3), associated with improvement of renal hemodynamic and excretory functions (1,3).

In saline-drinking rats, chronic infusion of angiotensin II (AII) causes severe hypertension accompanied by increased urinary excretion and renal synthesis of TXB$_2$ (6). This paper reviews the results of experiments aimed at examining the contribution of TXA$_2$ to high blood pressure and associated abnormalities of renal function in rats with AII-salt hypertension.

EFFECT OF CHRONIC AII INFUSION ON BLOOD PRESSURE AND
VASCULAR AND RENAL INDICES OF TXA$_2$ PRODUCTION

In rats drinking 1% NaCl, AII infused intraperitoneally at 125 ng/min causes progressive elevation of systolic blood pressure to levels in excess of 200 mmHg after 8 days (6). Rats with AII-salt hypertension of 12 days duration exhibit decreased renal blood flow and glomerular filtration rate, severe proteinuria and fibrinoid necrosis of small arteries in the kidney, heart and intestine. Table 1 contrasts the values of urinary TXB$_2$ excretion, and of net release of TXB$_2$ from rings of aorta and renal cortex slices incubated in Krebs solution, in normotensive rats and in rats with AII-salt hypertension of 12 days duration. Relative to the data in water-drinking rats without AII infusion, the urinary excretion of TXB_2 and the release of TXB_2 from aortic rings and renal cortex slices were significantly increased in AII-salt hypertensive rats. Collectively, these observations raise the possibility that augmentation of TXA_2 synthesis contributes to the pathogenesis of hypertension.

TABLE 1. Systolic blood pressure, urinary excretion of TXB_2 and net release of TXB_2 from rings of aorta and slices of renal cortex incubated in Krebs solution for 20 minutes.

Expmtl. Group	Blood Pressure (mmHg)	Urinary TXB_2 (ng/day)	TXB Release (pg/mg)	
			Renal Cortex	Aorta
Water-drinking Vehicle Infusion	129±3	5.4±0.9	71.3±6.7	28.8±2.9
Saline-drinking AII Infusion	217±12*	25.4±2.1*	121.1±4.4*	115.8±12.8*

Values are the mean±SE of observations in saline-drinking rats infused with angiotensin II (AII; 125 ng/min, ip, N=8), and in water-drinking rats infused with vehicle only (N=8), for 12 days. * indicates $P < 0.05$.

INFLUENCE OF TXA_2 ON BLOOD PRESSURE AND RENAL FUNCTION IN AII-SALT HYPERTENSIVE RATS

If augmentation of TXA_2 production by vascular and renal structures contributes to the pathogenesis of high blood pressure and depressed renal hemodynamics in rats with AII-salt hypertension, treatment of the hypertensive animals with thromboxane synthesis inhibitors or receptor blockers may be expected to lower blood pressure and improve renal blood flow. Accordingly, we investigated in rats with AII-salt hypertension of 12 days duration the effects on blood pressure and renal function of intravenous administration of UK38,485 (30 mg/kg followed by 15 mg/kg/h infusion) to inhibit thromboxane synthetase, or of SQ29,548 (5 mg/kg bolus followed by infusion at 5 mg/kg/h) to block TXA_2 receptors (6). One day prior to the experiment, the animals were instrumented with femoral arterial and venous cannulas to measure blood pressure and to infuse drugs, respectively, and with a bladder cannula for urine collection. Renal blood flow was calculated from the clearance of PAH and the hematocrit.

As shown in table 2, treatment with UK38,485 affected neither blood pressure nor renal blood flow, urine flow or the excretion of sodium and potassium. Confirming the effectiveness of UK38,485 to inhibit TXA_2 synthesis, we found that the concen tration of serum TXB_2 in AII salt hypertensive rats treated with UK38,485 was only 1.4% of the serum TXB_2 concentration in hypertensive rats without UK38,485 treatment. Contrasting with the lack of effect of UK38,485 on blood pressure and renal function in rats with AII-salt hypertension, the administration of SQ29,548 caused blood pressure to fall from 199±4 mmHg to 165±5 mmHg (P<0.05), associated with maintenance of renal blood flow due to reduction of renal vascular resistance, and with lowering of urine flow. In normal rats, treatment with SQ29,548 did not affect blood pressure or renal function but greatly inhibited the pressor effect of U46,619, a stable analogue of PGH_2 which interacts with the TXA_2 receptor (6). Accordingly, the effects of SQ29,548 in decreasing blood pressure and renal vascular resistance in AII-salt hypertensive rats may be attributed to blockade of the vascular actions of one or more endogenous pressor eicosanoids including TXA_2 and the prostaglandin endoperoxides. If so, pressor eicosanoids may be contributory factors in the pathogenesis of AII-salt hypertension in rats. That treatment with an inhibitor of thromboxane synthetase did not reduce blood pressure in rats with AII-salt hypertension does not exclude TXA_2 from playing such a role, as the functional consequence of a reduction in TXA_2 due to inhibition of TXA_2 synthesis may be obscured by the functional consequence of increased levels of prostaglandin endoperoxides which are capable of eliciting vasoconstriction.

TABLE 2. Effects of UK38,485 and SQ29,548 on renal function and mean arterial pressure in awake rats with AII-salt hypertension of 12 days duration.

Parameter	Control	UK38,485	Control	SQ29,548
Blood Pres. (mmHg)	185±4	181±6	199±4	165±5*
Renal Blood Flow (ml/min/100g BW)	2.39±0.26	2.13±0.13	2.14±0.09	2.17±0.22
Urine Flow (μl/min)	41±12	38±10	60±10	37±7*
Na Excretion (μEq/min)	5.6±1.6	5.4±1.3	10.2±1.3	7.3±1.5
K Excretion	1.0±0.2	1.2±0.1	1.2±0.1	1.1±0.1

Values are the mean ± SE of 6-7 experiments. For each experiment, the data from three consecutive clearance periods were averaged both before and during drug treatment. * indicates P<0.0t relative to control. UK38,485 was given as a 30 mg/kg bolus followed by iv infusion at 15 mg/kg/h; SQ29,548 was given as a 5 mg/kg bolus followed by iv infusion at 5 mg/kg/h.

SUMMARY AND CONCLUSION

Urinary TXB_2 excretion and the release of TXB_2 from vascular and renal cortical tissues are increased in rats with severe AII-salt hypertension. Treatment with an inhibitor of TXA_2 synthesis did not change the blood pressure of normotensive or of AII-salt hypertensive rats. Treatment with SQ29,548, a TXA_2 receptor antagonist, caused reduction of blood pressure and renal vascular resistance in AII-salt hypertensive but not in normotensive rats. We conclude that the SQ29,548-induced lowering of blood pressure and renal vascular resistance in AII-salt hypertensive rats is the result of blockade of the vascular actions of one or more pressor eicosanoids including TXA_2 and the prostaglandin endoperoxides. A corollary of this conclusion is that pressor eicosanoids may be contributory factors in the pathogenesis of severe AII-salt hypertension in rats.

ACKNOWLEDGEMENTS

Supported by USPHS Grants HL36670.

REFERENCES

1. Purkerson ML, Martin KJ, Kissane JM, et al. Hypertension 1986; 8:1113-1120

2. Konieczkowski M, Dunn MJ, Stork JE, et al. Hypertension 1983; 6:446-452

3. Purkerson ML, Joist JH, Yates J, et al. Proc Natl Acad Sci USA 1985; 82:193-197

4. Uehara Y, Tobian L, Iwai J, et al. Prostaglandins 1987; 33:727-738

5. Stahl RAK, Helmchen U, Paravocini M, et al. Am J Physiol 1984; 247:F975-F981

6. Mistry M, Nasjletti A Hypertension 1988; In press

Advances in Prostaglandin, Thromboxane, and Leukotriene Research, Vol. 19, edited by B. Samuelsson, P. Y.-K. Wong, and F. F. Sun, Raven Press, Ltd., New York ©1989.

Role of eicosanoids in regulation of vascular resistance

J. C. Frölich and U. Förstermann

Department of Clinical Pharmacology, Hannover Medical School, P.O. Box 610180, D-3000 Hannover 61, Germany, FRG

A. Introduction

There are powerful vasodilators (PGI_2, PGE_2) and vasoconstrictors (TxA_2, LTC_4) amongst the eicosanoids. This evidence stems from pharmacological studies in which eicosanoids were administered to whole animals, isolated vascular beds or isolated blood vessels. Furthermore, inhibitors of the action of some eicosanoids (LT-antagonists, TxA_2-antagonists) or of their synthesis (TxA_2-synthesis inhibitors) have shown, that they play a measurable and often clinically relevant role in the regulation of peripheral resistance. Results of studies obtained with inhibitors of cyclooxygenase are somewhat more difficult to interpret as they inhibit both vasoconstrictor as well as vasodilator eicosanoids. The picture is further complicated by the observation that in addition to direct vascular effects indirect effects of eicosanoids influence vascular resistance as eicosanoids are involved in the regulation of release of renin (1) and probably to a clinically less important degree of catecholamines. - The following discussion focusses on the local events as the indirect effects have been discussed recently (1, 2, 3). In addition this review forges a connection between the other important mediator of vascular tone, endothelial derived relaxing factor (EDRF), and shows that there are not only functional similarities between vasodilator eicosanoids and EDRF but that there may be biochemical links as well.

B. Production of eicosanoids and EDRF in the vascular wall

PGI_2 is the major cyclo-oxygenase product formed in large conduit arteries (4). Endothelial cells represent the main source of this prostaglandin, the smooth muscle layer has an about 10-times lower capacity to synthesize PGI_2 (5). Thus the intima produces about 40% of the total vascular PGI_2, although it only represents 5% of the vascular mass. This is due the higher activity of PGH synthase in endothelial cells, whereas 6 (9) oxycyclase activities were found to be the same in endothelial and smooth muscle cells (6). Nevertheless, synthesis of PGI_2 in smooth-muscle cells is far from being irrelevant. For example, in some rabbit arteries, bradykinin-induced relaxation are exclusively mediated by PGI_2 (and PGE_2) generated in subendothelial structures (7). Vascular tissue can also generate other prostaglandins, especially PGE_2 (8). It is interesting to note that this PGE_2 production increases relative to PGI_2 as vessel diameter decreases (9). Indeed, Gerritsen and colleagues have demonstrated that microvascular endothelial cells from certain areas are capable of releasing PGE_2 in excess of PGI_2 (9). Another, equally important vasodilator produced by endothelial cells is EDRF (10). EDRF is formed in all types of endothelial cells investigated so far, albeit in different quantities. During recent years, many vasodilators have been found to exert their relaxing action via EDRF. These compounds include acetylcholine, adenine nucleotides, substance P and various other peptides, histamine and thrombin (10). In general, the same compounds also enhance the production of PGI_2 in the vascular wall. Even compounds like the phospholipase activator, melittin, and the acyl-coenzyme A: lysolecithin acyltransferase inhibitor, thimerosal, stimulate the production of both PGI_2 and EDRF (11, 12). Interestingly, however, endothelial PGI_2 seems to play only a minor role in endothelium-dependent vasodilation, although its production is increased in parallel with EDRF (7). Also peptido-leukotrienes can be formed in vascular tissue under certain conditions (13, 14). The greatest amounts were released by adventitial tissue (13) whereas endothelial cell have not been reported to produce significant quantities of leukotrienes.

C. Effect of eicosanoids and EDRF on blood vessels

PGI_2, the major eicosanoid formed in large arteries, is generally considered a vasodilator (4). However, there are some exceptions to this rule, e. g. porcine coronary artery or rabbit femoral artery are slightly constricted by PGI_2. Also PGE_2, which is equally potent or even more potent than PGI_2 in reducing vascular resistance in vivo (15) is a constrictor in some blood vessels, such as human and bovine coronary arteries and rabbit femoral artery (8, 16). Peptido-leukotrienes are generally found to have vasoconstrictor properties in most isolated arteries (17). When administered to whole animals in vivo, they produce complicated bi- and triphasic blood pressure responses that involve reflex components and components mediated by cyclooxygenase products (17). LTC_4 and LTB_4, however, have been found to increase flow in the renal vascular bed of dogs (18) and, more recently, endothelium-dependent relaxation to LTD_4 has been demonstrated in canine renal and mesenteric arteries (19). In contrast to these somewhat heterogeneous vascular effects of the eicosanoids, EDRF is a vasodilator in all vascular tissues tested so far. The factor relaxes arteries as well as veins (20), and recently we and others have found that it is also active in the microvasculature (21, 22). Thus, EDRF could play an important role in the regulation of peripheral resistance, regional blood flow and blood pressure.

D. Inhibitors of eicosanoid synthesis and eicosanoid antagonists

a) Cyclooxygenase inhibitors block both vasodilator and vasoconstrictor eicosanoids. Nevertheless, most examples demonstrate enhanced vasoconstriction following cyclooxygenase inhibition. Most of these studies involve pathophysiological models such as post-traumatic states (23) in which inhibition of cyclooxygenase causes a significant increase in blood pressure due to a vasoconstrictor effect. In man, intravenous bolus administration of indomethacin also resulted in a 20% increase of total peripheral resistance in normal volunteers undergoing cardiac catheterization mainly due to increases in renal and splanchnic resistance (24). It is uncertain whether the magnitude of this increase reflects a change from true base line values or is of such impressive dimensions because cardiac catheterization induces a powerful stress with extremely elevated catecholamine levels (unpublished observation). Under truly basal conditions no effects on renal blood flow were observed in dog and man after inhibition of cyclooxygenase (25, 26). In contrast, under conditions of vasoconstrictor influence by angiotensin II, sodium depletion (27) or stress (23) PG synthesis is elevated and a reduction of renal blood flow by cyclooxygenase inhibition becomes apparent.

b) Thromboxane synthesis inhibitors

The dilemma posed by the non-specificity of cyclooxygenase inhibition is partially overcome by the recent development of specific thromboxane synthesis inhibitors. These substances would appear to provide the opportunity to test the hypothesis that certain disease states associated with enhanced vascular resistance are caused by vasoconstrictor action of thromboxane A_2. Indeed, a number of studies have shown that substances such as OKY1581, OKY046 or dazoxiben can ameliorate global myocardial ischemia (28), reduce infarct size (29), decrease vasospasticity in variant angina (30) or pulmonary hypertension during dialysis (31). On first sight these results might indicate that abolition of the vasoconstriction by thromboxane A_2 is the most proximal cause of there effects. On the other hand, inhibition of thromboxane synthesis has been claimed to lead to enhanced prostacyclin synthesis (32) which could by itself decrease vascular tone. Furthermore, inhibition of platelet aggregation might be an important feature and the mere mechanical factor possibly coupled with a decreased release of platelet derived vasoactive substances such as 5-hydroxytryptamine could significantly contribute to the observed effects.

We have recently studied this complex interaction between platelets and the vascular wall in the human coronary artery and discovered yet another facet (33). Epicardial human coronary arteries suspended in Krebs solution were exposed to washed human platelets. On aggregation these platelets caused vasodilation of intact arteries, but slight constriction when the endothelium was removed. The thromboxane synthesis inhibitor dazmegrel caused only modestly increased vasodilation in endothelium-intact arteries, even though U44069, a thromboxane A_2 analog, caused powerful contractions. This discrepancy between the lack of effect of a thromboxane synthesis inhibitor and the thromboxane analog was puzzling as during platelet aggregation large amounts of thromboxane A_2 were synthesized. Interestingly, dazmegrel inhibited this synthesis by more than 98%, but increased the synthesis of PGE_2 and $PGF_{2\alpha}$ by 79-fold and 31-fold, respectively. This is probably due to enhanced availability of the precursor endoperoxides. We therefore studied the effects of these two prostaglandins on vascular tone of human coronary arteries. Surprisingly, PGE_2 was found to contract these blood vessels. In effect thromboxane synthesis inhibition while abolishing thromboxane enhances concentrations of three cyclooxygenase dependent coronary vasoconstrictors: PGH_2, $PGF_{2\alpha}$ and PGE_2. These findings point to the limitations that are inherent in the approach to influence vascular tone by thromboxane synthesis inhibition.

c) Thromboxane A_2-receptor blockers

These drugs have the advantage over thromboxane synthetase inhibitors of leaving the synthesis of other prostanoids unaffected. They have been shown to have no effect on basal blood pressure but can prolong bleeding time and platelet aggregation to arachidonic acid, collagen and the thromboxane mimetics U46619 and U44069 (34, 35). Interestingly BM13177 and other thromboxane receptor blockers also block $PGF_{2\alpha}$-induced contractions of vascular smooth muscle. The thromboxane receptor antagonists BM13177 and BM13505 have been shown to reduce ischemic damage in experimental myocardial infarction (36). However, it is uncertain to what degree these effects are related to vascular and platelet effects, respectively.

d) Leukotrienes

More recently, the effects of leukotrienes (LT) on vascular tone have been studied. We have investigated the effect of LTC_4 on the isolated perfused kidney of the rat (37). LTC_4 caused a rapid increase in renal vascular resistance which lasted for over 60 min in a recirculating system and was blocked by the peptidoleukotriene receptor blocker FPL55712. When LTC_4 was given in a single-pass perfusion its vasoconstrictor effect lasted for only a few minutes, suggesting that in the recirculating system an active metabolite is formed. The effect of LTC_4 and/or its metabolite appeared to be independent of thromboxane or another cyclooxygenase product because neither OKY1581, a specific thromboxane synthetase inhibitor nor indomethacine changed the response to LTC_4. We found the potency of LTC_4 as compared to angiotensin II or norepinephrine much lower (1000 to 2000 resp. 10-20-fold).

We have further investigated the effect of i.v. bolus injections of LTB_4, LTC_4 and LTD_4 in the unaenesthetized freely moving rat (38, 39, 40). While LTB_4 showed no vascular effects in doses up to 51 nmole/kg LTC_4 and LTD_4 caused a dose dependent increase in blood pressure (BP) and decreased renal blood flow (RBF). Verapamil and the peptido-LT antgonist FPL55712 abolished the increase in BP while saralasine and indomethacine had no effect. However, under basal conditions, FPL55712 had no effect on BP or RBF suggesting that there is no basal release of peptidoleukotrienes that is high enough to affect these two parameters.

Nevertheless, synthesis of LTC_4, LTD_4 and LTE_4 has been shown to occur in various blood vessels including coronary arteries of dog, cat and man (13, 14, 41) showing that under some conditions LTC_4/D_4 can be released. Furthermore, the possibility of cells of the circulating blood migrating into vascular tissue has to be considered as a source of vasoconstrictor LTs. It is unclear at present whether in vivo synthesis of LTC_4/D_4 occurs at a rate that influences vascular resistance in man in vivo.

References

1. Frölich, J.C., Whorton, A.R., Walker, L., Smigel, M., Oates, J.A., France, R., Hollifield, J.W., Data, J.L., Gerber, J.G., Nies, A.S., Williams, W., Robertson, C.L.: Proceedings of the 7th Intern. Congress of Nephrology, Montreal (1978), Karger, Basel (1978), pp. 107-114
2. Hedquist, P.: Ann. Rev. Pharmacol. Toxicol. 17: 259-279, 1977
3. Frölich, J.C., Filep, J., Yoshizawa, M., Förstermann, U., Fejes-Toth, G.: Advances in Prostaglandin, Thromboxane and Leukotriene Research, Vol. 15 (ed. by. Y. Hayaishi and S. Yamamoto), Raven Press, New York, 1985, pp. 455-460
4. Moncada, S., Vane, J.R.: Pharmacol. Rev. 3: 293-331, 1979
5. Moncada, S., Herman, A.G., Higgs, E.A., Vane, J.R.: Thromb. Res. 11: 323-344, 1977
6. DeWitt, D.L., Day, J.S., Sonnenburg, W.K., Smith, W.L.: J. Clin. Invest. 72: 1882-1888, 1983
7. Förstermann, U., Hertting, G., Neufang, B.: Br. J. Pharmac. 87: 521-532, 1987
8. Förstermann, U., Hertting, G., Neufang, B.: Br. J. Pharmac. 81: 623-630, 1984
9. Gerritsen, M.E.: Biochem. Pharmacol. 36: 2701-2711, 1987
10. Furchgott, R.F.: Ann. Rev. Pharmacol. Toxicol. 24: 175-197, 1984
11. Förstermann, U., Neufang, B.: Am. J. Physiol. 249: H24-H19, 1985
12. Förstermann, U., Goppelt-Strübe, M., Frölich, J.C., Busse, R.: J. Pharmacol. Exp. Ther. 238: 352-359, 1986
13. Piper, P.J., Letts, L.G., Galton, S.A.: Prostaglandins 25: 591-599, 1983
14. Piomelli, D., Feinmark, S.J., Cannon, P.J.: J. Pharmacol. Exp. Ther. 241: 763-770, 1987
15. Förstermann, U., Neufang, B.: J. Pharm. Pharmacol. 35: 724-728, 1983
16. Needleman, P., Kulkarni, P.S., Raz, A.: Science 195: 409-411, 1977
17. Piper, P.J.: Physiol. Rev. 64: 744-761, 1984
18. Feigen, L.P.: J. Pharmacol. Exp. Ther. 225: 682-687, 1983
19. Secrest, R.J., Olsen, E.J., Chapnick, B.M.: Circ. Res. 57: 323-329, 1985
20. Ignarro, L.J., Byrns, R.E., Wood, K.S.: Circ. Res. 60: 82-92, 1987
21. Förstermann, U., Dudel, C., Frölich, J.C.: J. Pharmacol. Exp. Ther. 243: 1055-1061, 1987

22. Pohl, U., Dézsi, L., Simon, B., Busse, R.: Am. J. Physiol. 253: H234-H239, 1987
23. Terragno, N.A., Terragno, D.A., McGiff, J.C.: Circ. Res. 40: 590-595, 1977
24. Nowak, J, Wennmalm, A.: Acta Physiol. Scand. 102: 484-491, 1978
25. Fejes-Toth, G., Fekete, A., Walter, J.: Pfluegers Arch. 376: 67-72, 1978
26. Donker, A.J.M., Arisz, L., Brentjens, J.R.H., van der Hem, G.K., Hollemans, H.J.G.: Nephron. 17: 288-296, 1976
27. Rosenkranz, B., Wilson, T.W., Seyberth, H., Frölich, J.C.: Proc. Eight Int. Congress of Nephrology, Athen (1981), Karger, Basel, pp. 1045-1052
28. Lefer, A.M., Messenger, M., Okamatsu, S.: Naunyn-Schmiedeberg's Arch. Pharmacol. 321: 130-134, 1982
29. Burke, S.E., Lefer, A.M., Smith, G.M., Smith, J.B.: Br. J. Clin. Pharmac. 15: 97S-101S, 1983
30. Ohmori, M., Kuzuya, T., Kodama, K., Nanto, S., Kamada, T., Tada, M.: Jap. Circ. J. 51: 459-502, 1987
31. Cheung, A.K., Baranowski, R.L., Wayman, A.L.: Kidney Int. 31: 1072-1079, 1987
32. Yui, Y., Hattori, R., Takatsu, Y., Nakajima, H., Wakabayashi, A., Kawai, C., Kayama, N., Hiraku, S., Inagawa, T., Tsubojima, M.: Therapy and Prevention Thrombosis 70: 599-605, 1984
33. Förstermann, U., Mügge, A., Bode, S.M., Frölich, J.C.: Circ. Res. 62: 185-190, 1988
34. Bertelé, V., Falanga, A., Tomasiak, M., Dejana, E., Cerletti, C., de Gaetano, G.: Science 220: 517-519, 1983
35. Graesele, P., Deckmyn, H., Arnout, J., Lemmens, J., Janssens, W., Vermylen, J.: Lancet I: 991-994, 1984
36. Brezinski, M.E., Yanigisawa, A., Davins, H., Lefer, A.M.: Am. Heart J. 110: 1161-1167, 1985
37. Frölich, J.C., Yoshizawa, M.: Br. J. Pharmac. 92: 311-318, 1987
38. Fejes-Toth, G., Naray-Fejes-Toth, A., Ratge, D., Frölich, J.C.: Hypertension 6: 926-930, 1984
39. Filep, J., Rigter, B., Frölich, J.C.: Am. J. Physiol. 18: F739-F744, 1985
40. Filep, J., Földes-Filep, E., Frölich, J.C.: Br. J. Pharmac. 90: 431-439, 1987
41. Piper, P.J., Galton, S.A.: Prostaglandins 28: 905-914, 1984

Advances in Prostaglandin, Thromboxane, and Leukotriene Research, Vol. 19, edited by B. Samuelsson, P. Y.-K. Wong, and F. F. Sun, Raven Press, Ltd., New York ©1989.

THE ROLES OF RENAL PROSTAGLANDIN IN THE REGULATORY MECHANISM OF RENAL EXCRETORY FUNCTION AND BLOOD PRESSURE IN HYPERTENSION

Keishi Abe[1], Makito Sato[2], Kazuhisa Takeuchi[2], Kazuo Tsunoda[2], Minoru Yasujima[2] and Kaoru Yoshinaga[2].

[1]Department of Clinical Biology and Hormonal Regulation and [2]The Second Department of Internal Medicine, Tohoku University School of Medicine, Sendai 980, Japan.

The kidney is known to be involved in the regulation of blood pressure through the renin-angiotensin system and renal antihypertensive mechanism, including renal excretory function and renal vasodepressor hormones such as renal prostaglandin (PG) and kallikrein-kinin system.[1] The renal medulla and papilla are rich sources of prostaglandin synthetases. Recent studies using microdissected nephron segments and cultured renal cells have shown the localization in the generation of PGE_2, $PGF_{2\alpha}$, PGI_2, and thromboxane (TX) A_2 in the kidney.[2]-[7] Both PGE_2 and PGI_2 are vasodilatory substances thought to be involved in the regulation of blood pressure through peripheral arterial dilatation and water-sodium excretion in the kidney,[5]-[7] while TXA_2 is a vasoconstrictive and antidiuretic substance. Since non-steroidal antiinflammatory drugs (NSAIDs) inhibit PG synthesis in the kidney and in other organs via cyclooxygenase suppression, it should be considered that these drugs may affect renal function and blood pressure regulation in human and in animals.[8]-[11] The present study was done to investigate the roles of renal prostaglandin and kallikrein-kinin systems in the regulatory mechanisms of renal excretory function and blood pressure.

I. Effects of NSAIDs on PG generation in rat cultured cells.

In this experiment, PG was measured in rat renal glomerular mesangial cells, in renal papillary collecting tubule cells and in vascular smooth muscle cells before and after the administration of NSAIDs to investigate the role of PGs in the regulation of renal function and blood pressure. Renal glomerular mesangial cells, renal papillary collecting tubule cells and vascular smooth muscle cells of mesenteric artery were isolated from Sprague-Dawley rat (weight: 150-200 g) and were cultured in multiwell tissue culture plates.[12],[13] Cells were incubated in minimum essential medium (MEM) (Gibco Lab., Ohio, USA) for 30 minutes at 37 °C in an atmosphere of

5% CO_2–95% air in the absence or presence of aspirin (Sigma Chemical, St. Louis, USA), ibuprofen (Kaken Pharmaceutical Co., Tokyo, Japan), tiaprofenic acid (Roussel Medica Co., Tokyo, Japan), indomethacin or sulindac (sulfoxide) (both Banyu Pharmaceutical Co., Tokyo, Japan) at concentrations from 3.3×10^{-5} to 3.3×10^{-4}M, respectively. 6-keto-$PGF_{1\alpha}$ (a main hydrolysis product of PGI_2) or PGE_2 which was released into the media was measured by direct radioimmunoassay.

Main PG generated in vascular smooth muscle cells was PGI_2 and that in mesangial cells and collecting tubule cells was PGE_2. In all cells examined, aspirin, ibuprofen, tiaprofenic acid and indomethacin inhibited both basal and AA-stimulated 6-keto-$PGF_{1\alpha}$ synthesis in a dose dependent manner. Although sulindac inhibited both basal and AA-stimulated PGE_2 synthesis in renal papillary collecting tubule cells, it failed to inhibit basal 6-keto-$PGF_{1\alpha}$ synthesis in vascular smooth muscle cells and AA-stimulated PGE_2 synthesis in glomerular mesangial cells. Sulindac only at concentrations 10^{-4} and 3.3×10^{-4}M inhibited AA-stimulated 6-keto-$PGF_{1\alpha}$ synthesis in vascular smooth muscle cells and basal PGE_2 synthesis in glomerular mesangial cells. In glomerular mesangial cells and papillary collecting tubule cells, the stronger were the inhibitory effects of NSAIDs in the third incubation period, the higher were the values of AA-stimulated PGE_2 at the recovery period. In all cells examined, the order of potency for NSAIDs to inhibit PG synthesis was tiaprofenic acid, indomethacin > aspirin, ibuprofen > sulindac.

NSAIDs are well known to reduce glomerular filtration rate (GFR) in normal volunteers with volume depletion and in patients with renal diseases. The present study showed that PGE_2 was generated in renal glomerular mesangial cells and in renal papillary collecting tubule cells, and that NSAIDs besides sulindac inhibited PGE_2 synthesis in both cells, indicating that PGE_2 in renal glomerular mesangial cells is involved in the regulation of glomerular filtration and renal tubular function and that sulindac is renal sparing.

II. Effects of NSAIDs on renal function

In this study, changes in renal excretory function and urinary PGE_2 excretion were examined before and after the administration of sulindac and diclofenac sodium in patients with chronic glomerular diseases. Seven patients were hospitalized and given regular diet containing 10 g/day of salt. After 3 days of control period, sulindac (300 mg/day) was given for a week. Then it was withdrawn and diclofenac sodium (50 mg/day) was given for a week. Thus, effect of sulindac was compared with that of diclofenac sodium. Plasma samples and 24 hour's urine were collected at the end of control period and on days 3 and 7 of each medication period. Urine volume, urinary excretion of electrolytes and serum creatinine were not changed. Plasma renin activity (PRA) was reduced by sulindac on day 7 and by diclofenac sodium on days 3 and 7. Sulindac reduced urinary PGE excretion on day 7, while diclofenac sodium reduced it on day 3, but not significantly on day 7. Endogenous creatinine clearance was not decreased by sulindac, while it was decreased by diclofenac sodium on day 7 significantly. Sulindac did not affect urinary protein excretion, while diclofenac sodium decreased it.

III. Interactions among renal prostaglandins, kallikrein-kinin and renin-angiotensin systems in the pathogenesis of essential hypertension.

In this study, changes in blood pressure, urinary excretion of PGE_2 and sodium, and plasma angiotensin II concentration were examined before and after the administration of NSAIDs and captopril in patients with essential hypertension to investigate the interactions among renal PGs, kallikrein-kinin and renin-angiotensin systems in the pathogenesis of essential hypertension. Nine patients with essential hypertension were included in this study. Antihypertensive medication had been withdrawn for at least 2 weeks before the study. All patients were given a regular diet containing 10 g/day of sodium. After 5 days of a normal sodium diet, sodium intake was reduced to 5 g/day and maintained up to the end of the study. After 5 days of a low-sodium diet, indomethacin was given for 3 days (75 mg/day for the initial 2 days and 150 mg/day on the final day) and then withdrawn. After 5 day of recovery period, captopril was given for 4 days (37.5 mg/day for the initial 2 days and 75 mg/day for the subsequent 2 days). It was followed by the combined administration of captopril (75 mg/day) and indomethacin (150 mg/day) for 3 days. The sampling of blood was done in the morning after overnight fasting, and 24-hr urine was collected on the final day of each period.

Blood pressure was significantly lowered after dietary sodium deprivation. In contrast, it was notably elevated after the administration of indomethacin. Captopril lowered blood pressure as compared with dietary sodium deprivation alone. However, the combined administration of indomethacin with captopril induced a significant rise in blood pressure and consequently abolishd the hypotensive effect of captopril. Urinary excretion of sodium and PGE_2 was significantly decreased after the administration of indomethacin, while it was significantly increased after the administration of captopril. Plasma angiotensin II concentration was significantly decreased both after the administration of indomethacin and of captopril.

There was a negative correlation between changes in blood pressure and in urinary sodium excretion after the administration of indomethacin and of captopril. There was also a negative correlation between changes in blood pressure and in urinary excretion of PGE2 after the administration of indomethacin and of captopril. A reversed relation of changes in mean blood pressure and plasma angiotensin II concentraiton was found between the administrations of indomethacin and of captopril. There was a negative correlation between changes in blood pressure and plasma angiotensin II concentration after the administration of indomethacin despite a positive correlation after that of captopril.

The present study has clearly demonstrated that the inhibition of prostaglandin generation with indomethacin induced a significant rise in blood pressure associated with singificant decreases in urianry excretion of PGE and sodium. These data indicate that decreased prostaglandin generation in the nephron can elevate blood pressure by means of sodium retention caused by reduced renal excretory function, suggesting the involvement of renal tubular PGE2 in the regulation of blood pressure and in the pathogenesis of hypertension in human with defective renal prostaglandin synthesis.

Acknowledgement

We are grateful to Michiko Okamoto, Keiko Shiraishi and Naeko Nakagawa for excellent technical assistance and Junko Okazaki for secretarial assistance. This work was supported by a Research Grant for Cardiovascular Disease (61-A-1) from the Ministry of Health and Welfare and by a Grant-in-Aid (62870011) from the Ministry of Education, Science and Culture, Japan.

References

1) Abe, K.: The kinins and prostaglandins in hypertension, Clin. Endocrinol. Metab. 10, 577 (1981).

2) Schlondorff, D. et al.: Prostaglandin synthesis by isolated rat glomeruli: effect of angiotensin II. Am. J. Physiol. 249, F486 (1980).

3) Dunn, M. J. et al.: Characterization of prostaglandin production in tissue culture of rat renal medullary cells. Prostaglandins, 12, 37 (1976).

4) Petrulis, A. et al.: Prostaglandin and thromboxane

synthesis by rat glomerular epithelial cells. Kidney Int. 20, 469 (1981).

5) Abe, K. et al.: Renal kallikrein-kinin: Its relation to renal prostaglandins and renin-angiotensin-aldosterone in man. Kidney Int. 19, 869 (1981).

6) Stokes, J. B. et al.: Inhibition of sodium transport by prostaglandin E_2 across the isolated, perfused rabbit collecting tubule. J. Clin. Invest. 59, 1099 (1977).

7) Iino, Y. et al.: Influence of prostacyclin (PGI_2) on transepithelial potential difference (PD) in isolated perfused rabbit cortical collecting tubule (CCT). Kidney Int. 16, 822 (1979).

8) Ciabattoni, G. et al.: Renal effects of anti-inflammatory drugs, Eur. J. Rheum. Inflam. 31, 210 (1980).

9) Berg, K. J. et al.: Acute renal effects of sulindac and indomethacin in chronic renal failure. Clin. Pharmacol. Ther. 37, 447 (1985).

10) Kramer, H. J., et al.: Prostaglandins and renal sodium excretion in man: Prostaglandins and Membrane ion transport. edited by P. Braquet et al., Raven Press, New York, 253 (1984).

11) Dibona, G. F.: Prostaglandins and nonsteroidal antiinflammatory drugs. Effects on renal hemodynamics. Am. J. Med. 80(1A):12, (1986).

12) Sato, M., et al.: Atrial natriuretic factor and cyclic guanosine 3', 5'-monophosphate in vascular smooth muscle. Hypertension, 8, 762 (1986).

13) Scharschmidt, L. et al.: Prostaglandin synthesis by rat glomerular mesangial cells in culture. J. Clin. Invest. 71, 1756 (1983).

*Advances in Prostaglandin, Thromboxane, and
Leukotriene Research*, Vol. 19, edited by
B. Samuelsson, P. Y.-K. Wong, and F. F. Sun,
Raven Press, Ltd., New York ©1989.

SYNTHESIS OF LEUKOTRIENES C_4, D_4, E_4 AND 20-CARBOXY-B_4 BY THE ISOLATED PERFUSED KIDNEY

J.P. Merab[*], S.J. Feinmark[*+] and P.J. Cannon[*]

Departments of Medicine[*] and Pharmacology[+],
Columbia University, New York, New York, USA

The peptide-containing leukotrienes (LT) are potent effectors in the kidney where they induce the constriction of efferent arterioles and of mesangial cells. The net hemodynamic result produced by these activities is a fall in the glomerular filtration rate (1). While circulating leukocytes are considered to be a major source of leukotriene production, several recent reports provide evidence for the synthesis of leukotrienes in the kidney (2,3). We describe studies of the synthesis and metabolism of leukotrienes and report the characterization of 20-carboxy-LTB_4 as a major renal metabolite along with LTC_4, LTD_4 and LTE_4.

METHODS

Kidneys were isolated from New Zealand white rabbits and perfused according to the method of De Mello and Maack (4). The perfusate consisted of Krebs-Henseleit buffer with added bovine serum albumin (7.5%), glucose (0.1%), creatinine (0.05%) and amino acids. The perfusate was continuously gassed with 95% O_2/5% CO_2. Kidneys were perfused until free of blood and then equilibrated for 25-30 min by recirculation with fresh perfusate. At the end of the equilibration period, the test agent was injected intra-arterially and venous effluent was collected into methanol (1:3; v/v). Tracer amounts of [^{3}H]LTC_4 were added as an internal standard. The protein precipitate was removed by filtration and the filtrate was evaporated under vacuum. After reconstitution with 20 ml of water the pH was adjusted to 11 with sodium hydroxide and the sample was incubated at 37°C for 30 min. The sample was then acidified to pH 5.8 and a solid phase extraction was performed using an Alltech Maxi-Clean C18 cartridge. The lipid extract was fractionated by reversed-phase HPLC and LT were identified by UV spectrometry using a diode array detector (5). LTC_4 and LTD_4 were quantified by enzyme immunoassay.

RESULTS AND DISCUSSION

Isolated rabbit kidneys (n=3) were perfused with [^{3}H]arachidonic acid for 30 minutes and then washed to remove unincorporated label. After the prelabelling period, A23187 was injected intra-arterially. Lipids extracted from the venous effluent were fractionated by reversed-phase HPLC and radioactivity in the effluent was analyzed by liquid scintillation counting. This analysis demonstrated the release of several radioactive products from the kidney. Peaks were detected at the retention times of standard LTC_4 and LTD_4. In addition, a broad early peak of radioactivity was observed which probably contained 20-carboxy-LTB_4, as well as other unidentified components. Of note, in none of these experiments was a peak identified at the retention time of LTB_4.

In order to confirm that the radioactive peaks detected in the first series of experiments were actually LT, kidneys were perfused with [^{3}H]LTA_4. HPLC analysis of the lipids extracted from the venous effluent demonstrated the presence of radiolabelled products at the retention times of 20-carboxy-LTB_4, LTC_4 and the nonenzymatic LTB_4 isomers (which obscure the presence of LTD_4).

Intra-arterial administration of A23187 to isolated perfused kidneys (n=4) resulted in the release of 20-carboxy-LTB_4, LTC_4, LTD_4 and LTE_4 into the venous ef-

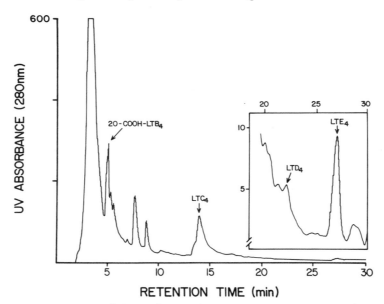

Figure 1. HPLC detection of LT from A23187 stimulated rabbit kidneys.

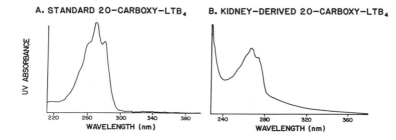

Figure 2. UV spectrum of 20-carboxy-LTB$_4$: standard compound (panel A) compared to kidney-derived material (panel B).

fluent. These compounds were detected in lipid extracts fractionated by reversed-phase HPLC and identified by retention time (Fig 1) and UV spectrometry.

Further confirmation of the identity of the 20-carboxy-LTB$_4$ was obtained by normal-phase HPLC analysis of the partially purified material after its conversion to the dimethyl ester. In this case, the kidney-derived material eluted at the retention time of standard 20-carboxy-LTB$_4$ dimethyl ester.

Enzyme immunoassay was performed on the LTC$_4$ and LTD$_4$ fractions from control, A23187 and LTA$_4$ perfusions (n=4). This quantification revealed that significantly more of these peptide-containing LT were released by perfusion of LTA$_4$ than were detected in the basal state or after stimulation with A23187 (Table 1).

TABLE 1. Immunoreactive LTC$_4$ and LTD$_4$ release.

	LTC$_4$ (pg/ml)	LTD$_4$ (pg/ml)
Kidney/A23187	786 ± 225	98 ± 22
Kidney/LTA$_4$	28802 ± 11246	2820 ± 1061

n=4
LTA$_4$ (45 nmol bolus injected intra-arterially followed by a 100 ml perfusion).
A23187 (15 ul of a 2.5 mM solution injected intra-arterially followed by a 100 ml perfusion).

These data demonstrate a large excess in the capacity of the kidney to convert LTA$_4$ to bioactive metabolites compared to the ability of this organ to generate LTA$_4$. In view of recent reports demonstrating in-vitro transcellular metabolism of LTA$_4$ (5,6) our results suggest that similar transcellular synthesis could occur in the kidney.

Our finding of 20-carboxy-LTB$_4$ release by the kidney is interesting in light of previous reports concerning renal LTB$_4$ production. In studies of the rat, Wong, et al. were able to detect LTB$_4$ synthesis in addition to the peptide-containing LT but found the enzymatic activity resided primarily in the renal cortex (3). Cattell, et al. (7) noted the presence of LTB$_4$ immunoreactivity in HPLC fractions with retention times that differed from LTB$_4$. We propose that LTB$_4$, a powerful leukocyte chemoattractant is rapidly oxidized within the renal circulation of the rabbit. This may occur by either the recently described isomerase pathway (8) followed by oxidation, or by initial oxidation as suggested in this report.

ACKNOWLEDGMENTS

The authors wish to thank Dr. Robert Sciacca for statistical analyses and Ms. Nooshin Ismail-Beigi for her excellent completion of the EIA. This work was supported by a grant from the NIH (HL 14148).

REFERENCES

1. Badr, K, Brenner, B, Ichikawa, I. Am. J. Physiology. 1987; 253:239-243.

2. Ardaillou, R, Baud, L, Sraer, J. Am. J. Med. 1986;81:12-22.

3. Wong, PY-K, Chao, PH-W, Spokas EG. In: Hayaishi, O, Yamamoto, S, eds. Advances in Prostaglandin, Thromboxane, and Leukotriene Research, vol 15. New York: Raven Press, 1985;423-426.

4. De Mello, C, Maack, T. Am. J. Physiology. 1976;231:1694-1701.

5. Feinmark, SJ, Cannon, PJ. J. Biol. Chem. 1986;261:16466-16472.

6. Feinmark, SJ, Cannon, PJ. Biochim. Biophys. Acta. 1987;922:125-35.

7. Cattell, V, Smith, J, Cook, HT, Moncada, S, Salmon, JA. Kidney International. 1986;29:339.

8. Breuer, O, Hammarstrom, S. Biochem. Biophys. Res. Comm. 1987;142(3):667-673.

Advances in Prostaglandin, Thromboxane, and Leukotriene Research, Vol. 19, edited by B. Samuelsson, P. Y.-K. Wong, and F. F. Sun, Raven Press, Ltd., New York ©1989.

EFFECTS OF ESTRADIOL ON PROSTAGLANDIN E_2 BIOSYNTHESIS AND PROSTAGLANDIN METABOLIC ENZYME ACTIVITY IN RAT KIDNEYS

Wen-Chang Chang

Department of Pharmacology, College of Medicine, National Cheng Kung University, Tainan, Taiwan, R.O.C.

We have been interested in systematically studying the effects of estradiol on the arachidonate cascade at the blood-vessel interface. Using rats as an experimental medel, we have found that estradiol inhibits the formation of arterial thrombosis induced by electric shock (1). A plausible biochemical explanation for the anti-thrombogenic effect of estradiol was provided by the finding that estradiol stimulates selectively prostacyclin synthesis in vascular wall, but not thromboxane formation in platelets (2).

In the systemic circulation, the kidney is responsible for the elimination of most nonvolatile waste products of metabolism from the body. The renally produced prostaglandin E_2 is vasodilator for stimulating the renal afferent arterioles. In the present study, the effects of estradiol on renal biosynthesis of PGE_2 and renal NAD^+-dependent 15-hydroxyprostaglandin dehydrogenase (15-PGDH) activity were investigated.

METHODS

Treatment with sex steroids

Male and female Wistar rats aged 3 months were used. The ovariectomized animals were used 2 weeks after the operation. Depo-estradiol cypionate or depo-testosterone cypionate, in cotton seed oil, was administered subcutaneously. Drug treatment was repeated at intervals of 3-4 days.

Prostaglandin biosynthetic activity assay

Each assay tube contained: arachidonic acid, 5 μg; hemoglobin, 1 μM; epinephrine, 1 mM; and appropriate amount of renal microsomal fraction in 1 ml of 50 mM Tris-HCl buffer, pH 7.5. Incubation was carried out at 37°C for 5 min. The reaction was stopped by acidification with 1 N HCl. Products were extracted with ethyl acetate and evaporated with nitrogen gas. The prostaglandin fraction was separated by passing through Sep-Pak cartridge according to the method described (3). The content of PGE2 was measured by a specific radioimmunoassay developed in our laboratory (4).

15-PDGH activity assay

The 15-PGDH activity in supernatant of kidney homogenate after centrifugation at 27,000 g for 20 min was determined by measuring the transfer of tritium from 15(S)-[³H]PGE2 to glutamate by coupling with glutamate dehydrogenase as described by Tai (5).

RESULTS

Effect of estradiol on renal PGE2 biosynthetic activity

As indicated in Table 1, the renal biosynthesis of PGE2 was significantly increased by estradiol treatment.

TABLE 1

Group	No. of rats	PGE2 formed (ng/mg protein)	
Control	6	8.2 $\pm$ 0.84	
Estradiol	6	14.1 $\pm$ 1.25	$P < 0.01$

The ovariectomized rats were injected at 3- to 4-day intervals with 0.5 mg estradiol/kg body weight for 4 weeks. Kidneys were removed, homogenized and assayed for PGE2 biosynthetic activity. Values were mean $\pm$ S.E.M.

Change in renal 15-PGDH activity with sex difference

The enzyme activity in female rats was lower than that in male rats, and was significantly increased by ovariectomy (Fig. 1).

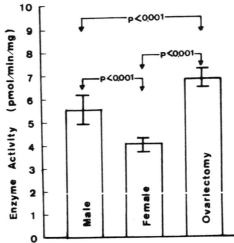

FIG. 1. Effect of sex and ovariectomy on renal 15-PGDH activity. Five rats were used in each group.

Effect of sex steroids on renal 15-PGDH activity

Since female rats showed lower 15-PGDH activity than male rats, effect of estradiol and testosterone on the enzyme activity in ovariectomized animals was then studied. As indicated in Table 2, estradiol significantly inhibited the enzyme activity, while testosterone showed no effect.

TABLE 2

Group	Dose (mg/kg body wt.)	Enzyme Activity PGE2 oxidized (pmol/min/mg)	Inhibition (%)	
Control		8.14 ± 0.33		
Estradiol	0.5	5.78 ± 0.22	29	P < 0.01
Testosterone	1	8.10 ± 0.65	0	
Testosterone	10	8.00 ± 0.39	2	

The ovariectomized rats were treated with a single injection of sex steroids. Animals were sacrificed 2 days after treatment. Values of enzyme activity represent mean ± S.E.M. from five individual animals of each group.

Decay of renal 15-PGDH activity in cell-free system

In order to see the decay of the enzyme in cell-free system, the crude enzyme was incubated for a peroid of time and then assayed for the enzyme activity. The enzymes from both two groups decayed at the same rate. The regression slope for the enzymes from control and estradiol-treated groups was not statistically different (Fig. 2).

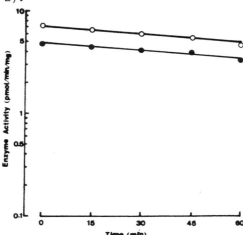

FIG. 2. Decay of renal 15-PGDH activity in cell-free system. Kidneys from single treatment of 0.5 mg estradiol/kg body weight were used.

DISCUSSION

In the present investigation, we found that the renal biosynthesis of PGE_2 is significantly increased by estradiol treatment. Stimulation of the renal PGE_2 biosynthesis by estradiol indicated that estradiol treatment might stimulate either fatty acid cyclooxygenase activity or PGE_2 isomerase activity. PGE_2 isomerase is a constitutive enzyme since its enzyme activity is at least 20 folds higher than the fatty acid cyclooxygenase activity in rat kidney (6). Therefore, stimulation of the renal PGE_2 biosynthesis might be due to the stimulation of renal fatty acid cyclooxygenase activity by estradiol treatment.

We also found that the renal 15-PGDH activity in female rats is lower than that in male rats, and the enzyme is significantly increased by ovariectomy. The results indicated that the renal enzyme activity might be regulated by the endogenous sex steroids. For studying the effect of sex steroids on enzyme activity, we found that estradiol significantly inhibits the renal enzyme activity, while testosterone does not show any significant effect. The results indicated that estradiol is the major endogenous sex steroid regulating the renal 15-PGDH activity. Since the enzymes from control and estradiol-treated groups decay at the same rate, the inhibitory effect of estradiol on the renal enzyme might be due to the inhibition of the enzyme biosynthesis.

ACKNOWLEDGMENTS

I am greatly indebted to Ms. Y.L. Suen and Ms. G. S. Fang for their excellent technical assistance. This research was supported in part by the National Science Council of the Republic of China (NSC75-0412-B006-13 and NSC76-0412-B006-15).

REFERENCES

1. Ohtsu A. Saitoh N, Okada N, Chang WC, Murota S. Thromb. Res. 1983; 32: 567-574.

2. Chang WC, Nakao J, Neichi T, Orimo H, Murota S. Biochim. Biophys. Acta 1981; 664: 291-297.

3. Chang WC. Prot. Leuk. Med. 1988; in press.

4. Powell WS. Prostaglandins 1980; 20: 947-957.

5. Tai HH. Biochemistry 1976; 15: 4586-4592.

6. Sheny WY, Wyche A. Lysz T, Needleman P. J. Biol. Chem. 1982; 257: 14632-14634.

Advances in Prostaglandin, Thromboxane, and Leukotriene Research, Vol. 19, edited by B. Samuelsson, P. Y.-K. Wong, and F. F. Sun, Raven Press, Ltd., New York ©1989.

INTRACELLULAR MECHANISMS OF THE EFFECT OF THROMBOXANE A_2 ON WATER TRANSPORT

B. Escalante and J.L. Reyes

Department of Pharmacology
Centro de Investigación y de Estudios Avanzados
del Instituto Politécnico Nacional
Apartado Postal 14-740 MEXICO D.F. 07000

It has been demonstrated that the toad urinary bladder synthesizes Thromboxane A_2 (TxA_2) and that its synthesis can be stimulated by vasopressin. Imidazole, an inhibitor of thromboxane synthesis was found to inhibit both vasopressin-stimulated TxB_2 synthesis and water flow while increasing vasopressin PGE_2 synthesis (1). Thus, those studies can be reconciled with the hypothesis that PGE_2 acts as negative modulator of vasopressin-stimulated water flow. However Ludens and Taylor (2) found that U44069, (15S)-hydroxy-9α, 11α (epoxymethanol)prosta-5Z, 13e-dienoic acid, a thromboxane synthetase inhibitor and thromboxane-like agonist also inhibited vasopressin-stimulated water flow. But PGE_2 and TxB_2 syntheses were not assessed in those experiments. Based on these observations it has been hypothesized that TxA_2 acts as a possible mediator of vasopressin-stimulated water flow. The extreme lability of TxA_2 precludes direct testing of its effects on water flow. Thus, stable compounds that mimic its actions must be sought to test the hypothesis. The stable prostaglandin endoperoxides analogs U44069 and 15(S) hydroxy-11α, -9α(epoxy-methanol)prosta 5Z, 13e-dienoic acid (U46619) possess biological activity that mimics the action of TxA_2 and/or the prostaglandin endoperoxides in platelets and aortic strips (3). Thus, the present study was designed to determine the effects of thromboxane analog U46619 on water flow in MDCK cells and urinary frog bladder.

METHODS

Measurement of water flow. MDCK monolayers grown onto nylon meshes coated with collagen or urinary frog bladder were mounted as a diaphragm between two Ussing-type hemichambers (7). Each compartment contained 2.5 ml either DMEM without serum or saline Ringer and the total exposed area was 0.1 cm^2. An adequate stirring of the media was achieved by the use of magnetic bars placed in each compartment, rotated by magnetic stirring plate. All the experiments were carried out at 36.5°C with air 5% CO_2 atmosphere. To determine the water fluxes, tritiated water (1 $\mu Ci/ml$) was added to one of the chambers at the beginning of the period and samples of 100 μl were taken each 2 minutes from the opposite chamber and the volume withdrawn was replaced with fresh solution. In some experiments the urinary frog bladder was incubated with colchicine (10 μM) trifluoperazine (10 μM) and verapamil (10 μM).

Intracellular calcium measurements. MDCK cells were loaded by incubation with Quin 2/AM in HEPES-buffered at 37°C (8), our usual procedure was to add 50 μM Quin 2/AM to cell suspension containing 10^6 cell/ml and incubate for 20 minutes, then dilute tenfold and continue incubation for further 40–60 minutes. After loading, the cells were centrifuged at 1000 g for 3–4 minutes and resuspended in tris HEPES-buffered at 1.5 x 10^7 cells/ml and kept at room temperature. For measurement of fluorescence 1 ml of this stock suspension was centrifuged at 14,000 g in a microcentrifuge for 1 minute and the cells resuspended in 2 ml simplified medium at 37°C and transferred to the cuve. Fluorescences were recorded in Perkin Elmer spectrophotometer at 339 nm excitation and 490 nm emission.

RESULTS

U46619 markedly increased the water flow in MDCK cells from 24.3 $\pm$ 26 to 164 $\pm$ 14 $\mu l/min/cm^2$, the water flow increased within 1–2 min after U46619 and remained elevated for 2–4 minutes and then returned to stable baseline. U46619 also increased the water in urinary frog bladder (table 1); this effect of U46619 on the water flow in urinary frog bladder was markedly inhibited by treatment of the bladder with either the calmodulin inhibitor trifluoroperazine or the inhibitor of cytoskeletal elements, colchicine (table 1). Neither the calcium entry blocker verapamil nor the calcium free medium affected the U46619 stimulated water flow in the urinary frog bladder (table 1). U46619 increased cytosolic calcium from 114 $\pm$ 14 to 265 $\pm$ 15 nM in the MDCK cells at the same concentration that stimulated the water flow (10^{-6}M).

TABLE 1

Water Flow
($\mu l/min/cm^2$)

	Control	U46619
Control	33 + 16	65 + 27
Colchicine	40 + 18	36 + 10
Trifluoperazine	63 + 15	72 + 17
Verapamil	50 + 9	109 + 47

DISCUSSION

Arachidonic acid metabolites have been shown to modulate vasopressin stimulation of water permeability in the toad urinary bladder. PGE_2 acts as a negative modulator (4) while TxA_2 appears to act as a positive modulator or mediator (5). Since TxA_2 is a short-lived intermediate of arachidonic acid metabolism direct demonstration of its effects in the toad bladder is technically difficult. Thus, in the present studies, the effects of stable endoperoxide/TxA_2-like agonist, U46619, was assessed on the water flow response of frog bladder or MDCK cells. U46619 stimulated water flow in both epithelia that were not pretreated with cyclooxygenase inhibitors. That the active arachidonic acid metabolite in the MDCK cells or the urinary frog bladder is TxA_2 and not the endoperoxides is supported by the previous observations that the thromboxane synthetase inhibitors decreased vasopressin-stimulated water flow (5) while the concentration of the endoperoxides would not have changed. The present study suggests that thromboxane causes increase in the water flow by a calcium dependent mechanism since U46619 thromboxane analog increases cytoplasmic calcium in the MDCK cells at the same concentration that stimulates the water flow, however, extracellular calcium seems not to be important since treatment with calcium entry blocker or calcium free medium did not affect the U46619 effect on stimulated water flow in urinary frog bladder. Our observations suggest that thromboxane increases cytoplasmic calcium and probably activates calmodulin and cytoskeletal elements, maybe in a similar way to that described for ADH effect (6) on transepithelial osmosis in urinary bladder.

Further studies are required to elucidate the possible role of thromboxane A_2 in the water and sodium reabsorption and to elucidate which transepithelial mechanism is affected by TxA_2.

REFERENCES

1. Burch RM, Knapp DR, Halushka PV. J Pharm Exp Ther 1979; 210: 344-348.

2. Ludens J, Taylor CJ. Fed Proc 1979; 38: 1060.

3. Malmsten C. Life Sci 1976; 18: 169-178.

4. Zusman RM, Keiser HR, Handler JS. J Clin Invest 1977; 60: 1339-1347.

5. Burch RM, Knapp DR, Halushka PV. Am J Physiol 1980; 239: F160-F166.

6. Dibona DR. Epithelial ion and water transport, New York Raven Press, 1981: 241-255.

7. Martínez F, Reyes J. J Physiol 1984; 347: 533-543.

8. Tsien RY, Pozzan T, Rink TJ. J Cell Biol 1982; 94: 325-334.

Advances in Prostaglandin, Thromboxane, and Leukotriene Research, Vol. 19, edited by B. Samuelsson, P. Y.-K. Wong, and F. F. Sun, Raven Press, Ltd., New York ©1989.

LEUKOTRIENE D4 (LTD4)/LEUKOTRIENE B4 (LTB4) INTERACTIONS

IN THE PATHOPHYSIOLOGY OF EXPERIMENTAL GLOMERULONEPHRITIS

Kamal F. Badr

Division of Nephrology, Vanderbilt University
School of Medicine, Nashville, TN, 37232, U.S.A.

INTRODUCTION

We have recently established the presence of specific receptors for LTD4 on cultured cells of glomerular mesangial origin. These cells are smooth muscle-like mesenchymal cells located in the intercapillary spaces of the glomerular tuft. They carry out a number of functions, among which is the dynamic control of the capillary surface area available for filtration (1). The concerted contractile action of mesangial cells under the influence of locally or systemically released vasoactive autacoids and hormones is currently thought to result in "derecruitment" of a number of capillary loops from the glomerular tuft, thereby reducing glomerular capillary surface area (S). This will result in a decrease in single nephron (SN) GFR since S is a component of the glomerular capillary ultrafiltration coefficient, K_f, an important determinant of the magnitude of SNGFR (2). In fact, intrarenal administration of LTD4 to normal rats results in a significant fall in K_f (3).

In experiments performed in the anesthetized rat, we investigated the role of LTD4-induced mesangial cell contraction in the pathogenesis of the diminished glomerular filtration rate which accompanies inflammatory glomerular injury (glomerulonephritis). (4)

EXPERIMENTS AND RESULTS

Acute glomerulonephritis was induced in the rat by the intravenous administration of rabbit anti-rat glomerular basement membrane antibody (nephrotoxic serum, NTS). The dose of NTS administered was titrated to result, two hours after its administration, in a significant reduction in GFR from 1.07 ± 0.05 in vehicle-treated control rats (Group 1) to 0.61 ± 0.07 ml/min in NTS-treated animals (Group 2). Micropuncture measurements revealed that this fall in GFR was due mainly to a major reduction in K_f which averaged 0.020 ± 0.003 nl/(s.mmHg) in NTS-treated animals as compared to 0.070 ± 0.009 nl/(s.mmHg) in control rats (p<0.05). Histologic examination of kidneys from control and NTS-treated animals revealed marked glomerular pathology in the latter, expressed as infiltration of the glomeruli with polymorphonuclear leukocytes (PMN), and electron microscopic examination revealed focal detachment of glomerular endothelial cells from the underlying basement membrane. In a third group of rats (Group 3), NTS was administered in the same dose as that used in Group 2, but animals were concomitantly treated with the specific LTD4 receptor antagonist, SK&F 104353. This compound is a structural analog of LTD4 which competes for binding to the LTD4 receptor in a number of tissues, including the glomerular mesangial cells in culture (1). Additionally, it effectively blocks LTD4-induced inositol triphosphate generation in these cells (1). In this group of animals, NTS administration was not associated with significant reductions in GFR or Kf, despite persistent PMN infiltration (PMN counts were not different in the two groups).

In Groups 2 and 3, NTS administration was associated with increases in pre- and post-glomerular resistances, with a resultant rise in total renal vascular resistance and fall in renal plasma flow (RPF). These changes were not modified by LTD4 antagonism. The restoration of GFR in Group 3 rats despite a persistent reduction in glomerular perfusion was due to the elevated level of intraglomerular capillary pressure, and hence, net transcapillary hydraulic pressure difference across the glomerular capillary into Bowman's space,Δ P. This increase in Δ P was attributed to the proportionately greater rise in efferent, as compared to afferent, arteriolar resistance.

In view of the above, we tested the role of LTB4 in potentially exacerbating the PMN-associated, NTS-induced fall in GFR. GFR, RPF, and glomerular PMN counts (250 glomeruli examined/group) were again performed two hours after the administration of NTS in three groups of rats: Group 1 (n=5) received 0.4 ml of rabbit serum; Group 2 (n=5) 0.4 ml of NTS, a dose titrated to achieve a mild reduction in GFR; Group 3 (n=5) 0.4 ml NTS, but functional measurements were preceded by a 10-min intrarenal infusion of LTB4 (0.5 ug/kg/min). Results: $\pm$ SEM.

	GFR	RPF	FF	PMN/glom.
Gp 1:	1.19±0.09	4.24±0.37	0.29±0.03	0.74±0.06
Gp 2:	0.86±0.07[a]	4.27±0.25	0.21±0.02[a]	0.87±0.10
Gp 3:	0.46±0.08[ab]	2.82±0.37[ab]	0.18±0.04[a]	1.39±0.12[ab]

[a] $p<0.025$ vs Gp 1.
[b] $p<0.025$ vs Gp 2.

Regression analysis of values for GFR vs PMN counts revealed a strong inverse correlation, demonstrating dependence of the fall in GFR on the increase in PMNs/glomerulus (r^2=0.75, $p<0.01$).

DISCUSSION

These experiments demonstrated the capacity of a specific LTD4 receptor antagonist to prevent the fall in Kf during inflammatory glomerular injury in the rat despite persistent PMN

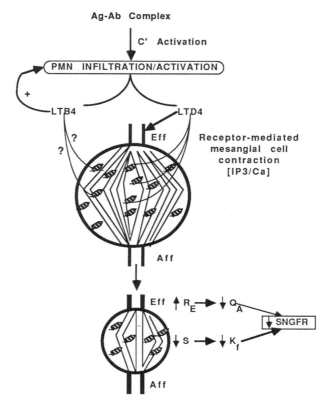

FIG. 1. Proposed mechanism for the role of leukotrienes (LTs) in the pathophysiology of immune-mediated glomerular injury. Antigen (Ag)-antibody (Ab) interactions within the glomerulus are associated with complement (C') activation and polymorpho-nuclear (PMN) cell infiltration/activation. The latter results in the local release of LTB4 and LTD4. LTD4 constricts efferent (Eff) arterioles (Ref. 3) and occupies specific receptors on the surface of smooth muscle-cntaining mesangial cells (Ref. 1). Receptor activation in these cells is associated with the intracellular release of inositol triphosphate (IP3), an increase in intracellular Ca, and cell contraction. Mesangial cell contraction results in a reduction in the number of patent capillary loops, thereby decreasing glomerular size and filtering surface area (S), a component of the glomerular capillary ultrafiltration coefficient, Kf. The increase in efferent (R_E), as well as afferent (R_A), arteriolar resistances results in a fall in single nephron plasma flow rate (Q_A). The combined reductions in Q_A and Kf conspire to depress single nephron glomerular filtration rate (SNGFR). LTB4 amplifies these responses through its chemoattractant and PMN activator properties.

infiltration.   This observation is consistent with the hypothesis that the presence of PMNs within the glomerulus per se is
not a major route of functional impairment.   Rather, the local
release from these cells of potent vasoactive mediators is at
the root of the observed deterioration of filtration function.
The crucial determinant of GFR which is compromised under these
conditions is the glomerular capillary ultrafiltration coefficient, Kf.   This mathematical parameter represents the product
of glomerular capillary hydraulic permeability and total
capillary filtering surface area (S).   The mechanism of its
reductions in this model of injury appears to be a fall in S
mediated through the contraction of glomerular mesangial cells.
Our studies strongly suggest a role for LTD4 in the mediation of
this contraction.   These studies, however, do not rule out the
possibiilty that LTD4 could be affecting the hydraulic permeability through some toxic effect on endothelial cell function,
as suggested by electron microscopic findings.

   Our experiments further suggest that the local release of
LTB4 may amplify the observed LTD4-induced functional derange-
ments, through the recruitment and activation of PMNs.   The
latter are thought to be the principal source of intraglomerular
LTD4 release in this model of injury.   These interactions are
schematized in Figure 1.

REFERENCES

1.   Badr KF, Mong S, Hoover RL, et al (submitted).

2.   Schlondorff D.   <u>FASEB J</u> 1987;272-281.

3.   Badr KF, Brenner BM, Ichikawa I.   <u>Amer J Physiol</u>
     1987;22:F239-F243.

4.   Badr KF, Schreiner GF, Wasserman M, Ichikawa I.   <u>J Clin
     Invest</u> 1988 (in press).

Advances in Prostaglandin, Thromboxane, and Leukotriene Research, Vol. 19, edited by B. Samuelsson, P. Y.-K. Wong, and F. F. Sun, Raven Press, Ltd., New York ©1989.

STIMULATION OF DE NOVO SYNTHESIS OF
PROSTAGLANDIN G/H SYNTHASE IN ENDOTHELIAL CELLS

K. K. Wu, S. S. Lo, A. C. Papp
and H. N. Vijjeswarapu

Center for Vascular and Thrombosis Research and
Department of Medicine, University of Texas
Health Science Center at Houston, Houston, TX 77225

Biosynthesis of eicosanoids is tightly controlled at several enzymatic steps in the arachidonic acid metabolism (1). Phospholipases (A and C) cleave arachidonic acid from the membrane phospholipids and the substrate availability is considered to be an important rate-limiting step in eicosanoid synthesis. Conversion of arachidonic acid into eicosanoids, in turn, depends on a number of enzymes of which prostaglandin G/H synthase occupies a central position. It catalyzes the conversion of arachidonic acid into several biologically important metabolites, such as prostacyclin (PGI_2), thromboxane A_2 (TXA_2), prostaglandin E_2 and $F_{2\alpha}$ (PGE_2 and $PGF_{2\alpha}$). Prostaglandin G/H synthase is a heme-containing glycoprotein, a homodimer reported to have one mole of heme per subunit of 70-kDa (2-4). The molecule has 2 enzyme activities (5,6), a dioxygenase (cyclooxygenase) activity catalyzing the formation of PGG_2 and a hydroperoxidase activity involved in the reduction of PGG_2 to PGH_2. Prostaglandin G/H synthase is rapidly inactivated upon the conversion of PGG_2 to PGH_2. Autoinactivation of the enzyme by oxidants leads to irreversible degradation of the enzyme (7-10). It is, hence, the rate limiting enzyme in prostanoid synthesis. Vascular endothelial cells are capable of synthesizing eicosanoids via the cyclooxygenase and the lipoxygenase pathways. One such metabolite, prostacyclin, plays a crucial role in maintaining the homeostasis of hemostasis and vascular reactivity (11). Prostacyclin production is stimulated by a number of agonists such as thrombin, histamine, bradykinin and calcium ionophore. When cultured endothelial cells are stimulated by these agonists, they undergo a burst of prostacyclin and eicosanoid synthesis but the stimulation dwindles rapidly within 30 min following the addition of the agonist (12-14). The self-limitation in prostanoid synthesis is probably due to autoinactivation of prostaglandin G/H synthase (12). In an attempt to understand the mechanism by which synthesis and degradation of this crucial enzyme is regulated, we have investigated the effects of cytokines on endothelial cell eicosanoid synthesis.

METHODS AND RESULTS

Eicosanoid Synthesis. We observed that interleukin 2 (IL-2) increased prostacyclin synthesis by cultured endothelial cells (15). In contrast to the self-limited stimulation of prostanoid synthesis by the commonly known agonists, the time course of IL-2 stimulation revealed a lag of 2 h and then followed by a steady increase in PGI_2 synthesis (15). PGI_2 stimulation was abolished by cycloheximide and actinomycin D suggesting that IL-2 stimulation requires continuous gene expression and protein synthesis. Since protaglandin G/H synthase occupies a central position in endothelial cell prostacyclin production and that it is the key rate limiting enzyme in converting arachidonic acid into prostanoids, we prostulated that continuous synthesis of prostaglandin G/H synthase is required for IL-2 induced sustained synthesis of PGI_2. To test this hypothesis, we determined the influence of IL-2 on the synthesis of the 70-kDa subunit of prostaglandin G/H synthase by Western blot and by a reverse immunoblot to detect newly synthesized cyclooxygenase in HUVEC metabolically labeled with L-[^{35}S] methionine.

Immunoblot. To determine the effects of IL-2 on the synthesis of prostaglandin G/H synthase in HUVEC, we incubated HUVEC (2×10^6 cells/flask) with medium in the presence and absence of IL-2. At designated time points, medium was removed, HUVEC were lysed by phosphate buffered saline (PBS) containing 0.1% Triton X-100, 1 mM PMSF, 0.01% EDTA and 0.03% leupeptin. The lysates were boiled for 3 min and centrifuged at 15,000 rpm for 10 min. The supernatant which contained the solubilized prostaglandin G/H synthase was concentrated and 50 μl of the sample was applied to an 8% SDS polyacrylamide gel. After electrophoresis, the proteins were transferred to nitrocellulose sheets and the 70-kDa subunit was identified by an affinity purified antibody. The 70-kDa band was detectable in HUVEC incubated in medium alone without stimuli. The 70-kDa band was enhanced by incubating HUVEC with IL-2. Enhancement of the 70-kDa band was abolished by cycloheximide. These studies indicate that IL-2 induces accumulation of prostaglandin G/H synthase in HUVEC. We then carried out additional experiments to determine the influence of IL-2 on de novo synthesis of prostaglandin G/H synthase. HUVEC metabolically labeled with 50 μCi of L-[^{35}S] methionine were incubated with medium in the presence and absence of IL-2. At specified times, cells were lysed and the solubilized fraction was applied to nitrocellulose discs pretreated with specific antibody against prostaglandin G/H synthase or with nonspecific immunoglobulins. After repeated washing, the discs was placed in scintillation fluid and the radioactivity was determined. The preliminary results showed that the radioactive counts in HUVEC incubated in medium alone in the absence of IL-2 was approximately 2-fold higher than the background counts determined on nitrocellulose membranes pretreated with nonspecific immunoglobulins (Table 1). IL-2 caused a substantial increment in the radioactive counts over the medium control (Table 1). Cycloheximide treatment of the medium- and IL-2 treated HUVEC reduced the counts to the background. Together with the Western blot data, our findings demonstrate that IL-2 stimulates de novo synthesis of prostaglandin G/H synthase. This represents a novel mechanism by which endothelial cells can undergo sustained synthesis of eicosanoids. The newly synthesized enzymes replenish the autoinactivated enzymes to convert arachidonic acid into biologically important eicosanoids.

TABLE 1. L-[^{35}S] methionine incorporation in endothelial cell prostaglandin G/H synthase

	2 h	4 h
	cpm (10^{-3})	
Medium Specific Ab*	9.4	10.2
Nonimmune Ig*	4.6	5.1
Blank	5.1	5.4
IL-2 Specific Ab	19.2	24.3
Nonimmune Ig	6.3	6.9
CH + Medium + Specific Ab	5.3	5.6
CH + IL-2 + Speicific Ab	5.9	6.3

Each value represent mean of 2 experiments. * Ab antibody, Ig, immunoglobulin, CH Cycloheximide (10 µg/ml).

Functional Recovery. Aspirin irreversibly inhibits the cyclooxygenase activity. Aspirin-treated cells can no longer convert arachidonic acid into prostanoids until new enzymes are synthesized. We have utilized this aspirin property to investigate the functional recovery of prostaglandin G/H synthase as influenced by IL-2. BAEC were incubated with medium containing aspirin (500 µM) for 30 min at 37°C. Cells were washed and incubated with medium in the presence and absence of IL-2. At specific times, cells were washed and treated with arachidonic acid (10 µM) for 1 h at 37°C. The medium was collected and assayed for 6-keto-PGF$_{1\alpha}$ by RIA. Aspirin-treated BAEC without IL-2 stimulation failed to convert arachidonic acid even after the cells have been free of aspirin for 24 h (15). By contrast, IL-2 stimulation led to rapid recovery of the ability of the cells to convert arachidonic acid. Following a 2-h lag period, there was a sustained increase in converting arachidonic acid into PGI_2 consistent with the notion that IL-2 stimulates de novo synthesis of prostaglandin G/H synthase.

CONCLUSION

We have shown that IL-2 induces sustained prostacyclin synthesis by vascular endothelial cells by stimulating de novo synthesis of prostaglandin G/H synthase. Stimulation of this important enzyme represents a novel regulatory mechanism for circumventing the rapid turnover of the enzyme activity (16) Since actinomycin D and cycloheximide abolish the stimulatory effect of IL-2, we postulate that IL-2 acts at the level of gene transcription. We postulate that IL-2 interacts with a specific IL-2 receptor on endothelial cells leading to activation of intracellular signal transduction. The signal(s) then mediates the upregulation of gene expression. Work is now in progress in our laboratory to test this hypothesis.

ACKNOWLEDGMENTS

The work is supported by NIH Programs Project Grant NS-23327.

REFERENCES

1. Needleman P, Turk J, Jakschik BA, Morrison AR, Lefkowith, JB. Anni Rev. Biochem. 1986;55:69-102.

2. Miyamoto T, Ogino N, Yamamoto S, Hayaishi O. J. Biol Chem. 1976;251:2629-2639.

3. Hemler M, Lands WEM, Smith WL. J. Biol. Chem. 1976; 251:5575-5579.

4. Van der Ouderaa FJ, Buytenhek M, Nugtren DH, Van Dorp DA. Biochim. Biophys. Acta 1977;487:315-331.

5. Ohki S, Ogino N, Yamamoto S, Hayachi O. J. Biol. Chem. 1979;254:829-836.

6. Pagels WR, Sach RJ, Murnett LJ, DeWitt DL, Day JS, Smith WJ. J. Biol. Chem. 1983;258:6517–6523.

7. Smith WL, Lands WEM. Biochem. 1972;11:3276–3285.

8. Egan RW, Paxton J, Kuehl FA. J. Biol. Chem. 1976;251:7325–7335.

9. Hemler ME, Lands WEM. J. Biol. Chem. 1980;255:6253–6261.

10. Marshall PJ, Kulmacz RJ, Lands WEM. J. Biol. Chem. 1978;262:3510–3517.

11. Moncada S, Vane JR. In: Berti F, Velo GP, eds. The Prostaglandin system. Endoperoxides prostacyclin and thromboxane New York: Plenum Press, 1981;203–2221.

12. Baenziger NL, Fogerty FJ, Mertz LF, Chernuta LF. Cell, 1981;24:915–923.

13. McIntyre TM, Zimmerman GA, Satoh K, Prescott SM. J. Clin. Invest. 1981;24:915–923.

14. Clark, MA, Littlejohn D, Meng S, Crooke ST. Prostagl. 1986;31:157–166.

15. Hall ER, Papp AC, Seifert WE Jr., Wu KK. Lymphokine Res. 1986;5:87–96.

16. Fagan JM, Goldberg AL. Proc. Natl., Acad. Sci. USA 1986;83:2771–2775.

Advances in Prostaglandin, Thromboxane, and
Leukotriene Research, Vol. 19, edited by
B. Samuelsson, P. Y.-K. Wong, and F. F. Sun,
Raven Press, Ltd., New York ©1989.

ENDOTOXIN STIMULATES THE PRODUCTION OF PROSTACYCLIN BY CULTURED HUMAN ENDOTHELIAL CELLS

Kentaro Watanabe, Timothy M. McCaffrey,
Babette B. Weksler, and Eric A. Jaffe

Division of Hematology-Oncology, Department of
Medicine, Cornell University Medical College,
New York, NY, 10021, USA

Endotoxin both in vivo and in vitro induces alterations in multiple physiologic systems. It has been shown that endotoxin induces the synthesis and secretion of plasminogen activator inhibitor (1), and IL-1 (2), suppresses thrombomodulin expression (3), increases the adhesion of PMN and lymphocytes to endothelial cells (4-6), and increases the cell surface expression of tissue factor (7). Endotoxin has also been shown to increase the synthesis of prostacyclin (PGI_2) by bovine aortic endothelial cells (8), although previous studies by others have failed to show an effect of endotoxin on PGI_2 production by human umbilical vein endothelial cells (HUVEC) (9).

We have now shown that endotoxin (10 ng/ml - 10 μg/ml for 4 to 24 hr) induced a 6-fold, dose- and time-dependent increase in unstimulated PGI_2 production by HUVEC. PGI_2 production induced by thrombin or histamine over a wide range of concentrations was also increased up to a maximum of 3-fold. These changes were not the result of endotoxin-induced cytotoxicity because LDH release by endotoxin-treated HUVEC was unchanged from that of controls. In contrast to its effect on PGI_2 production, endotoxin decreased thrombin- and histamine-induced rises in intracellular calcium by 80% though endotoxin did not change unstimulated, basal intra-cellular calcium levels. Endotoxin did not alter thrombin-induced rises in ^{3}H-arachidonate release and thrombin-induced IP_3 release was decreased only 11%. However, when endotoxin-treated HUVEC were incubated with arachidonate, they synthesized 10-fold more PGI_2 than non-endotoxin-treated HUVEC. In contrast, endotoxin-treated HUVEC incubated with PGG_2 or PGH_2 synthesized the same amount of PGI_2 as non-endotoxin-treated HUVEC. Measurement of cyclo-oxygenase antigen by ELISA using specific antibody showed that endotoxin treatment did no alter the amount of cyclooxygenase antigen within the cells. These results suggest that endotoxin may increase PGI_2 synthesis by increasing the activity of cyclooxygenase and thus altering the pattern of prostaglandin synthesis.

ACKNOWLEDGMENTS

Supported by NIH grant HL-18828.

REFERENCES

1. Colucci M, Paramo JA, Collen D J Clin Invest 1985;75:818-824.

2. Libby P, Ordovas JM, Auger KR, Robbins AH, Birinyi LK, Dinarello CA Am J Pathol 1986;124:179-185.

3. Moore KL, Andreoli SP, Esmon NL, Esmon CT, Bang NU J Clin Invest 1987;79:124-124.

4. Pohlman TH, Stanness KA, Beatty PG, Ochs HD, Harlan JM J Immunol 1986;136:4548-4553.

5. Schleimer RP, Rutledge BK J Immunol 1986;136:649-654.

6. Yu CL, Haskard D, Cavender D, Ziff M J Immunol 1986;136:569-573.

7. Colucci M, Balconi G, Lorenzet R, et al J Clin Invest 1983;71:1893-1896.

8. Nawroth PP, Stern DM, Kaplan KL, Nossel HL Blood 1984;64:801-806.

9. Harlan JM, Harker LA, Striker GE, Weaver LJ Thromb Res 1983;29:15-26.

Advances in Prostaglandin, Thromboxane, and Leukotriene Research, Vol. 19, edited by B. Samuelsson, P. Y.-K. Wong, and F. F. Sun, Raven Press, Ltd., New York ©1989.

A KALLIKREIN INDUCED NEW PEPTIDE STIMULATING PROSTACYCLIN

PRODUCTION BY VASCULAR ENDOTHELIAL CELLS

S.Murota, I.Morita and T.Kanayasu

Tokyo Medical and Dental University, 1-5-45, Yushima, Bunkyo-ku, Tokyo 113, Japan

INTRODUCTION

Endothelial cells were isolated from bovine carotid artery and cultured in a medium containing 10% fetal bovine serum. The cells had a high capacity for converting exogenous arachidonic acid to prostacyclin. This high activity was kept constant up to 40 to 50 passages. Kallikrein has been clinically used to improve peripheral circulation. We found kallikrein stimulating prostacyclin production by the endothelial cells (1). The cells were exposed to various doses of kallikrein for 1hr, and then the 6-keto-prostaglandin F_{1a} content in the medium was measured by radioimmunoassay (2). The cells produced a remarkable amount of prostacyclin in response to kallikrein.

RESULTS AND DISCUSSION

Fig.1 shows the time course of the stimulatory effect of kallikrein on arachidonic acid release and prostacyclin production. In the presence of kallikrein, the production of prostacyclin by the cells continued to increase in a linear fashion for at least 24h. On the other hand, the increase in prostacyclin production due to bradykinin leveled off after 6h. Although there was not so much difference in the value of radioactivity released (Fig.1, left), analysis of the released radioactivity showed that in the kallikrein treated cultures the radioactivity was mainly due to ^{14}C-prostacyclin, while in the bradykinin treated cultures, the radioactivity was mostly due to ^{14}C-arachidonic acid. These data suggests the possibility that some constant activation of prostacyclin synthesizing system may take place in the kallikrein treated cells.
There was another big difference between kallikrein and bradykinin in their stimulatory effect on the prostacyclin release

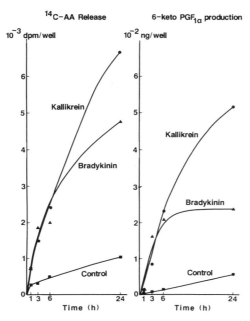

Fig.1. Kinetics of radioactivity release from ^{14}C–arachidonic
acid pre–labeled endothelial cells (left) and prostacyclin production by endothelial cells in culture (right)

from the endothelial cells. Thus, the effect of bradykinin was
blocked by cycloheximide, while that of kallikrein was not
(Fig.2). These data suggest that the stimulatory effect of

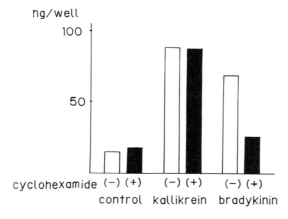

Fig.2. Effect of cycloheximide on 6–keto PGF_{1a} production
by kallikrein and bradykinin treated endothelial cells
in culture

kallikrein on prostacyclin synthesis is not associated with any
protein synthesis.

During the course of the investigation, we found a very interesting phenomena that serum content in the culture medium could
affect the stimulatory effect of kallikrein. When the cells were
cultured in a medium containing 10% serum, kallikrein clearly
stimulated their prostacyclin production. But when the cells
were cultured in a serum free medium, the effect of kallikrein
was completely abolished (3). These results suggest that kallikrein shows its effect through some unknown factor which may be
produced from serum by kallikrein. Fractionation of the serum by
ammonium sulfate showed that the precipitate of the 40-50% saturation fraction was the most active substrate for kallikrein.
Moreover, the analysis using centricon-10 showed that the molecular size of this factor should be less than 10,000 (3). The
stimulatory effect of kallikrein was abolished soon after the
addition of aprotinin, an inhibitor of kallikrein, to the medium
suggesting that the half life of the unknown factor must be very
short. The stimulatory effect of kallikrein was immediately
abolished when the cell layer was washed and exposed to a kallikrein free medium (Fig.3). These data suggest that the binding
capacity of the cells to the unknown factor is not strong. To
show its effect, it seems to be necessary for kallikrein to be
present in the medium all the time and keep producing the unknown
factor.

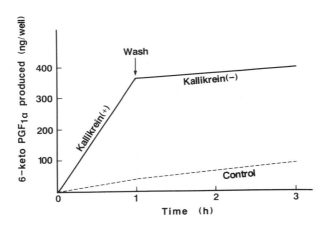

Fig.3. The stimulatory effect of kallikrein is abolished soon
       after the removal of kallikrein from the medium

The 40-50% ammonium sulfate serum fraction was incubated with
kallikrein for 1h at 37C. The reaction mixture was then subjected to centricon-10 analysis and the low molecular region was
purified by HPLC. Five new peaks were obtained, but none of
these peaks was detected in the absence of kallikrein. Each peak
was further purified by HPLC and identified the structure. Each

peak could be fractionated into 1 or 2 peaks and some of them were chemically identified. All of them were peptide consisted of 4-7 amino acids. Then we chemically synthesized these peptides and assayed for their biological activity on the cultured endothelial cells. Unfortunately, however, none of those peptides was active on the cells in terms of prostacyclin production. There are possibilities that the real factor is present elsewhere in other peaks which have not yet been identified, or those peptides might be breakdown products of the real factor. Because there is possibility that ammonium sulfate fractionation brought about concentration of some proteases in the serum as well as concentration of the substrate of kallikrein. Now we are reconsidering and trying to purify the substrate first. The 40-50% ammonium sulfate serum fraction was further analyzed by HPLC. As shown in Fig.4, the actual substrate protein for kallikrein was found to be located in the resion of peak 3-4. Identification of the unknown factor is now under way in our laboratory.

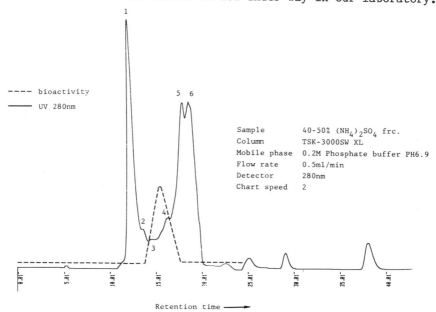

Fig.4. Substrate protein for kallikrein----Further fractionation of the 40-50% (NH$_4$)$_2$SO$_4$ fraction of serum protein by HPLC

REFERENCES

1. Morita, I., Kanayasu, T., and Murota, S. (1984): Biochim. Biophys. Acta, 792:304-309
2. Murota, S., Matsuoka, K., Mitsui, Y., Morita, I., and Kurata, M. (1983): Adv. PG. TX. LT. Res., 12:319-325
3. Murota, S., Morita, I., and Kanayasu, T. (1987): Adv. PG. TX. LT. Res., 17:569-572

Advances in Prostaglandin, Thromboxane, and Leukotriene Research, Vol. 19, edited by B. Samuelsson, P. Y.-K. Wong, and F. F. Sun, Raven Press, Ltd., New York ©1989.

LOW DENSITY LIPOPROTEIN-MEDIATED ENDOTHELIAL CELL PERTURBATION: EFFECTS ON ENDOTHELIAL CELL EICOSANOID METABOLISM

J.M. Miano, J.A. Holland, K.A. Pritchard Jr., N.J. Rogers, and M.B. Stemerman

Department of Medicine, New York Medical College, Valhalla, New York, 10595

INTRODUCTION

An elevation in serum low density lipoprotein (LDL) is considered a major risk factor in the pathobiology of atherosclerosis (1). Although the mechanism(s) remain unknown, atherosclerosis likely involves endothelial cell (EC) perturbation. The endothelium has been found to play an increasingly important role in modulating numerous vascular functions including relaxation (2), permeability (3), and hemostasis (4). The discovery of prostacyclin (PGI_2) production by aortic microsomes (5) and its subsequent localization to EC (6) has underscored the importance of EC in maintaining a thromboresistant barrier. PGI_2 exerts a powerful platelet anti-aggregation effect and is a potent vasodilator (5). In contrast, thromboxane (TXA_2) is known as an important platelet aggregator and vasoconstrictor (7). The effect of PGI_2 on platelet aggregation is mediated by stimulating adenyl cyclase and increasing the level of cyclic AMP (cAMP) (8). The discovery of these compounds led to the theory that a critical biosynthetic balance is maintained between PGI_2 and TXA_2 (9). Table 1 summarizes many of the EC types and their principal eicosanoid following stimulation.

EC INJURY

Endothelial cell perturbation (or dysfunction) is considered of notable importance in the development of atherosclerosis (10). Stemerman and Ross formulated the "response to injury hypothesis" describing that EC loss leads to smooth cell proliferation (11). The response to injury hypothesis has been modified to include more subtle, non-desquamating forms of EC injury (10,12). For example, moderate hypercholesterolemia is associated with an increase in the number of high permeability foci (13). The areas of heightened permeability show little evidence of EC morphologic change. In subsequent studies, using autoradiography, Stemerman and colleagues (14) demonstrated that the high permeability foci of the rabbit endothelium contained up to 47 times more LDL than control regions.

LDL OXIDATION

Although the pathogenetic link between LDL and atherosclerosis is unclear, it is speculated to be associated with LDL oxidation (15). There is some dispute concerning the physiologically important sight of oxidation of the particle. With oxidation, the apolipoprotein B (Apo-B) moiety undergoes fragmentation. This alteration in Apo-B correlates with the amount of lipid peroxidation and is inhibited by metal chelation or anti-oxidants (16). Oxidized LDL can induce cytotoxicity for cultured EC (17), smooth muscle cells (18) and fibroblasts (19). The LDL cytotoxicity is independent of receptor-mediated endocytosis (20), and is inhibited by high density lipoprotein (HDL) (20) or other proteins (17). The LDL cytotoxic effect is inhibited by general free radical scavengers suggesting that LDL induced cytotoxicity involves a free radical-mediated process (21). A positive correlation between cytotoxicity and the levels of malondialdehyde a by-product of lipid peroxidation, provides additional evidence that the cytotoxic effect of LDL is due to its oxidation (22).

In vitro, LDL free radical oxidation can be induced by a number of cell types including human umbilical vein EC (HUVEC) (23), SMC (24), monocytes (25), neutrophils (25), macrophages (26) and rabbit aortic EC (27). The LDL oxidation is attended by a number of chemical and physical alterations such as an increased electrophoretic mobility and depressed sterol content (23), an increase in density (27), a decrease in reactivity of the lysine residues of the apo-B moiety (28), and the degradation of phosphatidylcholine to lysophosphatidylcholine (29). In addition to its cytotoxic effect, oxidized LDL has been shown to be chemotactic for human monocytes (30), to inhibit the release of an EC PDGF-like protein (31), and to be taken up by the scavenger receptor (27). Whether a similar modification of LDL and its effect(s) occur in vivo is not known. However, the work of Raymond and colleagues (32) indicates that a modified form of LDL from rabbit inflammatory fluid exhibits an increased electrophoretic mobility and is recognized by the scavenger receptor. Recently, a similar form of LDL was isolated from atheroslerotic plaques of human carotid arteries (33). Whether oxidized LDL has an important pathologic effect is unclear, since it would imply widespread cellular injury and degeneration rather than the proliferation of intimal components as seen in an atherosclerotic plaque.

LDL AND EC EICOSANOID BIOSYNTHESIS

Another mechanism for LDL-induced EC dysfunction may be the effect of LDL on EC eicosanoid metabolism. EC incubated with LDL have been reported to both augment (34) or to have no effect (35) on PGI_2 biosynthesis. Oxidized LDL has been shown to enhance the PGI_2 production by human saphenous vein EC (36). In aortic slices from rat or superfused bovine coronary arteries, the

effect of LDL was inhibitory to PGI_2 biosynthesis (37). This observation indicates that LDL serves as a carrier of lipid peroxides which subsequently can inactivate arterial prostacyclin
synthetase. In this system, however, the relative effect of LDL
on the different cell types (EC, SMC) are not distinguishable.
In contradistinction to LDL, HDL has generally been demonstrated
to augment EC PGI_2 biosynthesis. HDL-mediated increase in
PGI_2 biosynthesis by EC may be due to a lipid transfer
protein that effectively shuttles arachidonic acid (AA) from
HDL to EC membrane phospholipids (38).

RECENT OBSERVATIONS

The conflicting reports of LDL-mediated changes in EC PGI_2
biosynthesis could be a result of the variability in the chemical
nature of the LDL molecule due to its isolation or utilization:
lipid peroxides may stimulate or suppress the activity of
cyclooxygenase and/or lipoxygenase (39). We have studied the
effects of long term LDL exposure on HUVEC function; especially
eicosanoid generation. To date, the isolation of LDL or its
subsequent incubation with various cells has resulted in the
chemical (23) or biological (40) modification of the lipoprotein.
Further, incubations of EC with LDL have lasted for only short
periods of time (48 hours) (17) and, in general, were at concentrations (60 mg/dl) (22) far below those associated with the
risk of accelerated atherosclerosis. We have developed a cell
culture system where HUVEC are maintained in the presence of LDL
(180-330 mg/dl) for periods up to 28 days (41). Large quantities
of unoxidized LDL were rapidly isolated by a novel method recently developed in this laboratory (42). Using this system, no
overt LDL cytotoxic effect was found using lactate dehydrogenase,
^{51}Cr release, trypan blue exclusion and cell counts as measures
of cell toxicity (43).
Despite the lack of any overt cytotoxicity, several metabolic
perturbations have thus far been identified. EC incubated with
LDL showed both a dose and time dependent increase in PGI_2 (44).
Similarly, the levels of TXA_2 and HETE products were augmented by
exposure to LDL; in contrast, PGE_2, PGD_2, and PGA_2 were
depressed (45). The increase in HETE products and the decrease
in cyclooxygenase metabolites suggest a shift in eicosanoid
biosynthesis.
In summary, we have observed several metabolic perturbations
associated with the culture of HUVEC in the presence of LDL at
concentrations associated with premature atherosclerotic heart
disease. A significant increase in PGI_2 was noted in cells
incubated with atherogenic levels of LDL. This increase was
maintained over a 12 day period compared with control cells where
PGI_2 progressively decreased (44). The increase in PGI_2 was not
apparent until 60 minutes following exposure to LDL (44). The
change in PGI_2 production appears to be an index of a profound
shift in eicosanoid production in the EC which effects the EC
homeostatic mechanism favoring atherogenesis.

TABLE I

THE PRINCIPAL PROSTAGLANDIN SYNTHESIZED
BY VARIOUS STIMULATED ENDOTHELIAL CELLS

Source	Stimulant	Principal PG
HUVEC	BK(46), A23(46), AA+EPA(47) H(48), Et-OH(49), T(50)	$17\text{-}6KETOPGF_{I\alpha}$(47) $6\text{-}KETO\text{-}PGF_{1\alpha}$
HSVEC	BK(46), A23(46)	$PGF_{2\alpha}$
BCVEC	BK(46), A23(46)	$PGF_{2\alpha}$
Baboon AEC	BK(46), A23(46)	$PGF_{2\alpha}$
BAEC	BK(46), A23(46), AA(51), ADP(52), LTC4, LTD4(53)	$6\text{-}KETO\text{-}PGF_{1\alpha}$
RAEC	BK(46), A23(46)	$6\text{-}KETO\text{-}PGF_{1\alpha}$
RCEC	BK(46), A23(46), AA(46)	$PGE_{2\alpha}$
HFSMVEC	A23(54)	$PGF_{2\alpha}$
BPAEC	BK(55), AA(56)	$6\text{-}KETO\text{-}PGF_{1\alpha}$
HPAEC	H(48)	$6\text{-}KETO\text{-}PGF_{1\alpha}$
Piglet AEC	AA(57), Steroid (58)	$PGF_{2\alpha}$
Fetal Bovine Heart EC	AA(59)	$6\text{-}KETO\text{-}PGF_{1\alpha}$
Porcine EC	BK(60), A23(60), T(61), AA(62)	$6\text{-}KETO\text{-}PGF_{1\alpha}$ $PGF_{2\alpha}$(62)
Bovine Carotid EC	Kallikrein (63)	$6\text{-}KETO\text{-}PGF_{1\alpha}$
Bovine Coronary AEC	BK, A23, T, AA(64)	$6\text{-}KETO\text{-}PGF_{1\alpha}$
Rabbit Coronary MVEC	AA(65)	$PGE_{2\alpha}$

References in parenthesis

Abbreviations:

AEC	Aortic EC	HFSMVEC	Human foreskin microvessel EC
AA	Arachidonic Acid	HPAEC	Human pulmonary artery EC
A23	A23187	HSVEC	Human saphenous vein EC
BCVEC	Baboon cephalic vein EC	HUVEC	Human umbilical vein EC
BAEC	Bovine aortic EC	RAEC	Rat aortic EC
BPAEC	Bovine pulmonary artery EC	RCEC	Rat capillary EC
BK	Bradykinin	T	Thrombin
EPA	Eicosapentaenoic acid		
H	Histamine		

Acknowledgements

The authors are indebted to Sue Murphy and Linda Miano for assistance in the preparation of this manuscript. This work was supported by National Institutes of Health Grant HL-33742.

References

1. Brown, M.S. and Goldstein, J.L. Scientific American 251(5):58-66, 1984.

2. Mullane, K.M. and Pinto, A. FASEB 46:54-62, 1987.
3. Ramirez, C.A., Colton, C., Smith, K.A., et al. Arteriosclerosis 4:283-291, 1984.
4. Jaffe, E.A., Hoyer, L.W. and Nachman, R.L. Proc.Natl.Acad.Sci. USA 71:1906-1909, 1974.
5. Moncada, S., Gryglewski, R., Bunting, S., et al. Nature 263:663-665, 1976.
6. Weksler, B.B., Marcus, A.J. and Jaffe, E.A. Proc.Natl.Acad.Sci. USA 74:3922-3926, 1977.
7. Hamberg, M., Svensson, J. and Samuelsson, B. Proc.Natl.Acad.Sci. USA 72:2994-2998, 1975.
8. Best, L.C., Martin, T.J., Russell, R.G.G., et al. Nature 267:850-852, 1977.
9. Moncada, S. Prostacyclin and Thromboxane A2 in platelet vessel wall interactions. In: Proceedings of the fifth international symposium on atherosclerosis, edited by Gotto, A.M., Smith, L.C. and Allen, B. New York: Springer-Verlag, 1980, p. 426-441.
10. Stemerman, M.B., Colton, C. and Morell, E. Perturbations of the endothelium. In: Progress in Hemostasis and Thrombosis, edited by Spaet, T.H. New York: Grune & Stratton, 1984, p. 289-324.
11. Stemerman, M.B. and Ross, R. J.Exp.Med. 136:769-789, 1972.
12. Ross, R. New England Journal of Medicine 314:488-500, 1986.
13. Stemerman, M.B. Arteriosclerosis 1:25-32, 1981.
14. Stemerman, M.B., Morell, E., Burke, K.R., et al. Arteriosclerosis 6:64-69, 1986.
15. Henriksen, T. Eur.Surg.Res. 16:Suppl. 2:62-67, 1984.
16. Schuh, J., Fairclough, G.F., Jr. and Haschemeyer, R.H. Proc.Natl.Acad.Sci. USA 75:3173-3177, 1978.
17. Henriksen, T., Evensen, S.A. and Carlander, B. Scand.J.Clin.Lab.Invest. 39:361-368, 1979.
18. Hessler, J.R., Robertson, A.L. and Chisolm, G.M., III. Atherosclerosis 32:213-229, 1979.
19. Evensen, S.A., Nilsen, E. and Galdal, K.S. Scand.J.Clin.Lab.Invest. 42:285-290, 1982.
20. Henriksen, T., Evensen, S.A. and Carlander, B. Scand.J.Clin.Lab.Invest. 39:369-375, 1979.
21. Evensen, S.A., Galdal, K.S. and Nilsen, E. Atherosclerosis 49:23-30, 1983.
22. Hessler, J.R., Morel, D.W., Lewis, L.J., et al. Arteriosclerosis 3:215-222, 1983.
23. Morel, D.W., DiCorleto, P.E. and Chisolm, G.M., III. Arteriosclerosis 4:357-364, 1984.
24. Heinecke, J.W., Baker, L., Rosen, H., et al. J.Clin.Invest. 77:757-761, 1986.
25. Cathcart, M.K., Morel, D.W. and Chisolm, G.M., III. J.Leukocyte Biol. 38:341-350, 1985.
26. Parthasarathy, S., Printz, D.J., Boyd, D., et al. Arteriosclerosis 6:505-510, 1986.
27. Steinbrecher, U.P., Parthasarathy, S., Leake, D.S., et al. Proc.Natl.Acad.Sci. USA 81:3883-3887, 1984.

28. Steinbrecher, U.P., Witztum, J.L., Parthasarathy, S., et al. Arteriosclerosis 7:135-143, 1987.
29. Parthasarathy, S., Steinbrecher, U.P., Barnett, J., et al. Proc.Natl.Acad.Sci. USA 82:3000-3004, 1985.
30. Quinn, M.T., Parthasarathy, S., Fong, L.G., et al. Proc.Natl.Acad.Sci. USA 84:2995-2998, 1987.
31. Fox, P.L., Chisolm, G.M., III. and DiCorleto, P.E. J.Biol.Chem. 262:6046-6054, 1987.
32. Raymond, T.L., Reynolds, S.A. and Swanson, J.A. Inflammation 11:335-344, 1987.
33. Shaikh, M., Quiney, J.R., Baskerville, P., et al. Atherosclerosis 69:165-172, 1988.
34. Spector, A.A., Scanu, A.M., Kaduce, T.L., et al. J. Lipid Res. 26:288-297, 1985.
35. Nordoy, A., Killie, J.E., Badimon, L., et al. Atherosclerosis 50:307-323, 1984.
36. Triau, J.E., Meydani, M., Libby, P., et al. Fed.Proc. 45:347-347, 1985.
37. Szczeklik, A. and Gryglewski, R.J. Artery 7:488-495, 1980.
38. Pomerantz, K.B., Fleisher, L.N., Tall, A.R., et al. J. Lipid Res. 26:1269-1276, 1985.
39. Lands, W.E. J.Free Radic.Biol.Med. 1:97-101, 1985.
40. Henriksen, T., Mahoney, E.M. and Steinberg, D. Proc.Natl.Acad.Sci. USA 78:6499-6503, 1981.
41. Holland, J.A., Pritchard, K.A., Jr. and Stemerman, M.B. FASEB 46:829, 1987.
42. Pritchard, K.A., Jr., Holland, J.A., Rogers, N.J., et al. manuscript submitted 1988.
43. Holland, J.A., Pritchard, K.A., Jr. and Stemerman, M.B. Arteriosclerosis 6:540a-541a, 1986.
44. Holland, J.A., Pritchard, K.A., Jr., Rogers, N.J., et al. manuscript submitted 1988.
45. Pritchard, K.A., Jr., Holland, J.A., Wong, P.Y.-K., et al. Clin.Res. 35:1987.
46. Taylor, L., Foxall, T., Auger, K., et al. Atherosclerosis 65:227-236, 1987.
47. Bordet, J-C., Guichardant, M. and Lagarde, M. Biochem.Biophys.Res.Commun. 135:403-410, 1986.
48. Johnson, A.R., Revtyak, G. and Campbell, W.B. FASEB 44:19-24, 1985.
49. Landolfi, R. and Steiner, M. Blood 64:679-682, 1984.
50. de Groot, P.G., Brinkman, H-J.M., Gonsalves, M.D., et al. Biochim.Biophys.Acta 846:342-349, 1985.
51. Ingerman-Wojenski, C., Silver, M.J. and Smith, J.B. J.Clin.Invest. 67:1292-1296, 1981.
52. Van Coevorden, A. and Boeynaems, J.M. Prostaglandins 27:615-626, 1984.
53. Clark, M.A., Littlejohn, D., Mong, S., et al. Prostaglandins 31:157-166, 1986.
54. Charo, I.F., Shak, S., Karasek, M.A., et al. J.Clin.Invest. 74:914-919, 1984.

55. Hahn, G.L. and Polgar, P.R. <u>Atherosclerosis</u> 51:143-150, 1984.
56. Menconi, M., Hahn, G. and Polgar, P. <u>J.Cell</u> <u>Physiol.</u> 120:163-168, 1984.
57. Ody, C., Seillan, C. and Russo-Marie, F. <u>Biochim.Biophys.Acta</u> 712:103-110, 1982.
58. Seillan, C., Ody, C., Russo-Marie, F., et al. <u>Prostaglandins</u> 26:3-12, 1983.
59. Ali, A.E., Barrett, J.C. and Eling, T.E. <u>Prostaglandins</u> 20:667-688, 1980.
60. Whorton, A.R., Collawn, J.B., Montgomery, M.E., et al. <u>Biochem.Pharmacol.</u> 34:119-123, 1985.
61. Whorton, A.R., Young, S.L., Data, J.L., et al. <u>Biochim.Biophys.Acta</u> 712:79-87, 1982.
62. Neichi, T., Chang, W-C., Mitsui, Y., et al. <u>Artery</u> 11:47-63, 1982.
63. Morita, I., Kanayasu, T. and Murota, S-I. <u>Biochim.Biophys.Acta</u> 792:304-309, 1984.
64. Revtyak, G.E., Johnson, A.R. and Campbell, W.B. <u>Am.J.Physiol.</u> 254:8-19, 1988.
65. Gerritsen, M.E. and Cheli, C.D. <u>J.Clin.Invest.</u> 72:1658-1671, 1983.

Advances in Prostaglandin, Thromboxane, and Leukotriene Research, Vol. 19, edited by
B. Samuelsson, P. Y.-K. Wong, and F. F. Sun,
Raven Press, Ltd., New York ©1989.

REGULATION OF POLYMORPHONUCLEAR LEUKOCYTE LEUKOTRIENE

SYNTHESIS BY ENDOTHELIAL CELL CYCLOOXYGENASE PRODUCTS

S.J. Feinmark[*+], J. Edasery[*], and P.J. Cannon[*]

Departments of Pharmacology[+] and Medicine[*], Columbia
University, New York, NY 10032

Leukotriene (LT)C_4 is a potent vasoconstricting autacoid which also has the ability to increase vascular permeability (1). Production of LTC_4 is primarily associated with inflammatory cells including mast cells, macrophages and granulocytes (2). Recent studies have detailed a prominent transcellular pathway for LTC_4 synthesis within the circulation (3-5). Although endothelial cells (EC) are unable to generate LT from arachidonic acid, it has been shown that polymorphonuclear leukocytes (PMNL) can transfer the unstable LT intermediate, LTA_4, to EC as substrate for LTC_4 synthesis (3). Similar results have been reported for porcine vascular smooth muscle cells (4) and human platelets (5). This pathway has been examined in vitro using the calcium ionophore, A23187, as the initiating stimulus for LT synthesis. The results of further experiments which use a more physiologically relevant leukocyte activator, fMLP, as the initiator of LT synthesis are described in this report.

METHODS

PMNL were prepared from human peripheral blood, after the removal of platelet rich plasma, by dextran sedimentation, hypotonic lysis and Lymphoprep density gradient centrifugation (6). EC were cultured from intimal scrapings of porcine aortae and subcultured up to passage 10. Monolayers were grown on 25 cm^2 flasks and coincubated with PMNL (20 x 10^6 PMNL in 1 ml) in Dulbecco's phosphate-buffered saline with 1% bovine serum albumin (PBS/BSA). Some EC were preincubated with acetylsalicylic acid (ASA; 0.2 mM) for 30 min and then washed. After adding the PMNL suspension to the EC, the cells were incubated with arachidonic acid (10 uM) for 1 min followed by fMLP (1 uM) for 30 min. The media were recovered and tracer amounts of [^{3}H]LTC_4 were added in ice cold methanol (1:1.5; vol/vol). LTC_4 was purified from the media by reversed-phase HPLC and fractions containing the tracer were subsequently analyzed by radioimmunoassay (3).

5-HETE was analyzed by GC/MS using a stable isotope dilution assay modified from (7). HPLC-purified 5-HETE was reduced by hydrogen gas in the presence of rhodium (5% on alumina) and converted to the corresponding pentafluorobenzyl ester, tert-butyldimethylsilyl ether. This derivative was analyzed on an HP5987A GC/MS in the negative ion mode. Data were collected for m/z 441, the derivatized 5-HETE ion and m/z 445 which is the doubly oxygen-18 labelled internal standard. Quantification was done after the construction of a standard curve.

RESULTS AND DISCUSSION

Previous studies of LTC_4 synthesis during PMNL/EC interactions have demonstrated the transfer of LTA_4 from PMNL to EC where it is converted to LTC_4 (3). This transcellular metabolism results in a substantial increase in the LTC_4 produced by the mixed cells compared to PMNL alone. For example, in a series of paired incubations, with A23187 (5 uM) as the stimulus mixed PMNL/EC produced over 12-fold more LTC_4 than PMNL alone (Table 1). To test whether the physiologic leukocyte activator, fMLP, was able to stimulate similar transcellular metabolism, mixed PMNL/EC and PMNL alone were incubated with arachidonic acid (10 uM) and then fMLP (1 uM) for 30 min. Contrary to the observation of increased LTC_4 synthesis induced by A23187, the fMLP-induced synthesis was nearly 70% lower in mixed PMNL/EC than in PMNL alone (Table 1).

TABLE 1.   LTC₄ production by PMNL mixed with EC.

	LTC_4 Production (pmol/10⁷ PMNL)	
	A23187[a]	20:4 + fMLP
PMNL	1.2 ± 0.8*	1.7 ± 0.9
PMNL + EC	15.9 ± 6.1*	0.5 ± 0.3

* $p < 0.05$, n=3. a: A23187 (5 uM); 20:4 (10 uM) for 1 min followed by fMLP (1 uM) for 30 min.

A previous report by Ham, et al. had demonstrated that certain prostaglandins could block fMLP-induced LTB_4 synthesis in cytochalasin B-treated PMNL suspensions (8). This suggested to us that EC-derived prostacyclin (PGI_2) might be responsible for the observed decrease in LT synthesis by the fMLP-stimulated mixed cell incubations. The production of PGI_2 was quantified in these experiments by enzyme-linked immunoassay (7). PMNL alone produced 0.2 ± 0.1

pmol/10^7 PMNL while mixed PMNL/EC generated 12.2 $\pm$ 4.7 pmol/10^7 PMNL-flask. These data confirm the presence of a biologically active cyclooxygenase product derived from the EC under these incubation conditions.

To directly test the importance of cyclooxygenase metabolism in this system, a second series of incubations was completed which compared LTC_4 production by PMNL alone, PMNL plus EC and PMNL plus ASA-treated EC using the fMLP stimulation protocol described above. If the EC-dependent inhibition of LTC_4 synthesis is caused by PGI_2, then it should be abolished by ASA treatment and the expected transcellular augmentation should reappear. Mixed PMNL/EC produced barely detectable levels of LTC_4 (Fig. 1, panel A) while PMNL plus ASA-treated EC produced nearly 10-fold more (panel B).

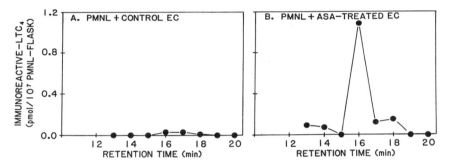

FIG. 1. RIA measurement of HPLC purified LTC_4.
Panel A: PMNL + EC; Panel B: PMNL + ASA-treated EC

Data from several experiments are summarized in Table 2. LTC_4 production was inhibited by 68% when PMNL were incubated with EC as compared to PMNL alone. However, when the EC were treated with ASA prior to the incubation, the mixed cells produced 2.2-times the amount of LTC_4 generated by PMNL alone and 7.2-times that produced by PMNL mixed with control EC.

TABLE 2. Effect of ASA on LTC_4 synthesis by PMNL/EC.

Cell-type	Drug	LTC_4 Production (pmol/10^7 PMNL)
PMNL	---	0.75 $\pm$ 0.39
PMNL + EC	---	0.23 $\pm$ 0.08[*]
PMNL + EC	ASA	1.66 $\pm$ 0.44[**]

* p<0.05 vs. PMNL, n=5. ** p<0.01 vs. PMNL, n=5.

In order to determine whether this EC-dependent inhibition of PMNL LT synthesis occured at or before the 5-lipoxygenase, the levels of 5-HETE were quantified as well. In agreement with the LTC_4 synthesis data, these results demonstrated that 5-HETE production was significantly greater in the mixed PMNL/ASA-treated EC incubations than in the control (3.6 ± 0.4 pmol/10^7 PMNL versus 2.8 ± 0.3 pmol/10^7 PMNL; $p<0.05$, n=4). These data suggest that the EC-dependent inhibition of PMNL LT synthesis is mediated by a cyclooxygenase product, presumably PGI_2. Furthermore, since both 5-HETE and LTC_4 synthesis are inhibited in the presence of EC, the regulated step is likely to be the 5-lipoxygenase itself or the phospholipase which must be activated to provide arachidonic acid to the lipoxygenase as substrate. It is noteworthy that both enzymes are calcium dependent (9). In addition, fMLP has been shown to stimulate a rapid increase in PMNL intracellular calcium levels via a receptor-mediated mechanism (10). These observations and the data presented above suggest that PGI_2 may act to modulate fMLP-induced calcium fluxes in the PMNL. Studies to confirm this hypothesis are in progress.

We thank Dr. R. Sciacca for statistical analyses and for helpful discussions. The technical assistance of Lucyna Olkowska and Nooshin Ismail-Beigi is gratefully acknowledged. This work was supported by grants from the NIH, HL21006 and HL14148. Dr. Feinmark was an investigator of the NY Heart Association.

REFERENCES

1. Piper PJ. Physiol Rev. 1984;64:744-61.
2. Samuelsson B. Science. 1983;220:568-75.
3. Feinmark SJ, Cannon PJ. J Biol Chem. 1986;261: 16466-72.
4. Feinmark SJ, Cannon PJ. Biochim Biophys Acta. 1987;922:125-35.
5. Maclouf J, Murphy RC J Biol Chem. 1988;263:174-81.
6. Claesson H-E, Feinmark SJ. Biochim Biophys Acta. 1984;804:52-7.
7. Westcott JY, Chang S, Balazy M, et al. Prostaglandins. 1986;32:857-73.
8. Ham EA, Soderman, DD, Zanetti, ME, Dougherty, HW, McCauley, E, Kuehl, FA, Jr. Proc Natl Acad Sci USA. 1983;80:4349-53.
9. Rouzer CA, Samuelsson B. Proc Natl Acad Sci USA. 1985;82:6040-4.
10. Korchak HM, Wilkenfeld C, Rich AR, Vienne K, Rutherford LE. J Biol Chem. 1984;259:7439-45.

Advances in Prostaglandin, Thromboxane, and Leukotriene Research, Vol. 19, edited by B. Samuelsson, P. Y.-K. Wong, and F. F. Sun, Raven Press, Ltd., New York ©1989.

PLATELETS AND ENDOTHELIAL CELLS CONTRIBUTE TO THE PRODUCTION OF LTC$_4$ BY TRANSCELLULAR METABOLISM WITH NEUTROPHILS

Jacques Maclouf[1], Robert C. Murphy[2] and Peter M. Henson[3]

[1]Unite 150 INSERM, Hopital Lariboisiere, 75475, Paris Cedex 10, France. [2]University of Colorado Health Sciences Center, Department of Pharmacology, Denver, Colorado, 80262, USA. [3]National Center for Immunology and Respiratory Medicine, Denver, Colorado, 80206.

The synthesis of peptido leukotrienes (LTs) results from the action of a 5-lipoxygenase on arachidonic acid to generate LTA$_4$ which is subsequently transformed into LTC$_4$ by a specific glutathione-S-transferase (1). Due to their pharmacological effects on the vessel and on smooth muscle tone, LTC$_4$ and its metabolite, LTD4 are suspected to play an important role in inflammatory, allergic or cardiovascular disorders (2). The cellular origin of these mediators has been ascribed mainly to eosinophils, mast cells, basophils as well as monocytes/macrophages (3). Although other potential sources are suspected, no clear cut evidence has emerged for the identification of another cell possessing the complete biosynthetic capacity of LTC$_4$ from arachidonic acid. However, recent reports have described the ability of porcine aortic endothelial cells (4), smooth muscle cells (5) as well as human umbilical endothelial cells (6) to synthesize LTC$_4$ from either exogenously added LTA$_4$ into LTC$_4$ or LTA$_4$ originally synthesized within neutrophils. Recently, we have demonstrated that human platelets exhibit a high capacity to transform exogenously added LTA$_4$ into LTC$_4$ (7). In addition, with cellular coincubations, we could also demonstrate that LTA$_4$ derived from neutrophils could be further metabolized into LTC$_4$ by platelets. The possibility that LTC$_4$ can be generated by transcellular metabolism adds an alternative mechanism for the production of this pathophysiological mediator under conditions where cell-cell cooperations are known to be important such as in inflammatory or cardiovascular processes (2,3).

In this report, we have investigated whether the combination of two recipient cells (i.e. human platelets or endothelial cells from different species and vascular origins) along with donor cells (i.e. neutrophils) could enhance the production of LTC$_4$.

MATERIALS AND METHODS

Washed human platelets were prepared according to Patscheke (8) and incubated at 0.3 x 10^9 cells/ml. Human neutrophils were prepared using a plasma percoll gradient (9) and incubated at 5 x 10^6 cells/ml. Human umbilical vein (HUVEC) porcine aorta (PAEC), and porcine pulmonary artery (PPEC) endothelial cells were cultured on 35 mm wells and were characterized morphologically as well as using biochemical and immunocytochemical criteria. All incubations were carried out in Hank's buffer (1 ml, pH 7.4) containing 0.4% bovine serum albumin.

The cells were challenged either alone or in combination with 5uM calcium ionophore A 23187. After 20 min., the reaction was quenched by the addition of 1 vol of ice cold methanol and centrifugation. The supernatant was analyzed for LTC_4 by an enzyme immunoassay (10) using an antiserum kindly provided by Dr. E. Hayes (Merck, Rahway, NJ).

RESULTS AND DISCUSSION

As can be seen on Figure 1, the synthesis of LTC_4 by ionophore challenged neutrophils alone was very low; this "basal" production could be due to the presence of eosinophils as well as to the unavoidable contamination of neutrophil suspensions by a small number of platelets.

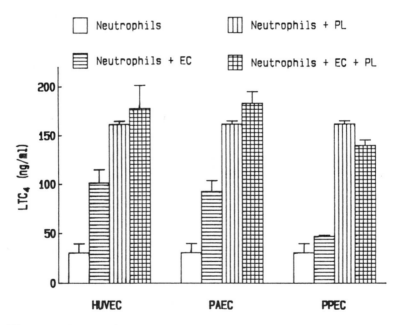

Figure 1: Leukotriene biosynthesis in neutrophils in the presence or in the absence of platelets and endothelial cells. Neutrophils (5×10^6) were stimulated with calcium ionophore A23187 (5uM) in the absence or presence of endothelial cells (5×10^5 per 35 mm well) and/or platelets (0.6×10^9/ml) for 30 min at 37°C. The LTC_4 content was analyzed as described in Materials and Methods. (Mean ± SEM from 2-3 experiments run in triplicate)

The addition of neutrophils either to endothelial cells or to human platelets greatly enhanced the production of LTC_4 from 31 ± 9 ng/ml to 101 ± 14, 92 ± 11, 47 ± 1 in the presence of human umbilical vein, porcine aortic and porcine pulmonary artery endothelial cells respectively or to 161 ± 3 ng/ml in the presence of platelets. It should be noted that the quantity of LTC_4 was considerably higher when neutrophils were combined with platelets as compared to neutrophil coincubation with endothelial cells. Approximately the same amount of LTC_4 was attained using endothelial cells from the human umbilical vein and porcine aorta suggesting that these endothelial cells tested in this set of experiments possess the same capacity to generate LTC_4 from the neutrophil-derived LTA_4 in spite of their different vessel and specie origin. There was some indication that less LTC_4 was produced by the pulmonary artery-derived endothelial cells. However, the coincubation of platelets and endothelial cells with neutrophils did not result in a further enhancement in the production of LTC_4 as compared to that observed with platelets in any of the experiments. This supports our previous suggestion that LTA_4 availability for transcellular metabolism may be limited.

The calcium ionophore is a potent stimulus for the synthesis of LTs by neutrophils, but it bypasses important receptor mediated signal transduction events which occur at the membrane level. It can be anticipated that using less drastic inducers of neutrophil activation such as complement fragments, IgG and/or phagocytosis to generate LTA_4, the availability of LTA_4 to recipient cells i.e. vicinal platelets and endothelial cells will be somewhat reduced. Yet, it should be mentioned that chronic stimulation of the neutrophil could lead to suicide inactivation of LTA_4-hydrolase (12) and thus a decreased metabolism of LTA_4 into LTB_4 by the neutrophil with consequently an enhanced availability of LTA_4 for export even when produced by such mild neutrophil activators. Under pathological situations such as inflammation, allergy, and ischemia, multiple interactions between neutrophils, platelets and vascular cells are known to occur and the production of LTC_4 by transcellular metabolism could represent an important mechanism in the generation of mediators known to profoundly influence vascular tone as well as capillary permeability.

ACKNOWLEDGEMENTS

This work was supported, in part, by grants from the National Institutes of Health (AI20774 and HL34303).

REFERENCES

1.   Murphy RC, Hammarstrom S, Samuelsson B, Proc Natl Acad Sci USA, 1979; 76:4275-4279.

2. Samuelsson B, Dahlen S-E, Lindgren JA et al., <u>Science</u>, 1987; 237:1171-1176.

3. Lewis RA, Austen KF, <u>J Clin Invest</u>, 1984; 73:889-897.

4. Feinmark SJ, Cannon PJ, <u>J Biol Chem</u>, 1986; 261:16466-16472.

5. Feinmark SJ, Cannon PJ, <u>Biochim Biophys Acta</u>, 1987; 922:125-135.

6. Claesson H-E, Haeggstrom J, In: Samuelsson B, Paoletti R, Ramwell P, eds. <u>Adv Prostaglandins Thromboxane and Leukotriene Research</u>, vol 17 New York; Raven Press, 1987; 115-119.

7. Maclouf J, Murphy RC, <u>J Biol Chem</u>, 1988; 263:174-1981.

8. Patscheke H, <u>Haemostasis</u>, 1981; 10:14-27.

9. Haslett C, Guthrie L, Kopaniak MM et al., <u>Am J Pathol</u>, 1985; 119:101-110.

10. Pradelles P, Grassi J, Maclouf J, <u>Anal Chem</u>, 1985; 57:1170-1173.

11. Harlan JM, <u>Blood</u>, 1985; 65:513-525.

12. McGee J, Fitzpatrick FA, <u>J Biol Chem</u>, 1985; 260:12832-12837.

Advances in Prostaglandin, Thromboxane, and Leukotriene Research, Vol. 19, edited by B. Samuelsson, P. Y.-K. Wong, and F. F. Sun, Raven Press, Ltd., New York ©1989.

INTERACTIONS BETWEEN PLATELETS AND NEUTROPHILS IN THE EICOSANOID PATHWAY

Aaron J. Marcus, Lenore B. Safier, Harris L. Ullman, Naziba Islam, M. Johan Broekman, J.R. Falck, Sven Fischer, M. Teresa Santos, Juana Valles, and Clemens von Schacky

Divisions of Hematology-Oncology, Departments of Medicine, New York Veterans Administration Medical Center, and the Specialized Center of Thrombosis Research, Cornell University Medical College, New York, NY 10010 (A.J.M., L.B.S., H.L.U., N.I., M.J.B., M.T.S, J.V.), Department of Molecular Genetics, University of Texas Health Science Center, Dallas, Texas (J.R.F.), and the Medizinische Klinik Innenstadt der Universitat Munchen, F.R.G. (S.F., C.v.S.)

EICOSANOID PRODUCTION AS A RESPONSE TO INJURY

Blood vessel injury or necrotic alterations resulting from atherosclerosis culminate in exposure of subendothelial components, such as collagen, which is a known agonist for platelet adhesion and activation (1). Activated platelets promote coagulation by serving as a catalytic surface for assembly of coagulation factors. Since platelets, endothelial cells and leukocytes possess active eicosanoid-producing mechanisms, autacoids with significant biological properties result from platelet, endothelial cell and neutrophil stimulation and interaction.

As the hemostatic, thrombotic and inflammatory processes evolve, component cells are brought into close contact, a phenomenon which provides the opportunity for biochemical interchange of eicosanoid precursors, intermediates and end products (2-4). Such interactions are actually classifiable in an orderly fashion (5).

INTERACTIONS BETWEEN PLATELETS AND NEUTROPHILS IN THE LIPOXYGENASE PATHWAY

The major lipoxygenase product produced in stimulated human platelets is 12-hydroxyeicosatetraenoic acid (12-HETE). We have been studying the metabolism of this eicosanoid for several years as an intracellular messenger which is produced in abundance under conditions of aspirin administration. Unstimulated neutrophils can metabolize 12-HETE released from platelets to 12,20-dihydroxyeicosatetraenoic acid (12,20-DiHETE). We demonstrated that this reaction occurred via an omega-hydroxylation step of the cytochrome P-450 type (4). Very recently, during a time-course study, we found that 12,20-DiHETE was metabolized by an NAD-dependent dehydrogenase mechanism in

the unstimulated neutrophil to a new and previously unidentified
eicosanoid 12-hydroxyeicosatetraen-1,20-dioic acid
(12-HETE-1,20-dioic acid) (6).

PLATELET-NEUTROPHIL "COMMUNICATION"

When platelets are stimulated, they lipoxygenate free
arachidonic acid in the C-12 position. This lipoxygenation takes
place in the presence or absence of aspirin or other
non-steroidal anti-inflammatory compounds. If an unstimulated
neutrophil is in close proximity to the platelet, 12-HETE will be
metabolized. The resulting compound, 12,20-DiHETE forms via a
cytochrome P-450 omega-hydroxylation process (4). We have now
ascertained that 12,20-DiHETE is further oxidized by unstimulated
neutrophils to 12-HETE-1,20-dioic acid.

We also compared 12-HETE-1,20-dioic acid formation to the
metabolism of the leukocyte eicosanoid, leukotriene B_4 (LTB_4).
It is well known that following neutrophil stimulation, LTB_4 is
produced, and this compound is one of the most proinflammatory
eicosanoids yet described. We determined whether the enzyme
complex responsible for catalyzing conversion of 12,20-DiHETE to
12-HETE-1,20-dioic acid might also be somehow involved in the
metabolism of LTB_4. The trihydroxy acid, 20-hydroxy-LTB_4 (which
is the omega-hydroxylated metabolite of LTB_4) can be further
processed to the dioic acid form, 20-carboxy LTB_4 by human
neutrophils (8-11). We carried out experiments in which
20-hydroxy-LTB_4 was added to incubates of neutrophils and
12,20-DiHETE. In this manner, we could observe effects on
12-HETE-1,20-dioic acid formation, and we did indeed determine
that partial inhibition had occurred. The results, therefore,
suggested that the two substrates (20-OH-LTB_4 and 12,20-DiHETE)
were actually in competition for the same enzyme. We already
knew that there was competition by LTB_4 for the
12-HETE-omega-hydroxylase in the unstimulated neutrophil (4).
We, therefore, concluded that platelet 12-HETE and its
metabolites were capable of exerting a modulating influence on
the metabolism of LTB_4, which is a neutrophil-derived,
biologically active substance.

CONCLUDING REMARKS

In this paper, we have described reactions which represent a
novel extension of previous research. We had demonstrated that
in the eicosanoid pathway, interactions can occur between
different cell types, such as platelets, neutrophils and
endothelial cells (5), at least in vitro. When stimulated
platelets synthesize 12-HETE, it is initially transformed by
unstimulated neutrophils to 12,20-DiHETE – a novel eicosanoid
which neither cell can synthesize alone. In our recent
classification of cell-cell interactions, this category would be

classified as Type IIB (5). We now have demonstrated that the neutrophil continues to metabolize 12,20-DiHETE to 12-HETE-1,20-dioic acid. It is also known that during hemostasis, thrombosis and the inflammatory response, platelets and neutrophils function in close physical apposition. Thus, metabolic interchange of biochemical substances generated by these cells may serve to modulate mechanisms of host defenses.

REFERENCES

1. Marcus, AJ. In: Wyngaarden, JB, Smith, LH, eds. Cecil

    textbook of medicine, 18th edition. Philadelphia: Saunders,

    1988;1042-1060.

2. Marcus, AJ, Weksler, BB, Jaffe, EA, Broekman, MJ. J Clin

    Invest 1980;66:979.

3. Marcus, AJ, Safier, LB, Ullman, HL, et al. Proc Natl Acad

    Sci USA 1984;81:903.

4. Marcus, AJ, Safier, LB, Ullman, HL, Islam, N, Broekman, MJ,

    von Schacky, C. J Clin Invest 1987;79:179.

5. Marcus, AJ. In: Coller, BS, ed. Progress in hemostasis and

    thrombosis. New York: Grune & Stratton, 1986;127-142.

6. Marcus, AJ, Safier, LB, Ullman, HL, et al. J Biol Chem

    1988;263:2223.

This work was supported by grants from the Veterans
Administration, National Institutes of Health HL-18828-12 SCOR
(to A.J.M., M.J.B., and C.v.S.), HL-29034 (to M.J.B.), GM-31278
(to J.R.F.), the Edward Gruenstein Fund, the Sallie Wichman Fund,
and SM Louis Fund (to A.J.M.), the Deutsche
Forschungsgemeinschaft (to S.F. and C.v.S.), and HL-36919 (to
M.T.S. and J.V.).

Advances in Prostaglandin, Thromboxane, and Leukotriene Research, Vol. 19, edited by B. Samuelsson, P. Y.-K. Wong, and F. F. Sun, Raven Press, Ltd., New York ©1989.

PROSTACYCLIN, ENDOTHELIUM-DERIVED RELAXING FACTOR AND VASODILATATION

G. Siegel[1], F. Schnalke[1], G. Stock[2], and J. Grote[3]

[1] Institute of Physiology, Biophysical Research Group, The Free University of Berlin, D-1000 Berlin 33, Germany
[2] Cardiovascular Pharmacology, Research Laboratories of Schering AG, D-1000 Berlin 65
[3] Institute of Physiology, The University of Bonn, D-5300 Bonn 1, Germany

Vasodilatation in vascular smooth muscle of the canine carotid artery can be evoked by numerous effector influences: slight decrease in external K^+ concentration, acidification of the pH value, application of prostacyclin or reduction of the O_2 partial pressure in the blood substitute solution [4-6,8,10]. The diminution in tone of the smooth muscle cells is mediated by a hyperpolarization of their cell membranes, which leads to a fall of the intracellular Ca^{2+} activity via a decrease in open state probability of a second category of Ca^{2+} channels, which are closed voltage-dependently between -40 and -80 mV [1,5,9]. The cause of the hyperpolarization can be an increase of passive K^+ permeability, a decrease of passive Na^+ permeability, or an increase of the active, electrogenic outward Na^+ transport.

EFFECTS OF PROSTACYCLIN ON MEMBRANE POTENTIAL AND TENSION

The present contribution deals with the electrophysiological correlate to vasodilatation often observed under prostacyclin or O_2 deficiency. With regard to the extreme chemical instability of native prostacyclin, we used iloprost, a stable carbacyclin analogue [3,8]. In concentrations between 10^{-9} and 10^{-6} M, iloprost hyperpolarizes and relaxes the vessel strip in a dose-dependent manner (Figs. 1,2). The membrane potential of the vascular smooth muscle cells amounts to -63.4 mV. The maximum hyperpolarization is 7.4 mV, the maximum relaxation 0.703 g (coupling ratio 11.0 mV/g). Half-maximal effect is attained at a concentration of $2 \cdot 10^{-8}$ M. In the concentration step $3 \cdot 10^{-6}$ M a reversal of the iloprost effect is indicated, which can be found also in the

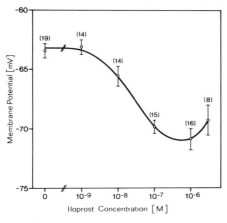

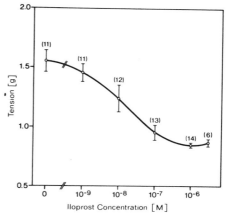

Fig. 1. Membrane potential of vascular smooth muscle in dependence on the iloprost concentration of the Krebs solution

Fig. 2. Dependency of the tension developed in isolated carotid segments on the iloprost concentration of the Krebs solution

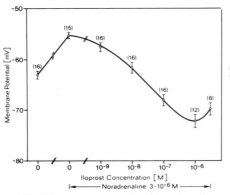

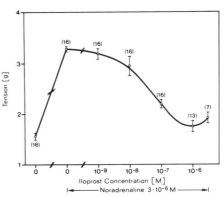

Fig. 3. Membrane potential of noradrenaline--depolarized vascular smooth muscle in function of the iloprost concentration in the Krebs solution. Application of iloprost 10 min at each concentration step

Fig. 4. Relation between developed tension and iloprost concentration in the Krebs solution of isolated carotid segments precontracted by noradrenaline. Addition of iloprost 10 min at each concentration step

experiments under noradrenaline [5,9]. In experiments without any additions, isolated vascular strips of the carotid artery were mounted isometrically with a pretension of 2 g. The various iloprost concentrations were applied 30 min each.

When a preparation fixed in such a way is precontracted additionally by $3 \cdot 10^{-6}$ M noradrenaline, the muscle cells depolarize to -55.2 mV with an increase in tension by 1.719 g (coupling ratio 4.6 mV/g). Iloprost re- and hyperpolarizes the resting potential by maximally 16.9 mV in a dose-dependent manner (Fig. 3). A close correlation (coupling ratio 10.4 mV/g) exists between potential course and force development: the hyperpolarization is parallelled by relaxation of 1.525 g of the vascular strip (Fig. 4). Under iloprost application, the noradrenaline contraction is abolished stepwise, the initial tone is almost reached [9]. Half-maximal effect on membrane potential and tension occurs with an iloprost concentration of $3 \cdot 10^{-8}$ M, that means, it is in good agreement with the experiments without noradrenaline treatment.

K^+ CHANNEL OPENING VS. CYCLIC NUCLEOTIDES

Eliminating the parameter iloprost concentration from the dose-response curves and plotting the developed tension against membrane potential [4], one obtains the stationary activation curves for the experiments without and with noradrenaline (Fig. 5). Both curves run parallel, the coupling ratio is identical. Thus, with application of the same iloprost concentrations,

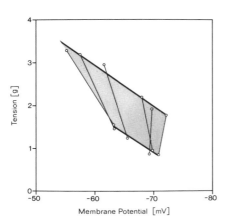

Fig. 5. Tension development in function of the membrane potential in isolated carotid segments (stationary activation curves). Change in membrane potential and tone by variation of the iloprost concentration in the Krebs solution as measured in preparations with normal tone (lower straight line) and preparations predepolarized by noradrenaline (upper straight line). Circles of identical iloprost concentration were connected. The dotted area represents the effect of noradrenaline

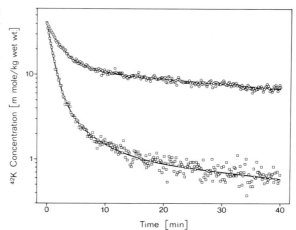

Fig. 6. ^{42} K$^+$ efflux in the carotid artery of the dog in Krebs solutions without (○) or with 10^{-6} M iloprost (□). The graph shows the time course of radioactive K$^+$ decrease within the preparations at intervals of 10 s in single experiments. The superimposed lines represent the optimal double-exponential functions found by computer fitting

the covered potential and tension range is much larger under noradrenaline. Considering further the activation curve for noradrenaline (left margin of the dotted area), one recognizes that the force developed under noradrenaline is reduced along quite a different path by iloprost. The potential difference required for abolition of the tension is much larger. This means that noradrenaline generates tension obviously also by mechanisms other than membrane potential, probably by a release of Ca^{2+} ions from intracellular storage sites [11]. Moreover, it seems presumable that iloprost effects vasorelaxation not only by hyperpolarization, but also by intracellular targets, e.g. by a rise in cAMP [2]. Fig. 5 suggests further that with an iloprost concentration of about 5·10^{-7} M (V ≈ -70 mV) the addition of noradrenaline (3·10^{-6} M) should generate force without any potential changes [cf. 11]. Conversely, one can calculate roughly that 65% of the relaxation under iloprost is to be attributed to membrane hyperpolarization, and 35% probably to an increase in cAMP.

These results lead to the question how prostacyclin effects hyperpolarization of the cell membrane. In Fig. 6, a ^{42} K$^+$ efflux experiment is represented without and with iloprost (10^{-6} M) with a time resolution of 10 s. Immediately, the much steeper course of the K$^+$ decay under iloprost can be recognized. After multiple exponential analysis and computation of a compartment model based on five experiments, we found an increase of passive K$^+$ efflux by 135% on an average under iloprost. Each time constant, especially the slowest, is diminished strongly. The calculation of membrane permeability for K$^+$ ions amounts to an increase of even 190% under iloprost [5,9]. Therefore, prostacyclin can be characterized as a 'K$^+$

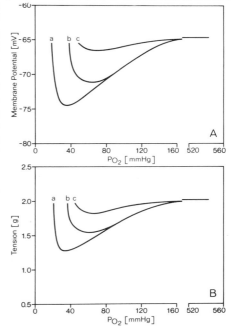

Fig. 7. Membrane potential (A) and tension (B) in isolated vascular strips of the *A. carotis communis* of the dog in dependency on the oxygen partial pressure of the Krebs solution. Mean values from five experiments. a: normal Krebs solution; b: Krebs solution with indomethacin (10^{-6} M); c: normal Krebs solution, endothelial layer of the carotid segments removed

channel opener' or 'K$^+$ agonist' [5,7,9,12].

ENDOTHELIUM-DERIVED HYPERPOLARIZING FACTOR

In the following we will report on experiments that were designed to elucidate the *in vivo* role of prostacyclin and endothelial dilator EDRF ('endothelium-derived relaxant factor'). Several authors presumed that hypoxic vasorelaxation could be evoked by prostacyclin. Recording membrane potential and tension in dependence on O_2 partial pressure, a dose-dependent hyperpolarization (ΔV = 9.8 mV) and relaxation (ΔT = 0.727 g) of vascular smooth muscle cells are observed with a reduction of P_{O_2} from 535 to 35 mm Hg (Fig. 7,a). Half-maximal effect is obtained with 87 mm Hg. A further decline of P_{O_2} reduces this hyperpolarization and relaxation, or even depolarization and contraction occur (P_{O_2} < 20 mm Hg).

In their extent, hyperpolarization and reduction in tone remind strongly of the influence of increasing iloprost concentrations. In fact, indomethacin (10^{-5} M) led to a 20% reduction of the hypoxia-dependent potential and tension alterations (Fig. 7,b). Moreover, the oxygen partial pressure with which maximal hyperpolarization and relaxation occur, is shifted to the significantly higher value of 64 mm Hg P_{O_2}. Only the complete removal of the endothelium prevents for the most part the hypoxic hyperpolarization and vasodilatation (Fig. 7,c). Decrease in oxygen tension down to a value of 70 mm Hg leads to a slight hyperpolarization of only 1.7 mV with simultaneous relaxation of 0.2 g. Below a P_{O_2} of 70 mm Hg again depolarization and vasoconstriction occur. Therefore, one can assume that about 80% of the effects in potential and tone under a decrease of oxygen tension is to be attributed to an endothelial dilator EDRF and 20% to the release of prostacyclin.

SUMMARY

In arterial smooth muscle with normal tone or predepolarized and precontracted by noradrenaline, prostacyclin (10^{-9} to 10^{-6} M) effects a dose-dependent hyperpolarization and relaxation. The hyperpolarization is due to K$^+$ channel opening. In hypoxic vasodilatation, which is likewise induced by membrane hyperpolarization, a share of 20% falls to prostacyclin and 80% to an endothelium derived hyperpolarizing factor.

REFERENCES

1. Loirand G, Pacaud P, Mironneau C, Mironneau J *Pflügers Arch* 1986;407:566-568.
2. Nicosia S, Oliva D, Bernini F, Fumagalli R. In: Greengard P, Robison GA, Paoletti R, Nicosia S, eds. *Advances in cyclic nucleotide and protein phosphorylation research*, vol 17. New York: Raven Press, 1984;593-599.
3. Schrör K, Darius H, Matzky R, Ohlendorf R *Naunyn-Schmiedebergs Arch Pharmacol* 1981;316: 252-255.
4. Siegel G *Physiol aktuell* 1986;1:31-52.
5. Siegel G, Bostanjoglo M, Thiel M, Adler A, Carl A, Stock G, Grote J. In: Betz E, ed. *Frühveränderungen bei der Atherogenese*. München: W Zuckschwerdt Verlag, 1987;91-101.
6. Siegel G, Kämpe Ch, Ebeling BJ. In: Cervó s-Navarro J, Fritschka E, eds. *Cerebral microcirculation and metabolism*. New York: Raven Press, 1981;213-226.
7. Siegel G, Litza B, Thiel M, Carl A, Stock G *Proc Chin Acad Med Sci* 1987;2:104.
8. Siegel G, Stock G, Schnalke F, Litza B. In: Gryglewski RJ, Stock G, eds. *Prostacyclin and its stable analogue iloprost*. Berlin Heidelberg New York: Springer-Verlag, 1987;143-149.
9. Siegel G, Thiel M, Schnalke F, Litza B, Adler A, Stock G. In: Strauer BE, Ehrly AM, Leschke M, eds. *Fortschritte in der kardiovaskulären Hämorheologie*. München: Münchner Wissenschaftliche Publikationen, 1987;107-114.
10. Siegel G, Walter A, Thiel M, Ebeling BJ *Adv Exp Med Biol* 1984;169:515-540.
11. Somlyo AV, Somlyo AP *J Pharmacol Exp Therap* 1968;159:129-145.
12. Weston AH, Abbott A *Trends Pharmacol Sci* 1987;8:283-284.

Advances in Prostaglandin, Thromboxane, and Leukotriene Research, Vol. 19, edited by
B. Samuelsson, P. Y.-K. Wong, and F. F. Sun,
Raven Press, Ltd., New York ©1989.

ENDOGENOUS NITRIC OXIDE AND THE VASCULAR ENDOTHELIUM

G.J. Dusting

Department of Physiology, University of Melbourne
Parkville, Victoria 3052, Australia.

The vascular endothelium produces potent local hormones that affect vascular tone and platelet function. This brief review focuses on two of these, prostacyclin and endothelium – derived relaxing factor (EDRF) which interact in platelets and vascular smooth muscle.

RELEASE OF NITRIC OXIDE FROM ENDOTHELIUM

Furchgott was the first to highlight the fact that acetylcholine relaxes isolated blood vessels only if the endothelium is present. It was subsequently shown that other agents also caused endothelium-dependent vasodilatation, and that this involved the release of a highly labile humoral factor known as endothelium-derived relaxing factor (1).

Endothelium-dependent vasodilatation is accompanied by activation of the soluble guanylate cyclase in the smooth muscle (1,2). It was also known that the nitrovasodilator drugs activate this enzyme, and they act by generating nitric oxide (NO, 2). This led Furchgott (3) and Ignarro (3) to speculate that EDRF was simply NO.

Palmer et al (4) subsequently provided evidence that NO release may indeed account for the biological activity of EDRF. Using bradykinin to release EDRF from porcine endothelial cells cultured on microcarrier beads, they showed that EDRF activity diminished, at the same rate as authentic NO, as it passed down a cascade of rabbit aortic strips. The activity of EDRF and NO was inhibited by haemoglobin and prolonged by superoxide dismutase (SOD), to the same extent (see below). But most important, they were able to detect NO released from the cells using a highly sensitive chemiluminescence technique, and showed that the amounts were sufficient to account for the relaxation of their bioassay tissues (4).

There is not universal agreement that endothelium-dependent vasodilatation results entirely from the production and release of the simple molecule NO. For example, we were able to distinguish the smooth muscle activity of authentic NO and EDRF released from bovine aortic endothelial cells (5).

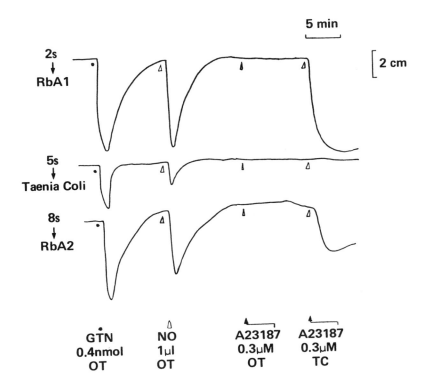

FIG. 1. Bioassay of EDRF and NO on rabbit aortic strips (RbA1, RbA2) and guinea-pig taenia coli. These strips were precontracted with phenylephrine (1µM) and carbachol (1µM). The effluent of a column of bovine endothelial cells, cultured on microcarrier beads, superfused the strips which were separated from the cells by delays of 2, 5 and 8s as shown. The tissues were calibrated with submaximal doses of glyceryl trinitrate (GTN) and NO (1µl of a saturated solution) given over the tissues (OT). A23187 has no direct effect OT, but releases EDRF when infused through the cells (TC). EDRF is less active than NO on the taenia coli.

Using a Vane cascade with the inclusion of non-vascular smooth muscles to allow a parallel pharmacological assay, we showed that the vasorelaxant activities of EDRF (released by bradykinin) and authentic NO were similar on rabbit aortic strips, but EDRF was less active than NO on the guinea-pig tracheal strip and taenia coli (Figure 1). Others have made similar observations (6). In addition, it has been reported that most of the EDRF activity released from bovine cells can be retained by freeze-drying (7), whereas free NO, being a gas, would be lost in this process. These discrepancies are yet to be resolved, but one possibility is that a "carrier" molecule for the NO moeity could be involved, at least in bovine endothelial cells. If that is the case, then the carrier molecule must break down faster than free NO is oxidized, for the stability of EDRF in cascades is similar to authentic NO (4,8). From all these studies it is clear that NO is the active end product of the EDRF biosynthetic pathway that has yet to be described.

INTERACTIONS OF EDRF AND PROSTACYCLIN ON SMOOTH MUSCLE AND PLATELETS

EDRF relaxes arteries, arterioles and veins from several species (1). In addition, it has powerful effects on platelets. EDRF inhibits aggregation induced in human and rabbit platelets by collagen, U46619, ADP, thrombin and platelet-activating factor (PAF), and causes platelet disaggregation (8,9). EDRF also inhibits adhesion of platelets to collagen fibrils, endothelial cell matrix and vascular endothelial cells (10). All of these actions in smooth muscle and platelets are due to stimulation of the intracellular "soluble" guanylate cyclase, leading to increases in intracellular cyclic-GMP (8,10).

Prostacyclin shares some of these activities. It relaxes most, but not all, blood vessels, and is a potent platelet disaggregator and inhibitor of platelet aggregation. However, the intracellular transmission of these actions is different from EDRF: prostacyclin activates membrane receptors coupled to adenylate cyclase, leading to elevation of cyclic-AMP (8). Prostacyclin is only a weak inhibitor of platelet adhesion.

EDRF and prostacyclin interact in the platelet. The anti-aggregating and disaggregating actions of EDRF and authentic NO are potentiated by prostacyclin (8,9). Conversely, the actions of prostacyclin as an inhibitor of platelet aggregation and an inducer of platelet disaggregation are potentiated by subthreshold concentrations of EDRF or authentic NO (8). Thus the very low concentrations of prostacyclin found in plasma may have a physiological effect in regulating platelet aggregability if acting on a background of NO release (8).

The synergy between EDRF and prostacyclin does not extend to platelet adhesion, for this appears to be regulated by cyclic-GMP but not by cyclic-AMP (10). Thus the physiological process of platelet adhesion to the vessel wall may proceed under circumstances in which both substances, acting in concert, are exerting a powerful anti-thrombotic (anti-aggregatory) action.

As in the platelet, there is evidence suggestive of a synergistic interaction between EDRF and activators of adenylate cyclase in blood vessels. In rat aortic smooth muscle, calcitonin-gene related peptide (CGRP), like isoprenaline and prostacyclin, activates adenylate cyclase (11). In rings of rat aorta, the vasorelaxant actions of these agents are amplified by the presence of endothelium, or by the stable analogue 8-bromo-cyclic GMP (12,13). In vessels with endothelium, methylene blue and haemoglobin partially inhibit the vasodilator action of isoprenaline and CGRP. All this is consistent with an augmentation of cyclic-AMP-mediated vasodilatation by EDRF (12), and suggests that there is synergy between the cyclic nucleotides in causing relaxation of this muscle. However, neither CGRP nor isoprenaline stimulated release of EDRF (12, 13). We suggested that EDRF was released spontaneously in the organ bath, and that the consequent elevation of cyclic-GMP explains the amplification of the vasorelaxation by the endothelium in this tissue (14). This synergy between the cyclic nucleotides may thus be further level of biological control of vascular smooth muscle tone, but the interaction between the nucleotides needs to be studied in other blood vessels.

INACTIVATION OF NITRIC OXIDE

Although EDRF can be transferred from isolated conduit vessels to detector bioassay tissues, it has not been possible to detect its release in the outflow of perfused organs. This raises the possibility that EDRF is actively degraded in the microvasculature. Indeed, our recent evidence indicates that even NO itself is oxidized rapidly in vascular beds such as the coronary circulation, to inactive nitrite and nitrate ions (15).

There are several known mechanisms capable of inactivating EDRF in vivo or in vitro. NO and EDRF are rapidly bound and inactivated by haemoglobin and haptoglobin/haemoglobin complex in plasma (1,5,8). Indeed the affinity of NO for haemoglobin is much greater than that of oxygen or carbon monoxide. Therefore, NO will not be transported in an active form in the bloodstream, although it may be passed from cell to cell through their membranes, for example, to platelets adhering to the vessel wall. In this respect NO may be regarded as the ultimate local hormone.

Molecular oxygen (O_2) will oxidize NO in aqueous solution to equal amounts of nitrite and nitrate ion. Superoxide anions (O_2-), which may be generated by endothelial cells or inflammatory cells, also inactivate EDRF or NO, but other oxygen-derived radicals do not (8). Thus superoxide dismutase (SOD) protects EDRF from breakdown in vitro (8, 16) and prevents the inhibition by oxygen radicals of vasodilatation in the microcirculation (17). The inactivation of EDRF by O_2- may be relevant in ischaemia or reperfusion injury, where O_2- is generated by invading inflammatory cells.

Both haemoglobin and methylene blue inactivate EDRF independently of O_2- production (5,8). Methylene blue may also directly inhibit the soluble guanylate cyclase (2).

DOES NITRIC OXIDE RELEASE ACCOUNT FOR ALL THE VASOACTIVITY OF THE ENDOTHELIUM ?

Other mechanisms have recently been proposed to participate in endothelial control of vessel tone. Activation of endothelial cells can induce hyperpolarization, which is transmitted to the smooth muscle (18,19). There is also direct communication between the vascular endothelium and smooth muscle: propagation via gap junctions may participate in acetylcholine or stretch-induced phenomena (19,20). None of these effects can be reproduced by NO or prostacyclin. Some vascular constrictions also appear to involve the endothelium, such as those produced by hypoxia and stretch (16,21,22). We also described an endothelium-dependent constrictor mechanism that is activated in the presence of the thromboxane analogue U46619 and appears to antagonise the actions of EDRF (23). There is now direct evidence for the generation and release by cultured endothelial cells of a vasoconstrictor peptide (called endothelin). This unusual peptide may act, like some neurotoxins, directly on ion channels in smooth muscle (24). Clearly, there is much more to learn about the regulation of vascular tone by the endothelium.

Supported by the National Health and Medical Research Council and National Heart Foundation of Australia.

REFERENCES

1. Furchgott RF, Ann Rev Pharmacol Toxicol, 1984; 24: 175-197.

2. Ignarro LJ, Kadowitz PJ Ann Rev Pharmacol Toxicol 1985; 25: 171-191.

3. Furchgott RF and Ignarro L In: Vanhoutte PM, ed. Mechanisms of Vasodilatation IV. Raven Press, New York 1988 (in press).

4. Palmer RMJ, Ferrige AG, Moncada S Nature 1987; 327: 524-526.

5. Dusting GJ, Read MA, Stewart AG Clin. Exp. Physiol. Pharmacol, 1988; 15: 83-92.

6. Shikano K, Ohlstein EH, Berkowitz BA Br. J. Pharmacol, 1987; 92: 483–485.

7. Cocks T, Angus JA, Grego B In: Rand MJ, Raper C, eds. Proceedings of the Tenth International Congress of Pharmacology, Amsterdam: Elsevier, 1987; 345–551.

8. Moncada S, Palmer RMJ, Higgs EA In: Verstraete M, Vermylen J, Lijnen HR, Arnout J (Eds) Thrombosis and Haemostasis Leuven University Press, Leuven, 1987; 597–618.

9. Macdonald PS, Read MA, Dusting GJ Thrombosis Research, 1988 (in press).

10. Radomski MW, Palmer RMJ, Moncada S Biochem Biophys Res Comm, 1987; 148: 1482–1489.

11. Kubota M, Moseley JM, Butera L, Dusting GJ, Macdonald PS, Martin TJ Biochem Biophys Res Comm, 1985; 132: 88–94.

12. Grace GC, Dusting GJ, Martin TJ, Kemp BE Br. J. Pharmacol, 1987; 91: 729–734.

13. Grace GC, Macdonald PS, Dusting GJ Eur. J. Pharmacol, 1988; 148: 17–24.

14. Dusting GJ, Macdonald PS, Read MA, Stewart AG In: Bevan JA, Majewski H, Maxwell RA, Story DF, eds. Sixth International Symposium on Vascular Neuroeffector Mechanisms, ICSU Press, 1988 (in press).

15. Amezcua JL, Dusting GJ, Palmer RMJ, Moncada S (submitted).

16. Vanhoutte PM, Rubanyi GM, Miller VM, Houston DS Ann Rev Physiol, 1986; 48: 307–320.

17. Loiacono RE, Dusting GJ, 1988 Submitted.

18. Feletou M, Vanhoutte PM Br. J. Pharmacol, 1988; (in press).

19. Olesen SP, Clapham DE, Davies PF Nature 1988; 331: 168–170.

20. Segal SS, Duling BR Science 1986; 234: 868–871.

21. DeMey JG, Vanhoutte PM J. Physiol, 1983; 335: 65–74.

22. Lansman JB, Hallam TJ, Rink TJ Nature 1987; 325: 811–813.

23. Dusting GJ, Macdonald PS In: Vanhoutte PM, ed. Mechanisms of Vasodilatation IV. Raven Press, New York 1988 (in press).

24. Yanagisawa M, Kurihara H, Kimura S et al. Nature 1988; 332: 411–415.

Advances in Prostaglandin, Thromboxane, and Leukotriene Research, Vol. 19, edited by
B. Samuelsson, P. Y.-K. Wong, and F. F. Sun,
Raven Press, Ltd., New York ©1989.

DIFFERENTIAL EFFECTS OF 17α AND 17β ESTRADIOL ON $PGF_{2α}$ MEDIATED CONTRACTION OF THE PORCINE CORONARY ARTERY.

Roberto Vargas, George Thomas, Barbara Wroblewska and Peter W. Ramwell

Department of Physiology & Biophysics, Georgetown University, Washington D.C. 20007.

Various steroids, particularly estrogens, affect both electrophysiological and contractile responses of excitable cells (1-4). Uterine smooth muscle cells, for example are particularly influenced by ovarian steroids (5). The treatment with estrogens depresses vascular responses of blood vessels and testosterone has the opposite effect (6). Although discrepancy between in vitro and ex vivo effects of steroids on vascular smooth muscle has been observed (2-4). The reasons for this discrepancy and the mechanism of action of steroids still remains unclear. It appears, however, that some of the effects of estrogens may represent direct non-genomic effects (7).

Estrogens have been suggested to affect membrane permeability to ions and smooth muscle contractility due to modulatory actions on the responses of the cells to several agonists (1-8). The purpose of our study was to investigate the differential, direct, non-genomic effects of 17α and 17β estradiol on the contractility of porcine left coronary artery (LAD) in vitro.

METHODS

Female domestic pigs (70-80 kg) were preanaesthetized with ketamine (5 mg/kg, i.m.) and Inovar (10 mg/kg, i.m.), and deep anaesthesia was induced with i.v. administration of pentobarbital (30 mg/kg). The heart was excised and stored in ice-cold Krebs bicarbonate buffer (pH 7.4) equilibrated with 5% CO_2 in oxygen. Epicardial vessels (LAD) were dissected and cleaned from surrounding tissue and cut into rings approximatly 4-6 mm long. Tissue segments were also prepared from thoracic aorta of male Sprague-Dawley rats (250-300 g). The intact segments of blood vessels were used for bioassay determination of contractile-relaxing responses (9) and for the radioimmunoassay determination of cyclic nucleotide content (10) using automated Gamma-Flow System (11). For the experiments performed in Ca^{++}-free buffer, 2.5 mM Ca^{++} was replaced with equimolar NaCl and 100 uM EGTA was added.

RESULTS

Both isomers of estradiol (17α and 17β) inhibited contractile responses of porcine left coronary artery (LAD) segments to $PGF_{2α}$ in a reversible manner. The effect of 17β estradiol (6 x 10^{-6}M) on contractility was more pronounced than that of 17α estradiol at the same concentration (FIG.1A).

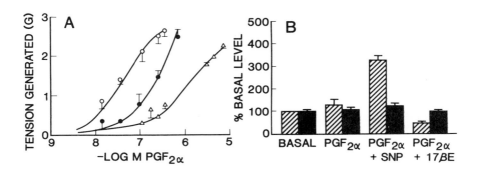

FIG.1   The effect of both isomers of estradiol on the   (A) contraction of pig coronary artery and (B) levels of cyclic nucleotides ;
o–o control, ●–● 17α, △–△ 17β estradiol, ▨ cGMP, ■ cAMP.

In the same vessel segments, the levels of cGMP stimulated with PGF₂ₐ (9 x 10⁻⁵M) and 5 x 10⁻⁵M sodium nitroprusside (SNP) were inhibited in the presence of 17β estradiol (4.9 x 10⁻⁵M). There was no significant change of cAMP level observed under our experimental conditions (FIG.1B). Control levels of cGMP and cAMP (measured in the presence of 100 μM phosphodiesterase inhibitor - IBMX) were 166.6 ± 38.3 and 32.5 ± 4.0 fmol/mg tissue protein, respectively.

Estradiol produced the same inhibitory effect on the contractile responses of rat thoracic aorta segments to phenylephrine (10⁻⁵M) in the presence of 2.5 mM Ca⁺⁺. However, after the removal of Ca⁺⁺ from the medium and in the presence of 100 μM EGTA, 17β estradiol (4.9 x 10⁻⁵M) did not attenuate contractile responses to phenylephrine (FIG.2).

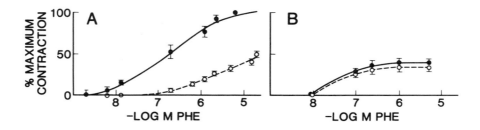

FIG.2   The responses of rat thoracic aorta to estradiol in the presence and absence of Ca⁺⁺; o–o control, ●–● 17β estradiol.

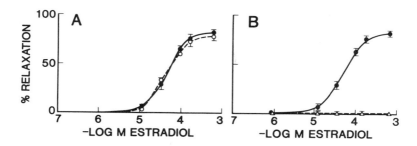

FIG.3   Relaxing responses of rat thoracic aorta to estradiol. (A) ●—● intact, O—O denuded; (B) ●—● 17β estradiol, △—△ 17α estradiol.

Estradiol applied directly to the vessel segments (prepared from rat thoracic aorta) precontracted with PGF$_{2\alpha}$ (1 x 10^{-6}M) caused relaxation (FIG.3) both in the presence and absence of the endothelium. Estradiol 17α under the same conditions did not have any relaxing effect.

DISCUSSION

The immediate actions of estrogens to increase electrical activity of the membrane of excitable cells (1-4) indicates a direct, non genomic effect which is not mediated by the classic steroid receptor which requires RNA and protein synthesis. This direct effect of estradiol can be blocked by specific calcium-transport inhibitors (12). Morgan et al. (13) have also shown that estradiol in micromolar concentrations inhibits the responses of the membrane potential to changes in extracellular Ca^{++}.

The effects presented above of estradiol on the contractile and relaxing responses of the left coronary artery and aorta indicate direct, non-genomic effects. The differential relaxing responses of precontracted vessel segments to 17 and 17β estradiol as well as the stronger inhibitory effect of 17β form on contraction indicate the specificity of this response. The inhibitory effect of estradiol on the contractile responses to PGF$_{2\alpha}$ in porcine coronary arteries was pronounced, and changed both the sensitivity and the maximal contraction. This effect was also reversible and occurred after a very short time, indicating that classical steroid receptors are not involved in this process. The relaxing effect of estradiol and the inhibition of contractile responses to PGF$_{2\alpha}$ did not occure through the competition with prostaglandin receptors or inhibition of prostaglandin release. The same effect was observed in phenylephrine-precontracted vessel segments. Similarly, blocking effects of estradiol on the contractions caused by several other agonists have been shown for guinea-pig ileum muscles (14).

The inhibitory effect of estradiol on contractile responses of studied blood vessel segments appears to be a calcium-dependent mechanism and was abolished in the presence of Ca^{++}-free medium.

The involvement of cyclic nucleotides in the effects of estradiol on the contractile mechanisms in blood vessels is still unclear. It has been suggested that rapid action of steroids may occur through increased levels of cAMP. However, in most of the tissues investigated, changes in cAMP levels have not been observed (15). The results of the present study indicate that estradiol inhibits levels of cGMP stimulated by agonists and has no significant effect on the levels of cAMP.

In conclusion, our results indicate that estradiol has a direct, rapid effect on vascular smooth muscle. This effect of estradiol is reversible and stereo-specific. Direct regulation of contractile responses of blood vessels segments by estradiol is possibly mediated by affecting Ca^{++} movements.

BIBLIOGRAPHY

1.   De Beer EL, Keizer HA. Steroids 1982; 40:223-231.
2.   Altura BM. J Pharmacol Exp Ther 1975; 193:403-407.
3.   Roesch CB, Borowitz JL. Pharmacology 1981; 22:15-23.
4.   Kishi Y, Numano F. Mechanisms of ageing and Development. 1982; 18:115-123.
5.   Ishii K, Kano T, Ando J. Japan J Pharmacol 1986;41:47-54.
6.   Baker PJ, Ramey ER, Ramwell PW. Am J Physiol 1978; 235:H242-H246.
7.   Duval D, Durant S and Homo-Delarche F. Biochem Biophys Acta 1983; 737:409-442.
8.   Hava M. Arch Int Pharmacodyn 1972; 195:315-319.
9.   Cunard CM, Maddox YT, Ramwell PW. J Pharmacol Exp Ther 1986; 237:82-85.
10.   Harper JF, Brooker G. J Nucl Res 1976; 1:207-218.
11.   Brooker G, Teraki WL, Price MG. Science 1976; 194:270-276.
12.   Dufy B, Vincent JD, Fleury H et al. Nature 1979; 282:855-857.
13.   Morgan JJ, Bramhall JS, Britten AZ, Perris AD. Biochem Biophys Res Commun 1976; 72:663-672.
14.   Seamen I, Fontaine J, Famaey JP, Reuse J. Arch Int Pharmacodyn 1977; 230:340-343.
15.   Rosenfeld MG, O'Maley BW. Science 1970; 168:253-255.

Advances in Prostaglandin, Thromboxane, and Leukotriene Research, Vol. 19, edited by B. Samuelsson, P. Y.-K. Wong, and F. F. Sun, Raven Press, Ltd., New York ©1989.

INVOLVEMENT OF PROSTAGLANDINS IN ARTERIOLAR VASODILATION TO PEROXIDES

Michael S. Wolin, Edward J. Messina and Gabor Kaley

Department of Physiology, New York Medical College, Valhalla, New York 10595

Our laboratory has recently described the vasoactive actions of oxygen metabolites derived from the xanthine oxidase reaction in the rat cremasteric microcirculation (1,2). Suffusion of this vascular bed with xanthine oxidase (0.25–7.5 mUnits/ml) produces vasodilation of third order arterioles in a concentration–dependent manner. This vasodilation is abolished by catalase but not effected by superoxide dismutase, implicating H_2O_2 as the vasoactive metabolite (1). Furthermore, topical application of H_2O_2 elicits vasodilation in a concentration–dependent manner over the $10^{-7}M–10^{-4}M$ range (1). Vasodilation to xanthine oxidase and to H_2O_2 up to a concentration of $10^{-5}M$ is completely antagonized by indomethacin, suggesting a role for prostaglandins in the mediation of the response (1,2). Vasodilation to higher concentrations of H_2O_2 ($10^{-4}M–10^{-3}M$) is, however, not completely inhibited by indomethacin. On the other hand, pre-treatment with an antagonist of soluble guanylate cyclase activation, methylene blue, markedly inhibits the response to these higher concentrations of H_2O_2, implicating the involvement of cyclic GMP in the mechanism of the vasodilator action of peroxide (2). In contrast, peroxides have previously been reported to elicit vasoconstrictor responses in two other vascular beds through the generation of cyclooxygenase products (3,4). In the present study we examined further the participation of prostaglandins in the response to peroxides in the cremasteric microcirculation.

Effect of peroxides on arterioles

The effects of topical application of vasoactive agents on the diameter of third order arterioles in cremaster muscle were determined by in vivo television microscopy in rats anesthetized with 30 mg/kg pentobarbital, as previously described (1). As shown in Figure 1 (top), topical application of 100µl aliquots of t-butylhydroperoxide (t-BuOOH) to the cremaster muscle produced a concentration–

dependent increase in arteriolar diameter over the $10^{-6}-10^{-4}$ M concentration range.   Also shown in Figure 1 (top), are vasodilator responses to topical application ($100\mu l$) of arachidonic acid (AA) and adenosine.   After the preparation was treated with continuous suffusion of indomethacin ($10\mu g/ml$), the vasodilation to every dose of t-BuOOH and AA was completely antagonized, whereas, the response to adenosine was not affected by this inhibitor of prostaglandin synthesis.   Other peroxides that have been studied include 15-hydroperoxyeicosatetraenoic acid (15-HPETE), which produces vasodilation over the 10^{-7} to 10^{-5}M concentration range.   Vasodilation to 15-HPETE was found to be similar to H_2O_2, in that indomethacin completely antagonized the increases in arteriolar diameter to low concentrations of 15-HPETE whereas responses to higher concentrations were only partially blocked (5).   The prostaglandin-independent portion of responses to 15-HPETE, however, were further inhibited by methylene blue.

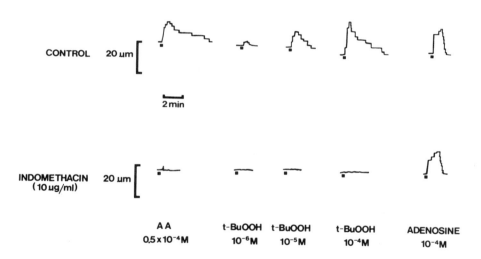

Figure 1.·   Dilator responses to t-butylhydroperoxide (t-BuOOH), arachidonic acid (AA) and adenosine of a single third order cremasteric arteriole (diameter= $20\mu M$) before and after inhibition of prostaglandin synthesis by indomethacin (2ml/min suffusion on tissue).   An upward deflection on record denotes an increase in diameter.   Dot marks the point of topical administration ($100\mu l$) of all agents.

Hypothesis for mechanisms of peroxide elicited arteriolar dilation

The actions of peroxide on cremasteric arterioles suggest the involvement of at least two mechanisms for vasodilation which are depicted in Figure 2. Since indomethacin inhibits a large part of the response to all the peroxides which have been examined, they appear to elicit the generation of vasodilator prostaglandins (6,7) such as PGI_2 and/or PGE_2. We speculate that endothelial cells are the major source of vasoactive prostaglandins. Also, peroxides have been reported previously to stimulate prostaglandin release from endothelium (8). Hydrogen peroxide and 15-HPETE also produce a prostaglandin-independent vasodilation that is inhibited by the antagonist of soluble guanylate cyclase activation, methylene blue, an agent which blocks increases in the intracellular mediator of relaxation, cGMP. There are currently two known mechanisms through which peroxides may activate guanylate cyclase, either via the production of an endothelium-derived relaxing factor (9), which appears to be nitric oxide (10) or via a mechanism mediated through the metabolism of intracellular peroxide by catalase within the vascular smooth muscle cell (11).

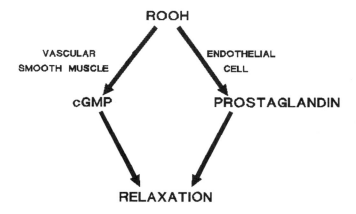

Figure 2. Hypothetical scheme for microvascular responses to peroxides.

Acknowledgements

We wish to thank Professor P.Y-K. Wong for the purified 15-HPETE employed in this study, Ms. J.M. Rodenburg for her expert technical assistance and Annette Ecke for preparation of the manuscript. This study was supported by USPHS grant HL 37453.

References

1. Wolin, M.S., Rodenburg, J.M., Messina, E.J. and Kaley, G. Am. J. Physiol. 1987; 252:H1159–H1163.

2. Wolin, M.S., Rodenburg, J.M., Messina, E.J. and Kaley, G. In: Tsuchiya et al., eds. Microcirculation–an Update, vol. 1, New York: Elsevier Science Publishers, 1987; 731–734.

3. Gurtner, G.H., Knoblauch, A., Smith, P.L., Sies, H. and Adkinson, N.F. J. Appl. Physiol. 1983; 55:949–954.

4. Rosenblum, W.I. and Bryan, D. Stroke 1987; 18:195–199.

5. Wolin, M.S., Rodenburg, J.M., Wong, P.Y–K, Messina, E.J. and Kaley, G. FASEB J. 1988; 2:A944.

6. Messina, E.J. and Kaley, G. Adv. Prost. Thromboxane Res. 1980; 7:719–722.

7. Messina, E.J., Rodenburg, J.M., Slomiany, B.L., Roberts, A.M., Hintze, T.H. and Kaley, G. Microvasc. Res. 1980; 19:288–296.

8. Harlan, J.M. and Callahan, K.S. J. Clin. Invest. 1984; 74:442–448.

9. Rubanyi, G.M. Free Radicals Biol. Med. 1988; 4:107–120.

10. Palmer, R.M.J., Ferrige, A.G. and Moncada, S. Nature 1987; 327:524–526.

11. Burke, T.M. and Wolin, M.S. Am. J. Physiol. 1987; 252:H721–H732.

Advances in Prostaglandin, Thromboxane, and Leukotriene Research, Vol. 19, edited by B. Samuelsson, P. Y.-K. Wong, and F. F. Sun, Raven Press, Ltd., New York ©1989.

POTENTIAL MECHANISM OF PULMONARY ARTERIAL RELAXATION AND GUANYLATE CYCLASE ACTIVATION BY 15-HYDROPEROXY-EICOSATETRAENOIC ACID

Michael S. Wolin, Theresa Burke-Wolin, Lisa A. Cohn and Peter D. Cherry.

Department of Physiology, New York Medical College, Valhalla, New York 10595.

Our laboratory has recently described a novel mechanism of activation of soluble guanylate (G) cyclase, obtained from bovine pulmonary arteries, by nanomolar levels of H_2O_2 which is mediated through peroxide metabolism by catalase (1,2). This mechanism of G-cyclase activation appears to mediate bovine pulmonary arterial smooth muscle relaxation to H_2O_2, since relaxation is inhibited by the antagonist of G-cyclase activation, methylene blue, and is associated with changes in tissue levels of cGMP (1). In addition, modulation of G-cyclase by H_2O_2 appears to function as an O_2 sensor in this artery, where H_2O_2 and cGMP appear to generate a tonic O_2-tension dependent relaxation which is not present under N_2 atmosphere (3). Since 15-hydroperoxyeicosatetraenoic acid (15-HPETE), which is not a substrate for catalase, was originally suggested to be involved in cGMP associated endothelium dependent relaxation (4) and has been reported to activate soluble G-cyclase in several tissue extracts and in myometrial smooth muscle (5), we investigated the mechanisms of modulation of bovine pulmonary arterial tone and purified lung G-cyclase by 15-HPETE.

Effects of 15-HPETE on pulmonary arterial tone. Isolated, endothelium intact, bovine pulmonary arteries (3-5mm), prepared as previously described (1), when submaximally (EC_{40}) contracted with 0.1µM serotonin (5-HT) show a relaxation of up to 60% over the concentration range of 0.1-10µM 15-HPETE. Relaxation to 15-HPETE is not significantly (ANOVA) affected by pretreatment with 10µM indomethacin (n=7) or by removal of the endothelium (n=7). In endothelium rubbed arteries, contracted to similar levels of force with 0.05-0.1µM 5-HT, relaxation to 15-HPETE was completely abolished by pretreatment with 10µM methylene blue (n=9). Relaxation was also inhibited ~50% under N_2 atmosphere (n=6, p<0.05, ANOVA). Pretreatment of arteries with reduced hemoglobin (10µM) enhanced relaxation to 15-HPETE when tone was in-

duced with 5-HT and abolished relaxations when tone
was induced by 30mM K$^+$. These observations suggest
that hemoglobin is converting 15-HPETE to metabolites that are not vasoactive, with simultaneous
co-metabolism of 5-HT. Both t-butylhydroperoxide and
15-HPETE generated by the addition of 0.1mM
arachidonic acid (AA) to 10μg/ml soybean lipoxygenase elicited responses similar to 15-HPETE.   In
summary, 15-HPETE appears to directly elicit pulmonary arterial smooth muscle relaxation through a
mechanism that appears to be dependent on oxygen and
G-cyclase activation.

Effects of 15-HPETE on G-cyclase. The effect of
15-HPETE and related agents of G-cyclase was examined, employing heme-containing bovine lung enzyme
purified and assayed as previously described (6), in
the presence of 0.1mM GTP and 25μM dithiothreitol.
As shown in Figure 1, G-cyclase is not activated by
15-HPETE using either the purified peroxide or endogenously generated 15-HPETE by soybean lipoxygenase
(10μg/ml) and 10μM AA. G-cyclase is activated by AA
in a manner that in not inhibited by glutathione
peroxidase plus glutathione (unpublished observations), but is inhibited by its metabolism via
lipoxygenase. The addition of reduced or methemo-
globin does not restore G-cyclase activation, as
shown in   Figure 2. The experiments in this figure
were conducted in the presence of 10μg/ml superoxide
dismutase to demonstrate catalase elicited G-cyclase

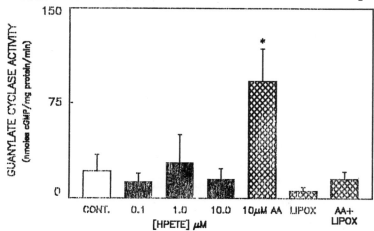

Figure 1. Effects of 15-hydroperoxyeicosatetraenoic
acid (HPETE), arachidonic acid (AA) and HPETE generated by AA plus soybean lipoxygenase (10μg/ml,
LIPOX) on purified G-cyclase activity.

activation, because this process appears to be both
dependent on H_2O_2 from the autooxidation of dithiothreitol and simultaneously inhibited by superoxide
anion, also generated by autooxidation (unpublished
observation). At the concentration shown in Figure
2, 15-HPETE inhibits G-cyclase activation by catalase. Results similar to those described above were
also found employing unpurified pulmonary arterial
smooth muscle G-cyclase preparations (unpublished
observations) and as described in Ref.2, similar results were found with t-butylhydroperoxide. In summary, 15-HPETE does not appear to directly activate
G-cyclase.

**Hypothesis for the mechanism of pulmonary
arterial relaxation and G-cyclase modulation by 15-
HPETE.** The results of this study suggest that the
activation of G-cyclase appeared to mediate arterial
relaxation to 15-HPETE, however, G-cyclase was not
found to be directly activated by 15-HPETE. Since,
relaxation to 15-HPETE is inhibited by lowering O_2
tension and O_2 tension appears to elicit a tonic relaxation associated (3) with increased tissue levels
of cGMP and intracellular H_2O_2 metabolism by catalase, we hypothesize that under O_2 atmosphere 15-
HPETE is shunting endogenous H_2O_2 metabolism from
glutathione peroxidase to catalase (see Figure 3).
Intracellular arterial levels of H_2O_2 are decreased
under N_2 atmosphere (3), which would reduce the

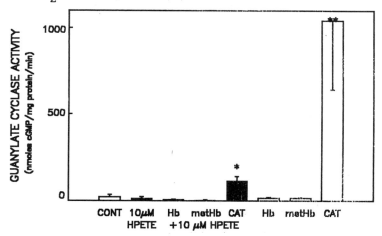

Figure 2. Effects of 15-hydroperoxyeicosatetraenoic
acid (HPETE) in the presence and absence of reduced
hemoglobin (0.5μM, Hb), metHb (0.5μM) or catalase
(1μM, CAT) on purified G-cyclase activity. *$p<0.05$
vs. control (CONT) and CAT, **$p<0.05$ vs. CONT.

amount of H_2O_2 available for shunting to catalase and inhibit both G-cyclase activation and relaxation.

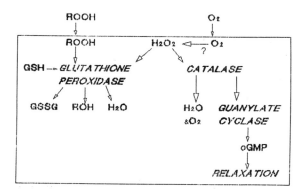

Figure 3. Proposed scheme for a mechanism of pulmonary arterial relaxation and G-cyclase activation by 15-HPETE and related peroxides. ROOH=15-HPETE, t-butylhydroperoxide, H_2O_2.

ACKNOWLEDGEMENTS. We wish to thank Professor P. Y-K. Wong for the purified 15-HPETE employed in this study. This research was supported by USPHS grant HL31069 and the American Heart Association with funds contributed from the Westchester/Putnam Affiliate Chapter.

REFERENCES

1.   Burke, T.M. and Wolin, M.S. <u>Am</u>. <u>J</u>. <u>Physiol</u>. 1987; 252:H721-H732.

2.   Wolin, M.S. and Burke, T.M. <u>Biochem</u>. <u>Biophys</u>. <u>Res</u>. <u>Comm</u>. 1987; 143:20-25.

3.   Burke-Wolin, T.M. and Wolin, M.S. <u>FASEB</u> <u>J</u>. 1988; 2:A723.

4.   Furchgott, R.F., Zawadzki, J.V. and Cherry P.D. In: Vanhoutte, P.M. and Leusen, I., eds. <u>Vasodilitation</u>, New York: Raven Press, 1981; 49-65.

5.   Leiber, D. and Harbon, S. <u>Molec</u>. <u>Pharmacol</u>. 1982; 21:654-663.

6.   Wolin, M.S., Wood, K.S. and Ignarro, L.J. <u>J</u>. <u>Biol</u>. <u>Chem</u>. 1982; 257:13312-13320.

Advances in Prostaglandin, Thromboxane, and Leukotriene Research, Vol. 19, edited by B. Samuelsson, P. Y.-K. Wong, and F. F. Sun, Raven Press, Ltd., New York ©1989.

VASOSPASM AND INJURIES OF CEREBRAL ARTERIES INDUCED BY ACTIVATION OF PLATELETS IN VIVO : IT MAY BE DUE TO THROMBOXANE A$_2$

Hiroh Yamazaki, Tsukasa Fujimoto*, Hidenori Suzuki, Yoshiharu Fukushima*, and Kenjiro Tanoue

Department of Cardiovascular Research, The Tokyo Metropolitan Institute of Medical Science, 3-18-22, Honkomagome, Bunkyo-ku, Tokyo 113, and Department of Neurosurgery, Showa University, Fujigaoka Hospital, 1-30, Fujigaoka, Midoriku, Yokohama, Kanagawa, 227*, Japan

When platelets are activated, several vasoactive substances including thromboxane A$_2$ (TXA$_2$) are released from the platelets. Those substances may affect blood vessels locally in vivo. However, there have been a few reports that induced platelet aggregation may initiate injuries of vascular walls (1-3). We have previously reported the appearance of vascular contraction and injuries in pulmonary and cerebral arteries induced by intravascular aggregation of platelets in rabbits (4, 5). In this paper, we describe the ultrastructural details of vascular changes induced by platelet aggregation in vivo and have analyzed a role of TXA$_2$ in the vascular injuries.

MATERIALS AND METHODS

In 34 male rabbits, a polyethylene catheter was inserted into a lingual artery, and its tip was advanced to the carotid bifurcation under anesthesia. Using this method, we injected a platelet aggregating substance into the cerebral arteries without disturbing the blood flow of the internal carotid artery. After heparinization, adenosine diphosphate (ADP, Sigma, 40 mg/kg, concentration of 40 mg/ml) was injected through the catheter into the right carotid artery within one min. In 10 rabbits, after clamping at the paroximal part of the right common carotid artery, warm (37°C) physiological saline was injected through the catheter under a pressure of 120 mm H_2O for 10 sec to wash out the blood in the right carotid and cerebral arteries. Then the same dose of ADP was injected into the catheter. During the injection and until one min after, vessels were continuously irrigated with saline and the clamp was released. Immediately after and 5 and 60 min after the ADP injection, the animals were decapitated and brains were removed. Several pieces of the middle cerebral artery in the subarachnoid space were resected and observed under an electron microscope (JEM-100S, JEOL). In 9 rabbits, blood levels of TXB_2 and 6-keto-$PGF_{1\alpha}$ were measured before and 3 and 60 min after the ADP injection, using radioimmunoassay.

RESULTS

When blood was present in the vessel, immediately after the ADP injection, small aggregates of platelets were seen in the vascular lumen on the injection side. Platelets showed slight shape change. However, the vascular wall showed a normal appearance. Five min later, intracytoplasmic vacuole formation (0.5 - 1 μm in diameter) was seen in the endothelial cells (Fig. 1). Tortuosity of internal elastic lamina suggesting vasospasm was also observed. There was also vacuole formation in the muscular and subendothelial layers. After 60 min, abundant intracytoplasmic vacuole formation and remarkable tortuosity of internal elastic lamina were seen. Deendothelialization was partially observed, and platelets adhered to such regions (Fig. 2). Edematous changes in the subendothelial layer and smooth muscle cells also were observed. The endothelial junctions were preserved. In some parts, a large number of platelet thrombi were found at the deendothelialized area. These vascular changes were observed only in the injection side. On the other hand, when the blood was replaced with saline before the ADP injection, the vascular wall was intact not only immediately after but also at 60 min after the ADP injection.

Before the ADP injection, the blood level of TXB_2 was 0.364 ± 0.143 ng/ml (mean ± SD). Three min after the injection, it increased significantly (p < 0.02) to 1.266 ± 0.741 ng/ml. Sixty min after, it returned to 0.460 ± 0.294 ng/ml, similar to the preinjection level. The level of 6-keto-$PGF_{1\alpha}$ was 0.833 ± 0.403 ng/ml before the injection. It increased significantly to 5.427 ± 1.521 ng/ml at 3 min after (p < 0.001). Sixty min after, it returned to 1.342 ±

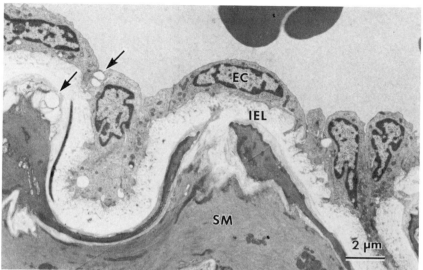

Fig.1   Middle cerebral artery 5 min after an injection of ADP. Tortuous internal elastic lamina (IEL), vacuole formation (arrows) in endothelial cells (EC), subendothelial layer and smooth muscle cells (SM) are revealed.

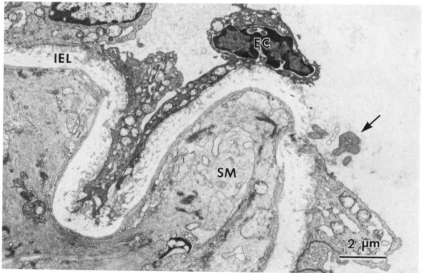

FIG.2   Middle cerebral artery one hr after an injection of ADP. Vacuolation in endothelial cells is remarkable. Note the adhesion of platelets (arrow) at the area of deendo-thelialization.

0.707 ng/ml.

DISCUSSION AND CONCLUSION

In this observation, we have found the characteristic vascular injuries after the ADP injection. The phenomenon was observed in middle and large sized cerebral arteries, such as middle cerebral artery, and not in cappilaries, venules and arterioles. The vascular injuries and vasospasm appeared concomitantly. When the blood was washed out with saline, the injuries and vasospasm were not observed during the experimental time. The blood level of TXB_2 increased to about four times the preinjection level at 3 min after the ADP injection. In other rabbits, we found that OKY-046, a specific inhibitor of TXA_2 synthetase, protected against these vascular injuries. Also we used horseradish peroxidase as a tracer and observed that the vesicular transportation in endothelial cells was not related to the genesis of vacuole formation(5). Swelling of mitochondria or endoplasmic reticulum would be related to their genesis. In a mechanism of the platelet-induced vascular injuries, the vasospasm may play an important role. TXA_2 released from the activated platelets may be one of the causative agents in the vascular injuries.

REFERENCES

1. Hughes A, Tonks RS. J Pathol 1962;84:370-390.
2. Jørgensen L, Hovig T, Rowsell HC, Mustard JF. Am J Pathol 1970;61:161-176.
3. Jørgensen L, Rowsell HC, Hovig T, Glynn WF, Mustard JF. Lab Invest 1976;17:616-644.
4. Yamazaki H, Motomiya T, Fujimoto T. Acta Haematol Jap 1980;43:208-216.
5. Fujimoto T, Suzuki H, Tanoue K, Fukushima Y, Yamazaki H. Stroke 1982;16:245-250.

*Advances in Prostaglandin, Thromboxane, and
Leukotriene Research*, Vol. 19, edited by
B. Samuelsson, P. Y.-K. Wong, and F. F. Sun,
Raven Press, Ltd., New York ©1989.

VESSEL WALL REACTIVITY AND 13-HYDROXY-OCTADECADIENOIC ACID SYNTHESIS

M.R. Buchanan[1], E. Bastida[2], G. Escolar[2], T.A. Haas[1], and E. Weber[1]*

[1]Department of Pathology, McMaster University, Hamilton, Canada and [2]Servicio
de Hemoterapia y Hemostasia, Universidad de Barcelona, Barcelona, Spain

Platelet/vessel wall interactions following injury are fundamental both
in hemostasis and thrombosis, and to the development of atherosclerosis (1-4).
In the past, considerable attention has been focussed on arachidonic acid
metabolism in platelets and vessel wall cells. Thromboxane A_2 (TxA_2) and
prostacyclin (PGI_2), the principle cyclo-oxygenase-derived arachidonic acid
metabolites in platelets and vessel wall cells respectively, are thought to be
important in regulating both hemostasis and thrombosis (Figure 1). TxA_2
promotes platelet aggregation and vaso-constriction (5,6). PGI_2 inhibits
platelet aggregation and promotes vaso-dilation (7,8).

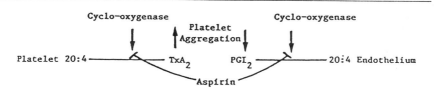

Figure 1. Metabolism of 20:4 in platelets and endothelium by cyclo-oxygenase:
effect of aspirin.

It has also been postulated that PGI_2 contributes (9), to the
thromboresistant property of the endothelium under normal conditions. More
recently, Radomski and his colleagues (9) have suggested that endogenous
endothelial cell-derived relaxant factor (EDRF) acts synergistically with PGI_2
to regulate platelet/vessel wall interactions. This hypothesis is supported
by the observations that inhibition of PGI_2 by endothelial cells facilitates
the adhesion of thrombin-stimulated platelets to the endothelial cell surface
(10) and that inhibition of PGI_2 in vivo results in enhanced thrombus
formation (11,12). However, a number of other observations have challenged
the hypothesis: 1) Curwen et al (14) found that pretreatment of endothelial
cells with low dose aspirin inhibited platelet adhesion to the endothelial
cell surface; 2) Buchanan and Hirsh (14) reported that aspirin in a dose
which inhibited both PGI_2 and TxA_2, was antithrombotic while high dose aspirin
was prothrombotic. Furthermore, the salicylate moiety of aspirin, which has

*Present Address: Jst-di Anatomia Umana Normale
U. Del Leterino 8
S3100 Sienna, Italy

been shown to inhibit the peroxidation of monohydroxyl fatty acids (15), enhanced thrombosis, (15). This latter effect was associated with an increase in PGI_2; and 3) Buchanan et al (16) in other unrelated studies, found that pretreatment of unstimulated endothelial cells with lipoxygenase-inhibitors blocked the basal adhesion of leukocytes to the endothelium while inhibition of the cyclo-oxygenase pathway (PGI_2 production) had no effect. Evidence that vessel wall cells have an active lipoxygenase pathway was first observed by Greenwald et al (17) who reported that vascular tissue synthesized a 12-HETE-like substance. All of these observations are consistent with the hypothesis, that under homeostatic conditions, i.e. under unstimulated conditions, PGI_2 is of little importance to platelet/leukocyte/vessel wall biocompatability, and rather, a unidentified lipoxygenase-derived metabolite influences endothelial cell reactivity. Therefore, we initiated a number of studies to investigate the possibility that a lipoxygenase-derived metabolite, synthesized under basal conditions in the endothelial cell, regulated in part, the thrombo-resistance of the vascular endothelium.

ENDOTHELIAL CELL METABOLISM OF LINOLEIC ACID

A number of in vitro studies were performed to investigate the metabolism of fatty acids endothelial cells under different conditions. Human umbilical endothelial cells were grown to confluence in M199 supplemented with 20% pooled human inactivated sera. The cells were stimulated by trypsin, thrombin, calcium ionophore, IL1 or fMLP. These cells were subsequently extracted into methanol and their endogenous fatty acid metabolite profiles were measured. We found that human endothelial cells synthesized 12-17ng of 13-hydroxy-octadecadienoic acid (13-HODE)/10^6 cells under basal conditions. All of the 13-HODE was associated with the endothelial cell, and we were unable to detect any 13-HODE or any other monohydroxy derivative of arachidonic acid or any other fatty acid within the cells or released into their supernatant (18-20). These latter observations were in contrast to a number of other studies in which endothelial cells were shown to preferentially synthesized exogenous arachidonic acid to 15-hydroxy-eicosatetraenoic acid (21,22). To address the apparent inconsistencies in the metabolism of fatty acids in the endothelium, we performed additional experiments and found that in competitive experiments, endothelial cells preferentially metabolized linoleic acid to arachidonic acid at equal linoleic acid:arachidonic acid ratios, but when the ratio of arachidonic acid:linoleic acid exceeded 3:1, the endothelial cells preferentially metabolized arachidonic acid (23). Thus, the addition of exogenous arachidonic acid, as seen in the studies of Hopkins et al (21,22) most likely resulted in the alteration in the ratio of available free substrates (linoleic and arachidonic acids) within the endothelial cells, and in so doing, facilitated 15-HETE production. It should be emphasized that cultured endothelial cells, grown under normal conditions, have not been shown to metabolize endogenous arachidonic acid to 15-HETE (18,19,23).

We also found that the interaction of platelets and tumor cells to intact unstimulated endothelial cells was inversely proportional to the amount of 13-HODE present within the endothelium. When endothelial cells were pretreated with low dose aspirin (which totally inhibited PGI_2 production), 13-HODE production was increased 67% and platelet adhesion was decreased significantly (18). Alternatively, pretreatment of the endothelial cells with sodium salicylate resulted in a 75% inhibition of 13-HODE production, and a significant increase in PGI_2 production. [This latter effect was also seen in vivo (14)]. The decrease in 13-HODE production was associated with enhanced adhesion of platelets to the endothelial cells.

Similar results were also found in vivo. We measured ^{3}H-adenine platelet accumulation onto intact endothelium and onto de-endothelialized carotid arteries in rabbits pretreated with salicylate. In sham-operated animals, we found no platelet accumulation. We also found that there was no initial platelet accumulation onto the denuded vessel wall when the endothelium was selectively removed by air-injury (25). However, this thromboresistant property of the exposed basement membrane was transient and with time, platelets accumulated onto the surface, reaching a maximum thrombogenic response within 12 to 18 hr (24). When the animals were pretreated with salicylate (which inhibited 13-HODE production in vitro) platelet accumulation onto the injured vessel wall was increased two-fold, and 13-HODE production was decreased 67 ± 4% (25). In contrast, in more recent experiments in collaboration with Dr. W. Eisert and his colleagues (Thomae, Biberache, Germany), we have found that pretreatment of the animals with dipyridamole resulted in a 40 ± 10% increase in vessel wall 13-HODE production and a 48 ± 5% decrease in vessel wall thrombogenecity. The overall correlation between in vivo 13-HODE production and platelet/vessel wall reactivity was r-0.9969, p < 0.001.

These data provide direct in vivo evidence that 13-HODE present in endothelial cells not only influences the thromboresistant property of the intact endothelium itself, but also influences vessel wall thrombogenecity following injury. One possibility to explain the latter effect is that 13-HODE is released from the abluminal side of endothelial cells into the endothelial cell basement membrane, perhaps blocking reactive sites. A number of in vitro studies support this possibility. Thus, we have demonstrated that the thrombogenecity of the basement membrane underlying endothelial cells also contains 13-HODE, the amount of which dramatically influences the degree of basement membrane thrombogenecity (27,28).

In a number of other studies, we have found that the relative amounts of 13-HODE present in the endothelium also influences the interaction of tumor cells with the endothelium. Thus, Bastida et al (20) demonstrated that stimulation of endothelial cells with increasing doses of fMLP, resulted in dose-related decreases in endothelial cell 13-HODE, which in turn, was associated with an increased adhesion of tumor cells to the endothelial cell surface. Furthermore, we have demonstrated that stimulation of endothelial cells with fMLP or interleukin-1 results in the decreased production of 13-HODE, and an increased expression of adhesive moieties onto the endothelial cell surface in association with the increased tumor cell adhesion (26, 27). Preincubation of the endothelial cells with the RGDS peptide blocked this adhesive response. As a consequence, Buchanan and Bastida (28) have postulated that 13-HODE acts as an internal regulator of the expression of adhesive moieties on the external endothelial cell surface.

LOCALIZATION OF 13-HODE IN THE ENDOTHELIUM

It was of interest to us that the contribution of 13-HODE to the vessel wall thromboresistance was associated with the presence of 13-HODE within the endothelium and not with 13-HODE being released from it into the fluid surroundings. Therefore, we performed a number of studies to identify the localization of 13-HODE within the endothelium. A polyclonal antibody to 13-HODE was raised in rabbits using a 13-HODE-albumin conjugate (30). We then used a double antibody-histoimmunofluorescent technique to identify 13-HODE in the endothelial cells. 13-HODE was distributed inside specific vesicles adjacent to the endothelial cell plasma membrane (Figure 2). It was necessary to permeabilize the membrane of endothelial cells to detect 13-HODE, similar to the detection of vWF. However, 13-HODE was found in vesicles in a pattern distinctly different from the widespread distribution of the Palade-Weibal bodies in which von Willebrand's factor is found (30). Furthermore, we have also been able to detect 13-HODE in the basement membrane of endothelial cells by histoimmunofluorescence (26). The detection of 13-HODE in the endothelial cells is completey blocked by authentic 13-HODE. 12-, 5- or 15-HETE had no effect. Finally, we have demonstrated that 13-HODE does not bind to nor directly influence the adhesion of platelets, leukocytes on tumor cells to the endothelial cell surface (31). These latter studies provide further evidence that 13-HODE functions biologically from the inside of the endothelium and does not have any relevant biological effect exogenously.

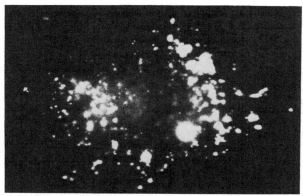

Figure 2.   Histoimmunofluorescent localization of 13-HODE in one human cultured endothelial cell (magnification 1250X). Endothelial cells were permeabilized before fluorescence was detectable, indicating intracellular vesicle localization.

CONCLUSIONS AND IMPLICATIONS

In conclusion, we have demonstrated that under basal i.e. homeostasis, endothelial cells continuously synthesize linoleic acid via the lipoxygenase pathway into 13-HODE. 13-HODE appears to be contained with in specific vesicles within endothelial cells, and appears to influence, in part, vessel wall thrombogenecity and tumor cell reactivity. In addition, 13-HODE appears to be released from the endothelial cell into the endothelial basement membrane, also influencing basement membrane reactivity. Thus, we conclude that 13-HODE contributes to the thromboresistance property of both the intact vessel wall and to the basement membrane following vessel wall injury. However, the thromboresistance property of the latter effect is transient presumbly due to the degradation of 13-HODE. We conclude therefore that although the cyclo-oxygenase derived products from the arachidonic acid pathway, perhaps in concert with EDRF, may influence hemostatic and thrombotic events following stimulation or injury, the metabolism of linoleic acid to 13-HODE in the intact endothelial cell under basal conditions, plays a more important role in contributing to the non-reactivity of the vessel wall under homeostasis and subsequent cell/cell adhesive events following vessel wall injury.

ACKNOWLEDGEMENTS

These studies were supported by grants from the Medical Research Council of Canada, the Ontario Heart and Stroke Foundation and the the Comision Asesora Cientifica y Tecnica in Spain.

REFERENCES

1. Jorgensen L, Hovig T, Rowsell HC, and Mustard JF (1970): Adenosine diphosphate-induced platelet aggregation and vascular injury in swine and rabbits. Amer J Path 61:161-170.
2. Stemerman MB (1973): Thrombogenesis of the rabbit arterial plaque. Amer J Path 73:7-26.
3. Baumgartner HR (1973): The role of blood flow in platelet adhesion, fibrin deposition, and formation of mural thrombi. Microvas Res 5:167-179.
4. Mustard JF, Packham MA and Kinlough-Rathbone R (1978): Platelets, thrombosis and atherosclerosis. Adv Exp Med Biol 104:127-144.
5. Hamberg M, Svensson J, Samuelsson B (1975): Thromboxanes. A new group of biologicall active compounds derived from prostaglandin endoperoxides. Proc Nat Acad Sci USA 72:2294-2998.
6. Hamberg M, Samuelsson B (1974): Prostaglandins, endoperoxides. Novel transformation of arachidonic acid in human platelets. Proc Nat Acad Sci USA 71:3400-3404.
7. Moncada S, Vane SR (1979). Arachidonic acid metabolites and the interactions between platelets and blood vessel walls. N Eng J Med 300:1142-1147.
8. Moncada S, Herman AG, Higgs EA, Vane JR (1977). Differential formation of prostacyclin (PGX or PGI$_2$) by layers of the arterial wall. An explanation for the antithrombotic properties of vascular endothelium. Thromb Res 11:323-344.
9. Radomski MW, Palmer RMJ and Moncada S (1987). Comparative pharmacology of an endothelium-derived relaxing factor, nitric oxide and prostacyclin in platelets. Brit J Pharmac 92:181-187.
10. Czervionke RL, Hoak JL, Fry GL (1978). Effect of aspirin on thrombin-induced adherence of platelets to cultured cells from the blood vessel wall. J Clin Invest 62:847-856.
11. Buchanan MR, Dejana E, Gent M, Mustard JF, Hirsh J (1981). Enhanced platelet accumulation onto injured carotid arteries on rabbits after aspirin treatment. J Clin Invest 67:503-508.
12. Kelton JG, Hirsh J, Carter CJ, Buchanan MR (1978). Thrombogenic effect of high dose aspirin in rabbits. Relationship to inhibition of vessel wall synthesis of prostaglandin I$_2$-like activity. J Clin Invest 62:892-895.
13. Curwen KO, Gimbrone MA, Handin RI (1980): In vitro studies of thromboresistance: the role of prostacyclin (PGI$_2$) in platelet adhesion to cultured normal and virally transformed human vascular endothelial cells. Lab Invest 42:366-374.
14. Buchanan MR, Hirsh J (1984): The effects of aspirin and salicylate in platelet/vessel wall interaction in rabbits. Athersclerosis 4:403-406.
15. Siegal MI, McConnell RT, Cuatrecasas P (1979): Aspirin-like drugs interfere with arachidonate metabolism by inhibition of the 12-hydroperoxy-5,8,10,14-eicosatetraenoic acid peroxidase activity in the lipoxygenase pathway. Proc Nat Acad Sci USA 76:3774-3778.
16. Buchanan MR, Vazquez MJ, Gimbrone MA Jr (1983): Arachidonic acid metabolism and the adhesion of human polymorphonuclear leukocytes to

cultured vascular endothelial cells. BLOOD 62:889–901.

17. Greenwald JE, Bianchine JR, Wong LK (1979): The production of the arachidonate metabolite HETE in vascular tissue. Nature 281:588–589.

18. Buchanan MR, Butt RW, Magas Z, Van Ryn J, Hirsh J, Nazir JD (1985): Endothelial cells produce a lipoxygenase derived chemorepellant which influences platelet/endothelial cell interactions: effect of aspirin and salicylate. Thromb Haemost 53:306–311.

19. Buchanan MR, Haas T, Lagarde M, Guichardant M (1985). 13-Hydroxy-octadecadienoic acid is the vessel wall chemorepellant, LOX. J Biol Chem 260:16056–10659.

20. Bastida E, Almirall L, Buchanan MR, Haas TA, Lauri D, Orr FW (1987). Effects of 13-HODE and HETEs on tumor cell/endothelial cell interactions. Thromb Haemost 58:315.

21. Hopkins NK, Oglesky TD, Bundy GL, Gorman RR (1984): Biosynthesis and metabolism of 15-hydroperoxy 5-, 8-, 11-, 13-eicosatetraenoic acid by human umbilical vein endothelial cells. J Biol Chem 259:14048–14058.

22. Kuhn H, Ponick K, Halle W, Wiesner R, Schewe T, Forster W (1985): Metabolism of (1-^{14}C)-arachidonic acid by cultured calf aortic endothelial cells and evidence for the presence of a lipoxygenase pathway. Prost, Leuk, Med 17:291–303.

23. Buchanan MR, Nakamura K, Haas TA, Hullin F (1987): Endothelial blood cell interactions; role of fatty acid metabolites. In BIOLOGY OF ICOSANOIDS IN BLOOD AND VASCULAR CELLS. M. Lagarde (ed.) INSERM Symposia, Brussels, Vol 152:247–258.

24. Buchanan MR, Richardson M, Haas T, Hirsh J, Madri J (1987): The basement membrane underlying the vascular endothelium is not thrombogenic. Thromb and Haemostas 58:698–704.

·25. Weber E, Haas TA, Richardson M, Hirsh J, Buchanan MR (1987): Interazioni Tra La Parete Vascolare e Le Piastrine: Aspetti Ultrastructurali Influenza del 13-HODE e del Trattamento con salicilato. Proc Cong Del Soc Italiana di Anat, Siena.

26. Buchanan MR, Bastida E, Aznar-Salatti J, de Groot P (1987): Is the endothelial extracellular matrix thrombogenic or thromboresistant? Effect of Preparation and 13-HODE levels. Thromb Haemost 58:206.

27. Aznar-Salatti J, Bastida E, Haas TA, Escolar G, Ordinas A, de Groot PHG, Buchanan MR (1988): The reactivity of the extracellular matrix with platelets is dependant upon the method of its preparation. Submitted to Blood.

28. Buchanan MR, Bastida E (1988): Endothelium and underlying membrane reactivity with platelets, leukocytes and tumor cells: Regulation by the lipoxygenase-derived fatty acid metabolites, 13-HODE and HETE's. Med. Hypothesis. In Press.

29. Lauri D, Orr FW, Bastida E, Sauder D, Buchanan MR (1988): Interleukin-1 and fMLP increase human vascular enodthelium adhesivity for tumor cells. Lab Invest, In Press.

30. Escolar G, Aznar-Salatti J, Bastida E, Buchanan MR (1987): Histoimmuno-fluorescence localization of 13-HODE in endothelial cells. Blood 70(Suppl 1):401a.

31. Haas TA, Bastida E, Nakamura K, Hullin F, Almirall L, Buchanan MR (1988): Binding of 13-HODE, 5-, 12- and 15-HETE to endothelial cells and subsequent platelet neutrophil and tumor cell adhesion. Biochem Biophys Acta. In Press.

Advances in Prostaglandin, Thromboxane, and Leukotriene Research, Vol. 19, edited by B. Samuelsson, P. Y.-K. Wong, and F. F. Sun, Raven Press, Ltd., New York ©1989.

Isolation and Identification of Human Plasma Factor which Stimulates Prostaglandin I_2 Production and Its Changes in Patients with Acute Myocardial Infarction

Yasumi Uchida, Masami Tsukamoto, Tsuneaki Sugimoto, Masao Ohguchi, Toru Yokoyama, Masami Shiratsuchi

Second Department of Internal Medicine, University of Tokyo, Tokyo and Tokyo Research Laboratory, Tokyo, Japan

In 1978, MacIntyer[1] and Remuzzi[2] demonstrated exsistence of a factor which stimulates prostaglandin(PG) I_2 production in human plasma. Since then, it has been shown that the plasma factor is deficient in patients with hemolytic uremic syndrome[2], thromboic thrombocytopenic purpura[3], and sickle cell anemia[4]. Despite many trials to purify and identify the plasma factor, the chemical structure of the factor is not known. Therefore, this study was performed to isolate and identify the factor and to examine its changes in patients with ischemic heart diseases.

Methods

1. Measurement of PG I_2 Stimulating Activities of Human Plasma and Other Substances
   The aorta removed from Wister strain rat was cut into rings. The rings were incubated in a bath containing 50mM Tris- saline buffer(TBS). The medium was exchanged every 15 min for 6 times and the wasted aortic rings were obtained.[5] The PG I_2 produced in the presence of plasma or other substances during each incubation period was measured as 6-keto PG $F_{1\alpha}$ and was compared with that produced in the presence of TBS and the stimulatory activity(SA) was expressed as % of TBS.

2. Purification and Identification of the Plasma Factor
   Deproteinized plasma was obtained by ultrafiltration of venous blood from healthy volunteers. The plasma factor was purified by Sephadex G-10 and QAE-Sephadex A-25. The purified plasma factor was examined by ultraviolet and infrared absorption spectroscopy, ^1H nmr and ^{13}C nmr spectroscopy.

3. Measurement of the Plasma Factor in Patients with Ischemic Heart Diseases
   Seven patients admitted within 12 hours after the onset of acute myocardial infarction were used. Venous blood was obtained before any medical treatment. The SA was compared with that of

age-matched cotrol group. SA in patients with angina pectoris was also measured. Patients with diabetes mellitus were excluded.

Results

1. Isolation and Identification of the Plasma Factor

The SA of deproteininzed plasma was about 2 folds of the undiluted plasma(Fig. 1). The deproteinized plasma was lyophilized, suspended in potassium phophate buffer, applied to Sephadex G-10 colum and was run at a flow rate of 0.7ml/min. A strong peak of ultraviolet absorption at 280 nm was detected in the fractions 63-70. The SA coincided with ultraviolet absorption fractions. The SA of fractions 63-70 was almost the same with that of fractions 10-35. The fractions 63-70 were subjected to QAE-Sephadex A-25$HCO_3^-$and was eluted with ammonium bicarbonate at 0-0.5M gradient. After this maneuvoir, only one peak was detected by ultraviolet absortion. The SA was recognized only in fractions having ultraviolet absorption. The active fractions were applied to Sephadex G-10 and were eluted with acetic acid. Each fraction was evaporated and lyophilized. The peak of ultraviolet absorbance of the eluate coincided with SA. Finally, 2.1 mg white powder was obtained from 220 ml deproteinized plasma. The ultraviolet absorption of the powder was with the maxima at 194, 235, and 291 nm; $E^{1\%}_{1cm}$ were 1900, 573, and 719 in water. In infrared absorption, a strong absorption was assigned to C=O. No signal was detected by ^1H nmr, while signals were detected at 102.70, 154.68, 163.49 and 165.83 ppm by^{13}C spectroscopy(Fig. 2). These phisicochemical properties coincided with those of uric acid. The SA of the purified plasma factor was coincided with that of arthentic uric acid. Uric acid-free deproteinized plasma was obtainoy adding uricase. The SA of uric acid-free deproteinized plasma was about a half of that of the deproteinized plasma(Fig. 1). Although tried to purify other acitve substances, it was difficult to purify them due to dispersion.

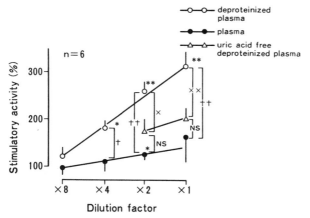

Fig.1. Stimulatory activities of plasma and deproteinized plasma at various dilution factors.
*P<0.05, ** P<0.01
x8 vs x4, x2 and x1.
X P<0.05, XX P<0.01.
+ P<0.05, ++ P<0.01.

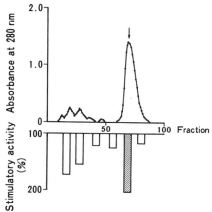

Fig. 2. Ultraviolet absorbance
and the stimulatory activity of
the fractions eluated by Sephadex G-10.

2. Changes in Plasma Factor and Uric Acid in Patients with
   Ischemic Heart Diseases

As shown in Fig. 3, the SA of the patients with acute myocardial infarction was significantly lower than that of the age-mat
ched control group. However, no significant difference in SA was
observed in other types of ischemic heart diseases. Plasma uric
acid concentration was measured in patients in whom acute myocardial infarction occurred during their admission to hospital. As
shown in Fig. 4, uric acid concentration was reduced on the day
of attack in all patients and it recovered gradually within a
few days.

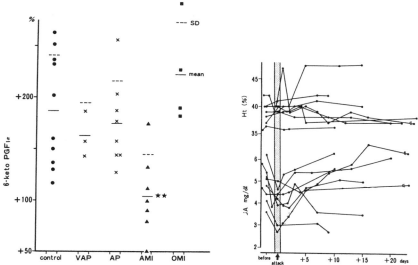

Fig. 3. Stimulatory activities
of deproteinized plasma in patients with ischemic heart diseases. AMI:acute myocardial infarction. AP: angina pectoris.

Fig. 4. Time course changes in
uric acid concentration in patients with acute myocardial
infarction. Ht: hematocrit.

The decrease in uric acid concentration was not related to hematocrit, BUN, creatinine, total protein or albumin concentration.

Discussion

It has been reported that the PG I_2 stimulating factor exists in human plasma. However, purification and identification of the factor has not been successful. In this study, isolation and identification of a major plasma factor could be made successfully, and it was revealed that the major factor is uric acid. Uric acid is different from the plasma factor described by McIntyer[1] and Remuzzi[2]. Also, uric acid is distinguished from platelet derived serum factor.[6] Ritter found dialysable heat-stable factor which is formed during coagulation.[7] Uric acid is dyalisable but not formed during coagulation. Although there is a possibility that uric acid is Ritter's factor and reciplocal coupling factor[8] is formed during coagulation and antagonizes the action of uric acid, the action of the coupling factor on uric aid was not examined. In this study, the PG I_2 stimulating factor in the deproteinized plasma and plasma uric acid were decreased on the day of attack in patients with acute myocardial infarction. In addition, uric acid concentration was recovered gradually after the attack. Although not examined whether uric acid decreases preceding the attack, there is a possibility that a decrease in the plasma factor, namely uric acid, accelerates the occurrence of acute myocardial infarction.

References

1. McIntyer DE, Pearson JD, Gordon JL: Nature 279: 549, 1978.
2. Remuzzi G, Misiani R, Marchesi R, et al: The Lancet 21:871, 1978.
3. Hensby CN, Lewis PJ, Hilgrad P, et al: The Lancet 6: 748,1979.
4. Stuart MJ, Sills RH: Br J Haematol 48: 545, 1981.
5. Remuzzi G, Livio M, Cavenaghi AE, et al: Thrombosis Res 13: 531, 1978.
6. Seid JM, Johnes PBB, Russell RGG, et al: Clin Sci 64:387,1983.
7. Ritter JM, Orchard MA, Lewis PJ: Biochem Pharmac 31:3047,1982.
8. Hoult JRS, Moore PK: Br J Pharmac 74: 485, 1981.

Advances in Prostaglandin, Thromboxane, and Leukotriene Research, Vol. 19, edited by
B. Samuelsson, P. Y.-K. Wong, and F. F. Sun,
Raven Press, Ltd., New York ©1989.

EVIDENCE FOR 20 mg ASPIRIN (ASA) AS BEING OPTIMAL

H.SINZINGER*, IRENE VIRGOLINI*, R.EYB**,
P.FITSCHA+, and J.KALIMAN++,

*Atherosclerosis Research Group (ASF) Vienna,
Departemnts of **Orthopedics and ++Cardiology,
University of Vienna, and +2nd Department of
Internal Medicine, Policlinic, Vienna, Austria

ASA is quite an old drug now. However, a variety of possible mechanisms discovered recently and a plenty of clinical data using various dosages have led to increasing confusion. It has been shown, that the administration of low doses selectively affects platelet cyclooxygenase without inhibition of vascular prostaglandin (PG) I2-production, whereas high doses inhibit both platelet and vascular cyclooxygenase (1-3). Attempts to adjust the ASA according to these findings and the possible clinical impact are of key interest today. The different actions of ASA on coagulation parameters, platelet function and the PG-system resulted very quickly in a plenty of dose-recommendations.

MATERIAL AND METHODS

Healthy volunteers (21-39a) were randomly allocated to receive either a single daily dose of ASA (1,10, 20,50,100,150,300,500,1000 or 1500 mg, respectively) or placebo. Blood was drawn before as well as at various time intervals during a 3 weeks treatment-period.
Various platelet function and PG-tests such as malondialdehyde (MDA; photometrically), serum and plasma thromboxane B2 (TXB2; RIA), platelet sensitivity against antiaggregatory PGs (E1,I2,D2), circulating endothelial cells (CEC, counting under microscope), conversion of exogenous arachidonic acid (AA) to TXB2 and HHT (radiothinlayer chromatography; RTLC), platelet aggregation (ADP-induced), platelet half-life (t/2) and platelet uptake (PUR) over active atherosclerotic lesions (after 111-In-labelling of autologous platelets were performed.

RESULTS

Measurement of the residence time of 111-In-labelled platelets reveals 20 and 1000 mg ASA being equally potent (4,5), whereas the doses in between are significantly (p<0.01) less effective (Tab.1).

In parallel the platelet t/2 shows a comparable be-
haviour (20 mg: 69.4±5.5 vs 76.1±6.0 p<0.01; 1000
mg: 70.2±5.3 vs 75.4±6.8 p<0.01; placebo: 72.3±6.4
vs 73.4±6.7 hours).
MDA-formation drops (6) significantly (p<0.01) below 1 nM/10(9) platelets within the first 5 days of
treatment with 20 mg ASA.In volunteers treated with
the smallest dose of 1 mg /day only, the MDA-values
exhibit a reduction to 50% of prevalues. 20 mg ASA
induce a quick and significant (p<0.01) drop in
both plasma and serum TXB2 (Tab.1). A maximal suppression amounting about 95% of the initial values
is achieved after 7 days. Even a dose of as low as
1 mg ASA suppresses serum TXB2-formation by 50 ng/
ml, whereas vascular PGI2-formation is not effected
(7).

Tab.1 Summary of (alterations of) various laboratory parameters after
       daily ingestion of ASA at different dose rates for 3 weeks

	(n)	1	10	20	50	100	150	300	500	1000	1500
t/2 (hours)	6	3	-	7*	4*	1	-	-	-	5*	-
PUR	6	0.01	-	0.07*	0.02	0	-	-	-	0.05*	-
MDA (ng/10(9)pl.)	4	3.4	0.7	0.5	<0.5	<0.1	<0.1	<0.1	<0.1	<0.1	<0.1
TXB2 serum (ng/ml)	6	149±31*	76±11*	7±4*	-	-	-	<0.1	<0.1	<0.1	<0.1
TXB2 plasma (pg/ml)	6	6±3	3±2*	<0.1	<0.1	<0.1	<0.1	<0.1	<0.1	<0.1	<0.1
PS (ng/ml)											
PGI2	6	0.84*	0.93	1.09	1.06	1.14	-	-	1.10	1.04	1.12
PGE1	6	10.1*	13.7	14.5	14.1	13.9	-	-	14.6	13.5	12.6
RTLC (%)											
TXB2	6	20.2	14.4*	8.3*	-	2.4*	-	-	<0.1	<0.1	<0.1
HHT	6	20.3	16.3	13.7*	-	2.9*	-	-	<0.1	<0.1	<0.1
CEC (n/µl)											
NS	4	2.4	-	2.5	2.3	2.6	-	-	2.5	2.3	2.4
SM	4	26	-	10*	16*	14*	-	-	26	20	28

*) p<0.01 versus prevalue; - not determined; NS...non-smokers; SM...smokers

The conversion of exogenously added AA to TXB2 is
clearly diminished even by the lowest dose of 1 mg.
In volunteers treated with 20 mg a reduction to
about 10% of prevalues is observed. The platelet
sensitivity during 20 mg up to a dose of 1000 mg
exhibits no change. However, the administration of
doses lower than 20 mg (1, 10 mg) results in lower
amounts necessary to suppress platelet function,
thus rendering the platelets more sensitive to the
action of antiaggregatory PGs (4).In healthy volunteers, the number of CEC is low; ASA is not effective under these conditions in neither of the doses
examined. However, in smokers and/or patients with

clinically manifest atherosclerosis the number of CEC is increased (5).Ingestion of 1 mg or more than 250 mg ASA a day does not result in a significant depression in the number of CEC in these groups. However, for the doses of 20, 50,and 100 mg such an effect is observed. At this low doses the number of CEC is significantly ($p < 0.01$) depressed.

DISCUSSION

The opinions about the optimal dose of ASA as anti-thrombotic agent are still controversial. Since the aggregation response shows no correlation to the antithrombotic activity and the clinical outcome this test can no longer be an argument for dose calculations. Our findings demonstrate changes in various parameters of platelet function and TXB2-formation during very low-dose ASA-treatment. They are somewhat different concerning the optimal dose, however,20 mg ASA a day seems to be the most effective one. The data confirm the results of Patrono's group (8) showing that a dosage of as low as 20 mg ASA per day induced suppression of serum T XB2 to below 10 % of control values. Whereas conversion of 14C-AA, MDA-and TXB2-formation are affected by ASA in a dose-dependent manner, the platelet sensitivity to PGI2 is surprisingly increased by treatment with the lowest dosage only (4). Previously we have shown that ASA in a dose of 1 mg daily gradually increased the platelet sensitivity against PGI2 and PGE1 within a 10 weeks treatment-period indicating that long-term daily administration of this low dose modifies the platelet sensitivity (4). Other studies showed that platelet sensitivity against PGI2 after a single dose of 325 mg ASA was enhanced for up to 72 hours (10). Previously we have shown that a single dose of 50 mg ASA depressed platelet TXB2-formation as well as vascular PGI2-synthesis (7). Patrono et al. (3) also demonstrated that a single dose of 100 mg ASA a day causes a ceiling inhibitory effect on platelet TXB2-production suggesting that the doses used presently for anti-thrombotic therapy are supramaximal with respect to the antiplatelet effect of the drug. Beneficial effects of treatment with 100 mg ASA daily beginning from the first postoperative day have been reported after aortocoronary bypass surgery (10). It looks likely,that the clinical effective dose may decline further. Our results are consistent with the view that an alteration in platelet function parameters as well as inhibition of TXB2-formation may be an important property of ASA. Since "low-dose ASA-treatment" currently means doses in the wide range of 1 to 350 mg, and since the optimal dose regimen in human is under strong debate,controlled and randomized double-blind studies are performed at present to assess the clinical impact of this hypothesis.

ACKNOWLEDGEMENTS

We gratefully acknowlegde the valuable help by E.Imhof, M.D. (Zürich, Switzerland) in formulating the drug as well as by Sonja Reiter, Ing. for the laboratory work.

REFERENCES

1. Burch JW, Baenziger NL, Stanford N and Majerus PW. Proc Natl Acad Sci USA, 1978;75:5181-5184.

2. Preston FE, Whipps S, Jackson CA, French AJ, et al. New Engl J Med 1981;304:76-79.

3. Patrono C, Ciabottoni G, Pinca, E et al. Thromb Res 1980;17:317-327.

4. Sinzinger H, O'Grady J, Fitscha P and Kaliman J. New Engl J Med, 1984;18:1052.

5. Sinzinger H, Silberbauer K, Kaliman J and Fitscha P. VASA 1988;17:10-15.

6. Sinzinger H, O'Grady J and Fitscha P. Prostaglandins, in press

7. Kaliman J, Cromwell M and Sinzinger H. Wien Klin Wschr 1983; 95:615-617.

8. Patrono C and Patrignani P. New Engl J Med 1981;304:1174-1176.

9. Philp RB and Paul ML. Prostagl Leucotr Med 1983;11:131-142.

10. Lorenz RL, Schacky CV, Weber M, et al. Lancet 1984;i:1261-1264.

Advances in Prostaglandin, Thromboxane, and Leukotriene Research, Vol. 19, edited by B. Samuelsson, P. Y.-K. Wong, and F. F. Sun, Raven Press, Ltd., New York ©1989.

THERAPEUTIC EFFECTIVENESS OF PROSTAGLANDINS (PGs) IN PERIPHERAL VASCULAR DISEASE (PVD)

O. I. Linet and N. R. Mohberg

The Upjohn Company, Kalamazoo, MI 49001, USA

Beneficial effects of PGE_1 were reported in PVD patients in 1973 and since then, effectiveness of PGE_1, epoprostenol (prostacyclin, PGI_2) and a stable analog of PGI_2, iloprost, have been studied in PVD with variable results. We reviewed the pertinent literature on this subject in order to find out whether PGs have a clear benefit in PVD. Studies related to PVD caused by arteriosclerosis obliterans and Buerger's disease were employed; single case reports were not included. A total of 53 studies were identified. The number of patients exposed to PGE_1, PGI_2 and iloprost was 1347, 350 and 77, respectively. Patients fell into two major groups: those with intermittent claudication and those with tissue loss characterized by ischemic ulcers. The following clinical endpoints were used for evaluation of PG's efficacy: increase in walking distance, alleviation of rest pain, percentage of patients with complete healing of ulcers and percentage of patients ending with amputation.

TABLE 1. Description of Studies

No. of Studies	Controlled (C) Uncontrolled (U)		Route IV - Intravenous IA - Intraarterial		Infusion Continuous (C) Intermittent (I)		Dose (ng/kg/min) Length of Infusion
PGE_1* 32	C	11	IV	13	C	11	IV: 0.6 - 21 2 - 142 days
	U	23	IA	21	I	23	IA: 0.05 - 10 2 - 345 days
PGI_2 14	C	7	IV	10**	C	12	IV: 2.5 - 10 2-7 days
	U	7	IA	4	I	2	IA: 5-60 3 days
Iloprost 6	C	3	IV	6	C	4	IV: 0.5 - 8 1-12 days
	U	3	IA	-	I	2	-

*One report has both controlled and uncontrolled studies; one report describes two uncontrolled studies
**Two reports did not state the route of administration, but were considered as IV route

PGE1

Results of 4 controlled studies indicated that absolute claudication distance increased more for PGE$_1$-treated patients than for controls. This improvement ranged from 73% to 471%. Studies exploring the effectiveness of PGE$_1$ in patients with tissue loss were categorized as those with positive, negative and equivocal outcome. All uncontrolled trials were assigned this category since the ulcer healing and amputation rates were not different from placebo rates (Table 2). The placebo rates were calculated from placebo arms of four well-controlled, double-blind trials.

Table 2. Comparisons of Ulcer Healing and Amputation Rates Between Placebo Response and PGE$_1$ and PGI$_2$ Uncontrolled Studies

	Placebo	PGE$_1$	PGI$_2$
Ulcer healing %*	16-62 (30.1) N = 163	14-54 (22) N = 674	0-60 (39.2) N = 84
Amputation rates (% of patients)	14-23 (15.1) N = 139	16-64 (25.7) N = 657	31-67 (45.1) N = 113

*Percentage of patients with completely healed ulcers

Table 3 indicates that results of most of the studies with PGE$_1$ fall into the "equivocal" category.

Table 3. PGE$_1$ in Tissue Loss

		Outcome - Number of Studies		
Route	Infusion	Positive	Equivocal	Negative
IA	Intermittent	2	8	-
	Continuous	1	5	-
IV	Intermittent	1	6	1
	Continuous	-	3	2

Table 3 shows that 3 of 4 "positive" trials were done by the IA route, whereas all "negative" trials were done by the IV route.

Evaluation of rest pain data appear to support the contention that PGE_1 treatment alleviated pain beyond that observed with control treatments regardless of the effect on tissue loss.

PGI2

Only one controlled trial explored the effects of PGI_2 on intermittent claudication; the absolute claudication distance increased in PGI_2 patients by 41% and in placebo patients by 28%. Table 4 indicates the positive, negative and equivocal outcome in tissue loss trials. The number of "positive" and "negative" studies appears to be balanced; most of these were done by the IV route. The comparison between "equivocal", ie uncontrolled trials, and placebo response is summarized in Table 2.

Table 4. PGI_2 in Tissue Loss*

| Route | Infusion | Outcome - Number of Studies | | |
		Positive	Equivocal	Negative
IA	Intermittent	-	-	-
	Continuous	1	3	1
IV	Intermittent	-	1	1
	Continuous	3	3	1

*One report had a study both in intermittent claudication and tissue loss

ILOPROST

Three controlled trials show no benefit of iloprost on claudication; two uncontrolled studies suggest benefit on claudication distance in patients with tissue loss. In terms of ulcer healing and amputation rates, there are no controlled studies available. Amputation rates in two uncontrolled trials were 40% and 33%, respectively. The complete ulcer healing rate was given only in one out of three uncontrolled trials and it was 25%.

In conclusion, PGE_1 and PGI_2 appear to have therapeutic effect in patients with intermittent claudication; the need for parenteral infusion makes this treatment approach unattractive and possibly dangerous when given by the IA route. In addition, it appears that PGE_1 treatment reduces rest pain. In the tissue loss stage of PVD, the therapeutic benefit of PGs seems to be in doubt. There is a suggestion that PGE_1, when given by the IA route (Table 3), exerts a positive effect. However, many studies were done in an uncontrolled design and high placebo response makes the proof of efficacy even in controlled trials rather difficult. In addition, a meaningful improvement in ankle/brachial index was not reported in any of the studies reviewed. One may suspect that the outcome of tissue loss studies is much more related to the severity of the disease rather than to the drug effect. It cannot be excluded that patients in irreversible stages of the disease were quite often enrolled into these trials. In design of future studies, an attempt to define in a better way the patient population who may respond to PGs should be implemented.

A complete list of references is available from authors upon request.

Advances in Prostaglandin, Thromboxane, and Leukotriene Research, Vol. 19, edited by B. Samuelsson, P. Y.-K. Wong, and F. F. Sun, Raven Press, Ltd., New York ©1989.

CLINICAL BENEFITS OF ILOPROST, A STABLE
PROSTACYCLIN (PGI$_2$) ANALOG,
IN SEVERE PERIPHERAL ARTERIAL DISEASE (PAD)

H. Oberender, Th. Krais, M. Schäfer, and G. Belcher
Clinical Research, Schering AG, Berlin, Bergkamen
Federal Republic of Germany

PAD encompasses a number of disorders either of degenerative etiology such as peripheral atherosclerotic obliterative disease (PAOD) and diabetic angiopathy or of inflammatory/immunological origin (e.g. thromboangiitis obliterans or Raynaud's phenomenon secondary to systemic sclerosis). The management of the severe stages - rest pain and trophic lesions - remains an outstanding problem in patient care when vascular reconstruction and sympathectomy are inappropriate or have failed. To date no medical treatment, generally accepted as being efficacious, exists.

Since the discovery of prostacyclin in 1976 and the demonstration of its potent effects on platelets and the vessel wall, therapeutic potential has been investigated in several disorders within PAD. However, it soon became evident that the widespread use of PGI$_2$ was limited because of its chemical instability 8). Consequently, efforts were made to develop chemically stable derivatives.

At Schering AG these efforts resulted in the synthesis of iloprost 10).

Iloprost's efficacy in the treatment of the severe stages of PAOD, diabetic angiopathy and Raynaud's phenomenon secondary to systemic sclerosis have been investigated in individual clinical studies.

I. RANDOMIZED PLACEBO-CONTROLLED STUDIES
IN SEVERE LIMB ISCHEMIA DUE TO PAOD AND
DIABETIC ANGIOPATHY

Description of the Studies

Two controlled studies in patients with trophic lesions, one due to PAOD and another to diabetic angiopathy, were performed. A third controlled study was conducted in patients with rest pain, due to both PAOD and diabetic angiopathy (table 1). The principal aim of all these studies was to investigate iloprost's clinical efficacy.

Prior to the studies the therapeutic response had been defined in patients with trophic lesions as "par-

TABLE 1. Pivotal studies with iloprost in severe limb ischemia

Study No.	Diagnosis	N	Type of Study	Dosage and Regimen	Aim of Study	Published
1	trophic lesions in PAOD	101	randomized placebo-controlled	placebo or iloprost $\leq 2ng/kg/min$ i.v. for 6 hours/ day on 28 consecutive days	clinical efficacy (H_A-hypothesis 30% difference between the responder rates under iloprost and placebo; $\alpha = 0.05$; $\beta = 0.1$)	(3), (4)
2	trophic lesions in diabet. angiop.	109	multi-centre group comparison			(2), (4)
3	rest pain in PAOD or diabet. angiop.	113		placebo or iloprost $\leq 2ng/kg/min$ i.v. for 6 hours/ day on 14 consecutive days		(1), (6)

tial healing of the largest ulcer at the end of the treatment or complete healing during or at the end of treatment". Patients with rest pain were to be considered responders when "free of pain without any analgesics for a minimum of 5 consecutive days including the 3 days after ending the therapy".

Nonresponders were to be patients without improvement or deterioration of the symptoms during the treatment.

In all 3 studies, patients who had failed to respond to conventional treatment and without possibilities for any form of revascularisation but in stable clinical conditions were included. The groups within these studies were well matched in respect to demographic data, risk factors, concomitant diseases and medication, to angiographic data and peripheral Doppler pressures. There were no apparent advantages for the iloprost groups.

Results and Discussion

62 % of the patients treated with iloprost showed healing of ulcers or relief of rest pain, thus fulfilling the responder criteria. These results were obtained in both patients with PAOD and diabetic angiopathy and were quite similar for trophic lesions and

rest pain (table 2). The proportion of patients with trophic lesions responding to placebo was about 20 %. However, in patients with rest pain placebo response was distinctly higher, especially in patients with PAOD (table 2). A high placebo response has been found by other investigators too [6] and can be explained by the intensive hospital care, the treatment of concomitant diseases and a 2-week-infusion of saline solution resulting in mild haemodilution. Nevertheless, in patients with ischemic rest pain the difference in favour of iloprost was statistically significant.

TABLE 2. Clinical results with iloprost in severe limb ischaemia

Efficacy Criterion	Diagnosis	Iloprost			Placebo		
		Resp.	Nonresp.	Total	Resp.	Nonresp.	Total
			number (percentage) of patients				
Trophic lesions	PAOD (study 1)	32 (61.5)	20	52 (100)	8 (17)	39	47 (100)
		⌐———— p< 0.05 ————⌐					
	Diabet. Angiop. (study 2)	31 (62)	19	50 (100)	12 (23.5)	39	51 (100)
		⌐———— P< 0.05 ————⌐					
Ischemic rest pain (study 3)		30 (62.5)	18	48 (100)	23 (42.6)	31	54 (100)
		⌐———— p< 0.05 ————⌐					
	PAOD	19 (63.3)	11	30 (100)	18 (53)	16	34 (100)
	Diabet. Angiop.	11 (61.1)	7	18 (100)	5 (25)	15	20 (100)

Long-term benefit for trophic lesions was ascertained by reexamination or by telephone interviews with the patients who had been receiving individual therapies throughout the follow-up period of 1 year (median value). In PAOD, clinical benefit was generally maintained in 88 % of those patients who had shown a positive response to iloprost. However, nonresponders had a bad prognosis: 75 % underwent amputation within 4 months, an indication that subsequent conventional individual therapies in these patients were also ineffective.

Long-term benefit in diabetics with an initial response to iloprost was found in 59 %. Another 36 %, however, deteriorated or finally had to undergo amputation during the follow-up despite conventional therapies which were obviously not able to stabilize even the initially improved clinical status. In view of the initial response to iloprost, a second treatment cycle should be considered.

II. EXPLORATIVE STUDIES IN RAYNAUD'S PHENOMENON SECONDARY TO SYSTEMIC SCLEROSIS

Description of the Studies

In three studies, two uncontrolled and one controlled, in patients with Raynaud's phenomenon, all fulfilling the clinical, serological and capillaroscopic criteria for systemic sclerosis (table 3), the efficacy of short-term i.v. iloprost was evaluated.

Criteria for efficacy were healing of skin lesions and the subjective improvement in vasospastic pain attacks, i.e. reduction in frequency, duration and intensity.

Apart from the clinical aspects these investigations also considered (5, 7, 9) pharmacological effects on platelets and digital blood flow.

TABLE 3. Explorative studies in patients with severe Raynaud's phenomenon secondary to systemic sclerosis

Study No.	N	Type of Study	Dosage and regimen	Follow-up	Published
1	25	uncon-trolled	$\leq$ 4ng/kg/min i.v. 4-5 hours/day on 5 consec. days	6 weeks	(5)
2	13	uncon-trolled	$\leq$ 2ng/kg/min i.v. 8 hours/day on 3 consec. days	10 weeks	(9)
3	29	placebo-controll. cross-over	$\leq$ 2ng/kg/min i.v. 6 hours/day on 3 consec. days	6 weeks	(7)

Clinical Results and Comments

In study one, healing of skin lesions occurred in 6 of 11 patients, and a subjective improvement in pain attacks was reported by 21 of the 25 patients (84 %). In study two, the number of skin lesions was reduced from 26 to 7 and pain attacks were reduced in 9 of the 13 patients (69 %). In the placebo-controlled study no differences in respect to the healing of skin lesions between the groups were detectable. However, 12 of the 24 remaining patients (50 %) under iloprost reported relief from pain attacks, while only 5 of these 24 patients (21 %) improved under placebo. Clinical benefit lasted for approximately 6 weeks after the 3-5 day iloprost treatment. These results have encouraged further controlled studies in Raynaud patients.

III. SIDE EFFECTS

Side effects in all patients treated were comparable. Flush and headaches being the most frequent side effects were reported in about 70 % of the patients, nausea in 30 % and vomiting in 16 %. The majority of the less frequent events e.g. sedation, apathy, restlessness or sudden sweating were uncharacteristic, in some cases attributable to the condition being treated or to concomitant diseases.

Distinct differences in tolerability between patients do exist. However, in the individual patient the typical side effects could be shown to be dose-dependent. This has led to the recommendation of individual dose-titration during the first days of treatment up to the dose causing flush and mild headache. By using this regimen, gastrointestinal side effects can virtually be avoided and iloprost can be regarded as safe.

In conclusion, iloprost's clinical efficacy and safety has been demonstrated in severe disorders within PAD thus paving its way as a beneficial and generally accepted therapy in these indications.

REFERENCES

1. Balzer K, Bechara G, Bisler H, et al. VASA 1987; Suppl. 20:379-381.

2. Brock FE. angio archiv 1986; 12:72.

3. Diehm C. Klin Wochenschr 1987, Suppl. IX:38-39.

4. Diehm C. VASA 1987, Suppl. 20:382-383.

5. Keller J, Kaltenecker A, Schricker KTh, Krais Th, Schönberger A, Gevatter M, Hornstein OP. Dtsch. med. Wschr. 1984;109:1433-1438.

6. Lowe GDO, Dunlop DJ, Lawson DH, et al. Angiology 1982;33:46-50.

7. McHugh NJ, Csuka M, Watson H, et al. Ann. Rheum. Dis. 1988;47:43-47.

8. Mitchell JRA. Brit. Med. J. 1983;287:1824-1826.

9. Rademaker M, Thomas RHM, Provost G, Beacham JA, Cooke ED, Kirby JD. Postgrad. Med. 1987;63:617-620.

10. Skuballa W, Radüchel B, Vorbrüggen H. Prostacyclin and Its Stable Analogue Iloprost, ed. by RJ Gryglewski, G. Stock. Berlin/Heidelberg: Springer Verlag, 1987;17-24.

*Advances in Prostaglandin, Thromboxane, and
Leukotriene Research*, Vol. 19, edited by
B. Samuelsson, P. Y.-K. Wong, and F. F. Sun,
Raven Press, Ltd., New York ©1989.

LEUKOTRIENES AND THE MICROVASCULAR PERMEABILITY
OF ACUTE LUNG INJURY

A.J. Lonigro, R.S. Sprague, A.H. Stephenson,
T.E. Dahms, and D.A. Hayek

Departments of Medicine and Pharmacology
St. Louis University School of Medicine
St. Louis, Missouri 63104

Acute lung injury is characterized by increased permeability of the pulmonary microvaculature (1) as well as failure of pulmonary circulatory control mechanisms which match perfusion with ventilation (2). Arachidonic acid metabolites have been implicated both in the accumulation of extravascular lung water in acute lung injury (3,4) and the altered vascular reactivity (2,5,6). In the present work, we present evidence in support of the hypothesis which states that leukotrienes participate in the permeability changes of acute lung injury.

MATERIALS AND METHODS

Animal Models

Male mongrel dogs (20-25 kg), anesthetized with pentobarbital sodium, were ventilated with room air at 12-15 breaths/min with a tidal volume of 15 ml/kg. Two flow-directed catheters were advanced into the main pulmonary artery for continuous measurement of mean pulmonary arterial pressure (Ppa) and for obtaining mixed venous blood. Following thoracotomy, catheters were placed into the left atrium and into the aorta for measurements of mean left atrial pressure (Pla) and mean systemic arterial pressure (Psa), respectively. In the models of unilateral acute lung injury (7), an electromagnetic flow probe and external balloon-type vascular occluder were placed around the left main pulmonary artery. Right pulmonary blood flow was calculated as the difference between left and total pulmonary blood flow (cardiac output) measured by thermal dilution. Estimates of extravascular lung water (EVLW), made with a double-indicator (thermal-dye) dilution technique (7), were confirmed gravimetrically (3,5). In those models of unilateral acute lung injury, right lung EVLW was obtained by occluding the left main pulmonary artery during administration of the

317

thermal-dye bolus (7).

Bilateral acute lung injury was produced by either ethchlorvynol (ECV) at 15 mg/kg or phorbol myristate acetate (PMA) at 10-15 μg/kg or 20-30 μg/kg. For the ECV experiments, blood samples for leukotriene analyses were taken before and 120 min after ECV administration and pulmonary edema fluid was collected for assay. In unilateral acute lung injury, produced with ECV, a bronchoscope was wedged in the lower lobe of one lung. The lung segment was then lavaged. After recovery of the lavage fluid, the contralateral lung was lavaged. Unilateral acute lung injury was produced by interrupting blood flow to the left lung for 1-2 min during which time ECV (9 mg/kg) was administered, i.v. After two hours each lung was again lavaged. For bilateral injury produced with PMA, bronchoalveolar lavage was performed before and 60 min after the induction of acute lung injury.

Human Studies

Bronchoscopic lavage was performed on 32 control subjects and in 9 patients with the adult respiratory distress syndrome (ARDS). Patients were defined as having ARDS if, consequent to either sepsis, aspiration of gastric contents or hypertransfusion, they developed acute respiratory failure requiring mechanical ventilation, and exhibited bilateral pulmonary infiltrates, wedge pressure less than 15 mm Hg, total static pulmonary compliance less than 50 ml/cm H_2O and an arterial to alveolar PO_2 ratio less than 0.2.

Leukotriene Assay

Plasma, pulmonary edema, and bronchoalveolar lavage fluids were extracted as described previously (3,4). The leukotrienes were separated initially from more polar compounds by reverse-phase high-performance liquid chromatography (HPLC). The eluate corresponding to retention times of authentic leukotrienes was collected and rechromatographed with an isocratic solvent system (4). The eluates corresponding to the retention times of authentic leukotrienes were collected, evaporated to dryness and subjected to radioimmunoassay (3,4).

RESULTS

ECV-induced bilateral lung injury did not affect Ppa or Pla although cardiac output decreased by 37.6±3.8% (P<0.01) 120 min after ECV administration. Total EVLW was increased 164±31% (P<0.001) from a control of 6.4±1.1 ml/kg body wt. Systemic and pulmonary arterial plasma concentrations of LTC_4 were small and unaffected by the administration of ECV, whereas the concentration of LTC_4 in the pulmonary edema fluid was 35.2±10.8 pg/ml, nearly sevenfold that found in the arterial plasma. In six dogs, 120 min after ECV-induced unilateral lung injury, LTC_4 was elevated solely in the bronchoalveolar lavage fluid of the injured lung (Table 1). In two pilot experiments, nordihydroguaiaretic acid (NDGA) administered prior to ECV was associated with a 58% reduction in LTC_4 in bronchoalveolar lavage fluid and a 44% reduction in EVLW.

TABLE 1. Effect of ECV given unilaterally on extravascular lung water (EVLW) and on LTC_4 and protein concentrations in bronchoalveolar lavage fluid.

	EVLW (% increase)	LTC_4 (pg/ml)	Protein (mg/ml)
Uninjured lung	34±19	10.5±1.4	0.4±0.0
Injured lung	134±22[a]	24.2±3.4[a]	4.1±0.4[b]

[a]P<0.01, [b]P<0.05

PMA-induced bilateral acute lung injury, was used to evaluate further the role of leukotrienes in altered microvascular permeability. PMA, in contrast to ECV, is thought to be dependent on neutrophils to produce injury. Two doses of PMA, a "high" dose of 20-30 µg/kg and a "low" dose of 10-15 µg/kg were used. Although both doses of PMA were associated with decreases in the number of circulating white blood cells, it was only the "high" dose that was associated with increases in EVLW and leukotriene concentrations (Table 2).

In patients with ARDS, which is characterized in part by non-hydrostatic pulmonary edema, leukotrienes were found to be elevated in bronchoalveolar lavage fluid compared to normal control subjects (Table 3).

TABLE 2. Effect of "high" dose PMA on extravascular lung water (EVLW) and on leukotriene concentrations in bronchoalveolar lavage fluid.

	EVLW (ml/kg)	Leukotrienes (pg/lavage)		
		LTB_4	LTC_4	LTD_4
Control	6.5±0.6	379±259	169±40	73±22
PMA (20-30 µg/kg)	15.0±0.9	2284±920	663±272	171±48
Significance	P<0.05	P<0.05	NS	P<0.05

NS = not significant

DISCUSSION

When bilateral lung injury was induced with ECV, EVLW increased and leukotrienes were identified in edema fluid. When unilateral acute lung injury was produced with ECV, EVLW increased solely in the injured lung as did leukotrienes. In the latter model when leukotriene synthesis was attenuated with the lipoxygenase inhibitor, NDGA, the accumulation of EVLW was decreased. Similarly, in the case of PMA administration, only those doses which increased leukotriene concentrations were associated with increased EVLW. Finally, leukotrienes were identified in the bronchoalveolar lavage fluid of patients with ARDS and not in normal subjects. These results are, therefore, supportive of the hypothesis that leukotrienes participate in the altered microvascular permeability of acute lung injury.

TABLE 3. Leukotriene and protein concentrations in bronchoalveolar lavage fluid of patients with ARDS and in normal control subjects

	Leukotrienes (ng/lavage)			Protein (mg/lavage)
	LTB_4	LTC_4	LTD_4	
Control	0.7±0.1	1.1±0.2	1.2±0.5	15.9±1.6
ARDS	9.5±5.4	12.5±3.0	30.5±7.8	390.2±101.2
Significance	P<0.05	P<0.05	P<0.05	P<0.05

ARDS = adult respiratory distress syndrome

REFERENCES

1. Anderson, R.R., Holliday, R.L., Driedger, A.A., Lefcoe, M., Reid, B., and Sibbald, W.J. (1979): Am. Rev. Respir. Dis. 119:869-877.

2. Brigham, K.L. (1982): Clinics Chest Med. 3:9-24.

3. Stephenson, A.H., Sprague, R.S., Dahms, T.E., and Lonigro, A.J. (1987): J. Appl. Physiol. 62:732-738.

4. Stephenson, A.H., Lonigro, A.J., Hyers, T.M., Webster, R.O., and Fowler, A.A. (1988): Am.Rev. Respir. Dis. (In Press).

5. Sprague, R.S., Stephenson, A.H., Dahms, T.E., and Lonigro, A.J. (1986): J. Appl. Physiol. 61:1058-1064.

6. Sprague, R.S., Stephenson, A.H., Dahms, T.E., Asner, N.G., and Lonigro, A.J. (1987): Chest 92:1088-1093.

7. Stephenson, A.H., Sprague, R.S., Dahms, T.E., and Lonigro, A.J. (1984): J. Appl. Physiol. 56:1252-1259.

Advances in Prostaglandin, Thromboxane, and Leukotriene Research, Vol. 19, edited by B. Samuelsson, P. Y.-K. Wong, and F. F. Sun, Raven Press, Ltd., New York ©1989.

ROLE OF THROMBOXANE A$_2$ IN MYOCARDIAL ISCHEMIA AND CIRCULATORY SHOCK

Allan M. Lefer

Department of Physiology, Jefferson Medical College
Thomas Jefferson University, Philadelphia, PA 19107 U.S.A.

Evidence has been accumulating that TxA$_2$ is involved in the pathogenesis of circulatory shock and myocardial ischemia which leads to cell death and extension of myocardial cellular damage (1). TxB$_2$, the stable breakdown product of TxA$_2$, is found in the blood of animals and humans in circulatory shock (e.g., traumatic, endotoxic, hemorrhagic, splanchnic vascular occlusion, and cardiogenic shock), in myocardial ischemia and myocardial infarction, in coronary vasospasm (2, 3), and in unstable angina (4, 5). Nevertheless, TxB$_2$ is not always detected in hypoxic or ischemic states. This does not mean that TxA$_2$ is not involved in a particular disease state, because significant quantities of the TxA$_2$ can be produced by vascular smooth muscle, lung parenchyma, and cardiac tissue and therefore may remain in the extracellular fluid or lymph without reaching the circulating blood, despite exerting important local effects in the ischemic myocardium, edematous lung, or other site (3).

TxA$_2$ is reported to exert a variety of pathological actions. Specifically, TxA$_2$ strongly constricts blood vessels, sometimes to the point of vasospasm. This effect occurs in small and large vessels and in virtually all vascular beds tested. The vasoconstrictor effect of thromboxane A$_2$ is especially prominent in large coronary arteries as illustrated by Figure 1, which represents typical recordings in an isolated perfused cat coronary artery. The isolated cat coronary artery is perfused with Krebs–Henseleit solution under constant flow and coronary perfusion pressure is recorded. TxA$_2$ at 3 to 100 nM exerts a marked increase in perfusion pressure signifying a vasoconstriction. This can be washed out (W). In the presence of 300 nM PTA$_2$ (pinane thromboxane A$_2$), a thromboxane receptor antagonist, the usual constrictor effect of TxA$_2$ is blocked. Thus, thromboxane A$_2$ constricts coronary arteries via activation of the TxA$_2$/PGH$_2$ receptor.

Cat Coronary Artery

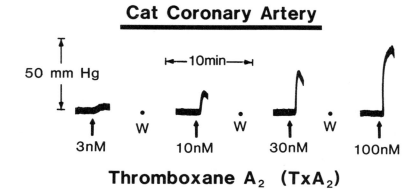

Thromboxane A$_2$ (TxA$_2$)

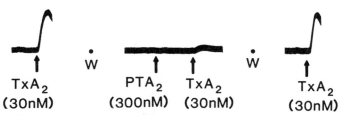

FIGURE 1. Representative recordings of perfusion pressure from an isolated constant flow perfused cat coronary artery. (From Smith, J.B. et al., Prostaglandins, 33:777-781, 1987).

Second, TxA$_2$ is a potent aggregator of blood platelets. This appears to be applicable in all species thus far tested. This aggregatory effect is so potent that it can lead to significant thrombosis. Indeed, sudden death by i.v. injection of arachidonic acid results from formation of TxA$_2$ and the subsequent pulmonary thrombosis (6, 7). Figure 2 illustrates the platelet aggregating effect of arachidonic acid (AA) given intravenously to a rabbit. This effect, which is due to formation of TxA$_2$, can be blocked by addition of a thromboxane receptor antagonist (i.e., SQ-29,548). SQ-29,548 also blocked platelet secretion as evidenced by the markedly reduced circulating ATP concentration following AA injection.

TxA$_2$ also is a powerful bronchoconstrictor. This effect may be of great significance in mediating arachidonate induced sudden death. The thromboxane-mimetic, U-46619, is a potent bronchoconstrictor in cat pulmonary parenchymal strips, and this effect is blocked totally by the thromboxane receptor antagonist BM-13,505 which is specific for TxA$_2$ and its mimetics and does not block the bronchoconstrictor effect of histamine or LTC$_4$ (8).

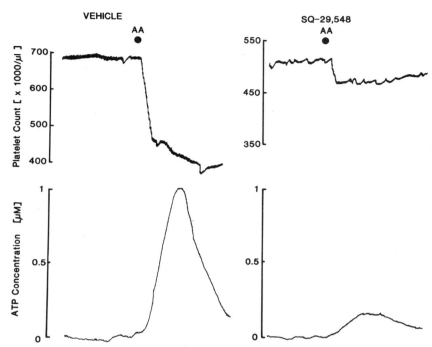

FIGURE 2. Reduction in circulating platelet count (thrombocytopenia) and elevation in circulating ATP concentration (platelet secretion) in an anesthetized rabbit given arachidonic acid (AA) intravenously in the presence and absence of a thromboxane receptor antagonist (SQ-29,548). (From Darius, H. and Lefer, A.M., J. Pharmacol. Exptl. Therap. 235:274-281, 1985).

Although it is not as well appreciated as the other effects of TxA_2, TxA_2 and its mimetics promote leakiness in lysosomal membranes (6). Recently TxA_2 was shown to cause leakiness of human and cat red blood cell membranes (9). This membrane lytic effect may serve to propagate the other effects of thromboxanes in disease states, particularly if this enhanced permeability effect is widespread in biological membranes.

Clearly, TxA_2 is present in a variety of ischemic disorders and exerts a constellation of deleterious effects that exacerbate these disease states. Thus, CTA_2 injected i.v. into cats in doses too low to alter systemic blood pressure or heart rate, dramatically enhances the cellular damage of the myocardium observed during acute myocardial ischemia. It is therefore not surprising that selective thromboxane synthetase inhibitors (10) (e.g., dazoxiben, CGS-13080, OKY-1581) and thromboxane receptor antagonists (e.g., PTA_2, SQ-29,548, BM-13505) have been developed to block the effects of TxA_2 (2). Some of the beneficial effects of thromboxane synthetase inhibitors may result from their redirection of endoperoxide substrate (11) to PGI_2, a prostaglandin which is cytoprotective and inhibits platelet aggregation.

In contrast, thromboxane receptor antagonists do not directly alter metabolism of arachidonic acid, rather they antagonize the TxA_2/PGH_2 receptor. None of the available thromboxane receptor antagonists distinguish between thromboxanes and endoperoxides (e.g., PGG_2 and PGH_2). Thus, this receptor is known as the thromboxane-endoperoxide receptor rather than solely as the thromboxane receptor (12). These antagonists may also be important because they also block the actions of TxB_2, which exerts significant biological effects when it accumulates to high concentrations. With these agents, one can effectively investigate the role of the thromboxanes in disease states.

Thromboxane receptor antagonists have been found to be particularly effective in preventing the extension of ischemic damage following permanent myocardial ischemia (13, 14, 15, 16). Moreover, this effect translates into an increase in survival in animals during acute myocardial ischemia (16). Recently, the thromboxane receptor antagonist BM-13505 was found to preserve myocardial integrity in a reperfusion model of myocardial ischemia in cats. In this experiment, LAD coronary artery occlusion was allowed to progress for two hours followed by reperfusion and observation for an additional four hours. Table 1 summarizes the area of ischemic damage (i.e., necrotic area). The area-at-risk was comparable but BM-13505, when given at a dose of 1 mg/kg one hour prior to reperfusion followed by an infusion of 1 mg/kg/h, reduced the necrotic area by half. This is clear cut evidence for an anti-ischemic effect of this thromboxane receptor antagonist in reperfusion-induced ischemic injury.

TABLE 1. Effect of BM-13505 on Reperfusion MI Injury

Group	N	% Area at Risk (AAR)	Necrotic Area (% AAR)
Sham MI + Vehicle	5	0 ± 0	0 ± 0
MI + Vehicle	7	26.4 ± 1.6	30.9 ± 3.1
MI + BM-13505	7	22.7 ± 1.3	$14.6 \pm 3.2*$

All values are means $\pm$ SEM. * $p<0.01$ from MI + vehicle.
N = number of cats.

REFERENCES

1.   Lefer AM. In: McConn R, ed. Role of Chemical Mediators in the Pathophysiology of Acute Illness and Injury, New York: Raven Press, 1982; 101-109.

2.   Lefer AM, Darius H. Drugs of the Future 1987; 12:367-373.

3.   Ribeiro LGT, Lefer AM. In: Chahine RA, ed. Coronary Artery Spasm, Mt. Kisco, New York: Futura Publishing, 1983; 39-63.

4.   Walinsky P, Lebanthal M, Smith JB, Lefer AM. In: Santamore WP, Bove AA, eds. Coronary Artery Disease, Baltimore: Urban and Schwarzenberg, 1982; 247-253.

5.   Fitzgerald DJ, Roy L, Catella F, Fitzgerald GA. New Eng J Med 1986; 315:983-989.

6.   Lefer AM, Smith EF III, Araki H, et al. Proc Natl Acad Sci USA 1980; 77:1706-1710.

7.   Lefer AM, Okamatsu S, Smith EF III, Smith JB. Thromb Res 1981; 23:265-273.

8.   Lefer DJ, Lefer AM. Med Sci Res 1987; 15:707-708.

9.   Brezinski ME, Lefer DJ, Bowker B, Lefer AM. Prostaglandins 1987; 33:75-84.

10.   Burke SE, Lefer DJ, Lefer AM. Arch Int Pharmacodyn Ther 1983; 265:76-84.

11.   Vermylen J, Deckmyn H. Br J Clin Pharmacol 1983; 15:17S-22S.

12.   Halushka PV, Mais DE, Saussay DL Jr. Fed Proc 1987; 46:149-153.

13. Schror K, Smith EF III, Bickerton M, Smith JB, Nicolaou KC, Magolda R, Lefer AM. Am J Physiol 1980; 238:H87-H92.

14. Brezinski ME, Yanagisawa A, Darius H, Lefer AM. Am Heart J 1985; 110:1161-1167.

15. Brezinski ME, Yanagisawa A, Lefer AM. J Cardiovasc Pharmacol 1987; 9:65-71.

16. Hock CE, Brezinski ME, Lefer AM. Eur J Pharmacol 1986; 122:213-219.

*Advances in Prostaglandin, Thromboxane, and
Leukotriene Research*, Vol. 19, edited by
B. Samuelsson, P. Y.-K. Wong, and F. F. Sun,
Raven Press, Ltd., New York ©1989.

MECHANISM OF ACTION OF ADRENERGIC AND CHOLINERGIC STIMULI ON
CARDIAC PROSTAGLANDIN SYNTHESIS

K.U. Malik, M.T. Weis and N. Jaiswal
Department of Pharmacology, College of Medicine, The University
of Tennessee, Memphis, 874 Union Avenue, Memphis, TN 38163, USA

Stimulation of adrenergic and cholinergic nerves promotes
prostaglandin (PG) synthesis in several tissues, including the
heart. These observations and the demonstration that PGs, particularly PGE_2 or PGI_2, inhibit release of the adrenergic and
cholinergic transmitters norepinephrine (NE) and acetylcholine
(ACh), respectively, and influence the postjunctional actions of
these neurotransmitters have led to the proposition that PGs act
as modulators of autonomic transmission (1, 2). However, the
mechanisms by which adrenergic and cholinergic stimuli promote
PG synthesis and PGs influence autonomic transmission have not
been established. The major site for PG synthesis in peripheral
tissues appears to be postjunctional effector cells because PG
synthesis, elicited by adrenergic and cholinergic stimuli, is
inhibited by agents that block postjunctional adrenergic receptors (3-5). Both adrenergic and cholinergic transmitters stimulate PG synthesis in various tissues by interacting with specific types of adrenergic and cholinergic receptors (3-5). Our
studies in the isolated rabbit heart perfused according to the
Langendorff technique at a constant flow rate (18 ml/min) with
Krebs-Henseleit buffer indicate that adrenergic stimuli promote
the output of 6-keto-$PGF_{1\alpha}$, the stable hydrolysis product of
PGI_2, via activation of beta-adrenergic receptors (3). Moreover, the demonstration that a beta-1 agonist dobutamine, but
not a beta-2 agonist isoetharine, enhanced the output of
6-keto-$PGF_{1\alpha}$ which was blocked by atenelol, a selective beta-1
antagonist, but not by butoxamine, a selective beta-2 antagonist, suggests that cardiac PG synthesis elicited by adrenergic stimuli is linked to activation of the beta-1 subtype of
adrenergic receptors (Fig. 1). Cardiac PG synthesis elicited by
activation of beta-adrenergic receptors was not the consequence
of alterations in mechanical function of the heart produced by
adrenergic agents. Phenylephrine, which increased coronary perfusion pressure and myocardial contractility, and isoetharine,
which produced coronary vasodilation and decreased coronary perfusion pressure, failed to alter 6-keto-$PGF_{1\alpha}$ output. The
increase in PG output produced by beta-receptor stimulation was
also not due to an increase in heart rate because when the heart
was paced by electrically stimulating the right atrium, the cardiac rate increased but the output of 6-keto-$PGF_{1\alpha}$ was unal-
tered. However, administration of isoproterenol during pacing
did not further augment the heart rate, but increased the output
of 6-keto-$PGF_{1\alpha}$.

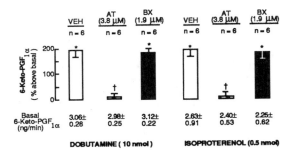

Fig. 1.   Effects of isoproterenol and dobutamine in the absence and presence of atenelol (AT) or butoxamine (BX) on immunoreactive 6-keto-PGF$_{1\alpha}$ in the isolated rabbit heart.   Bars in columns represent means ± S.E.M.   * denotes value significantly different from basal and † significantly different from vehicle group (P < 0.05).

Cardiac PG synthesis elicited by cholinergic stimuli is mediated via muscarinic receptors because it is stimulated by muscarinic agonists and is selectively blocked by atropine (1, 4). Our recent findings that in the isolated rabbit heart ACh and arecaidine propargyl ester (APE), a selective M-2 muscarinic receptor agonist, but not the M-1 agonist McN-A-343, enhanced PG synthesis and that both ACh- and APE-induced outputs of 6-keto-PGF$_{1\alpha}$ were inhibited by AF-DX-116, a selective M-2 antagonist, but not by the M-1 antagonist pirenzepine, suggest that cholinergically induced cardiac PG synthesis is mediated through the M-2 subtype of muscarinic receptors (Fig. 2) (4). Since M-2 receptors that are blocked by AF-DX-116 have been

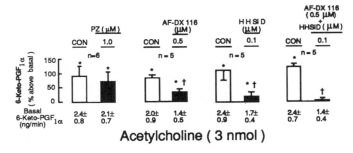

Fig. 2.   Effects of acetylcholine on the output of immunoreactive 6-keto-PGF$_{1\alpha}$ before (control, CON) and during infusion of pirenzepine (PZ), AF-DX-116 and HHSiD in the isolated rabbit heart.   Bars in columns are means ± S.E.M.   * denotes value significantly different from basal and † significantly different from that obtained before infusion of these agents.

classified as M-2 alpha, it would appear that M-2 receptors
linked to cardiac PG synthesis are of the M-2 alpha subtype of
muscarinic receptors. However, ACh- and APE-induced output of
6-keto-PGF$_{1\alpha}$ were also inhibited by a selective M-2 beta-
receptor antagonist HHSiD (hexhydro-sila-difendiol), and the
combination of AF-DX-116 and HHSiD was more effective than
either agent alone in inhibiting the output of 6-keto-PGF$_{1\alpha}$ in
response to APE or ACh (Fig. 2). These observations suggest
that cardiac PG synthesis elicited by cholinergic stimuli is
linked to both the M-2 alpha and M-2 beta subtypes of M-2 muscarinic receptors. The sites of the muscarinic and beta-adrenergic receptors involved in PG synthesis in the heart are not
known. Since coronary vasculature is believed to be the major
site of PGI$_2$ synthesis in the heart, M-2 alpha and M-2 beta muscarinic and beta-1 adrenergic receptors that are linked to PG
synthesis might be located predominantly in coronary vessels.

Activation of beta-adrenergic and muscarinic receptors in
various tissues, including the heart, is known to be associated
with distinct biochemical events. Therefore, it is possible
that the mechanisms of cardiac PG synthesis elicited by beta-
adrenergic and muscarinic receptors are also different. Inas-
much as activation of beta-adrenergic receptors is associated
with increased levels of cAMP, it is possible that cAMP, by
increasing the activity of protein kinase A directly or
indirectly, stimulates one or more lipase. However, in the rabbit heart, infusion of 8-(4-chlorophenylthio)cAMP or of agents
that increase levels of cAMP did not stimulate, but rather inhibited the isoproterenol-induced output of 6-keto-PGF$_{1\alpha}$ (6).
These observations suggest that cAMP does not mediate but rather
acts as an inhibitory modulator of cardiac PG synthesis elicited
by beta-adrenergic receptor stimulation. Activation of beta-1
adrenergic receptors in the heart and of muscarinic receptors in
nonvascular smooth muscles is known to increase the influx of
extracellular Ca^{++}. Therefore, it is possible that activation
of beta-adrenergic and muscarinic receptors promotes the influx
of extracellular Ca^{++}, which, by increasing the activity of one
or more lipases directly or by interacting with calmodulin, releases arachidonic acid for PG synthesis. Our findings that
isoproterenol-stimulated cardiac PG synthesis a) was positively
correlated with extracellular Ca^{++} concentration and b) was inhibited by the Ca^{++} channel blockers diltiazem and nifedipine
and by the intracellular Ca^{++} antagonist ryanodine but not by
calmodulin inhibitors suggest that beta-adrenergic receptor stimulation promotes the influx of extracellular Ca^{++} through vol-
tage-dependent Ca^{++} channels and increases the release of intracellular Ca^{++}, which in turn, by increasing the activity of a
Ca^{++}-sensitive but calmodulin-independent lipase, releases arachidonic acid from tissue lipids for PG synthesis (7). Although
the ACh-induced output of 6-keto-PGF$_{1\alpha}$ from the heart was also
dependent upon extracellular Ca^{++} concentration, it was not inhibited by Ca^{++} antagonists or calmodulin inhibitors (unpublished data). These observations indicate that muscarinic

receptor activation in the heart increases the influx of Ca^{++} through voltage-independent, probably receptor-operated, Ca^{++} channels, which in turn release arachidonic acid by activating a lipase independent of calmodulin.

The cardiac lipase(s) involved in the release of arachidonic acid for PG synthesis in response to beta-adrenergic and muscarinic receptor stimulation appear to be distinct from those present in some other tissues for the following reason. The phospholipase A_2 and C inhibitors mepacrine, parabromophenyl-acylbromide and dexamethasone, the phospholipase C inhibitor neomycin and the mono- and diglyceride lipase inhibitor RH-80267, which are known to attenuate the release of arachidonic acid or PG synthesis in various tissues did not alter the isoproterenol- or ACh-induced output of 6-keto-$PGF_{1\alpha}$ in the rabbit heart (data not shown). Our recent finding in the isolated rabbit heart prelabeled with 1-stearoyl, 2-[^{3}H]arachidonyl phosphatidylcholine, which is taken up by the heart and incorporated as an intact phospholipid, administration of isoproterenol but not ACh released radioactively labeled free fatty acid and lysophosphatidylcholine suggests that beta-adrenergic receptor stimulation activates both phospholipase A_1 and A_2 (8). Whether the failure of ACh to promote the breakdown of radiolabeled phosphatidylcholine incorporated into the heart is due to its uptake into cell types insensitive to ACh, to utilization by ACh-activated phospholipase A_2 of other phospholipids as substrates, or to activation by ACh of a different type of phospholipase A_2, phospholipase C or diglyceride lipase, remains to be determined.

REFERENCES

1. Hedqvist P. Ann Rev Pharmacol Toxicol 1977;17:259-279.

2. Malik, KU. Fed Proc 1978;39:203-207.

3. Shaffer JE, Malik KU. J Pharmacol Exp Ther 1982;223:729-735.

4. Jaiswal N, Malik KU. J Pharmacol Exp Ther 1988 (in press).

5. Cooper CL, Malik KU. J Pharmacol Exp Ther 1985;233:24-31.

6. Williams Jr JL, Malik KU. Fed Proc 1988;2:A382 (abstract).

7. Weis MT, Malik KU. J Pharm Exp Ther 1985;235:178-185.

8. Weis MT, Malik KU. Fed Proc 1987;46:873.

ACKNOWLEDGMENTS

Studies reported in this chapter were supported by U.S. Public Health Service Grant HL 19134 from the National Heart, Lung and Blood Institute.

Advances in Prostaglandin, Thromboxane, and Leukotriene Research, Vol. 19, edited by B. Samuelsson, P. Y.-K. Wong, and F. F. Sun, Raven Press, Ltd., New York ©1989.

SYNTHETIC STABLE ORALLY AND TRANSDERMALLY LONG–ACTING PROSTAGLANDIN E_2 (PGE$_2$) CONGENER (VIPROSTOL; CL 115,347) AND PROSTACYCLIN CONGENER (CL 115,999) AS ANTIHYPERTENSIVE AGENTS

Peter Cervoni and Peter S. Chan

American Cyanamid Company, Cardiovascular Biological Research, Medical Research Division, Lederle Laboratories Pearl River, New York 10965, U.S.A.

Despite the desirability of the hypotensive mechanism of PGE$_2$ and prostacyclin, today there is still no prostaglandin marketed as an antihypertensive agent. One reason is that natural PGE$_2$ given orally, even at high doses, cannot produce an appreciable lowering of blood pressure (BP). Only transient lowering of BP was observed after bolus intravenous (i.v.) injections of high doses of PGE$_2$. This is mainly due to its rapid metabolism by the pulmonary circulation. About 95% of PGE$_2$ is inactivated in one circulation. In addition, PGE$_2$ stimulates the smooth muscles of the gastrointestinal tract causing diarrhea and therefore lacks specificity. Prostacyclin is very unstable in acidic aqueous solutions and thus lacks oral antihypertensive efficacy. Its biological half–life in the blood is only several minutes. Therefore, the practical use of the natural PGE$_2$ and prostacyclin as antihypertensive agents is hampered by the lack of oral efficacy and ultrashort duration of action. Prosta-glandins possess a desirable antihypertensive mechanism, i.e., they cause direct vasodilatation of the resistance blood vessels. Furthermore, PGE$_2$ increases renal blood flow, induces diuresis and natriuresis, opposes the renin–angiotensin system and amplifies the kallikrein system (1). For these reasons, it has been an elusive and aspiring goal to synthesize analogs with oral efficacy, prolonged duration of antihypertensive action and tissue specificity. Degradation of the 15–hydroxyl group by 15–hydroxy–prostaglandin dehydroxylase renders all prosta-glandins inactive as antihypertensives. Attempts to protect the 15–hydroxyl group of PGE$_2$ by substitution of the 15–hydrogen with alkyl groups have met with some success (2). The discovery that moving the hydroxyl group from the 15– to the 16–position yielded compounds with oral efficacy and prolonged duration of antihypertensive action was crucial in the development of viprostol (15–deoxy–16–hydroxy–16–vinyl–PGE$_2$ methyl ester) by our team. The substitution of the hydrogen at the 16–position with alkyl or other groups greatly enhanced the activity and

331

prolonged the duration of antihypertensive action. Using direct BP measurement in conscious spontaneously hypertensive rats (SHR) for screening prostaglandin congeners for oral antihypertensive activity at 5 mg/kg, various 15-deoxy-16-hydroxy-PGE$_2$ congeners with the hydrogen at the 16-position substituted by varying groups were synthesized and tested. Thus, substitution with methyl (CL 112,731) or difluoromethyl (CL 115,789) group produced compounds with weak oral activity. Substitution with a propenyl (CL 115,747) group produced a compound with no significant activity. Substitution with ethynyl (CL 115,538) or allenyl (CL 115,972) resulted in increased potency while substitution with vinyl (CL 115,129) and its methyl ester, CL 115,347 (viprostol) or fluorovinyl (CL 116,171) produced the most potent compounds with excellent oral efficacy and prolonged duration of hypotensive effect. CL 115,789 was very active only following i.v. administration but not active following oral dosing. Various esters, such as ρ-acetamidophenyl ester (CL 116,217); isopentyl ester (CL 116,218) and m-acetylphenyl ester (CL 116,219) were found to retain the activity. Replacing the carboxylic acid group with alcohol or the hydroxymethylketone group decreased oral activity. After considering all of the efficacy data, viprostol was chosen for further development (Table 1) (3).

Similar treatments of the prostacyclin structure produced stable orally and transdermally very active prostacyclin congeners. CL 115,974 (5,6-dihydro-prostacyclin) at 1 and 5 mg/kg i.v. produced a 57 and 72 mmHg lowering of mean arterial blood pressure (MABP) lasting 45 and 60 min, respectively, in conscious SHR, but at 5 mg/kg orally, the antihypertensive effects were minimal (-10 mmHg). With the 15-deoxy-16-hydroxy-16-vinyl side chain kept constant, the 5,6-dihydro-prostacyclin congener (CL 116,000) was found to be less active (-30 and -42 mmHg at 1 and 5 mg/kg i.v., respectively) than CL 115,974, but the oral antihypertensive activity improved (-25 mmHg). When the hydrogen at the 5-position of CL 115,974 was substituted by iodine to yield CL 115,973, the oral antihypertensive activity was improved somewhat. Similar substitution with iodine in CL 116,000 to yield CL 115,999 which produced potent oral, i.v. and transdermal antihypertensive activity (-62, -59 and -49 mmHg lowering at 5 mg/kg p.o., 1 mg/kg i.v. and 1 mg/kg transdermally, respectively). Replacement of the carboxylic acid group of CL 115,999 by hydroxymethylketone and hydroxymethyldioxolane to yield CL 116,099 and CL 116,144, respectively, increased the duration of antihypertensive effect but the degree of MABP lowering was somewhat less. CL 115,999 (5-iodo-5,6-dihydro-15-deoxy-16-hydroxy-16-vinyl-prostacyclin methyl ester) was finally chosen for development (Table 2) (4).

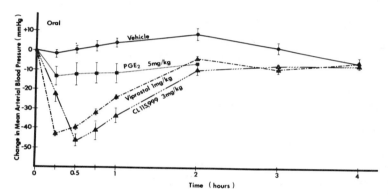

CL No.	R¹	R²	Orally (mg/kg) 1	5	Intravenous 1 mg/kg
			CONSCIOUS SHR MABP (Δ mmHg)		
115,347	-CH₃	-CH=CH₂	-52	-57	-56
115,129	-H	-CH=CH₂	-45	-50	-63
112,731	-H	-CH₃	-13	-13	
115,149	-H	CH₂-CH₂ \ CH		-10	
115,538	-H	-C≡CH		-29	
115,747	-CH₃	CH₃		+4	
116,171	-H	-CF=CH₂		-58	
115,789	-H	-CHF₂	-8	-16	-45
115,972	-H	-CH=C=CH₂		-40	-54

Compound CL Number	ORAL ADMINISTRATION			INTRAVENOUS ADMINISTRATION			Chemical Structures
	Dose mg/kg	Changes in MABP (Δ mmHg)	Duration of Action (Hr)	Dose mg/kg	Changes in MABP (Δ mmHg)	Duration of Action (Hr)	
115,974	5	-10	0.25	5 / 1	-72 / -57	1 / 0.75	15-OH
115,999	5	-62	2.5-3	1	-59	1	5-I 16-OH 16-Vinyl
116,000	5	-25	0.75	5 / 1	-42 / -30	0.5-0.75 / 0.5	16-OH 16-Vinyl

TABLE 1. Antihypertensive activity of 1-prostaglandin E_2 congeners in conscious SHR

TABLE 2. Antihypertensive activity of prostacyclin congeners in conscious SHR

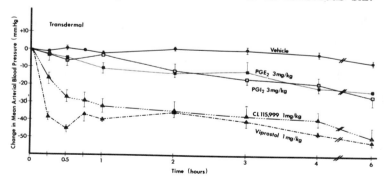

FIG. 1.   Comparison of the antihypertensive activity of 1-prostaglandin E_2 (PGE_2), viprostol and CL 115,999 following oral administration in conscious SHR

FIG. 2.   Comparison of the antihypertensive activity of PGE_2, prostacyclin (PGI_2), viprostol and CL 115,999 in conscious SHR

In comparing the antihypertensive effects of viprostol and CL 115,999 with l-PGE$_2$ and prostacyclin in conscious SHR, it was found that after oral dosing, l-PGE$_2$ at 5 mg/kg maximally lowered MABP 13 mmHg. At 30 mg/kg, l-PGE$_2$ lowered MABP 32 mmHg and the duration of action was about 45 min. Viprostol at 1 mg/kg achieved a 43 mmHg lowering of MABP that lasted about 120 min. CL 115,999 at 3 mg/kg exhibited the same degree of lowering as 1 mg/kg of viprostol (Figure 1). Following i.v. administration, l-PGE$_2$ at 2 mg/kg lowered MABP 39 mmHg and lasted about 20 min while viprostol at 2 mg/kg lowered MABP 50 mmHg that lasted about 90 min. CL 115,999 at 1 mg/kg i.v. lowered MABP 52 mmHg that lasted about 60 min. Following transdermal (topical) administration of l-PGE$_2$ and prostacyclin in petrolatum at 3 mg/kg decreased the MABP about 10 to 20 mmHg while viprostol and CL 115,999 at 1 mg/kg lowered MABP 40 to 50 mmHg and lasted more than 6 hr (Figure 2). Viprostol was found to be as potent as l-PGE$_2$ in relaxing the rabbit isolated ear central artery but viprostol was about 200 times less potent than l-PGE$_2$ in contracting the isolated gerbil colon. Therefore, viprostol appears to be more specific for vascular smooth muscle.

In conclusion, our team has succeeded in synthesizing stable congeners of l-PGE$_2$ and prostacyclin with potent oral and transdermal antihypertensive efficacy and prolonged duration of action.

Acknowledgements

The CL compounds were synthesized by Dr. M.J. Weiss and his colleagues from our company.

References

1. Chan PS, Cervoni P. Drug Development Res 1986;7:341-359.

2. Muchowski JM. Synthetic prostanoids. In: Willis LW, ed. CRC Handbook of Eicosanoids: Prostaglandins and Related Lipids, Vol. I, Part B. Boca Raton: CRC Press, 1987;19-153.

3. Chan PS, Cervoni P, Ronsberg MA, et al. J Pharmacol Exp Ther 1983;226:726-732.

4. Chan PS, Cervoni P, Ronsberg MA, et al. Federation Proc 1986;45:913.

Advances in Prostaglandin, Thromboxane, and
Leukotriene Research, Vol. 19, edited by
B. Samuelsson, P. Y.-K. Wong, and F. F. Sun,
Raven Press, Ltd., New York ©1989.

PULMONARY P-450-MEDIATED EICOSANOID METABOLISM AND REGULATION

IN THE PREGNANT RABBIT

B.S.S. Masters, R.T. Okita, A.S. Muerhoff,
M.T. Leithauser, A. Gee, S. Winquist, D.L. Roerig[*],
J.E. Clark, R.C. Murphy[x] and P. Ortiz de Montellano [‡]

Departments of Biochemistry, Anesthesiology[*], and
Pharmacology/Toxicology[*], Medical College of Wisconsin and
VA Medical Center[*], Milwaukee,WI 53226, USA. Department of
Pharmacology[x] The University of Colorado School of Medicine,
Denver, CO 80262, USA. Department of Pharmaceutical
Chemistry[‡], University of California, San Francisco, CA
94143, USA. Supported by USPHS GM 31296 to BSSM and RTO.

The hydroxylation of a number of endogenous compounds is
catalyzed by cytochromes P-450 localized in specific cell types
in a variety of tissues. Those oxygenations occurring on the
ultimate (ω) or penultimate (ω-1) carbons of fatty acids or
eicosanoids are being studied by several laboratories who
believe these products have physiological significance beyond
serving as intermediates in an excretory pathway (1-3).
Following the demonstration by Powell and Solomon (4) and
Powell (5) that pregnancy or progesterone treatment resulted in
a dramatic induction in rabbit lung microsomes of the ω-hydrox-
ylation of prostaglandins of the E and F series and of thromboxane B_2, our laboratory purified and characterized the
cytochrome P-450 (P-450$_{PG-\omega}$) responsible for this activity (6).
Simultaneously, Yamamoto, et al. purified the enzyme (7) and
cloned and sequenced the cDNA (8). Our laboratory has shown
recently that the gestational age dependence of this enzyme
activity parallels its levels of protein and of in vitro
translatable mRNA (9).

EXPERIMENTAL PROCEDURES

Lungs from New Zealand white rabbits were obtained from
whole animals (Smith's Rabbitry, Seymour, WI or Hickory Hill,
Inc., Flint, TX) or purchased frozen from Pel-Freez Biologicals
(Rogers, AR). The acetylenic substrates, 17-octadecynoic acid
(17-ODYA) and 12-hydroxy-16-heptadecynoic acid (12-HHDYA) were
synthesized as described (10,11). Isolated, perfused lung

335

experiments were performed (12) in an artificial thorax system in which physiological parameters were controlled. A 0.5 ml bolus of perfusate containing 2.5 µCi [^{3}H]-PGE$_1$ (60 pmol) was infused through an injection port connected to the arterial cannula and fractions were collected from the venous cannula at a rate of one per sec for the 45-sec duration of the single-pass experiments. Perfusion metabolites were identified by co-elution with enzymatically generated standards. The standards, produced from microsomal and/or cytosolic incubations, were purified by reverse phase HPLC and normal phase Sep-Pak and then identified by gas chromatography/mass spectrometry of their O-methoxime, trimethylsilyl ether, trimethylsilyl ester derivatives.

EXPERIMENTAL RESULTS AND DISCUSSION

Studies on the specificity of the P-450$_{PG-\omega}$ have revealed that several prostanoids and the lipoxygenase product, 15-HETE, are substrates. However, Okita, et al. (13) demonstrated that neither 5-HETE, 12-HETE, nor leukotriene B$_4$, are substrates, and proposed that an ω-6 hydroxyl group confers specificity. Also, our laboratory has found (unpublished observations) that P-450$_{PG-\omega}$ does not catalyze the ω-hydroxylation of long chain fatty acids at significant rates, contrary to the reports from Kusunose's laboratory (7,8). To elucidate the specificity of the pulmonary hydroxylases, acetylenic fatty acid mechanism-based inhibitors were applied to microsomal and reconstituted systems (11,14).

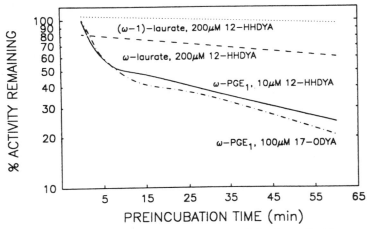

FIG. 1. Inhibition of the microsomal hydroxylations of laurate and PGE$_1$ by 12-HHDYA and 17-ODYA. Microsomes from lungs of pregnant rabbits were preincubated with the acetylenic inhibitors and then assayed for the activities indicated (6,11).

Fig. 1 shows a composite of data from experiments in which the acetylenic substrates 12-HHDYA (containing an ω-6 hydroxyl) and 17-ODYA were used as inhibitors of the hydroxylation of lauric acid and of PGE_1 by lung microsomes from pregnant rabbits (25-28 days of gestation). It can be seen that the microsomal hydroxylation of lauric acid at either the ω- or (ω-1)-position is only slightly inhibited by a high concentration (200 μM) of 12-HHDYA while only 10 μM 12-HHDYA is required for potent inhibition (> 80%) of PGE_1 ω-hydroxylation. For comparison, the curve for inhibition of PGE_1 metabolism by 17-ODYA at 100 μM is shown. These results indicate that the 12-HHDYA is at least 10-fold more potent in inhibiting PGE_1 ω-hydroxylation than 17-ODYA, reinforcing the suggestion that $P-450_{PG-\omega}$ is highly specific for substrates containing the ω-6 hydroxyl group.

To examine in situ the pregnancy-induced ω-hydroxylation of prostaglandins, an isolated, perfused lung system was utilized in which a bolus of $[^3H]-PGE_1$ was introduced into lungs from non-pregnant or pregnant (25-28 days of gestation) rabbits. Perfusate fractions were analyzed for metabolism of $[^3H]-PGE_1$. As shown in Fig. 2, the lungs of non-pregnant rabbits produced primarily (∿75%) the relatively nonpolar metabolite, 13,14-dihydro-15-keto-PGE_1, and only small quantities (∿25%) of polar compounds. In marked contrast, the lungs of pregnant rabbits produced only polar metabolites which have now been identified by mass spectrometry as 20-hydroxy-PGE_1 and 13,14-dihydro-15-keto-20-hydroxy-PGE_1.

These results indicate that in the pregnant rabbit, the $P-450_{PG-\omega}$ contributes significantly to the pulmonary metabolism

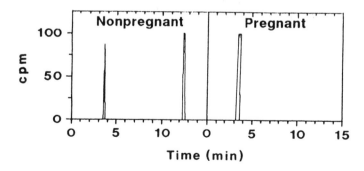

FIG. 2 Reverse phase HPLC profiles of metabolites collected 26 sec after injection of $[^3H]-PGE_1$ into isolated, perfused lungs of non-pregnant or pregnant rabbits. Elution times were ∿ 3.5 min for the polar metabolites and ∿ 12.5 min for the nonpolar. HPLC conditions: isocratic $H_2O/CH_3CN/CH_3COOH/C_6H_6$; 59.8/39.8/0.2/0.2, 0.7 ml/min, Bio-Sil ODS-5S.

of certain eicosanoids, in particular, those containing an ω-6 hydroxyl. The physiological role of this interesting cytochrome P-450 in pregnancy is not yet understood.

REFERENCES

1. Capdevila, J., Kim, Y.R., Martin-Wixtrom, C., Falck, J.R., Manna, S., and Estabrook, R.W. Arch Biochem Biophys 1985; 1:8-19.

2. Schwartzman, M.L., Abraham, N.G., Carroll, M.A., Levere, R.D., and McGiff, J.C. Biochem J 1986; 238:283-290.

3. Oliw, E.H. and Hamberg, M. Biochim Biophys Acta 1986; 879:113-119.

4. Powell, W.S. and Solomon, S. J Biol Chem 1978; 253:4609-4616.

5. Powell, W.S. Biochim Biophys Acta 1979; 575:335-349.

6. Williams, D.E., Hale, S.E., Okita, R.T., and Masters, B.S.S. J Biol Chem 1984; 259:14600-14608.

7. Yamamoto, S., Kusunose, E., Ogita, K., Kaku, M., Ichihara, K., and Kusunose, M. J Biochem (Tokyo) 1984; 96:593-603.

8. Matsubara, S., Yamamoto, S., Sogawa, K., et al. J Biol Chem 1987; 262:13366-13371.

9. Muerhoff, A.S., Williams, D.E., Leithauser, M.T., Jackson, V.E., Waterman, M.R., and Masters, B.S.S. Proc Natl Acad Sci USA 1987; 84:7911-7914.

10. Shak, S., Reich, N.O., Goldstein, I.M., and Ortiz de Montellano, P.R. J Biol Chem 1985; 260:13023-13028.

11. Williams, D.E., Muerhoff, A.S., Reich, N.O., Ortiz de Montellano, P.R., and Masters, B.S.S. 1988 (submitted).

12. Masters, B.S.S., Okita, R.T., Williams, D.E., et al. In: Burkitt, D.J., et al., eds. VIIth International Symposium on Microsomes and Drug Oxidations, London: Taylor and Francis, Ltd. 1988 (in press).

13. Okita, R.T., Soberman, R.J., Bergholte, J.M., Masters, B.S.S., Hayes, R., and Murphy, R.C. Mol Pharmacol 1987; 32:706-709.

14. Muerhoff, A.S., Williams, D.E., Ortiz de Montellano, P.R., et al. FASEB J 1988; 2: A1262.

Advances in Prostaglandin, Thromboxane, and Leukotriene Research, Vol. 19, edited by B. Samuelsson, P. Y.-K. Wong, and F. F. Sun, Raven Press, Ltd., New York ©1989.

CHARACTERISTICS OF THE HEPATIC CYTOCHROME P-450 CATALYZING OMEGA HYDROXYLATION OF PROSTAGLANDINS

David Kupfer and Karsten H. Holm

Worcester Foundation for Experimental Biology, Shrewsbury, Massachusetts 01545, U.S.A.

The observations that prostaglandins (PGs) are metabolized in vivo into dicarboxylic PG derivatives in several species (1), initiated an interest into the possible mode of formation of these products. The findings that guinea pig liver preparations catalyze the hydroxylation of PGA_1 at C-19 and C-20 (1), suggested that the formation of the dicarboxylic PG metabolites may involve an initial hydroxylation at the terminal (ω-) position followed by further oxidation. This was further supported by the observations that hepatic and extrahepatic microsomes, in the presence of NADPH and molecular oxygen, hydroxylate also other PGs (2-4) and that liver cytosol of several species catalyzes the oxidation of 20-hydroxy-PGs into the corresponding dicarboxylic acids (4). While examining the hydroxylation of PGE_1, at two concentrations, with rabbit liver microsomes, we observed that the hydroxylation activities at C-19 and C-20 exhibit widely different affinities for the substrate, suggesting that different enzymes catalyze the two hydroxylations. Kinetic studies demonstrated that the Km for the ω-hydroxylase was markedly lower than that for the ω-1 hydroxylase (5). Indirect observations indicated that the microsomal enzymes catalyzing these reactions are cytochrome P-450s. In collaboration with Drs Coon, Vatsis and Koop, we showed that several forms (isozymes) of P-450 from rabbit liver microsomes exhibit overlapping but distinct regioselective hydroxylation of PGEs at ω-, ω-1 and ω-2 (6,7). More recently we isolated from rabbit liver a constitutive form of P-450, referred to as form 7 (60KDa), which hydroxylates PGEs solely at the ω- site (8). Table 1 depicts the activities of rabbit liver P-450s towards PGE_2. Interestingly, among rabbit liver P-450s, only LM2 and form 7 require cytochrome b_5 for significant activity. The reason for b_5 requirement is not understood. The high affinity of form 7 for PGE_2, Km being 6μM, suggests that this enzyme is responsible for the high affinity ω-hydroxylase in rabbit liver microsomes (5). Form 7 demonstrates a relatively high substrate specificity (Table 2); it does not catalyze the metabolism of typical substrates of P-450s, such as benzphetamine and ethylmorphine, and

339

TABLE 1. Hydroxylation of PGE_2 by cytochrome P-450 forms from rabbit liver microsomes

P-450 Form

Metabolite	2^a	4^a	6^b	7
		(pmol/min/nmol P-450)		
20-OH	14	0	0	650
19-OH	74	115	440	0
18-OH	0	0	250	0

Cytochrome b_5 is almost obligatory for forms 2 and 7.
[a] From Vatsis et al. (1982) J. Biol. Chem. 257:11221.
[b] From Holm et al. (1985) Arch. Biochem. Biophys. 243:135.

has no activity towards LTB_4. However, a low activity towards hydroxylation of benzo[a]pyrene was observed and hence this P-450 might be similar to P-450 LM_7, prepared by different procedures (9,10). Additionally, form 7 was found to exhibit a relatively high resistance to inhibition by alternate substrates

TABLE 2. Comparison of catalytic activities of liver microsomes from untreated rabbits with ω-hydroxylase (Form 7)

Substrate	Microsomes (nmol/min/mg protein)	ω-Hydroxylase[a] (nmol/min/nmol P-450)
PGE_2	0.02	0.46
LTB_4	N.Q.[b]	0
Benzoa[a]pyrene	0.24	0.06
Benzphetamine	5.0	0
Ethylmorphine	1.2	0

[a] Reconstituted with NADPH-P-450 reductase and cytochrome b_5
[b] Not quantitated: only a small peak with retention time of 19-OH-LTB_4

and inhibitors of monooxygenases (Table3). The finding that arachidonate is a strong inhibitor of PGE_2 hydroxylation, suggests that arachidonate might be a substrate for this enzyme. Recently, Ozols (11) described the isolation from rabbit liver microsomes of a 60KDa protein with high esterase activity. This protein has similar amino acid sequence to that of our form 7 for which 40 residues were sequenced. A notable difference is in amino acid 12 (lysine vs. histidine). Subsequently in collaboration with Dr. Pohl's group, we demonstrated that form 7 also has esterase activity towards p-nitrophenyl acetate (PNPA). This raised the question whether our preparation of 60KDa protein is composed of a single chain with two enzymatic activities (ω-hydroxylase and esterase) or contains a mixture which copurifies. Since form 7 preparations

TABLE 3. Effect of substrates of monooxygenases on the
hydroxylation of PGE_2 by rabbit liver P-450 form 7
(ω-hydroxylase)

Additions (µM)	Ratio of Added Compound to that of PGE2 (15µM)	20-OH-PGE_2 (% of control)
--- [a]	---	100[a]
Laurate (50)	3.3	106
(200)	13.3	82
Arachidonate (10)	0.67	52
(100)	6.7	0
LTB_4 (15)	1.0	99
Benzo(a)pyrene[b] (80)	5.3	81

[a] 172 mM ethanol; 100% control activity was 6.25 nmol
20-OH-PGE_2 per nmol form 7 per 25 min

[b] In 68 mM acetone; acetone alone yielded 89% of control of
20-OH-PGE_2
Reconstituted system: P-450 (40 nM), Reductase (80 nM) and 65
(60 nM); PGE_2 (15 µM)

have low specific P-450 content, we speculated that it contains
apo-P450, possibly generated during purification (8). Similar
conclusion was reached by others with respect to LM7 (9). It was
reported that apomyoglobin, but not myoglobin, exhibits esterase
activity (12). That activity is most likely due to imidazole
groups which are freed by heme removal. Subsequently, we observed that apohemoglobin has esterase activity (unpublished). These
findings raised the possibility that esterase activity in form 7
resides in the apo-P-450. Our findings that the addition of heme
(10µM) inhibits the esterase activity of apomyoglobin, of rabbit
liver microsomes and of form 7, supports that assumption. Of
additional interest is our observation that both microsomal and
form 7 esterase activities, but not that of apomyoglobin, are
inhibited by PGE_2. We observed that mercaptoethanol has
potent ester hydrolyzing activity towards PNPA, indicating that
sulfhydryl containing compounds could function as esterases.
Cytochrome P-450s have a thiol group as the 5th ligand of their
heme iron. In apo-P-450, the free thiol group could be available
for esterase activity. Our findings that disulfiram, which reacts with sulfhydryls, inhibits rabbit liver microsomal esterase
but not that of apomyoglobin, further suggests that free thiols
are involved in the catalytic activity of microsomal esterases.

In conclusion, rabbit liver microsomes contain a high affinity
cytochrome P-450 with ω-hydroxylase activity towards PGs. The
isolated protein(s) exhibits two enzymatic activities (ω-hydroxylase and esterase). Indirect evidence suggests that both activities reside on the same protein and that in the hemeprotein,
which functions as a monooxygenase, the esterase activity is sup-

pressed and is expressed only upon heme dissociation. However, the possibility that the two activities reside in different peptides was not ruled out. The resolution of that problem must await the sequencing of the protein and the cloning of the holo-P-450 with ω-hydroxylase activity.

Acknowledgement. This work was supported in part by a USPHS grant ES00834 from NIEHS. The sequencing of form 7 was carried out at the UCLA Protein Microsequencing Facility (Dr. Audree Fowler).

References

1. Samuelsson B, Granstrom E, Green K, and Hamberg M. Ann NY Acad Sci 1971;180:138-163.

2. Kupfer D, Navarro J, and Piccolo DE. J Biol Chem 1978;253:2804-2811.

3. Powell WS. J Biol Chem 1978;253:6711-6716.

4. Kupfer D. In:Schenkman JB, and Kupfer D, eds. Hepatic Cytochrome P-450 Monooxygenase System. New York: Pergamon Press, 1982;157-187.

5. Theoharides AD, and Kupfer D. J Biol Chem 1981;256:2168-2175.

6. Vatsis KP, Theoharides AD, Kupfer D, and Coon MJ. J Biol Chem 1982;257:11221-11229.

7. Holm KA, Koop DR, Coon MJ, Theoharides AD, and Kupfer D. Arch Biochem Biophys 1985;243:135-143.

8. Holm KA, and Kupfer D. J Biol Chem 1985;260:2027-2030.

9. Deutsch J, Leutz JC, Yang SK, Gelboin HV, Chiang YL, Vatsis KP, and Coon MJ. Proc Natl Acad Sci 1978;75:3123-3127.

10. Guengerich FP. J Biol Chem 1977;252:3970-3127.

11. Ozols J. J Biol Chem 1987;262:15316-15321.

12. Zemel H. J Am Chem Soc 1987;109:1875-1876.

Advances in Prostaglandin, Thromboxane, and Leukotriene Research, Vol. 19, edited by B. Samuelsson, P. Y.-K. Wong, and F. F. Sun, Raven Press, Ltd., New York ©1989.

PROSTAGLANDIN ω-HYDROXYLASE AND RELATED CYTOCHROME P-450

*M.Kusunose,*Y.Kikuta,*E.Kusunose,*+S.Matsubara, *+N.Yokotani,**I.Kubota,+K.Sogawa, and +Y.Fujii-Kuriyama

*Toneyama Institute for Tuberculosis Research, Osaka City University Medical School, Toyonaka, Osaka 560; +Department of Biochemistry, Cancer Institute, Japanese Foundation for Cancer Research, Toyoshima-ku, Tokyo, 170; and **Suntory Institute for Medical Research, Chiyoda, Gumma 370-05, Japan

Although both liver and adrenal cortex cytochrome P-450 (P-450) systems have been extensively investigated, the properties of the P-450 systems in other organs are still poorly understood. For the past several years, we have isolated a number of forms of P-450 from rabbit extrahepatic tissues (1-6). We found that the specific forms of P-450 highly active in the ω-hydroxylation of fatty acids or prostaglandins (PGs) are present at high levels in several extrahepatic tissues such as kidney cortex, small intestine, and lung. The cDNA and derived amino acid sequences for pulmonary PG ω-hydroxylase have been determined (7). Most recently, we have also isolated PG ω-hydroxylases from rabbit liver microsomes. In this report, we strongly suggest that various rabbit ω-hydroxylases constitute a new gene family in the P-450 superfamily.

RESULTS

Cloning and Characterization of cDNA for Pulmonary Prostaglandin ω-Hydroxylase (P-450p-2)

We have isolated a new type of P-450 (designated P-450p-2) from lung microsomes of rabbits treated with progesterone (2). P-450p-2 efficiently catalyzed the ω-hydroxylation of PGE_1,-PGE_2, $PGF_{2\alpha}$, PGD_2, PGA_1, and PGA_2 as well as the ω- and (ω-1)-hydroxylation of palmitate. Various metal ions and organic solvents were required for the maximum activity in a reconstituted system containing NADPH-P-450 reductase, cytochrome b_5 and phosphatidylcholine (Table 1). Williams et al.(8) have also isolated a very similar P-450 (P-450PGω) from lung microsomes of pregnant rabbits.

We have isolated cDNA clones of the mRNA for P-450p-2 by using synthetic oligonucleotide probes (7). The complete polypeptide contained 506 amino acids, with a molecular weight of 58,515. Whereas P-450p-2 showed less than 25% sequence simila-

TABLE 1.   *Effects of metal ions and organic solvents on PGE_1 ω-hydroxylation by P-450p-2*

Salts		Organic solvents		Activity (nmol/min/nmol P-450)	
				Exp. 1	Exp. 2
None				6.4	4.7
LiCl	100 mM	–		13.0	
NaCl	"	–		16.2	
KCl	"	–		16.4	12.5
RbCl	"	–		19.0	
NH_4Cl	"	–		20.4	
$MgCl_2$	10	–		15.2	
$CaCl_2$	0.5	–		10.0	
KCl	100	Methanol	10 µl		35.3
"	"	Ethanol	"		32.6
"	"	Propanol	"		22.6
"	"	Acetone	"		27.7
"	"	Ether	"		22.1
"	"	Benzene	"		27.3
"	"	Toluene	"		18.8
"	"	Dioxane	"		5.8

rity to other forms of P-450, it shared 74% similarity with rat hepatic lauric acid ω-hydroxylase (P-450LAω)(9). Northern blot analysis showed that either progesterone treatment or pregnancy increased the levels of mRNA hybridizable to the cDNA by about 100-fold in the lung.   Furthermore, the mRNA hybridizable to the cDNA was also detected to a significant level in the liver and placenta from pregnant rabbits, and the kidney from un-treated rabbits, suggesting the presence of P-450p-2 or very closely related proteins in these tissues.

Isolation and Characterization of Prostaglandin ω-Hydroxylases from Liver Microsomes of Pregnant Rabbits

Recently, we have highly purified PG ω-hydroxylase, desig-nated P-450LPGω, from the liver microsomes of pregnant rabbits. P-450LPGω was very similar to P-450p-2 (2) in its molecular weight, spectral properties, and catalytic activities.   P-450LPGω was very unstable on storage, while P-450p-2 was stable at $-80°C$ for one year.

Isolation and Characterization of Fatty Acid and Prostaglandin A ω-Hydroxylases from Kidney Cortex Microsomes

We have highly purified 4 different forms of P-450 (P-450ka-1, P-450ka-2, P-450kc, and P-450kd) from the kidney cortex mic-rosomes of untreated rabbits. Both P-450ka-1 and P-450ka-2 efficiently catalyzed the ω-hydroxylation of PGA_1 and PGA_2. P-450ka-1, P-450ka-2, P-450kc, and P-450kd were also very active in the ω- and (ω-1)-hydroxylation of fatty acids.   All these forms had no activity toward xenobiotics.

Isolation of Prostaglandin A ω-Hydroxylases from Liver Microsomes of Rabbits treated with DEHP

Furthermore, we have isolated two forms of PGA ω-hydroxylases (P-450LPGAω-1 and P-450LPGAω-2) from the liver microsomes of rabbits treated with DEHP. P-450LPGAω-1 and P-450LPGAω-2 were very similar to P-450ka-1 and P-450ka-2 in their molecular weights, spectral properties, and catalytic activities, respectively.

Immunochemical and Structural Relationship of Prostaglandin and Fatty Acid ω-Hydroxylases

Fig.1 shows that guinea pig antibody against P-450p-2 cross-reacts with nine forms of ω-hydroxylase, indicating that all these ω-hydroxylases are immunochemically related. In contrast, this antibody does not react with other forms of P-450 such as P-450kb, liver P-450 isozyme 2, and isozyme 4.

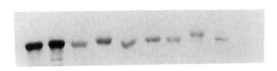

1 2 3 4 5 6 7 8 9 10

FIG.1. Western blot analysis of ω-hydroxylases with anti-P-450p-2 antibody. Purified P-450 (each 10 pmol) were electrophoresed. After electrophoretic transfer of the protein bands to nitrocellulose paper, immunnoperoxidase staining with the antibody to P-450p-2 was performed. 1,P-450p-2; 2,P-450LPGω; 3,P-450LPGAω-1; 4,P-450LPGAω-2; 5,P-450ka-1; 6,P-450ka-2; 7,P-450kc; 8,P-450kd; 9,P-450ia; 10,P-450kb.

Table 2 shows that six forms of ω-hydroxylase isolated in this laboratory have a great degree of N-terminal sequence homology. P-450p-2 and P-450LPGω have identical sequences. Moreover, the sequence of P-450kd is also identical with that of P-450p-2. P-450kd differs from P-450p-2 in its molecular weight, catalytic activities, and inducer. When these P-450 were subjected to limited proteolysis with V8 protease, P-450p-2 was found to be very similar to P-450LPGω, but slightly different from P-450kd in its peptide pattern. P-450LPGAω-1 and P-450ka-1 show 85% sequence homology with P-450p-2. P-450ka-2 shows at least 80% sequence homology with P-450p-2. This form is different from P-450ka-1 in its peptide pattern.

In summary, the present studies indicate that prostaglandin and fatty acid ω-hydroxylases from various tissues such as lung, liver, kidney, and small intestine constitute a new gene family in the P-450 superfamily.

Table 2. *N-terminal sequences of six forms of ω-hydroxylase*

No.	P-450p-2	P-450LPGω	P-450LPGAω-1	P-450ka-1	P-450ka-2	P-450kd
1	Ala	Ala	Ala	Ala	Ala	Ala
2	Leu	Leu	Leu	Leu	Leu	Leu
3	Ser	Ser	Asn	Asn	Ser	Ser
4	Pro	Pro	Pro	Pro	Pro	Pro
5	Thr	Thr	Thr	Thr	Thr	Thr
6	Arg	Arg	Arg	Arg	Arg	Arg
7	Leu	Leu	Leu	Leu	Leu	Leu
8	Pro	Pro	Pro	Pro	Pro	Pro
9	Gly	Gly	Gly	Gly	Gly	Gly
10	Ser	Ser	Ser	Ser	Ser	Ser
11	Leu	Leu	Leu	Leu	Phe	Leu
12	Ser	Ser	Ser	Ser	Ser	Ser
13	Gly	Gly	Gly	Gly	Gly	Gly
14	Leu	Leu	Leu	Leu	Phe	Leu
15	Leu	Leu	Leu	Leu	Leu	Leu
16	Gln	Gln	Gln	Gln	Gln	Gln
17	Val	Val	Ala	Ala	Ala	Val
18	Ala	Ala	Ala	Ala	Ala	Ala
19	Ala		Gly	Gly	x	Ala
20	Leu		Leu	Leu	Leu	Leu

REFERENCES

1. Ogita,K., Kusunose,E., Ichihara,K., and Kusunose,M. (1983) Biochem.Int., 6:191–198.
2. Yamamoto,S., Kusunose,E., Ogita,K.,Kaku,M., Ichihara,K., and Kusunose,M. (1984) J.Biochem., 96:593–603.
3. Kaku,M., Ichihara,K., Kusunose,E., Ogita,K., Yamamoto,S., Yano,I., and Kusunose,M. (1984) J.Biochem., 96:1883–1891.
4. Kaku,M., Kusunose,E., Yamamoto,S., Ichihara,K., and Kusunose, M. (1985) J.Biochem., 97:663–670.
5. Yamamoto,S., Kusunose,E., Matsubara,S., Ichihara,K., and Kusunose,M. (1986) J.Biochem., 100:175–181.
6. Yamamoto,S., Kusunose,E., Kaku,M., Ichihara,K., and Kusunose, M. (1986) J.Biochem., 100,1449–1455.
7. Matsubara,S., Yamamoto,S., Sogawa,K., Yokotani,N., Fujii-Kuriyama,Y., Haniu,M., Shively,J.E., Gotoh,O., Kusunose,E., and Kusunose,M. (1987) J.Biol.Chem., 262:13366–13371.
8. Williams,D.E., Hale,S.E., Okita,R.T., and Masters,B.S.S. (1984) J.Biol.Chem., 259:14600–14608.
9. Hardwick,J.P., Song,B.J., Huberman,E., and Gonzalez,F.J. (1987) J.Biol.Chem., 262:801–810.

Advances in Prostaglandin, Thromboxane, and Leukotriene Research, Vol. 19, edited by
B. Samuelsson, P. Y.-K. Wong, and F. F. Sun,
Raven Press, Ltd., New York ©1989.

CHARACTERIZATION OF HUMAN LIVER AND KIDNEY CYTOCHROME P-450-

DEPENDENT ARACHIDONIC ACID EPOXYGENASE

N.G. Abraham, K. Davis, and M.L. Schwartzman

New York Medical College, Valhalla, New York USA 10595

A novel human liver cytochrome P-450 (P-450) epoxygenase which catalyzes Arachidonic Acid (AA) epoxidation, has been purified to homogeneity. The NH_2-terminal sequence of 20-amino acid residues was compared to other known P-450 isozymes. The P-450-AA oxidized AA in a reconstituted system into the four regioisomeric epoxyeicosatrienoic acids (EETs) 5,6-, 8,9-, 11,12-, 14,15-EETs. We raised antibodies against P-450 epoxygenase used to characterize human kidney microsomes. We screened cortex microsomes from 6 post-mortem subjects for their ability to metabolize AA by P-450. Addition of anti-P-450-AA epoxygenase IgG inhibited formation of 11,12-EET without significant effect on $\omega/\omega-1$ hydroxylase products 19- and 20-HETEs. Interindividual variations were observed in the P-450-dependent AA metabolism and the activities ranged between 0.031 to 5.027 nmol AA converted/mg protein/30 min which is about a 150-fold difference. We conclude that the biologically active EETs and 19-,20-HETE are formed within the kidney. The P-450-AA metabolism may play a significant role in the susceptibility of certain individuals to develop clinical disorders such as essential hypertension.

INTRODUCTION

P-450 refers to a family of membrane-bound hemoproteins that oxidize a wide variety of structurally unrelated compounds. The substrates being transformed by P-450 range from endogenous substrates, such as fatty acids and steroids, to exogenous substrates such as drugs, hydrocarbons, and chemical carcinogens (3). Several isozymes of rat liver microsomal P-450 have been purified and characterized in addition to rabbit and mouse liver isozymes (8,9,11,14). Recently, several laboratories have verified the hypothesis that multiple forms of P-450 also exist in human tissues. Wang et al. (15) demonstrated the purification of eight isozymes from human liver, six of them fully characterized by substrate specificity, spectral changes, physical properties, and immunoreactivity to antibodies raised against known forms of

P-450 from rabbit, rat, and mouse (15,19,20). P-450-dependent monooxygenases have been demonstrated as vehicles to generate biologically active compounds from AA. The hepatic and renal P-450 systems from rabbits and rats have been shown to metabolize AA to monohydroxyeicosatetraenoic acids, ω- and ω-1-oxidation products and four regioisomeric EETs[1] which undergo hydrolysis by epoxide hydrolase to form the corresponding diol metabolites, DHTs (24,25). The EETs have been shown to stimulate secretion of hormones and to inhibit chloride transport in renal tubules (26).

Using immunochemical techniques, we were able to demonstrate involvement of human liver and kidney P-450-AA metabolism to biologically active metabolites.

RESULTS AND DISCUSSION

A summary of the purification of P-450-AA from human liver microsomes, which has been described (12), is shown in Table 1. These procedures are a modification of Wang et al. (15) and involve five purification steps. Solubilized human liver microsomes were applied to an octyl-Sepharose-CL-4B column. The elution profile was monitored by absorbance at 417 nm, and under these conditions the contaminating hemoproteins were separated with the first 1500 ml of elution buffer. A summary of the three other purification steps is seen in Table 1.

TABLE 1. Purification Of P-450-AA Epoxygenase From Human Liver

Step	Preparation	Volume	Total protein	P-450 content	Yield[a]
		ml	mg	nmol/mg protein	%
1	Microsomes	137	4076	0.33	100
2	Octyl Sepharose	134	473	1.37	48
3	Hydroxylapatite	50	23.50	7.45	13
4	Sephadex LH-20	10	12.30	8.29	7.5
5	Hydroxylapatite	5	1.00	10.72	0.8

[a]Calculated on the basis of all forms of P-450 present in the microsomes, except for step 5 which accounts only for P-450-AA.

The resulting purified protein appears to be a homogenous protein (12), with a molecular weight of about 53,100.

The NH_2-terminal sequence of 20-amino acid residues of P-450-AA is as follows:

1	2	3	4	5	6	7	8	9	10
ala	leu	pro	leu	val	phe	leu	val	leu	gly

11	12	13	14	15	16	17	18	19	20
phe	ile	ala	ala	val	leu	lys	leu	tryp	phe

Metabolites of AA formed by P-450-dependent enzyme(s) were defined as those metabolites whose formation was absolutely dependent on NADPH addition, and inhibited by IgG of P-450 (c) reductase, SKF-525A, an inhibitor of P-450-dependent enzymes via a type-I binding mechanism, and unaffected by indomethacin. AA was converted into P-450-derived metabolites by all the renal microsomal preparations. HPLC separation of AA metabolites formed by human cortical microsomes in the presence of NADPH is seen in Figure 1. Three major radioactive peaks were separated.

The GC/MS analysis of the P-450-dependent AA metabolites revealed at least two types of oxidation pathways represented by two or more isozymes epoxygenase activity which is represented by the formation of 11,12-EET (peak III) and its hydrolytic metabolites 11,12-DHT (peak I) and $\omega/\omega-1$ hydroxylase(s) which are represented by the formation of 19-HETE and 20-HETE (peak II).

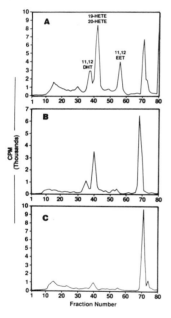

Fig. 1. Antihuman liver P-450-AA epoxygenase IgG (Fig. 1B) inhibits the formation of peaks I and III in the presence of NADPH (Fig. 1A). These metabolites were not formed in the absence of NADPH (Fig. 1C).

Antibodies raised against human P-450-AA epoxygenase (12) were used to distinguish between the activities of both epoxygenase and $\omega/\omega-1$ hydroxylase. As seen in Figure 1, antihuman liver P-450-AA epoxygenase IgG (Figure 1b) markedly inhibits the formation of peaks I and III in the presence of NADPH (Figure 1a). These metabolites were not formed in the absence of NADPH (Figure 1c). We examined several human kidney P-450 in AA metabolism. In six cortical P-450, a large variation existed between subjects: in both P-450(s), epoxygenase and $\omega/\omega-1$ hydroxylase. The range of activity of P-450-AA epoxygenase varied from 0.058 to 5.027 nmole/mg/30 min, which is about a 100-fold difference.

Although we observed identical qualitative patterns of AA metabolites by human cortical P-450, there were large quantitative differences in AA metabolites. Thus, there are individuals in which the relative concentration of AA metabolizing enzymes is higher than in others by a factor of 100.

Previous work has shown that epoxides derived from epoxygenase activity are potent secretagogues, vasodilators, and inhibit chloride transport in isolated collecting tubules (13,14,15,16) and recently it was found that $\omega/\omega-1$ hydroxylase product, 19(s) HETE, is a stimulator of renal $Na^+K^+ATPase$ (17). We demonstrated that in SHR, formation of 19-HETE is 5-10-fold higher than in normotensive rats (unpublished data). In the present report, we demonstrated that human kidney metabolized AA by two types of oxidation, epoxygenase and $\omega/\omega-1$ hydroxylases. We also reported that there are low and high metabolizers of AA to the epoxides and $\omega/\omega-1$ hydroxylated compounds.
HETE, is a stimulator of renal $Na^+K^+ATPase$ (17). We demonstrated that in SHR, formation of 19-HETE is 5-10-fold higher than in normotensive rats (unpublished data). In the present report, we demonstrated that human kidney metabolized AA by two types of oxidation, epoxygenase and $\omega/\omega-1$ hydroxylases. We also reported that there are low and high metabolizers of AA to the epoxides and $\omega/\omega-1$ hydroxylated compounds. It remains to be established whether a relationship exists between a pathological state such as hypertension and the activity of the hydroxylases and/or epoxygenase, as both metabolize AA to a product that may play an important role in the pathogenesis of hypertension. A large number of individuals grouped for age and sex as well as for normal and hypertensive have to be screened before an association between these isozymes activities and hypertension can be established.

REFERENCES

1. Conney AH. Cancer Res 1982;42:4875-4917.
2. Thomas PE, et al. J Biol Chem 1981;256:1044-1052.
3. Guengerich FP, et al. Biochemistry 1982;21:6019-6030.
4. Koop DR, et al. J Biol Chem 1981;256:10704-10711.
5. Wang PP, et al. Biochemistry 1983;22:5375-5383.
6. Distlerath LM, et al. J Biol Chem 1985;260:9057-9067.
7. Jaiswal AK, et al. Science 1985;228:80-83.
8. Oliw EH, et al. J Biol Chem 1982;257:3771-3781.
9. Capdevila J., et al. Proc Natl Acad Sci USA 1982;79:767-770.
10. Falck JR, et al. Biochem Biophys Res Commun 1983;114:743-749.
11. Schwartzman ML, et al. In:Samuelsson B, et al. eds. Advances in Prostaglandin, Thromboxane and Leukotriene Research, vol. 17. New York: Raven Press, 1987;78-83.
12. Schwartzman ML, et al. J Biol Chem 1988;263:2536-2542.
13. Schwartzman ML, et al. Biochem J 1986;238:283-290.
14. Carroll MA, et al. Eur J Pharmacol 1987;138:218-283.
15. Schwartzman ML, et al. Proc Natl Acad Sci USA 1987;84:8125-8129.
16. Capdevila J., et al. Endocrinology 1983;113:421-423.
17. Escalante B., Falck JR., et al. Bioch. Biophys. Res. Commun. 1988 (in press).

Advances in Prostaglandin, Thromboxane, and Leukotriene Research, Vol. 19, edited by B. Samuelsson, P. Y.-K. Wong, and F. F. Sun, Raven Press, Ltd., New York ©1989.

CORNEAL ARACHIDONATE METABOLISM VIA CYTOCHROME P450:

CHARACTERIZATION OF TWO NOVEL BIOLOGICALLY ACTIVE METABOLITES

Jaime L. Masferrer, Robert C. Murphy*, Nader G. Abraham and Michal Laniado-Schwartzman

Departments of Pharmacology and Medicine
New York Medical College, Valhalla, NY 10595 and
*Department of Pharmacology
University of Colorado, Denver, CO 80262

In addition to cyclooxygenase and lipoxygenase enzymes, arachidonic acid (AA) can be metabolized by cytochrome P450-dependent monooxygenases. Metabolism of AA via the cytochrome P450 enzymes includes I) formation of epoxyeicosatrienoic acids (5,6; 8,9; 11,12; 14,15 EETs) which can be enzymatically hydrolyzed by epoxide hydrolase to the corresponding diols (DHTs); II) oxidation that leads to the formation of monohydroxyeicosatetraenoic acids (HETEs); III) ω and $\omega-1$ hydroxylation to form the 20- and 19-HETEs (1,2). The initial description of biological activities of the P450-dependent AA metabolites arising from cytochrome P450 monooxygenases revealed similarities to prostanoids, i.e., they can act as secretagogues and local modulators of circulating hormones, and their activity is usually circumscribed to the microenvironment of the cell origin (3,4,5).

Human and bovine corneal epithelia possess an active cytochrome P450 system that specifically metabolizes arachidonic acid to novel oxygenated products separated by HPLC into four main compounds, A, B, C, D (6,7). The formation of these metabolites was NADPH-dependent, unaffected by indomethacin and inhibited by carbon monoxide and SKF-525A.

The structure of Compound C and D have been identified, and some of their biological activities characterized.

Compound C

We previously demonstrated that epithelial cells of the TALH segment generate a cytochrome P450-dependent AA metabolite that inhibits Na^+-K^+-ATPase (8). As the corneal epithelium possesses similar transport properties to those of the TALH, AA metabolites of the cytochrome P450 in this tissue may have an important role in the modulation of ion transport mechanisms that rely on the pump function. Therefore, the Na^+-K^+-ATPase activity of membrane fractions from the corneal epithelium was determined in the presence and absence of the corneal AA metabolites using ouabain as the reference standard. We found that only metabolite C inhibited Na^+-K^+-ATPase activity with a potency of 1000-fold greater than ouabain. The UV absorbance at 237 nm and the gas chromatography/mass spectrometric (GC/MS) analysis of compound C were indicative of a 12-hydroxy-5,8,10,14-eicosatetraenoic acid, 12-HETE structure (9). We further compared the effect of compound C on Na^+-K^+-ATPase activity to those of the chemically synthetized enantiomers 12(R)-HETE and 12(S)-HETE. As seen in Fig. 1, 12(R)-HETE was the only stereoisomer that inhibited Na^+-K^+-ATPase to the same degree as the purified compound C. The isomer, 12(S) HETE, formed by platelets, had no significant effect on Na^+-K^+-ATPase activity. We therefore concluded that the structure of compound C is 12(R)-HETE.

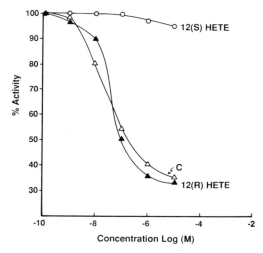

FIG. 1.   Effect of compound C 12(R) HETE and 12(S) HETE on the partially purified Na-K-ATPase from bovine corneal epithelium.

Compound D

The other biologically active metabolite of AA, compound D, showed no UV absorbance. Purification of this metabolite and further GC/MS analysis led us to the conclusion that compound D had the structure of 12-hydroxy-5,8,14-eicosatetrienoic. This compound has the ability to affect vascular resistance as tested in the isolated-perfused-rat-tail artery preconstricted with phenylephrine. In this preparation, compound D dose-dependently relaxes the tail-artery with an estimated EC_{50} of 1.5 µM. Acetylcholine and the 5,6 epoxide (a cytochrome P450 metabolite of AA) showed similar potency in this preparation with an estimated EC_{50}-5.2 µM (10). These results demonstrate that compound D

purified by HPLC is a vasodilator being 3-4-fold more potent
than acetylcholine on a molar basis.

Ocular effects of compound D, namely vasodilation, and effects
on permeability were examined in New Zealand albino rabbits, and
we found that topical application of a single drop (5 ng in 25μl)
on the conjunctiva over the superior rectus muscle resulted in a
prompt and sustained vasodilatation of the underlying anterior
ciliary blood vessels as seen in Fig. 2B. A single drop of 25 μl
of the buffer applied in a given manner failed to produce any
change in vessel caliber (Figure 2A).

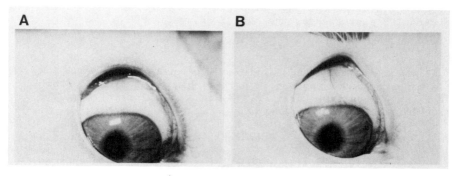

FIG. 2. Effect of topically applied compound D on the conjunc-
tival blood vessels of the rabbit eye.
   A) vehicle control, B) 5 ng of compound D in potassium buffered saline, pH 7.4

Protein content in the rabbit aqueous humor is normally low
and ranges between 30 and 70 mg %, indicating an intact blood
aqueous barrier. Exposure to compounds which compromise the integrity of the blood aqueous barrier results in an increase in
protein content of the aqueous humor. We tested the effects of
compound D on the blood aqueous barrier by injecting various concentrations of the compound through the cornea into the anterior
chamber and, after 15 min, removing 10 μl of aqueous humor for
measurement of protein concentration. Table I shows that injections of compound D into the anterior chamber produced a dose-
dependent increase in the amount of protein present in the aqueous humor without any detectable change in pupillary diameter.

The vasodilator and increased-permeability-producing properties of compound D indicate that it is a proinflammatory agent.
Vasodilation and breakdown of the blood-aqueous barrier are well-
known consequences of ocular diseases and injury. We hypothesize
that injury to the corneal epithelium stimulates the production
of compound D, resulting in the appearance of the classic signs
of acute inflammation.

TABLE 1. Effect of Intracameral Injections of Compound D on
Aqueous Humor Protein Levels

Intracameral Compound D (ng)	Aqueous Humor Protein (mg %) [a,b]
None	30 ± 5
1	40 ± 4
5	210 ± 24
10	1040 ± 310

[a]Samples of aqueous humor for protein determinations were removed 15 min after the injection.
[b]Results expressed as the mean ± SE, n=3.

ACKNOWLEDGMENTS

We thank Pam Blank and Sallie McGiff for typing and editing this manuscript. Supported in part by NIH grant EYO6513 from the National Eye Institute. M.L.S. is a recipient of Irma T. Hirschl Career Scientist Award.

REFERENCES

1. Capdevila J, Marnett LJ, Chacos N, Prough RA, Estabrook RW. Proc Natl Acad Sci USA 1982;79:767-770.

2. Oliw EH, Lawson JA, Brash AR, Oates RA. J Biol Chem 1981; 256:9924-9931.

3. Capdevila J, Chacos N, Falck JR, Manna S, Negro Villar A, Geela SR. Endocrinology 1983;113:421-423.

4. Snyder GD, Capdevila J, Chacos N, Manna S, Falck JR. Proc Natl Acad Sci USA 1983;80:3504-3507.

5. Fitzpatrick FA, Ennis MD, Bazi ME, Wynalda MA, McGee JE, Liggett WF. J Biol Chem 1986;261:15334-15338.

6. Schwartzman ML, Abraham NG, Masferrer J, Dunn MW, McGiff JC. Biochem Biophys Res Commun 1985;132:343-351.

7. Schwartzman ML, Abraham NG, Masferrer J, Dunn MW. Invest Ophthalmol Vis Sci 1987;Suppl 28(3):328.

8. Schwartzman ML, Ferreri NA, Carroll MA, Songu-Mize S, McGiff JC. Nature 1985;314:620-624.

9. Schwartzman ML, Balazy M, Masferrer J, Abraham NG, McGiff JC, Murphy RC. Proc Natl Acad Sci USA 1987;84:8121-8125.

10. Carroll MA, Schwartzman ML, Capdevila J, Falck JR and McGiff JC. Eur J Pharmacol 1987;138:281-283.

Advances in Prostaglandin, Thromboxane, and Leukotriene Research, Vol. 19, edited by
B. Samuelsson, P. Y.-K. Wong, and F. F. Sun,
Raven Press, Ltd., New York ©1989.

PAF-ACETHER (PLATELET-ACTIVATING FACTOR)

J. Benveniste

INSERM U.200, Université Paris-Sud, 92140 Clamart, France

DEFINITION AND CHARACTERIZATION OF PAF-ACETHER

Paf-acether is the first and only example of a phospholipid being a cell-to-cell mediator. When its release from immuno-globulin E-sensitized rabbit basophils was demonstrated in 1972, it was named platelet-activating factor (PAF) (1). Its human origin (2), its effect on human platelets, some physicochemical characteristics (2) and its glycero-phosphocholine backbone (3) were unveiled thereafter. Its structure was fully elucidated as being 1-O-alkyl-2-acetyl-sn-glycero-3-phosphocholine (4-6), hence the modern and structurally relevant paf-acether (paf) (Fig. 1). Stringent criteria distinguish it from other agonists : a) platelet activation in the presence of aspirin and ADP scavengers, b) elution pattern identical to synthetic paf from direct and reverse phase high pressure liquid chromato-graphy (HPLC) or gas chromatography with electron capture detection, c) inactivation by phospholipases (PL) A_2, C and D but not by Rhizopus arrhizus lipase (3), d) inhibition by specific paf antagonists and e) mass spectrometry.

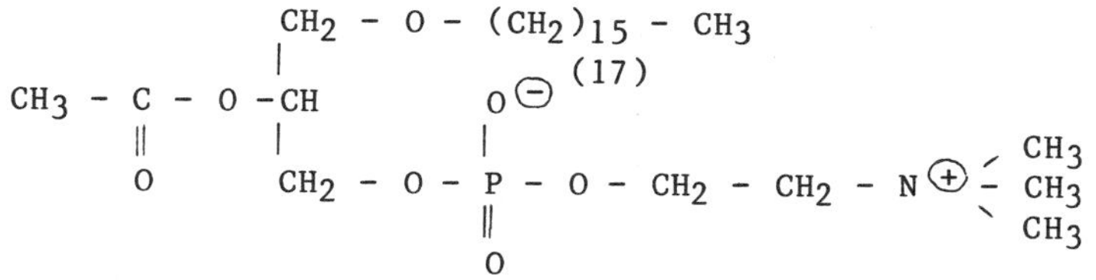

$$CH_3 - \overset{\overset{\textstyle O}{\|}}{C} - O - \overset{\overset{\textstyle CH_2 - O - (CH_2)_{15} - CH_3}{|}}{\underset{\underset{\textstyle CH_2 - O - \overset{\overset{\textstyle O^{\ominus}\ (17)}{}}{\underset{\underset{\textstyle O}{\|}}{P}} - O - CH_2 - CH_2 - N^{\oplus} \overset{CH_3}{\underset{CH_3}{\overset{-}{\smile}}} CH_3}{|}}{CH}}$$

Figure 1. Structure of paf-acether.

Recently some controversy arised on the molecular heterogen-eity of paf. Reverse phase HPLC and gas chromatography revealed that in most cells about 80 % of paf is composed of the C_{16} alkyl chain vs nearly 20 % of the C_{18} moiety. Other bizarre chain-lengths exist, not reaching 5 % of the activity. Some authors go as far as calling "paf" any phospholipid that, whatever the dose, activates platelets, including the 1-acyl analog and even those with other head groups than choline. In fact, paf is a well-defined molecule and the active near isomers differ only by 2 carbons at the first chain level.

ORIGIN, METABOLISM, EFFECTS AND PATHOLOGY OF PAF (Rev. in 7, 8)

This rather ubiquitous molecule originates from many organs and cells. Paf is formed and released by circulating basophils (1), murine macrophages and cultured but not peritoneal mast cells (9, 10), platelets, alveolar macrophages, blood monocytes, and, in high amount, neutrophils and eosinophils but not lymphocytes (11, 12). It was recently recovered from skin fibroblasts (submitted). One of the most remarkable source is the IL 1- and thrombin-stimulated endothelial cell. Paf might thus control neutrophil diapedesis (13, 14). High amounts of preformed paf and lyso paf (see below) are carried piggy-back on blood lipoproteins (15). Finally we found it in E. coli and other bacteria, a result of pathophysiologic (in bacterial infections) and phylogenic significance (16). It was recently proposed that in most cells paf is formed but not released. In fact, between 50 and 100 % of the formed paf is released (10, 11). Cell association of paf mainly results from technical artifacts of cell preparation and stimulation (17).

From 1-alkyl-2-acyl-sn-glycero-phosphocholine, an analog of phosphatidylcholine present in most cell membranes, PLA_2 activity yields 1-alkyl-2-lyso-glycero-phosphocholine (lyso paf) thus freeing both the paf precursor and fatty acids, among them arachidonic acid. Therefore interaction of one phospholipid with one enzyme results in the simultaneous triggering of the two main pathways generating inflammatory mediators. Lyso paf, in turn, is acetylated into paf by an acetyltransferase. The inactivation of paf depends on acetylhydrolase and acyltransferase activities. Paf can also be formed by enzymatic linkage of phosphocholine to 1-alkyl-acetyl-glycerol. Finally, paf might be released in large amount upon breakdown of plasma or cell lipoproteins (15).

Paf is a potent cell agonist active on many other cells than the original platelets. Among the most potent effect is neutrophil activation (chemotaxis, chemokinesis, degranulation). Paf attracts eosinophils in vitro as opposed to ECF-A and LTB_4 (18). Our early studies showed that paf increased vascular permeability. This was repeatedly documented since and in this function paf is again one of the most potent compound. Its hypotensive effect is observed in various species and it also triggers in vivo and in vitro a profound cardiac negative inotropic effect, decrease of coronary flow and arrhythmias. It was recently shown to act on the immune system. In our hands, paf modulated the expression of functionally crucial T cell antigens. It decreased

CD2 and CD3 antigen expression on human T cells, and markedly inhibited T cell proliferation to anti-CD3 or to the combination of anti-CD2 mAbs (19, 20). Paf also modulates c-fos and c-myc gene in human monocytes, indicating for the first time initiation of differentiation signals at the genetic level (21). Associated with a second signal such as bacterial endotoxin, paf markedly increased human monocyte IL 1 activity (submitted). All these effects are : 1) independent from cyclooxygenase activity, 2) occasionally linked to lipoxygenase-dependent arachidonate metabolites, 3) mediated via specific receptors, 4) inhibited by the newly developed paf receptor antagonists.

Paf has been implicated in many (too many ?) pathological effects, from inflammation to graft rejection, kidney immune disease, cardiac anaphylaxis, diabetes and parasitic diseases. A firm basis exists for its role in septic shock (22, 23) and gastro-intestinal damage (24, 25). Better than any other agonist, paf is able to mimick asthma : immediate bronchocons-triction, mucus generation, influx of eosinophils in the lung (26), and a striking non-specific bronchial hyperreactivity observed in man up to 2-3 weeks after one aerosol of paf (27). Yet, whatever remarkable these features are, one must not confuse coincidence and causality. In the past, histamine, prostaglandins, leukotrienes and many other substances have been suspected of being the culprit of e.g. asthma attacks. Only the clinical use of specific antagonists will allow to delineate the pathological role of paf. First encouraging answers are available but not yet definitive evidence.

REFERENCES

1. Benveniste J, Henson PM, Cochrane CG. J exp Med 1972;136: 1356-1377.

2. Benveniste J. Nature 1974;249:481-583.

3. Benveniste J, Le Couedic JP, Polonsky J et al. Nature 1977; 269:170-171.

4. Blank ML, Snyder F, Byers LW, et al. Biochem Biophys Res Commun 1979;90:1194-1200.

5. Demopoulos CA, Pinckard RN, Hanahan DJ. J Biol Chem 1979; 254: 9355-9359.

6. Benveniste J, Tencé M, Varenne P., et al. C R Acad Sc Paris 1979;289D:1037-1040.

7. Snyder F. Platelet-Activating Factor and Related Lipid Mediators, New York: Plenum Press, 1987.

8. Roubin R, Tencé M, Mencia-Huerta JM, et al. In: Pick E, ed. Lymphokines, vol 8. New York: Academic Press, 1983;249-276.

9. Mencia-Huerta JM, Benveniste J. Eur J Immunol 1979;9:409-415

10. Mencia-Huerta JM, Lewis RA, Razin E, et al. J Immunol 1983; 130:2958-2964.

11. Jouvin-Marche E, Ninio E, Beaurain G, et al. J Immunol 1984; 133:892-898.

12. Lotner GZ, Lynch JM, Betz SJ, et al. J Immunol 1980;124:676-684.

13. Camussi G, Aglietta M, Malavasi F. J Immunol 1983;131:2397-2403.

14. Zimmerman GA, MacIntyre TM, Prescott SM. J clin Invest 1985; 76:2235-2246.

15. Benveniste J, Nunez D, Duriez P, et al. FEBS Lett 1988;226:371-376.

16. Thomas Y, Denizot Y, Dassa E, et al. C R Acad Sc Paris 1986; 303(série III):699-702.

17. Benveniste J, Leyravaud S. J Immunol (letter to the editor) 1988;140:1711.

18. Wardlaw AJ, Moqbel R., Cromwell O, et al. J clin Invest 1986;78:1701-1706.

19. Dulioust A, Vivier E, Salem P, et al. J Immunol 1988;40:240-245.

20. Vivier E, Salem P, Dulioust A, et al. Eur J Immunol 1988;18:425-430.

21. Ho Y, Lee WMF, Snyderman R. J exp Med 1987;165:1524-1538.

22. Inarrea P, Gomez-Cambronero J, Pascual J, et al. Immunopharmacology 1985;9:45-52.

23. Terashita Z, Imura Y, Nishikawa K, et al. Eur J Pharmacol 1985;109:257-261.

24. Hsueh W, Gonzalez Crussi F, Arroyave JL. Am J Pathol 1986; 122:231-239.

25. Rosam AC, Wallace JL, Whittle BJ. Nature 1986;319:54-56.

26. Arnoux BA, Page CP, Denjean A, et al. Am Rev resp Dis 1988; 137:855-860.

27. Cuss FM, Dixon CMS, Barnes PJ. Lancet 1986;II:189.

Advances in Prostaglandin, Thromboxane, and
Leukotriene Research, Vol. 19, edited by
B. Samuelsson, P. Y.-K. Wong, and F. F. Sun,
Raven Press, Ltd., New York ©1989.

RECENT DEVELOPMENT OF PLATELET-ACTIVATING FACTOR ANTAGONISTS

T. Y. Shen[1], Isa Hussaini[1], San-Bao Hwang[2] and Michael N. Chang[2]

[1]Department of Chemistry, University of Virginia, Charlottesville, Virginia 22901 USA
[2]Medicinal Chemical Research, Merck Sharp and Dohme Research Laboratories, Rahway, New Jersey 07065 USA

Stimulated by the increasing significance of PAF in many biological systems (1,2), the development of PAF receptor antagonists has rapidly progressed beyond the discovery stage (3) and entered the realm of clinical applications. Following the initial reports on CV-3988 and kadsurenone, a variety of potent, specific and reversible PAF antagonists have been discovered in many laboratories (4). Their biological activities were generally characterized by a series of PAF induced cellular and in vivo responses. Recently, to seek greater therapeutic efficacy, additional considerations, such as pharmacokinetics, pharmacological profile and possible tissue specificity, have received further attention.

In various laboratory models, most of the early PAF antagonists appeared to have relatively short duration of action. In the case of kadsurenone, a detailed metabolic study (5) was carried out with its tritiated derivative, 9,10-[^{3}H]-dihydrokadsurenone, which has the same receptor binding characteristics and in vivo activity (6). Following i.v. administration to rhesus monkeys or incubation with rat liver microsomes, it was rapidly hydroxylated at the C-5 di[^{3}H]propyl side chain, and excreted mainly as glucuronides in the urine. Approximately half of the radiolabelled dose was thus recovered during the first 24 hours. Similar side-chain hydroxylations was observed with kadsurenone. Analogous to the development of synthetic prostaglandin derivatives, replacement of the metabolically labile allyl side-chain in kadsurenone with aryl or other hydrophobic groups might improve its pharmacokinetics.

The potency of several prototypes of PAF antagonists have been improved significantly by further structural modifications. For example, a methylsulfone analog (L-659,989) of the widely used antagonist L-653,731 was found to be ten times more potent (7). L-659,989 has a K_i of 1.1 nM in the rabbit platelet and PMN binding assays, and inhibits

PAF-induced guinea pig bronchoconstriction at 0.5 mg/kg p.o. (8). In accordance with the previously established stereospecificity of this class of lignans, L-659,989, with a trans configuration, is 200 times more active than its cis isomer. The levorotatory enantiomer of L-659,989 is 20-30 times more potent than the dextrorotatory one. This potency ratio is much greater than the 4-fold difference observed with (-) and (+) isomers of the symmetrically substituted L-652,731. Presumably the binding sites for the two substituted aryl groups in L-659,989 differ in steric tolerance and are not interchangeable.

9,10-[^{3}H]-dihydrokadsurenone

L-659,989

L-652,469

L-662,025

Regarding the pharmacological profile of PAF antagonists, in view of the involvement and interplay of multiple mediators in many inflammatory processes, an antagonist with a broader spectrum of action, affecting the function or synthesis of another mediator as well, might have greater efficacy in some clinical disorders. The feasibility of combining PAF antagonism with 5-lipoxygenase inhibitory activity was demonstrated with a lignan derivative, L-651,250 (3,9). Recently, a sesquiterpene isolated from Tussilago farfara L, L-652,469, was found to possess both PAF and calcium channel blocking activities at 1-10 μM (10). Although these activities are ca. 1000-fold weaker than the activity of reference standards, L-652,731 and nitrendipine, respectively, L-652,469 was comparable to L-652,731 in two rat assays, i.e. inhibitions of PAF-induced foot edema and the first phase of carrageenan-induced paw edema. As both PAF and calcium influx are involved in these pathophysiological responses, the dual inhibitory activities of L-652,469 appeared to act synergistically.

In the biochemical characterization of PAF receptor, the presence of high affinity binding proteins for PAF in brain tissues has been demonstrated in gerbil (11) and bovine (Hussaini and Shen, submitted) recently (Figure 1). Progress has also been made in the solubilization and partial purification of the binding proteins in the membrane of human platelets, PMN and bovine brain tissue (Hussaini and Shen, submitted). Specific binding of [³H]-PAF and PAF antagonists to a platelet protein of 65 kD was found (Figure 2). Further purification and characterization of these binding proteins is in progress.

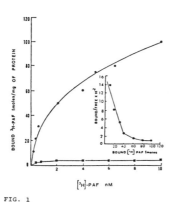

FIG. 1

Specific binding of [³H]-PAF binding to bovine cerebral (● - ●) and cerebellum (■ - ■) membrane preparations. Scatchard plot of [³H]-PAF to bovine cerebral membranes (inset).

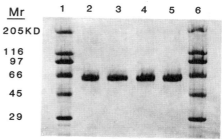

FIG. 2

Identification of a [³H]-PAF binding component in solubilized human platelet and mononuclear cell membranes. Gel-filtered membrane fractions corresponding to peaks of high radioactivity and specific binding were lyophilized and electrophoresed on 12% polyacrylamide gels. Lanes 1 and 6 are standard protein markers, lanes 2 and 3 are mononuclear cell membrane proteins (100μg) and lanes 4 and 5 are platelet membrane fractions (100μg).

As receptor probes, an azido derivative (L-662,025) of the lignan L-652,731 was synthesized and characterized as a photolabile, irreversible PAF antagonist (12). Before irradiation, L-662,025 inhibits the binding of [³H]-PAF to human platelet and PAF-induced aggregation in a competitive and reversible manner at 1-5 uM (Figure 3). Photoactivation of L-662,025 at wavelength >320 nm produced an irreversible inhibition of platelet aggregation and membrane receptor binding of PAF that was not reversed by increasing PAF concentration or washing, respectively (Figure 4). Photolysis of L-662,025 did not affect collagen or ADP-induced human platelet aggregation, thus indicating its specificity for the PAF receptor.

Another irreversible PAF-antagonist, futoxide, was isolated from a batch of haifenteng (Piper futokadsura) from Taiwan (Shen et al., unpublished). Futoxide inhibits the specific binding of [³H]-PAF to human platelet and leukocyte at 0.1 uM. It irreversibly inactivates the receptors in a concentration and time dependent manner. It has no effect on platelet aggregation induced by collagen or ADP. These reversible and irreversible antagonists are being used as molecular probes of the PAF receptor from different tissues.

Futoxide

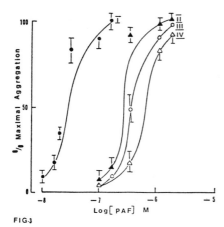

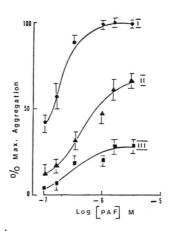

FIG.3

Shows the log dose - % maximal aggregation curves for PAF in the absence (I) and presence of L-662, 025, 6uM (II), 10uM (III) and 20uM (IV) before photoactivation (Control). Vertical bars are mean ± s.e. (n = 3).

FIG.4

Effect of L-662, 025, 6uM (I), 10uM (II) and 20uM (III) on PAF-induced human platelet aggregation after photoactivation (320 - 400nm) for 15 min. The control curve (without L-662, 025) for PAF is the same as shown in figure 3.

Acknowledgments.   This study was supported in part (I.H. and T.Y.S.) by grants from the Virginia Center for Innovative Technology and the Merck & Co. Foundation.

References

1. Benveniste, J. and B. Arnoux, eds., Platelet-Activating Factor and Structurally Related Ether-Lipids.   New York, Elsevier Sci. Pub., 1983.
2. Snyder F, ed. Platelet-Activating Factor and Related Lipid Mediators, New York: Plenum Pub. Corp., 1987.
3. Braquet, P., Touqui, L., Shen, T.Y., and Vargaftig, B.B., Pharmacol. Rev., 1987, 39, 97-145.
4. Shen, T.Y., Hwang, S.-B., Doebber, T.W. and Robbins, J.C., in reference 1, 153-190.
5. Thompson, K.L., Chang, M.N., Chabala, J.C. et al., Drug Metabolism and Disposition (in press).
6. Hwang, S.-B., Lam, M.-H., and Chang, M.N., Biochem. 1986, 261, 13720-13726.
7. U.S. Patent 4,539,332 (September 3, 1985).
8. Lam, M.-H., Hwang, S.-B., Alberts, A.W., Chabala, J.C., Bugianesi, R.L., Dallob, A.L. and Ponpipom, M.M., FASEB J., 1988, 2, A413.
9. Biftu, T., Gamble, N.F., Hwang, S.-B., Chabala, J.C., Doebber, T.W. Dougherty, H.W. and Shen, T.Y., Abstr. of 6th Int. Conf. on Prostaglandins and Related Compounds, June 3-6, 1986, Florence, Italy.
10. Hwang, S.-B., Chang, M.N., Garcia, M.L. et al., Europ. J. Pharmacol., 1987, 141, 269-281.
11. Domingo, M.T., Spinnewyn, B., Chabrier, P.E. and Braquet, P., Biochem. Biophys. Res. Comm., 1988, 151, 730-736.
12. Hussaini, I. and Shen, T.Y., FASEB J., 1988, 2, A411.

*Advances in Prostaglandin, Thromboxane, and
Leukotriene Research*, Vol. 19, edited by
B. Samuelsson, P. Y.-K. Wong, and F. F. Sun,
Raven Press, Ltd., New York ©1989.

TUMOR NECROSIS FACTOR-INDUCED BOWEL NECROSIS: THE ROLE OF PLATELET-ACTIVATING FACTOR.

Wei Hsueh and Xiaoming Sun

Department of Pathology, Children's Memorial Hospital,
Northwestern University Medical School,
Chicago, IL 60614. U.S.A.

In 1983, we reported an experimental model of ischemic bowel necrosis in the rat (1). The lesions were produced by injecting platelet-activating factor (PAF), or a combination of low doses of bacterial endotoxin (LPS) and PAF into the mesenteric vascular bed (1). It has recently been shown that injection of tumor necrosis factor (TNF-α) (2), (also named cachectin (3)), a macrophage product activated by LPS (2,3), also induced shock and necrotic lesion in the gastrointestinal tract (4). The marked similarity of the morphological features of TNF- and PAF-induced bowel necrosis suggested to us that PAF could be a secondary mediator of TNF or vice versa. In the present study, we demonstrated that the necrotizing effect of TNF on the bowel is exerted through mediation by PAF, and that TNF and LPS actuate synergistically to produce bowel lesions.

METHODS

Young male Sprague-Dawley rats (60-80 g) were catheterized via the carotid artery and the jugular vein for continous recording blood pressure and for withdrawing blood samples and injecting drugs. The animals were divided into three main groups to investigate: (a) the effect of varying doses of recombinant TNF-α (Genentech, Inc., South San Francisco, CA) on intestinal injury, (b) the possible synergism of TNF (0.5 mg/kg) and LPS (200 μg/kg, injected 1 hour later), and (c) the effects of a PAF antagonist, SRI 63-119 (5 mg/kg, Sandoz Research Institute, E. Hanover, NJ) on the TNF-induced bowel necrosis. The following parameters were examined:

systemic blood pressure, WBC count, hematocrit (Hct), extent of gross and microscopic intestinal lesions (1), and PAF content of the small intestine. Quantitation of PAF content was done according to our previously published method (5).

RESULTS AND DISCUSSION

TNF alone, at 0.5 mg/kg, did not cause shock or intestinal lesions throughout the experimental period (3 hours). Only mild leukopenia (WBC count: 3920 $\pm$ 540) was observed. Increasing the dose of TNF to 1 mg/kg resulted in hypotension (50.7 $\pm$ 13.8 mmHg), leukopenia (1910 $\pm$ 210) and mild (involvement of tip of villi only) or moderate (involvement of mucosa or submucosa) necrosis of the small intestine in 3 rats at the end of 3 hours. A further increase of the dose to 2 mg/kg resulted in severe shock and death within 2 hours in all 3 animals thus treated (one died within an hour), and examination of the intestine showed only mild necrosis. This is probably because a short survival time did not allow development of advanced lesions.

LPS alone, at the dose used (200 µg/kg), did not cause significant hypotension or intestinal injury. Only mild leukopenia (3070 $\pm$ 260) was observed at the end of the experiment. In contrast, a combination of TNF (0.5 mg/kg) and LPS (200 ug/kg) caused all 5 animals thus treated to develop focal bowel necrosis. The involvement varied from 10 to 60% of the small bowel, and microscopically, most of the animals (4 out of 5 rats) showed moderate degree of necrosis. The intestinal injury was accompanied by severe systemic hypotension (19.8 $\pm$ 5.4 mmHg), and marked leukopenia (1360 $\pm$ 180). As stated above, TNF alone, at 5 mg/kg, showed no effect. These observations indicate a synergism between TNF and LPS in inducing shock and intestinal injury.

To investigate if the TNF-induced bowel necrosis is mediated via PAF production, the PAF content of the small intestine was quantitated. Sham-operated animals produced only 0.08 $\pm$ 0.07 ng PAF/g tissue. Both LPS (200 µg/kg) and TNF (0.5 mg/kg) induced PAF production in the bowel tissue (1.28 $\pm$ 0.45 ng/g and 0.86 $\pm$ 0.31 ng/g respectively). The effects of LPS and TNF are additive: animals receiving a combination of TNF and LPS showed a significantly ($p < 0.05$) higher PAF production in the intestine (2.08 $\pm$ 0.44 ng/g) compared with those receiving LPS or TNF alone. Pretreatment of the animal with PAF antagonist, SRI 63-119, completely prevented the bowel necrosis induced by LPS and TNF (0.5 mg/kg). The hypotensive response was also partially ameliorated (B. P. at the end of 3 hrs: 62 ± 11); so was the leukopenic response (WBC count: 3010 ± 610). SRI 63-119 treatment also prevented the bowel necrosis induced by high dose of TNF (1 mg/kg). Hypotension and leukopenia were also totally or partially recovered. (B.P.: 111 ± 2.3; WBC count: 3850 ± 490).

We have previously shown that injection of LPS and PAF caused shock and ischemic bowel necrosis in the rat (1) and that PAF is the endogenous mediator for shock and bowel necrosis in endotoxemia (5). Since clinically, ischemic bowel necrosis is often associated with shock or infection, it is likely that PAF plays an important role in the pathophysiology of ischemic bowel necrosis. In the present study, we have shown that TNF, another endogenous mediator that causes shock and bowel necrosis (4), exerted its effect via endogenous PAF production, and the effect of TNF and LPS was synergistic.

The production of PAF is not the final answer to the pathogenesis of ischemic bowel necrosis, since the endogenous production of PAF was less than one tenth of that of the effective exogenous dose (7 μg/kg) required to produce bowel lesions. This discrepancy is probably due, at least in part, to a synergism between TNF and PAF. If the rat was pretreated with 0.2 mg/kg of TNF, 1 μg/kg of PAF was sufficient to induce bowel necrosis. We have already reported a synergism between LPS and PAF (1). In the present study we further showed a synergism between LPS and TNF, and between TNF and PAF. The pathogenesis of septic shock and ischemic bowel necrosis is obviously a complicated phenomenon that requires interaction of various mediators. It is possible that in sepsis, LPS activates macrophages to produce TNF, which acts additively with LPS to produce endogenous PAF. The produced PAF acts synergistically with LPS and TNF to cause bowel injury.

ACKNOWLEDGMENTS

This work is partly supported by NIH grant DK34574. We are grateful to Dr. H. M. Shepard at Genentech, Inc. for providing us with the recombinant human tumor necrosis factor-alpha, and to Sandoz Research Institute for giving us SRI 63-119.

REFERENCES

1. Gonzalez-Crussi F, Hsueh W. Am J Pathol 1983; 112:127-135.

2. Carswell EA, Old LJ, Kassel RL, Green S, Fiore N, Williamson B. <u>Proc Natl Acad Sci USA</u> 1975;72: 3666-3670.

3. Beutler B, Cerami A. <u>Nature (London)</u> 1986;320: 584-588.

4. Tracey KJ, Beutler B, Lowry SF, et al. <u>Science (Washington DC)</u> 1986;234:470-474.

5. Hsueh W, Gonzalez-Crussi F, Arroyave JL. <u>FASEB J</u> 1987;1:403-405.

Advances in Prostaglandin, Thromboxane, and Leukotriene Research, Vol. 19, edited by B. Samuelsson, P. Y.-K. Wong, and F. F. Sun, Raven Press, Ltd., New York ©1989.

CHEMISTRY AND PHARMACOLOGY OF PAF ANTAGONISTS. EVALUATION OF CHANGES AT POTENTIAL METABOLISM SITES ON ACTIVITY AND DURATION OF ACTIVITY

D.A. Handley, W.J. Houlihan, J.C. Tomesch, C. Farley
R.W. Deacon, J.M. Koletar, M. Prashad, J.W. Hughes, C. Jaeggi,

**Platelet Biology and Chemistry
SANDOZ RESEARCH INSTITUTE
East Hanover, New Jersey 07936**

Our understanding of the *in vitro* and *in vivo* properties of platelet activating factor (PAF) has been aided and paralleled by the development of PAF receptor antagonists. Antagonists with marked improvements in parenteral (1,2) and oral (3,4) activity have been developed and used to study the involvement of PAF in clinically relevant animal models. A potential limitation of such antagonists is their relatively short duration of biological activity. Although PAF is rapidly metabolized and cleared from the circulation ($t_{\frac{1}{2}}$ = 30-45 sec), it can produce an array of sustained hematological, circulatory, pulmonary and inflammatory effects that far exceed its biological half-life. Since the pathological effects of endogenously released PAF appear to involve its continuous release, the duration of action of PAF antagonists needs to be adequate to contain these PAF-related consequences.

In an effort to increase the *in vivo* duration of pharmacological activity of the PAF receptor antagonist SDZ 63-441 (5), we identified potential sites of metabolism that could account for loss of biological inhibition. We modified SDZ 63-441 [1] by preparing compounds that: block metabolism at the ω-1 site on the long alkyl chain [2,3]; inhibit or retard hydrolysis of the carbamate linkage [4,5]; hydrolysis of the phosphate [6]; or oxidation in the tetrahydrofuran ring [7]. One of these modifications resulted in 5-fold increase in biological duration of activity, when evaluated for inhibition of PAF-induced hemoconcentration (HC) and bronchoconstriction (BC) in the guinea pig. These structural modifications will be discussed in relation to the potential clinical advantages of PAF antagonists with extended duration of activity.

MATERIALS AND METHODS

The PAF-C_{18} used was synthesized according to reported methods (>98% pure). The PAF antagonist 63-441 [1] and compounds 2-7 were prepared at the Sandoz Research Insititute. Structures were confirmed by ^1H, ^{13}C, ^{31}P NMR, FAB (Mass Spectra) and elemental analysis. Compounds and PAF were dissolved in tris-Tyrode's buffer containing 1% BSA.

Guinea pigs (male, 300-350 gm) were anesthesized, tracheotomized, and the femoral artery catheterized for blood sampling. Animals were artificially ventilated and the starting hematocrit measured. At 100 ng kg^{-1} PAF i.v., the increase is 47 ± 7.9% (n=128) for HC and 48.2 ± 9.9% in BC (6). Compounds were given i.a 1 min before the PAF and the % inhibition calculated. The ED_{50} for inhibition (5-7 doses, n=3-6 animals per dose) of PAF-induced HC and BC was done first for compounds (1-7). For duration of activity, compounds were given at dose 1.5-15x their ED_{50} at t=0 hr to animals, which were tested at later times to establish % inhibition to PAF induced responses. The time periods were extended until about 50% inhibition remained. By subtracting the ED_{50} value (mg kg^{-1}) from the loading dose (mg kg^{-1}) and dividing by the time (min), it is possible to obtain a rate of loss of compound (μg kg^{-1} min^{-1}) (7).

RESULTS

The chemical structure of compounds 1-7 are shown in Fig. 1.

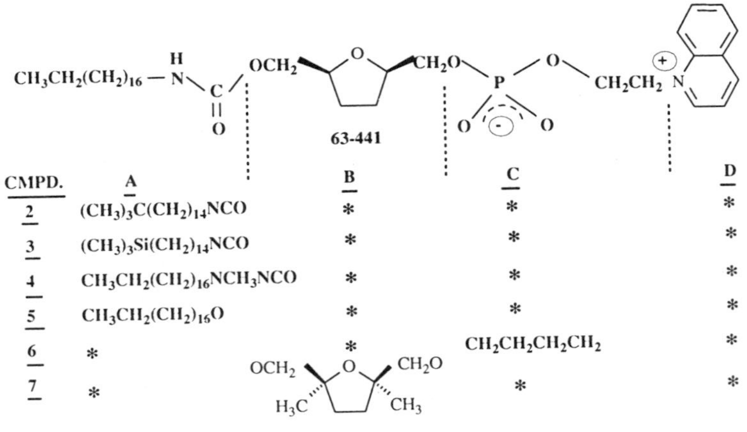
CH3CH2(CH2)16 — N — C(=O) OCH2 CH2O P O O CH2CH2 N
63-441
CMPD. A B C D
2 (CH3)3C(CH2)14NCO * * *
3 (CH3)3Si(CH2)14NCO * * *
4 CH3CH2(CH2)16NCH3NCO * * *
5 CH3CH2(CH2)16O * * *
6 * * CH2CH2CH2CH2 *
7 * OCH2 O CH2O H3C CH3 * *

Fig. 1. Structure and modifications of 63-441 (1). To block the ω-1 oxidation in the C_{18} alkyl chain of 1, two methyl groups were added at the ω-1 position (2) or the CH_2 at the ω-1 in 1 was replaced by a $Si(CH_3)_2$ (3). Inhibition of hydrolysis of the carbamate group was approached by making the N-CH_3 analog (4) and replacing the NHCO group by an ether (5). Hydrolysis of the phosphate group was eliminated by removing the PO_3 group and replacing it by a CH_2CH_2 group (6). Addition of two methyl groups at positions 2 & 5 of the tetrahydrofuran ring (7) blocks metabolism at those sites and may slow it at positions 3 & 4. (* = no modification).

The ED_{50} value and a representative loss of biological activity as a function of time for compound 3 are shown in Figs. 2 & 3.

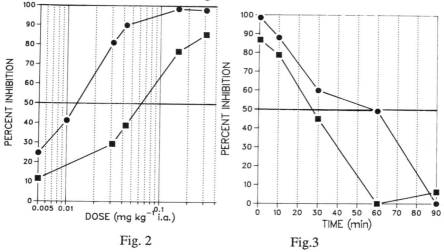

Fig. 2   Fig.3

Fig. 2 Dose-response inhibition by compound 3 of 100 ng kg^{-1} PAF-induced HC (●) and BC (■) in the guinea pig. ED_{50} values are 0.012 and 0.062 mg kg^{-1}, respectively. In Fig. 3 compound 3 was given at 0.156 mg kg^{-1} i.v. About 50% inhibition of HC and BC remains at t = 52 and 28 mins, respectively.

The ED_{50} and rate loss for compounds 1-7 for inhibition of 100 ng kg^{-1} PAF-induced HC and BC are shown on Table 1.

TABLE 1

COMPARATIVE IN VIVO POTENCIES AND DURATION OF
BIOLOGICAL ACTIVITIES FOR TEST COMPOUNDS

CMPD	Dose[a]	$ED_{50}HC$	Rate[b]	$ED_{50}BC$	Rate
1	180	12	10.50	37	16.80
2	339	30	7.14	70	5.83
3	156	12	2.61	62	3.35
4	156	25	8.73	100	5.16
5	143	90	11.41	90	17.66
6	180	40	12.23	50	16.25
7	85	17	7.55	24	9.38

a: all values are in µg kg^{-1}. b: rate= dose-ED_{50}/time for activity to decay to 50% remaining inhibition.

DISCUSSION

We have modified the PAF receptor antagonist SRI 63-441 in an attempt to extend duration of activity while maintaining potency. Clearly, no improvements in duration of activity were obtained by replacing the carbamate with an ether linkage (5) or by replacing of the PO_3 group with an ethylene group (6). There were obvious decreases in potency associated with these changes. Attempts to block metabolism of the tetrahydrofuran ring (7) improved slightly the duration of activity while maintaining similar potency. Blocking ω-1 oxidation in the alkyl chain (2) or inhibiting hydrolysis of the carbamate group (4) only slightly extended duration of activity, although there was a modest loss of potency. Only the substitution of a terminal $Si(CH_3)_3$ group (3) achieved a 4 to 5-fold improvement in duration of activity while maintaining comparable potency.

Improved duration of activity by chemical modification has been approached by other groups. When comparing CV-6209 (2) to a structural predecessor CV-3988 in our guinea pig model, CV-6209 is about 100 fold more potent and 30 fold longer acting (7). These changes in potency and duration of activity can be attributed to the replacement of the phosphorylethyl thiazolium group by a carbamoyl acetamidomethyl pyridinium group. Improvements in these areas allow reduction in the amount of compound needed to inhibit PAF involvement in disease states, afford more continual protection, and reduce potential side-effect problems.

REFERENCES

1.. Handley DA, Van Valen RG, Winslow CM, Tomesch JC, Saunders RN. Thromb Haemost 1987; 57:187-90.

2. Terashita ZI, Imura Y, Takatani M, Tsushima S, Nishikawa K. J Pharmacol Exp Ther 1987; 242:263-68.

3. Handley DA, Van Valen RG, Melden MK, Houlihan WJ, Saunders RN. J Pharmacol Exp Ther 1988; in press.

4. Casals-Stenzel J, Muacevic G, Weber KH. J Pharmacol Exp Ther 1987; 241:974-81.

5. Handley DA, Van Valen RG, Tomesch JC, Melden MK, Jaffe JM, Ballard FH, Saunders RN. Immunopharmacology 1987; 13:125-32.

6. Handley DA, Anderson RC, Saunders RN. Eur J Pharmacol 1987; 141:409-16.

7. Handley DA. Drugs Future 1988; 13:137-52.

Advances in Prostaglandin, Thromboxane, and Leukotriene Research, Vol. 19, edited by B. Samuelsson, P. Y.-K. Wong, and F. F. Sun, Raven Press, Ltd., New York ©1989.

EFFECT OF CHRONIC ADMINISTRATION OF PLATELET-ACTIVATING FACTOR (PAF) IN THE GUINEA-PIG AND THE RAT

Bernadette Pignol, Caroline Touvay, André Pfister*, Jean-Michel Mencia-Huerta and Pierre Braquet

Institut Henri Beaufour Research Labs.
1 avenue des Tropiques, 91952 LES ULIS, France.
*Laboratoire d'Anatomo-Pathologie, Université Paris V,
169 rue de Vaugirard, 75015 PARIS, France.

Asthma is characterized by a non specific increase in airway reactivity to various agonists such as histamine and methacholine. Studies in asthmatic patients have shown that cell infiltration, including mast cells and eosinophils (1), within lung parenchyma is frequently associated with bronchial smooth muscle hyperplasia. The precise mechanisms leading to bronchial hyperreactivity and smooth muscle cell hyperplasia are presently unknown. Over the past 10 years numerous mediators, including PAF, have been incriminated as playing a major role in allergic diseases. Indeed, PAF is released at the time of antigen stimulation of isolated perfused guinea-pig lungs and intravenous injection of this mediator induces a potent bronchoconstriction associated with cell infiltration in lung tissue. Since the discovery of specific and potent PAF antagonists, further evidences strengthened the pivotal role of this mediator in such processes.

PAF is also generated by various cell types including macrophages (2). Besides their classical role in inflammatory reactions, macrophage are also involved in the regulation of the immune response. Recently, works from our laboratory have demonstrated that PAF modulates interleukin 1 (IL1) and interleukin 2 (IL2) production in vitro (3, 4). However, the possibility that PAF could play a role in vivo in the regulation of the immune response was not yet determined.

The aim of the present study was to determine on the one hand the effect of chronically administered PAF on airway reactivity, cell recruitement and lung morphology in the guinea-pig and, on the other hand, IL1 and IL2 production in the rat. The specificity of the effect of the phospholipid mediator was determined using the PAF antagonist, BN 52021.

371

METHODS

IMPLANTATION OF OSMOTIC MINIPUMS

Minipumps (Alzet, London UK) were loaded with defined quantities of PAF in 0.25 % bovine serum albumin (BSA) in saline (saline-BSA) or solvent alone. The minipumps were connected to the jugular vein of Sprague Dawley rats (300 g) or Hartley guinea-pigs (400 g) and placed under the skin of the back.

EXPERIMENTAL PROTOCOL

- The guinea-pigs received over a 15-day period a total amount of 7.2 mg PAF/kg in a final volume of 0.2 ml saline-BSA. As a control group, animals were implanted with minipumps loaded with 0.2 ml saline-BSA. In selected experiments, guinea-pigs were implanted with PAF- containing minipumps and were given 15 mg/kg BN 52021 orally in suspension in arabic gum (0.2 ml/100 g), twice a day for 15 days.

- The rats received over a 7-day period a total amount of 1 µg, 4.5 µg, 9 µg or 28 µg PAF in 10 % ethanol in 0.15 M NaCl. Control rats were implanted with minipumps containing 10 % ethanol solution in 0.15 M NaCl. In selected experiments, rats were implanted with PAF- containing minipumps and were treated intraperitoneally with BN 52021, twice a day at the dose of 5 mg/kg. Treatments with BN 52021 were given for 7 days, starting from the day of minipumps implantation.

ASSESSMENT OF PULMONARY REACTIVITY TO HISTAMINE

At the end of the 15-day period guinea-pigs were artificially ventilated via a tracheal cannula and pulmonary inflation pressure (PIP) was recorded by the mean of differential pressure transducers. Bronchial reactivity was assessed by intravenous injections of increasing doses of histamine (0.2 µg to 100 µg/kg). In selected experiments, PAF- and saline-BSA-treated guined-pigs were killed and the in vitro reactivity of lung parenchymal strips to histamine was assessed as previously described (5).

HISTOLOGICAL TECHNIQUES

Lung fragments from PAF-treated and control animals were fixed in Bouin's solution prior to be processed for inclusion in paraffin. The specimens were cut and stained with 1) Hematein - eosin - safran to study the general aspect of lung tissue, 2) Biedrich's ecarlate stain to detect eosinophils according to the luna technique (6), and 3) toluidine blue to characterize mast cells. The results are expressed as the number of cells per 0.045 μm^2.

ASSESSMENT OF IL1 AND IL2 PRODUCTION FROM RAT SPLENOCYTES

At the end of the 7-day period, rats were killed and the spleens were removed. The mononuclear cells were isolated by centrifugation on Ficoll hypaque cushions. The cell population collected at the interface was composed of approximatively 80 - 90 % lymphocytes and 10 - 20 % monocytes. Monocytes were separated by adherence on plastic petri dishes for 1 hr, the monolayers were removed and counted and then cultured in RPMI 1640 containing 5 % Fetal calf serum (FCS) (7) at a final concentration of 1×10^6 cells/ml. The cells were incubated at 37° C for 24 h in the presence or absence of 20 µg/ml lipopolysaccharide (LPS) and the supernatants were collected. The activity in these supernatants was referred to as the released IL1 activity. One ml of fresh medium was added to the cell pellet and the samples were frozen at - 20° C. After 3 cycles of freezing/thawing, the supernatants were referred to as the cell-associated IL1 activity. All samples were stored at - 70° C prior to measurement of IL1 production. For the assessment of IL2 production, mononuclear cells from Ficoll hypaque cushions were resuspended in RPMI 1640 supplemented with 10 % FCS and IL2 production was initiated or not by the addition of Con A (15 µg/ml). Cultures were incubated at 37° C for 24 h before the cell-free supernatants were harvested and stored at - 70° C prior to measurements of IL2 activity.

IL1 AND IL2 ASSAY

The IL1 content in the samples was assessed using the mouse thymocyte proliferation assay (8). The IL2 activity in the cell-free supernatants from spleen lymphocytes was determined by the proliferation assay using the IL2-dependent murine CTLL cell line (9).

RESULTS

IN VIVO REACTIVITY TO HISTAMINE OF PAF- AND SALINE BSA- TREATED GUINEA-PIGS

Guinea-pigs treated with PAF for two weeks exhibited an increased in bronchopulmonary response to intravenous injections of histamine (Table 1). PAF-infused guinea-pigs treated with BN 52021 demonstrated a response to histamine significantly lower as compared to that of guinea-pigs receiving PAF alone (Table 1).

The doses of histamine inducing an increase in PIP of 100 % were respectively, 5.5 µg/kg in animals receiving BSA; 2.2 µg/kg for those receiving PAF, 4.0 µg/kg for those receiving BSA and treated with BN 52021 and 7.0 µg/kg for those receiving PAF and treated with BN 52021.

Table 1 - Pulmonary reactivity to histamine.

Histamine doses μg/kg IV	Treatment of the guinea-pig			
	none (n = 8)	BN 52021 (n = 8)	PAF (n = 8)	PAF + BN 52021 (n = 8)
0.2	0	0	0	0
0.5	6.1 ± 4.3	6.9 ± 3.2	15.2 ± 5.5	4.3 ± 4.3
1	28.0 ± 6.0	19.6 ± 6.4	40.0 ± 10.1	14.1 ± 9.5
2	68.4 ± 9.0	59.6 ± 14.0	93.0 ± 19.5	35.6 ± 16.4 *
5	137.6 ± 18.6	119.0 ± 26.3	176.6 ± 30.3	85.3 ± 20.9 *
10	165.1 ± 15.7	166.3 ± 29.3	231.8 ± 32.4	121.9 ± 23.1 *
20	200.6 ± 14.6	222.3 ± 40.6	277.8 ± 33.5	154.4 ± 29.5 *
50	266.0 ± 23.1	275.0 ± 41.9	361.7 ± 40.4 a)	215.0 ± 37.5 *
100	254.0 ± 28.1 d)	302.8 ± 54.4	385.8 ± 49.6 b)	245.6 ± 38.7 * c)

a) n = 7   b) n = 6   c) n = 5   d) n = 4

* $p < 0.005$ by comparison to PAF-treated animal.

IN VITRO REACTIVITY TO HISTAMINE OF LUNG PARENCHYMAL STRIPS

The contractile responses to histamine (300 μg) were similar for strips from PAF-infused guinea-pigs treated or not with BN 52021 and control animals (Data not shown).

CELL RECRUITEMENT AND LUNG MORPHOLOGY

In guinea-pigs receiving PAF for 15 days, the numbers of eosinophils infiltrating lung tissue and mast cells in the peribronchial zones were significantly increased by 53 % and 75 %, respectively. After long-term infusion with PAF, lungs from guinea-pigs exhibited a congestive appearance as compared to those from control animals and in most of the cases, a marked hyperthrophy of the Reissessen muscles was noted. Lung alterations and cell infiltration were not observed when the animals receiving PAF were simultaneously treated with BN 52021.

IL1 AND IL2 PRODUCTION IN THE RAT

Monocytes from rats treated 7 days with 9 μg PAF exhibited a 91.2 % increase of LPS-induced IL1 production of (Table 2). However when the rats were administered with 28 μg PAF, a marked and significant decrease in the ex vivo LPS-induced IL1 production was observed (Table 2).

As compared to Con A-stimulated spleen lymphocytes from controls animals, those from rats receiving 1 µg or 4.5 µg PAF exhibited an increased capability to produce IL2 (Table 2).

Table 2 - Effect of in vivo administration of PAF on the IL1 and IL2 production from rat splenocytes.

Treatment of the rats	^{3}H thymidine incorporation (cpm)	
	IL1 production	IL2 production
Vehicle alone	4674 ± 898	1319 ± 174
PAF 1 µg	4716 ± 423	4444 ± 938**
PAF 4.5 µg	7123 ± 1610	3163 ± 1799*
PAF 9 µg	8937 ± 1869*	1987 ± 381
PAF 28 µg	1782 ± 373**	1774 ± 540

** $p < 0.01$; * $p < 0.005$ by comparison to control animals.

Administration of BN 52021 during treatment with 28 µg PAF totally reversed the effect of the mediator on IL1 production. As well, treatment of the PAF-infused rats with BN 52021 markedly reversed by 81 % the effect of 1 µg PAF on the IL2 production.

DISCUSSION

The present data demonstrate that long-term infusion of PAF in the guinea-pig induces an increased bronchopulmonary response to histamine as compared to control animals receiving the vehicle alone. This increased response to histamine is rather characterized by the extent of the response than by a higher sensitivity of the tissue to the agonist. This PAF-induced increase in bronchial hyperresponsiveness is prevented by the specific PAF antagonist, BN 52021. In contrast to what was observed in vivo, the reactivity of lung parenchymal strips to histamine in vitro is not altered in PAF-infused guinea-pigs. This result indicates that the in vivo hyperresponsiveness to histamine is related to complex mechanisms rather than to a higher sensitivity of airway smooth muscle to the agonist. The hypertrophy of bronchial Reissessen muscle, associated with the eosinophil infiltration occuring within 15 days of PAF infusion is similar to the alterations observed in lungs from asthmatic patients. It is thus reasonable to speculate that the bronchopulmonary hyperresponsiveness observed in PAF-treated animals is related to the alterations of lung architecture.

The present data also demonstrated that PAF may play a critical role in the in vivo regulation of IL1 and IL2 production. The opposite effect of PAF on the IL1 production suggests that this mediator may either act on two different monocyte populations or on two receptor classes present on the same or different cell types. PAF also regulates IL2 production, maximal increase being observed with the lowest dose of the autacoid used. From the present experiments, it is not possible to determine whether or not the action of the mediator on monocytes and lymphocytes is direct or indirect. However, the effect of PAF appears to be mediated via specific binding sites since BN 52021 reverses the PAF-induced decrease in IL1 production and the increase in IL2 release. This further supports the concept that PAF is not only a mediator of the acute allergic and inflammatory reactions but also probably contribute to long-term processes such as chronic diseases involving immuno-competent cells.

REFERENCES

1. Frigas E and Gleich GJ. J. Allergy Clin. Immunol. 1986; 77:527-537.
2. Mencia-Huerta JM and Benveniste J. Eur. J. Immunol. 1979; 9:409.
3. Rola-Pleszczynski M, Pignol B, Pouliot C and Braquet P. Biochem. Biophys. Res. Commun. 1987; 142:754.
4. Pignol B, Henane S, Mencia-Huerta JM, Rola- Pleszczynski M and Braquet P. Prostaglandins 1987; 33:931.
5. Touvay C, Vilain B, Carre C, Mencia-Huerta JM and Braquet P. BBRC in presse 1988.
6. Luna LG. Manual of histologic staining methods of the armed forces institut of plathology, 3 rd Ed. New York, MC. Graw-Hill. 1968; 258.
7. Chu E, Rosenwasser LJ, Dinarello CA, Lareau M and Geha RS. J. Immunol. 1984; 132:1311.
8. Mizel SB, Oppenheim JJ and Rosenstreich DL. J. Immunol. 1978; 120:1504.
9. Gillis S, Ferm M, W Ou and Smith KA. J. Immunol. 1978; 120:2027.

Advances in Prostaglandin, Thromboxane, and Leukotriene Research, Vol. 19, edited by
B. Samuelsson, P. Y.-K. Wong, and F. F. Sun,
Raven Press, Ltd., New York ©1989.

PLATELET-ACTIVATING FACTOR IN ORGAN

TRANSPLANT REJECTION

M.L. Foegh*, E. Chambers, B.S. Khirabadi, T. Nakanishi, and
P.W. Ramwell, *Georgetown University Medical Center, Department of Surgery,
Division of Transplantation and Department of Physiology & Biophysics,
Washington, D.C., USA

INTRODUCTION

The involvement of platelet-activating factor (PAF) in cell mediated rejection is a novel discovery. There are number of reasons for such a proposal. Firstly, Camussi and collaborators, (1984) showed an increase of PAF in plasma, in a rabbit model of hyperacute rejection. This type of rejection occurs shortly following perfusion of the transplanted organ and is due to preformed humoral antibodies against the allograft (6). A unique feature of hyperacute rejection is platelet thrombi formation causing cessation of blood flow through the allograft. Thus with the involvement of platelets in this rabbit model it is conceivable that PAF might be released and contribute to hyperacute rejection.

In contrast to hyperacute rejection, cell mediated rejection takes place within the first week following transplantation and is characterized by activation of lymphocytes and their response to foreign antigens of the allograft. The foreign antigens are processed and presented to the lymphocytes by monocytes and macrophages as shown in Figure 1. Platelets are not generally thought to play a major role in cell mediated rejection; however, platelets are deposited in the allograft during rejection and are released into the circulation following infusion of the antiplatelet drug, prostacyclin (8). PAF is released from platelets and macrophages upon stimulation and a lymphocyte cell line has also been shown to release PAF (2). This may not occur with human peripheral blood lymphocytes (7). A characteristic effect of PAF is increased vascular permeability and this is a consistent feature of rejection. In addition PAF stimulates arachidonate metabolism, the products of which are known to modulate immune responses (3) including allograft rejection (4,5).

Platelets and PAF possess many properties which are related to cell mediated transplant rejection. An initial event in lymphocyte proliferation is calcium influx. PAF promotes calcium influx. A further step in lymphocyte activation in addition to antigen presentation as shown in Figure 1 is an increase in interleukin-1 (IL-1) (9). The initiation of lymphocyte proliferation is dependent on IL-1 production, but the continuation of lymphocyte proliferation requires interleukin-2 (IL-2). Initial in vitro experiments showed inhibition of IL-2 by PAF but a recent in vivo study (10), showed that PAF administered in vivo increases (IL-2) formation in spleen cells and thus may promote clonal expansion. The biologically activity of PAF related to transplant rejection is summarized in Table 1.

A major problem in cardiac transplantation is the development of accelerated coronary atherosclerosis. This has become the major cause of graft loss after the first three months following transplantation. Transplant atherosclerosis does not correlate with the known risk factors for atherosclerosis such as cholesterol, HDL-cholesterol, and LDL- cholesterol (1). Furthermore, no correlation has been found between known

TABLE I

EFFECT OF PAF RELATED TO TRANSPLANTATION

PAF
VASCULAR PERMEABILITY ↑
Ca⁺⁺ FLUX ↑
VASODILATION OR CONSTRICTION
IL - 1 ↑
IL - 2 ↑ (*in vivo*) ↓ (in vitro)

TABLE II

EFFECT OF PAF ANTAGONIST ON
RABBIT ASCENDING AORTA

TRANSPLANT ATHEROSCLEROSIS		
	NATIVE %	GRAFT %
CONTROL (N=4)	22.4±10.1	95.2±2.1
BN52021 (N=4)	18.7±2.7	62.9±20.9

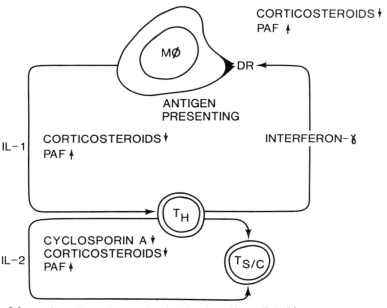

Fig. 1 Macrophage-lymphocyte interaction in cell-mediated immune responses and its modulation by platelet activating factor (PAF), cyclosporin A and corticosteroids.

Mø	=	macrophage
IL-1	=	Interleukin - 1
IL-2	=	Interleukin - 2
TH	=	T-helper lymphocyte
Ts/c	=	T-suppressor/cytotoxic lymphocyte
DR	=	HLA - DR antigen expression

immunological events and the degree of transplant atherosclerosis such as numbers of rejection episodes and degree of cellular infiltrates in myocardial biopsies.

Since PAF may be involved in cell mediated rejection and because of its thrombotic effects and spectrum of hemodynamic properties we chose to explore the putative causal role of this lipid by use of a specific antagonist. We have studied, therefore, the effect of the PAF antagonist, BN 52021 on transplant atherosclerosis. We selected the rabbit heterotopic cardiac transplant model and evaluated the degree of atherosclerosis in the ascending aorta of the graft compared to the native ascending aorta.

METHODS

Dose Evaluation

Preliminary dose-ranging studies were done in rabbits in order to determine the in vivo dose of BN 52021 needed for maximum inhibition of PAF-induced platelet aggregation ex vivo. Two different doses of BN 52021 (20 mg/kg/d and 100 mg/kg/d) were administered intramuscularly for ten days to white New Zealand rabbits. Platelet aggregation was studied prior to treatment and on day five and day ten following treatment with BN 52021 (20 mg/kg/d, i.m.) which was administered twice daily. The platelet aggregation studies showed that a dose of 20 mg/kg/d was as effective as 100 mg/kg/d in inhibiting platelet aggregation induced by PAF. Consequently, the dose of 20 mg/kg/d of BN 52021 was chosen for studying the effect of a PAF antagonist on transplant atherosclerosis. This was, therefore, done in a heterotopic cardiac transplant model using the same strain of rabbit.

The Accelerated Transplant Atherosclerosis Model

Eight white New Zealand male rabbits were divided into two groups. Group 1 (N=4) was the control group and Group 2 (N=4) received BN 52021 (20 mg/kg/d i.m.) in two divided doses. Both the donor and the recipient rabbits were fed a 0.5% cholesterol diet one week prior to transplantation. At the day of transplantation, the recipients received cyclosporin A (10 mg/kg/d i.m.) until sacrifice six weeks later. In addition Group 1 received DMSO the vehicle for BN 52021 while the other group, (Group 2) received BN 52021. The recipients continued their cholesterol diet. After sacrifice, the extent of atherosclerosis in the native and graft ascending aorta was determined. The vessels were stained with oil-o-red and the area of lipid deposition was traced. The lipid deposition was determined as a percentage area of total vessel area. The tracing was done using a computer software developed by Dr. Friedman, Georgetown University Medical Center. The software allows the data from the tracing to be stored directly in an IBM computer where the total areas of lipid deposition are summed. The results express the percentage area of lipid deposition compared to total vessel area.

RESULTS

The PAF-induced aggregation of platelets removed from rabbits treated with BN 52021 was significantly inhibited. No difference was observed between 20 and 100 mg/kg/d. The data are shown in Figure 2. In Figure 3 is shown the effect of the

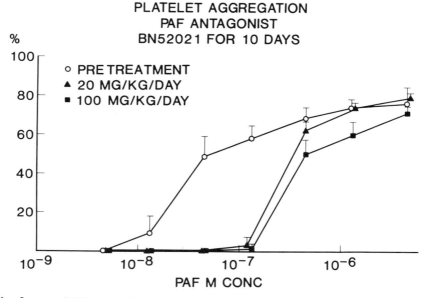

Fig. 2   PAF-induced rabbit platelet aggregation and its inhibition by <u>in vivo</u> treatment with two different doses of a PAF antagonist, BN 52021. Similar inhibition is obtained with 20 and 100 μg/kg of BN 52021.

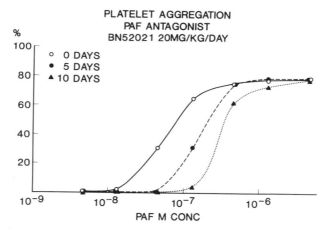

Fig. 3   Increased inhibition of PAF-induced platelet aggregration with duration of <u>in vivo</u> treatment with the PAF antagonist, BN 52021.

duration of treatment with BN 52021 (20 mg/kg/d) on platelet aggregation induced by PAF. The longer the duration of treatment the greater was the dose of PAF required to obtain the same degree of aggregation.

BN 52021 inhibited both native and graft atherosclerosis as determined by lipid deposition. However, this protective effect of BN 52021 did not achieve significance. The area of lipid deposition also underwent severe cell proliferation. Cell proliferation in the graft was more extensive than cell proliferation in the native ascending aorta.

Cyclosporine A (10 mg/kg/d) prevented cell mediated rejection. Some mononuclear cell infiltration was noticed. Two of the hearts in the control group stopped beating due to complete occlusion of the coronary arteries by accelerated atherosclerosis.

DISCUSSION

Inhibition of PAF-induced platelet aggregation was achieved by treatment of rabbits with BN 52021. This confirms a previous study of the same nature with BN 52021. However, it is of interest that the inhibitory effect of BN 52021 increases with duration of treatment so that following ten days a larger dose of PAF is required for platelet aggregation than after five days of treatment. The effect of different doses of BN 52021 on platelet aggregation showed that a dose of 20 mg/kg/d was as effective as 100 mg/kg/d. Thus the subsequent studies on transplant atherosclerosis in the rabbits were carried out with a dose of 20 mg/kg/d of BN 52021.

These data, although not significant indicate decreased lipid deposition and intimal hyperplasia in the graft ascending aorta and the native ascending aorta by BN 52021. The inhibitory effect of BN 52021 on coronary artery atherosclerosis was significant but will be reported in full elsewhere. The mechanism by which the PAF antagonist may exert such an effect is uncertain and needs to be explored. Some of the mechanisms may relate to attenuation of formation of leukorienes and thromboxane by inhibition of PAF-induced release of arachidonate. Other mechanisms may be inhibition by PAF antagonists of PAF-induced chemotaxis. PAF may also be involved in smooth muscle cell proliferation but there is no information of such an effect.

The involvement of PAF in cell mediated rejection and in transplant atherosclerosis was initially suggested from our findings that BN 52021 and other PAF antagonists act synergistically with cyclosporin A in significantly prolonging cardiac allograft survival. Mechanisms of action are unclear, but in vitro and in vivo data support the suggestion that PAF antagonist will inhibit both IL-1 and IL-2 release and thereby attenuate the cell mediated response. In addition, PAF may exert some specific actions related to transplant atherosclerosis.

REFERENCES

1. Billingham, M.E. (1987): Transpl. Proc. 19(4): 19-25.

2. Bussolino, F., Foa, R., Malarasi, F., Ferrando, M.L., and Camussi, G. (1984): Exp. Hematol. 12:988-993.

3. Foegh, M.L., Alijani, M.R., Helfrich, G.B., Khirabadi, B.S., Lin, K., and Ramwell, P.W. (1986): Transpl. Proc. 18 (4): 20-24.

4.   Föegh, M.L., Hartmann, D.P., Rowles, J.R., Khirabadi, B.S., Alijani, M.R., Helfrich, G.B., and Ramwell, P.W. (1987): Adv. Prostaglandins, Thomboxane, Leukotriene Res. 17:140-146.

5.   Foegh, M.L., Khirabadi, B.S., Rowles, J.R., Braquet, P., and Ramwell, P.W.(1986): Transplantation 42:86-88.

6.   Ito, S., Camussi, G., Tetta, C., Milgrown, F., and Andres, G. (1984): Lab. Invest. 51:148-161.

7.   Jouvin-Marche, E., Nimo, E., Beaurain, G., Tencé, M., Niandet, P., and Benveniste, J. (1984): J. Immunol. 133:892-898.

8.   Leithner, C., Sinzinger, H., and Schwartz, M. (1981): Prostaglandins 22:783-788.

9.   Pignol, B., Henane, S., Mencia-Huerta, J.M., Rola-Pleszczynski, M., et al. (1987): Prostaglandins 33:931-939.

10. Pignol,B., Henane,S., Sorlin,B. (1988): In: New trends in lipid mediates research, edited by P. Braquet, pp. 38-43. Karger, Basel.

Advances in Prostaglandin, Thromboxane, and Leukotriene Research, Vol. 19, edited by B. Samuelsson, P. Y.-K. Wong, and F. F. Sun, Raven Press, Ltd., New York ©1989.

RECENT STUDIES ON ICOSANOIDS AND PAF-ACETHER MODULATION

OF SOME CENTRAL NEUROSECRETIONS IN THE RAT

F. Dray, K. Gerozissis, V. Fafeur,
A. Wisner, M.C. Bommelaer-Bayet, M. Saadi, C. Rougeot,
C. Tiberghien and M.P. Junier

INSERM U 207, URIA, Institut Pasteur, 28 Rue du Dr Roux,
75724 Paris Cedex 15, France

The possibility that prostaglandins (PGs) might act within the central nervous system and particularly within neuroendocrine structures has been a subject of great interest for more than 15 years [1]. Whereas the importance in the brain of PGs like PGE_2 and PGD_2 has been emphasized [2-4], new arachidonate metabolites issued from the lipoxygenase [5-9] or epoxydase [10] pathways and the ethero-phospholipid, Platelet-Activating Factor (PAF-acether) have recently focused attention [11-13].

We present here some results of studies that we carried out confirming this aspect.

LUTEINIZING HORMONE-RELEASING HORMONE (LHRH) SECRETION

Several eicosanoids and PAF-acether have been found to alter the in vitro secretion of LHRH from rat median eminence (ME) : PGE_2, 12-and 5-HETEs, leukotrienes (LT) C_4 and D_4 stimulated whereas PAF-acether inhibited LHRH release. The pattern of the effects varied from one compound to another, as observed in the following events.

Profile of dose-response curves

The response to increasing concentrations followed a saturation curve (maximum at 10^{-6} M) for PGE_2 and 12-HETE, a biphasic curve for 5-HETE and LTD_4 (maximum at 10^{-8} M), a bimodal curve for LTC_4 (two maxima at 10^{-16} and 10^{-8} M) and a biphasic curve for PAF-acether (maximum at 10^{-14} M).

Relations with the catecholaminergic systems

Norepinephrine (NE) and dopamine (DA), which are known to stimulate LHRH release, enhanced the synthesis of PGE_2 and

12-HETE but not LTs. However, DA inhibited Ca^{2+} ionophore (A 23187)-induced LTC_4 production and LHRH release. Furthermore, PGE_2 inhibited K^+-evoked $[^3]NE$ release from hypothalamus slices but had no effect on K^+-evoked $[^3H]DA$ release. The other eicosanoids tested (12-HETE and LTs) had no effect. The relations of PAF-acether with NE and DA systems have not yet been studied.

Specific binding to membrane preparations

The presence of specific binding sites was demonstrated in different parts of the brain and particularly in the hypothalamus for PGE_2 and PAF-acether, confirmed for LTC_4, but not observed for 12-HETE or LTD_4.

PGE_2 binding sites

A specific binding of $[^3H]PGE_2$ was demonstrated in synaptosome preparations from hypothalamus. Scatchard plot analysis revealed the existence of two binding site populations, of high (R_H) and low (R_L) affinities. The two states of PGE_2 receptor were interconvertible ; their ratio depended on guanine nucleotides suggesting the coupling of the receptor to a guanine nucleotide-protein N-adenylate cyclase complex. Furthermore, a good correlation existed for PG analogues between their binding capacity and two related pharmacological effects : stimulation of LHRH release and inhibition of $[^3H]NE$ release. The PGE_2 receptor was independent from α_2 pre- and α_1 post-synaptic noradrenoreceptors which mediate the inhibitory effect of NE on $[^3H]NE$ release and its stimulatory effect on LHRH release. All these results suggest that PGE_2 is a synaptic modulator of LHRH secretion.

LTC_4 binding sites

Their presence has already been demonstrated in the rat and guinea pig brain [14]. We confirmed this binding in hypothalamus membranes. However, the analysis of competition binding data revealed a composite profile of several events, excluding any calculation of affinity constant(s) and questioning the notion of LTC_4 hypothalamic receptor(s).

PAF-acether binding sites

We demonstrated the existence of two binding site populations for $[^3H]PAF$-acether, both in whole brain and in hypothalamus : $K_{D1} = 2.14+0.32$ nM, $n_1=25.4\pm3.2$ fmoles/mg protein, $K_{D2} = 61.6\pm16.4$ nM, $n_2 = 146.2\pm47.5$ fmoles/mg protein, respectively. A neuronal distribution of $[^3H]PAF$-acether binding was observed with the greatest number of binding sites found in the telencephalic structures. The absence of displacement of $[^3H]PAF$-acether binding and the absence of effect on LHRH release with lyso-PAF and 1-O-hexadecyl-sn-glycerol prove the specificity of this binding and strengthened the reality of PAF-acether receptor(s) in the hypothalamus.

GRF/SRIF/GH SECRETIONS

The secretion of growth hormone (GH) is under the control of two hypothalamic releasing peptides = GH releasing factor (GRF) and GH releasing inhibitory factor (SRIF). PGE_2 stimulated basal and partially GRF-induced GH secretion. This effect seems to be mediated through specific PGE_2 receptor(s) which have the same binding properties as described with hypothalamus membranes. 12-HETE and LTC_4 had no effect on basal and GRF-induced GH secretion. However, a slight stimulatory effect of 10^{-8} M PAF-acether on basal GH release was observed but no specific binding for $[^3H]$PAF-acether was found in pituitary membranes. Furthermore, GRF was found to stimulate specifically the synthesis of PGE_2 and 12-HETE.

GRF/β ENDORPHINE/ACTH SECRETIONS

PAF-acether increased corticotropin releasing factor (CRF) and β endorphin secretion from rat ME incubated in standard conditions. A saturation curve was obtained with a plateau from 10^{-9} M. These results were in contrast with those obtained with LHRH and SRIF release presented previously. The relation between $[^3H]$PAF-acether binding and stimulation of CRF and β endorphin release has not yet been elucidated.

MELATONIN SECRETION

Melatonin is the main known hormone of the pineal. The daily rhythm of its synthesis is mediated by NE, through α_1 and β adrenoceptors, which operate in a synergistic manner on N-acetyl transferase activity and on melatonin release. A role of arachidonate metabolites in mediating NE-induced melatonin release has been proposed since both cyclooxygenase and lipoxygenase inhibitors have been reported to decrease NE-induced melatonin release. Furthermore, we found that 12- and 15-lipoxygenase activities were predominent in rat pineal compared to different structures in rat brain and that 12-HETE, with its two derivatives hepoxilin A and B and 15-HETE were the major arachidonate metabolites produced by rat pineal incubated for 6 hours in the presence of $[^{14}C]$arachidonate. The addition of 12-hydroperoxyeicosatetraenoic acid (12-HPETE) and 15-HPETE stimulated both N-acetyl transferase activity and melatonin release while 5-HPETE or hydroxyderivatives of these compounds (12-, 15- and 5-HETEs) were ineffective. These results and those recently published [12] describing a stimulatory effect of LTC_4 on melatonin release strengthen the predominance of the lipoxygenase pathway in the regulation of melatonin synthesis and release, and emphasize the involvement of hydroperoxy derivatives in the regulation of secretory processes.

REFERENCES
1. Cardinali OP, Ritta MN. Neuroendocrinology 1983;36:152-160.

2. Ojeda SR, Urbanski HF, Katz KH, Costa ME and Conn PM. Proc. Natl. Acad. Sci. USA 1986;83:4932-4936.

3. Malet C., Scherrer H, Saavedra JM, Dray F. Brain Research 1982;236:227-233.

4. Watanabe Y, Yamashita A, Tokumoto H, Hayaishi O. Proc. Natl. Acad. Sci. USA 1983;80:4542-4545.

5. Hulting AL, Lindgren JA, Hökfelt T, et al. Proc. Natl. Acad. Sci. USA 1985;82:3834-3838.

6. Gerozissis K, Vulliez-Le Normand B, Saavedra JM, Murphy RC, Dray F. Neuroendocrinology 1985;40:272-276.

7. Gerozissis K, Saadi M, Dray F. Brain Research 1987;416:54-58

8. Vacas MI, Keller-Sarmiento MI, Etchegoyen GS, Peyreyra EN, Gimeno MF, Cardinali OP. Neuroendocrinology 1987;46:412-416.

9. Sakai K, Fafeur V, Vulliez-Le Normand B, Dray F. Prostaglandins 1988 (in press)

10. Capdevila J, Chacos N, Falck JR, Manna S, Negro-Vilar A, Ojeda SR. Endocrinology 1983;113:421-423.

11. Bussolino F, gremo F, Tetta C, Perscarmona GP, Camussi G. 6th International Conference on Prostaglandins and Related Compunds, Florence, Italy, 1986:333

12. Spinnewyn B, Blavet N, Clostre F, Bazan N, Braquet P. Prostaglandins 1987;34:337-347.

13. Junier MP, Tiberghien C, Rougeot C, Fafeur V, Dray F. Endocrinology 1988 (in press)

14. Cheng JB, Townley RG. Biochem. Biophys. Res. Commun. 1984;119: 612617.

Advances in Prostaglandin, Thromboxane, and Leukotriene Research, Vol. 19, edited by B. Samuelsson, P. Y.-K. Wong, and F. F. Sun, Raven Press, Ltd., New York ©1989.

SYNTHESIS AND FUNCTIONS OF CYCLOOXYGENASE AND LIPOXYGENASE PRODUCTS IN BRAIN: NEW FINDINGS AND AN APPRAISAL

L. S. Wolfe, L. Pellerin, K. Rostworowski and H. M. Pappius
Montreal Neurological Institute, McGill University,
3801 University Street, Montreal, Québec, Canada H3A 2B4.

In the basal resting state in most tissues of the body including all regions of the brain, arachidonic acid is normally esterified rapidly by coenzyme A dependent acylation to the 2-acyl position of phospholipids. Thus, the tissue levels of free arachidonic acid and its enzymatically formed oxygenated metabolites are present locally at very low levels. A wide range of stimuli initiate arachidonic acid release and initiate reactions catalysed by fatty acid cyclooxygenase and lipoxygenases. Immune reactions, platelet activation and the action of platelet activating factor, inflammation, peptides, neurotransmitters and their agonists, growth factors, tumor promoters, electrical stimulation of brain and nerves, seizures, trauma, hypoxia, hypoglycemia and ischemia are but a few of the agents which initiate arachidonic acid release and metabolism (1,2). Prostaglandins, thromboxane A_2, leukotrienes and hydroxyperoxyeicosatetraenoic acids bioregulate tissue responses to second messengers and may in certain circumstances act themselves as second messengers. In the brain the biosynthesis of prostaglandins and thromboxane A_2 in vitro and following pathological responses is now well documented (1,3). Currently a subject of much interest is the realization that in the nervous system lipoxygenase reactions can form leukotrienes (LTB_4, LTC_4) and monohydroxyperoxy eicosatetraenoic acids which form the monohydroxy acids (HPETEs and HETEs) (4,5). This short paper addresses briefly three subjects. The metabolism of prostaglandin D_2 (PGD_2) in human brain, the stimulation of the synthesis by specific neurotransmitters of lipoxygenase products and the functional disturbances caused by focal brain injury which involve the intermediacy of arachidonic acid metabolites.

METABOLISM OF PROSTAGLANDIN D_2 IN HUMAN CEREBRAL CORTEX BY AN NADPH-DEPENDENT 11-KETOREDUCTASE

Studies largely from the laboratory of Professor Osamu Hayaishi at Osaka Medical College, Japan indicate that PGD_2 acts as a neuromodulator in the rat brain and it also has other interesting properties in rat brain and human tissues (6-8). These are summarized in Table 1.

An important difference between rat and human cerebral cortex is that PGD_2 could be found in only very small amounts after tissue incubations (9). Recent studies have shown that during incubations of homogenates of human temporal cortex (obtained by biopsy during the surgical treatment of epilepsy) added PGD_2 is actively metabolized to $9\alpha11\beta$-PGF_2 (11-epi-PGF_2) in the presence of an NADPH-generating system by an 11-keto-reductase. The quantification of the amounts of

TABLE 1.   Properties of prostaglandin D_2

Rat	Human
Most abundant PG in rat brain	Formed by mast cells
Induces sedation and sleep	Increased in mastocytosis
Produces hypothermia	Bronchoconstrictor
Potentiates barbiturate hypnosis	Releases inflammatory
Acts as an anticonvulsant	mediators
Antinociceptive	Released in acute allergic
Induces cataleptic state	reactions
Depresses sympathetic neurotransmission	Metabolized by an 11-
Augments serotonin turnover	keto-reductase in liver,
Releases luteinizing hormone from	lung and brain
pituitary gland	

$9\,\alpha11\beta$ -PGF_2 formed was determined by capillary column mass fragmentography as the trimethylsilyl ether methyl ester derivatives with monitoring of ions of m/z 423 and 429 (the tetradeuterated $9\,\alpha11\alpha$ -PGF_2 added as internal standard). The amount of $PGF_2\alpha$ formed was determined as the n–butylboronate derivatives monitored at m/z 435 and 439 by the method of Pace-Asciak and Wolfe (10,11) and subtracted from the total PGF_2 isomers formed. The relative intensities to the base peak, m/z 191, of the 423 ion in the two PGF_2 isomers did not differ more than 5 per cent. These results are illustrated in Figure 1 and the metabolism of PGD_2 to the 11-epi-PGF_2 and other possible isomers is shown in Figure 2.

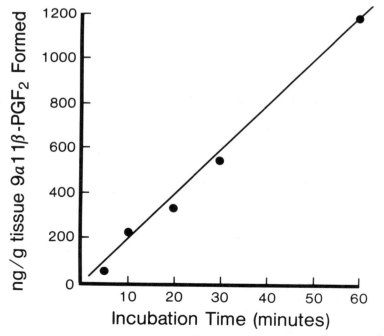

FIG. 1. Formation of $9\,\alpha11\beta$ -PGF_2 by human temporal cortex after addition of 5μ PGD_2 and an NADPH-generating system.

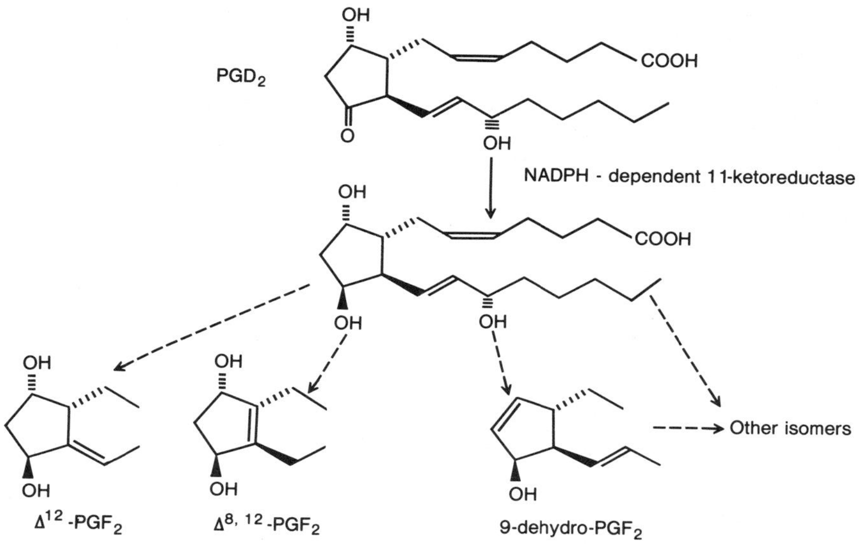

FIG.2. Pathways in the metabolism of PGD_2 (see also Ref. 12).

We conclude that PGD_2 is indeed formed in human brain but is rapidly metabolized by an NADPH-dependent 11-ketoreductase as has been found in other human tissues. The isomer has important biological activities such as inhibition of platelet aggregation induced by ADP and thrombin, disaggregates platelets and is a vasoconstrictor as well as a bronchoconstrictor. Its formation in human brain must be considered along with other eicosanoids when pathophysiological situations such as brain injury and ischemia are considered.

LIPOXYGENASE PATHWAYS IN RAT BRAIN: THE EFFECTS OF NEUROTRANSMITTERS

Recent studies have shown that brain can form leukotrienes (LTB_4, LTC_4) by a 5-lipoxygenase and as well as other hydroxyeicosatetraenoic acids (HETEs) can be formed by 12- and 15-lipoxygenases (4,5,13). We have found that incubations of intact physiologically active rat brain cortical slices can synthesize significant amounts of 12-HETE upon stimulation with the calcium ionophore A23187. When exogenous arachidonic acid is supplied, 5-,12- and 15-HETE synthesis increases with time but 12-HETE is the predominant product formed. The amounts of 12-HETE formed was considerably greater than the prostaglandins. The identity of 12-HETE formed was determined by mass spectrometry of the hydrogenated compound.

We examined then the effects of a series of neurotransmitters or their agonists on HETE formation. The results are shown in Figure 3. Glutamate and norepinephrine (NE) increased 12-HETE formation. The glutamate receptor agonist N-methyl-D-aspartate (NMDA) but not kainate stimulated 12-HETE formation. The effect of NE was mediated by alpha receptors since no stimulation occurred with isoproterenol. Of considerable interest is that at the same time Piomelli and coworkers (14,15) found that 12-HPETE and 12-HETE were formed in <u>Aplysia</u> sensory neurones and activated specific potassium channels. Thus the 12-HPETE or other metabolites may act as second messengers not only in <u>Aplysia</u> but also in specific NMDA receptors in brain (16). We conclude that lipoxygenase products particularly 12-HETE or its hydroperoxy precursor might be important bioregulators in the central nervous system, modifying neuron responsiveness through interaction with signal transduction mechanisms and/or ion channels and in long term potentiation.

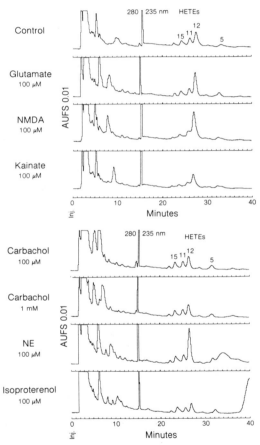

FIG. 3. HPLC chromatographic separations of HETEs formed in intact rat cerebral cortex pieces and the effects of various neurotransmitters and agonists.

INVOLVEMENT OF ARACHIDONIC ACID METABOLITES AND BIOGENIC AMINES IN BRAIN INJURY

A small focal freezing lesion to the rat cerebral cortex induces a widespread decrease in cortical local cerebral glucose utilization (LCGU) which has been interpreted as a reflection of a functional brain depression. It was found that the non-steroidal anti-inflammatory drugs indomethacin and ibuprofen significantly diminished the injury induced changes in LCGU thus implicating arachidonic acid metabolites in the modification of function in traumatized brain (17). Indeed the release of arachidonic acid and the formation of prostaglandins has been clearly demonstrated in these studies and indomethacin was shown to inhibit prostaglandin synthesis (Table 2).

Subsequently it was shown that the serotonergic system is activated unilaterally in the cortex of the injured hemisphere (18). Table 3 summarizes these results. The functional involvement of serotonin in the injury associated depression was demonstrated when inhibition of serotonin synthesis by p-chlorophenylalanine normalized the LCGU in cortical areas of the injured hemisphere (19,20). Studies are in progress to establish a relationship between the prostaglandin effects on serotonin formation in injured brain and ion channels. PGD_2 has already been shown to affect serotonin turnover and release in brain (21). Our hypothesis is that prostaglandins, serotonin and noradrenaline but not dopamine are intermediates in processes involved in the development of the functional disturbances in injured brain.

Acknowledgements

This research was supported by grants from the Medical Research Council of Canada (MT-1345 and MT-3021) and the Donner Canadian Foundation. We wish to thank Dr. A. Sherwin and Neurosurgeons of the Montreal Neurological Hospital for providing the human brain material and Marie Clark for her expert preparation of the manuscript.

References

1. Wolfe LS. J Neurochem 1982;28:1-14.

2. Nishizuka Y. Science 1984;225:1365-1367.

3. Saunders R, Horrocks LA. Neurochem Path 1987;7:1-22.

4. Lindgren JA, Hokfelt T, Dahlen S-E, et al. Proc Natl Acad Sci USA 1984;81:6212-6216.

5. Adesuyi SA, Cockrell CS, Gamache DA, et al. J Neurochem 1985;45:770-776.

6. Hayaishi O. Reports of Special Project Research 56222006, Ministry of Education, Science and Culture of Japan 1984:1-288.

Table 2.   Arachidonic acid release and prostaglandin formation
            in rat cerebral cortex in traumatized brain

Conditions	AA μg/g tissue	PGF$_{2\alpha}$	PGE$_2$ ng/g tissue	PGD$_2$
Control hemisphere				
Untreated	2.6 ± 1.4 (20)	1.4 ± 1.0 (8)	1.1 ± 0.1 (4)	2.0 ± 1.8 (4)
Indomethacin	3.3 ± 2.6 (3)	N.D.	N.D.	N.D.
Lesioned area				
Untreated	15.4 ± 7.1 (13)	57.5 ± 19.8 (6)	29.5 ± 12.4 (4)	111.5 ± 13.0 (3)
Indomethacin	10.4 ± 5.6 (6)	1.8 ± 0.3 (3)	-	-

Results are means ± S.D. Number of experiments in brackets. Prostaglandins determined by GC/MS with tetradeuterated internal standards. N.D. is not detectable.

Table 3.   Serotonin and 5-hydroxy indole acetic acid content of rat fronto-parietal
            cerebral cortex with time after a focal freezing lesion

Conditions	5-HT pmoles/g tissue	5-HIAA
Normal (13)	1964 ± 316	895 ± 140
Lesioned hemisphere Time after lesion		
4 hours (5)	1901 ± 357	1314 ± 328
1 day (18)	1569 ± 242*	1670 ± 668*
3 days (21)	1971 ± 405	1366 ± 436*
8 days (3)	2035 ± 81	827 ± 70

Results are means ± S.D. Number of animals in brackets. * $p < 0.01$. Measurement made by HPLC with electrochemical detection.

7. Shimizu T, Mizuno N, Amano T, et al. Proc Natl Acad Sci USA 1979;76:6231-6234.

8. Bhattacharya SK, Mohan Rao PJR. J Pharm Pharmacol 1987;39:743-745.

9. Wolfe LS, Pappius HM. In: Bes A, Braquet R, Paoletti R, Siesjo BK, eds. Cerebral Ischemia, Amsterdam: Elsevier Science Publishers B.V. 1984;223-231.

10. Pace-Asciak C, Wolfe LS. J Chromatogr 1971;56:129-133.

11. Watanabe K, Iguchi Y, Iguchi S, et al. Proc Natl Acad Sci USA 1986;83:1583-1587.

12. Wendelborn DF, Seibert K, Jackson Roberts II L. Proc Natl Acad Sci USA 1988;85:304-308.

13. Pellerin L, Wolfe LS. Trans Amer Soc Neurochem 1988;19:76.

14. Piomelli D, Volterra A, Dale N, et al. Nature 1987;328:38-43.

15. Piomelli D, Shapiro E, Feinmark SJ, et al. J Neurosci 1987;7(11):3675-3686.

16. Collingridge G. Nature 1987;330:604-605.

17. Pappius HM, Wolfe LS. J Cerebr Blood Flow Metab 1983;3:448-459.

18. Pappius HM, Dadoun R. J Neurochem 1987;49:321-325.

19. Pappius HM, Wolfe LS. In: Baethmann A, Go KG, Unterberg A, eds. Mechanisms of Secondary Brain Damage, New York: Plenum Press, 1986; 151-167.

20. Pappius HM, Dadoun R, McHugh M. J Cerebr Blood Flow Metab 1988 (in press).

21. Hollingsworth EG, Patrick GA. Pharm Biochem Behav 1985;22:371-375.

Advances in Prostaglandin, Thromboxane, and
Leukotriene Research, Vol. 19, edited by
B. Samuelsson, P. Y.-K. Wong, and F. F. Sun,
Raven Press, Ltd., New York ©1989.

PROSTAGLANDIN E_2 IN THE PATHOGENESIS OF PYROGEN FEVER: VALIDATION OF AN INTERMEDIARY ROLE

F. Coceani, I. Bishai, J. Lees, and S. Sirko

Research Institute, The Hospital for Sick Children,
Toronto, Ontario M5G 1X8, Canada

During recent years, there has been considerable debate on
whether prostaglandin(PG) E_2 is an intermediary in the
central action of pyrogens and, by extension, is essential in
the onset of fever (1). An additional point of contention has
been whether PGE_2 acts alone or in concert with another
cyclooxygenase product, possibly thromboxane(TX) A_2. So far,
resolution of either issue has been precluded not only by the
conflicting data in the literature, but also by uncertainties
on the site of action of blood-borne pyrogens and lack of
information on the changes in prostaglandin synthesis occurring
in the hypothalamus during fever. In addressing these
questions we have therefore used a comprehensive approach,
combining diverse methodologies and lines of investigation.
All experiments were conducted in the cat.

PROSTAGLANDIN E_2 AS A CENTRAL MEDIATOR OF FEVER

Conventionally, identification of any substance with a
neural mediator entails verification of several conditions,
foremost among them being the demonstration of a causal
relationship between synthesis and biological response.
Validation of the latter condition in the case of the "PGE_2
mediator" concept had been clouded by much controversy (1) and
required a fresh approach. This was achieved by monitoring
prostaglandin levels, and any change caused by pyrogen fever,
in the cerebrospinal fluid (CSF) and locally in the
hypothalamus.

Prostanoids in Cerebrospinal Fluid

PGE_2 and the TXA_2 byproduct, TXB_2, were normally found
in CSF collected from the third ventricle, respective levels
being about 40 and 500 pg/ml (2). The relatively low content
of PGE_2 reflects the basal rate of synthesis rather than
catabolic breakdown of the compound in the tissue, because no
evidence was obtained for the occurrence of 15-keto-13,14-
dihydro PGE_2.
Intravenous administration of pyrogen, whether bacterial or
leucocytic (natural or recombinant interleukin-1; IL-1),
increased PGE_2 levels severalfold (2). Furthermore, the
PGE_2 rise preceded the onset of the fever and was sustained

for as long as body temperature remained elevated.
Significantly, endotoxin was more effective than IL-1 in
promoting PGE_2 synthesis, implying a more direct, or diffuse,
action for that pyrogen. The response to IL-1, on the other
hand, was the same in naive and endotoxin-conditioned animals.
Both such findings have implications for the pathogenetic
mechanism of fever (see below). Pyrogens also stimulated
PGE_2 synthesis when injected into the third ventricle and, as
in the case of the blood-borne pyrogen, their effect was
already manifest during the latent phase of the fever (2).
With either route of administration, PGE_2 elevation occurred
only with doses of pyrogen above threshold for the fever.

Unlike PGE_2, TXB_2 content of the CSF remained unchanged
during the fever to intravenous endotoxin or IL-1. Both pyrogens stimulated instead thromboxane synthesis by the intracerebroventricular route, but this response was short-lived and
did not extend beyond the uprise phase of the fever (2,3).

In brief, this study supported the idea of PGE_2 being a
central mediator of fever. No evidence was obtained for an
equivalent role of TXA_2. However, prostaglandin levels in
the CSF may or may not reflect events in the thermoregulatory
region. For this reason, subsequent experiments addressed the
specific question of changes in prostaglandin synthesis
occurring locally in the hypothalamus in the course of fever.
A corollary aim was to define the location of any such change
and hence obtain information on the site of action of
blood-borne pyrogens.

Local Release of Prostanoids in the Hypothalamus

Formation of PGE_2 and TXB_2 was monitored at discrete
hypothalamic sites, using a "push-pull" perfusion procedure
that had been appropriately modified to limit damage to the
tissue. In the absence of fever, PGE_2 release was steady
from the second hour of perfusion onwards, while TXB_2 release
tended to decline with time. Their relative release rate
accorded with the results of CSF measurements, with TXB_2
exceeding PGE_2 values two- to fivefold (0.15 - 0.43 vs.
0.08 - 0.12 pg/min).

Basal release of the two compounds was similar in the
anterior hypothalamic/preoptic region (AH/POA) and the
tuberal-posterior hypothalamus (PH/Tu). Likewise, both
compounds were formed in higher amounts (two- to tenfold
increase) at either site after injecting locally endotoxin. In
contrast, intravenous administration of endotoxin or IL-1
stimulated selectively the formation of PGE_2, though the
response itself did not differ between AH/POA and PH/Tu.
Significantly, PGE_2 release was particularly high from
posterior sites abutting the median eminence. In either
region, the degree of enhancement in PGE_2 release correlated
with the magnitude of the fever. In addition, values of PGE_2
release tended to be greater with endotoxin than IL-1.

In sum, "push-pull" perfusion experiments proved that hypothalamic tissue forms both PGE$_2$ and TXA$_2$ under physiologic conditions; however, only PGE$_2$ formation could be linked to the occurrence of fever. Accelerated formation of PGE$_2$ during the febrile state is not confined to the AH/POA, nothwithstanding the importance of that region for thermoregulatory adjustments.

SITE OF ACTION OF PYROGENS

It is generally believed that diverse noxae, specifically infectious noxae (e.g. endotoxin), elicit the release of IL-1 from mononuclear phagocytes. Blood-borne IL-1, in turn, is regarded as a general stimulus for host reactions, including fever. Any scheme involving PGE$_2$ in the genesis of fever has to be reconciled, on one hand, with the apparent inability of pyrogens to cross the blood-brain barrier and, on the other hand, with the occurrence of cyclooxygenase activation within the confines of brain. Two possibilities were examined in the attempt to overcome this apparent inconsistency, that is, (i) the likelihood that blood-borne endotoxin, or rather an active fragment formed in the circulation, may elicit the appearance of IL-1 in the CNS by acting directly on neural tissue or by promoting IL-1 synthesis at the interface between blood and brain, and (ii) the feasibility of the cerebral micro-vasculature to function as a source of fever-producing PGE$_2$.

Work on the first topic (4) proved that neither endotoxin nor IL-1 promoted the appearance of IL-1 activity in the CSF when administered intravenously. Endotoxin, however, caused measurable activity by the intracerebroventricular route. Therefore, the idea of IL-1 crossing the blood-brain barrier or being formed ex novo within the substance of the brain was not borne out by these experiments, though it was confirmed that neural tissue (glial cells?) is intrinsically capable of IL-1 synthesis. The alternative possibility of the vasculature releasing PGE$_2$ into the brain interstitium upon pyrogen challenge was verified in isolated cerebral microvessels (5). This vascular preparation, consisting predominantly of capillaries, produced PGE$_2$ and 6-keto-PGF$_{1\alpha}$ (hence PGI$_2$), their respective release rate being about 60 and 500 pg/mg protein/min. Endotoxin stimulated selectively PGE$_2$ formation (two- to threefold increase) at an appropriately low concentration, while IL-1 was without effect.

From the foregoing it is concluded that blood-borne IL-1 may only act at central sites lacking a blood-brain barrier. Conversely, endotoxin can exert a direct effect on the cerebral vasculature in addition to the IL-1-mediated effect.

CONCLUSION

Our study proves that under normal conditions PGE$_2$ is formed in the CNS at an exceedingly low rate. PGE$_2$ formation is stimulated by pyrogens and the activation pattern conforms with a causative role of the compound in the onset and progression of fever. No such role can be ascribed to TXA_2. The sequence of events leading to accelerated formation of PGE_2 differs in some respects depending on the pyrogen and its route of administration. Blood-borne IL-1 acts at a discrete site, or rather sites, lacking the blood-brain barrier, one of which is identified with the organum vasculosum laminae terminalis (OVLT) in light of data implicating this structure in the genesis of fever (6,7). The median eminence and possibly other circumventricular organs may also function as targets for blood-borne IL-1. The mechanism by which IL-1 action in the OVLT is translated into stimulation of PGE_2 synthesis remains speculative. OVLT neurons projecting to the AH/POA (8) might be involved in this process. The alternative possibility of reticuloendothelial cells in the OVLT being the source of PGE_2 (7) is inconsistent with our finding that endotoxin-conditioned animals behave as naive animals in response to the pyrogen challenge. Our work also suggests that endotoxin may act on the CNS both directly and through the intermediacy of IL-1, hence explaining its greater effectiveness in promoting PGE_2 synthesis. Unlike blood-borne pyrogens, intracerebro-ventricularly injected pyrogens have free access to the brain parenchyma and stimulate PGE_2 production diffusely. The multiplicity of targets for pyrogens is conceivably important in sustaining fever and fever-related events, specifically the sequence of coordinated events marking the host defence against infection.

ACKNOWLEDGEMENT

This work was supported by the Medical Research Council of Canada.

REFERENCES

1. Coceani F, Bishai I, Lees J, Sirko S, Yale J Biol Med 1986; 59:169-174.
2. Coceani F, Lees J, Bishai I, Am J Physiol 1988; 254:R463-R469.
3. Coceani F, Bishai I, Dinarello CA, Fitzpatrick FA, Am J Physiol 1983; 244:R785-R793.
4. Coceani F, Lees J, Dinarello CA, Brain Research (in press).
5. Bishai I, Dinarello CA, Coceani F, Can J Physiol Pharmacol 1987; 65:2225-2230.
6. Blatteis CM, Intern J Neuroscience 1988; 38:223-232.
7. Stitt JT, Yale J Biol Med 1986; 59:137-149.
8. Phillips MI, Camacho A. In: Gross PM, ed. Circumventricular organs and body fluids, vol 1. Boca Raton: CRC Press, 1987; 158-169.

Advances in Prostaglandin, Thromboxane, and Leukotriene Research, Vol. 19, edited by B. Samuelsson, P. Y.-K. Wong, and F. F. Sun, Raven Press, Ltd., New York ©1989.

POSITRON EMISSION TOMOGRAPHY STUDIES USING [11C]ESTER OF PROSTAGLANDIN D2

Y. Watanabe[1,2], B. Långström[3], C.-G. Stålnacke[3], P.G. Gillberg[3], P. Gullberg[3], H. Lundqvist[3], S.-M. Aquilonius[3], U. Pontén[3], G. Sperberg[3], K. Hamada[1], Y. Watanabe[1], N. Yumoto[1], M. Hatanaka[1], H. Hayashi[1], and O. Hayaishi[1]

[1] Hayaishi Bioinformation Transfer Project, JRDC, Kyoto 601, [2] Department of Neuroscience, Osaka Bioscience Institute, Osaka 565, Japan, and [3] Uppsala University, 751 21 Uppsala, Sweden.

Arachidonic acid metabolites, prostaglandin(PG)s and leukotrienes, exert various neurophysiological functions such as sleep induction (1,2), modulation of senses——pain (3) and olfaction (4)——and of autonomic functions (5), neuroendocrine roles (5), and anticonvulsive effects (5). The localization of PG systems in the central nervous system has been investigated, namely, with respect to PGD2 synthetase (6), NADP-dependent PGD2 15-hydroxydehydrogenase (7), and the receptor proteins for PGD2, E2, and F2α (7-10), to unveil the novel roles of PG's in CNS. The regional distribution of the specific binding sites for PGD2, E2, and F2α has been demonstrated in postmortem human brain (11) and the precise localization in the nucleus level was obtained in monkey brain by *in vitro* autoradiography (9,10).

The study in combination with the neurophysiological experiments revealed close relationships between the localization of PG receptors (12) and known functions of PG's and also the novel roles such as the modulation by PGD2 of the olfactory stimulus-response (4). However, little is known concerning the role of arachidonate metabolites in the higher brain functions. Only the clinical data concerning the PG levels in the plasma and cerebrospinal fluid in the patients with psychological disorders are available. Higher brain functions could be approached in human and primates using the noninvasive techniques such as positron emission tomography (PET).

We succeeded in the synthesis of [11C]methyl ester (Me) of PG's (13) and reported the results of PET study using [11C]Me of PGD2 and its 9-epimer (14). In that experiment, we found 2.3-fold higher uptake of the radioactivity into the monkey brain by the use of [11C]Me of PGD2 than that using [11C]Me of 9β-PGD2.

The major argument against the use of the epimer for the control study is sometimes concerning the difference of the physicochemical properties between the epimers. From this reason, [11C]Me of the enantiomer of PGD2 was synthesized as discribed by us (13) and was employed in this study. Their chemical structures are shown in Scheme 1. The radiochemical purity after the purification using Sep-pak C_{18} cartridge was more than 95%. The specific radioactivity was in the order of 0.9

GBq/μmol (ca. 24 Ci/mmol). The dose of [¹¹C]esters injected was around 120 MBq (ca. 3.6 mCi) without any dilution by nonradio-active esters, the dose corresponding to 0.13 μmol (ca. 6 μg/kg).

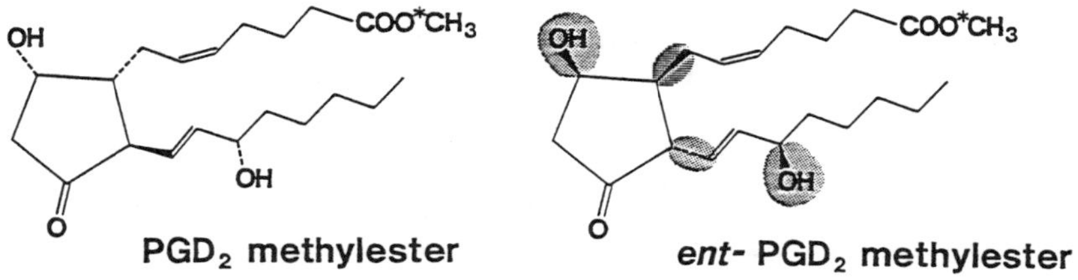

PGD₂ methylester   *ent-* **PGD₂ methylester**

Scheme 1. Structure of PGD₂-[¹¹C]Me and ent-PGD₂-[¹¹C]Me

Experimental protocols were as follows: Female rhesus monkey, weighing 6.8 kg, was employed. The first experiment was per-formed using [¹¹C]methyl ester of total enantiomer (ent-PGD₂-[¹¹C]Me) and the second one was using PGD₂-[¹¹C]Me at 1.5-h interval. At 15-min point in the second exp., unlabeled PGD₂ (0.2 mg/kg *i.v.*) was injected for the displacement study.

For autoradiographical study, a rhesus monkey was anesthetized with ketamine HCl and perfused with cold phosphate-buffered saline via left ventricle of the heart for the exclusion of the blood component from the brain. The brain was rapidly removed, cut into 5-mm slices, and frozen on dry-ice. The frozen sagittal sections of the brain with 80-μm thickness were prepared in a cryostat and collected onto the gelatin-coated glass slides (ca. 7 X 11 cm). The slide-mounted sections were preincubated in two changes of 1 l of 50 mM Tris/HCl (pH 7.4) containing 0.1 M NaCl (Buffer A) at 4°C for 30 min each. The sections were then incu-bated with 10 ml of 10 nM PGD₂-[³H]Me or 10 nM ent-PGD₂-[³H]Me in Buffer A at 4°C for 30 min. After the incubation, the sections were washed four times in 300 ml each of Buffer A at 4°C for 15 sec each, splashed by distilled water, and dried on a hot-plate at 60°C. After being further dried in the cold room with dessi-cant, the sections associated with [³H]microscale (Amersham) were juxtaposed tightly with ³H-Hyperfilm (Amersham) at 4°C for 4 weeks. The autoradiograms thus obtained were analyzed by an image processing system (10).

Fig. 1 shows the time course of the uptake of ent-PGD₂-[¹¹C]Me and PGD₂-[¹¹C]Me into the brain and temporal muscle. The uptake value into the temporal muscle was also around 1.0 in both cases, but the uptake into the brain was different: the uptake after the injection of ent-PGD₂-[¹¹C]Me reached its maximum at around 2 min and at the value of 1.72 and then decreased gradually; the uptake after the injection of PGD₂-[¹¹C]Me reached its maximum at around 3 min and at the value of 2.05 and plateaued for several min and then decreased. The distribution of the radioactivity taken up into the brain by using ent-PGD₂-[¹¹C]Me was rather diffuse compared with that by using PGD₂-[¹¹C]Me. The concentrated region was observed by using PGD_2-$[^{11}C]$Me and the highest uptake was observed in the structure of lateral basal ganglia containing amygdala (Fig. 1 LBG), while little difference was seen between the uptake values into the whole brain and LBG in the case of ent-PGD_2-$[^{11}C]$Me. When the displacement study was attempted by the *i.v.* injection of excess amounts (0.2 mg/kg) of unlabelled PGD_2 15 min after the original injection, there was no significant changes of the pattern of the uptake. The blood curves were almost the same in these two experiments (the uptake value into the venous blood at 15 min point = 2.0 and 2.1, using ent- and PGD_2-$[^{11}C]$Me, respectively). The half life of the ester form in the plasma was ca. 1.5 min in both experiments.

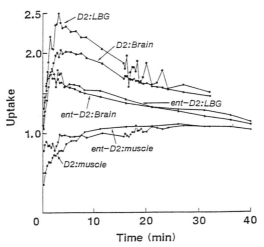

FIG. 1 The time course of the uptake of ent-PGD_2-$[^{11}C]$Me and PGD_2-$[^{11}C]$Me into the brain, temporal muscle, and the structure containing lateral basal ganglia /amygdala area (LBG).

The present study demonstrated the difference between the uptake values into the brain after the injection of PGD_2-$[^{11}C]$Me and its stereoisomers. This difference could be interpreted by several possibilities, the difference of the metabolism containing the susceptibility to esterase, the difference of the cerebral blood flow caused by the injection of PG, the different action toward a transport system for blood-brain barrier, and the stereospecific binding to some molecule(s) in the brain. Since PGD_2 is rather resistent to the metabolism in the lung, compared with PGE_2 and $PGF_{2\alpha}$, the rate of the hydrolysis of the ester moiety might be rate-limiting in this case. Although extensive studies on the metabolites using the stereoisomers have not so far performed, no great difference of the decay rate of the radioactivity remaining in the ether-extracted fraction (the radioactivity not deesterificated) was observed between the experiments using the stereoisomers. This suggests a lower possibility of the difference of the susceptibility to esterase between the stereoisomers.

The dose of PGD_2-[^{11}C]Me and its stereoisomers used in the present study was around 6 $\mu g/kg$ body weight. It has not so far been checked if this dose of PGD_2-Me could change the regional cerebral blood flow or not. However, this dose had no significant effects on the peripheral blood pressure, heart rate, and respiratory rate, when the autonomic behavior was measured in ketamine-anesthetized rhesus monkey by the injection of PGD_2 and its methyl ester.

The difference between the uptake values into the brain of ent-PGD_2-[^{11}C]Me and PGD_2-[^{11}C]Me could be explained by the results of *in vitro* autoradiography using ent-PGD_2-[^{3}H]Me and PGD_2-[^{3}H]Me. The difference of the binding activities of both isomers was obtained. The dense stereospecific binding was observed in the hippocampus, amygdala, cerebral and cerebellar cortices.

[References]
1. Ueno R, Honda K, Inoué S and Hayaishi O. <u>Proc Natl Acad Sci USA</u> 1983;80:1735-1737.
2. Onoe H, Ueno R, Fujita I, Nishino H, Oomura Y and Hayaishi O. <u>Proc Natl Acad Sci USA</u> 1988;85:in press.
3. Horiguchi S, Ueno R, Hyodo M and Hayaishi O. <u>Eur J Pharmac</u> 1986;122:173-179.
4. Watanabe Y, Mori K, Imamura K, Takagi SF and Hayaishi O. <u>Brain Res</u> 1986;378:216-222.
5. Wolfe LS. <u>J Neurochem</u> 1982;38:1-14.
6. Urade Y, Fujimoto N, Kaneko T, Konishi A, Mizuno N and Hayaishi O. <u>J Biol Chem</u> 1987;262:15132-15136.
7. Watanabe Y, Yamashita A, Tokumoto H and Hayaishi O. <u>Proc Natl Acad Sci USA</u> 1983;80:4542-4545.
8. Yamashita A, Watanabe Y and Hayaishi O. <u>Proc Natl Acad Sci USA</u> 1983;80:6114-6118.
9. Watanabe Y, Watanabe Y and Hayaishi O. In: Hayaishi O, Torizuka K, eds. <u>Biomedical Imaging</u> New York: Academic Press, 1986:227-238.
10. Watanabe Y, Watanabe Y and Hayaishi O. <u>J Neurosci</u> 1988; in press.
11. Watanabe Y, Tokumoto H, Yamashita A and Hayaishi O. <u>Brain Res</u> 1985;342:110-116.
12. Watanabe Y, Långström B, Watanabe Y, et al. <u>NY Acad Sci</u> 1988; in press.
13. Gullberg P, Watanabe Y, Svärd H, Hayaishi O and Långström B. <u>Appl Radiat Isot</u> 1987;38:647-649.
14. Watanabe Y, Långström B, Stålnacke C-G, et al. <u>Adv PG TX LT Res</u> 1987;17:939-941.

Advances in Prostaglandin, Thromboxane, and Leukotriene Research, Vol. 19, edited by
B. Samuelsson, P. Y.-K. Wong, and F. F. Sun,
Raven Press, Ltd., New York ©1989.

BIOSYNTHESIS OF CYSTEINYL-LEUKOTRIENES
BY HUMAN BRAIN TISSUE IN VITRO

Thomas Simmet, Werner Luck,
*Wolfgang K. Delank and B.A. Peskar

Department of Pharmacology and Toxicology and
*Department of Neurosurgery, Ruhr-University Bochum,
D-463o Bochum (F.R.G.)

INTRODUCTION

Previously we have shown that rat brain tissue has the capacity to synthesize cysteinyl-leukotrienes (LT) in vitro (1). These results have been extended and confirmed by others (2). In addition to the in vitro production of cysteinyl-LT by rat brain tissue after ionophore A23187 stimulation, various pathophysiological conditions such as ischemic insult, concussive injury, subarachnoid hemorrhage, and seizures (3,4,5,6) have been demonstrated to induce biosynthesis of cysteinyl-LT in gerbil brain tissue in vivo. With regard to possible physiologic functions in the central nervous system there is evidence that lipoxygenase products might have a role as second messengers in neurons or might be modulators in central nervous activity and neuroendocrine events (7,8,9,1o). Since so far it is not known whether human brain tissue has the capacity to synthesize cysteinyl-LT, we investigated cysteinyl-LT formation by human brain tissue slices from non-pathological grey and white matter.

MATERIALS AND METHODS

Human brain tissue was obtained at neurosurgery from patients subjected to resection of brain tumors. After resection the brain tissue was immediately placed in ice-cold Tyrode solution and was rapidly transported to the laboratory. Non-pathological grey and white matter was manually cut into slices which were washed in ice-cold saline. Aliquots of 1oo to 15o mg of tissue slices were incubated at 37°C in 2.0 ml of oxygenated Tyrode solution and were adapted to in vitro conditions for 6o min with buffer changes every 3o min. After an additional preincubation period of 3o min the buffer was removed and fresh buffer containing ionophore A23187 (1o.o µM) or its solvent dimethylsulfoxide (DMSO) was added for 3o min. At the end of the incubation periods the supernatants were decanted and proteins were pelleted by rapid centrifugation after boiling for 4 min. When brain tissue slices were incubated in the presence of enzyme inhibitors such as indomethacin (2.8 μM) or nordihydroguaiaretic acid (NDGA, 1o μM), the compounds were present throughout the experiment. After incubation the tissue samples were examined histologically and were found to consist of non-pathological tissue only.

Aliquots of 2.o ml of fresh human blood were either allowed to clot spontaneously or in the presence of ionophore A23187 (1o.o μM) at 37° C for 3o min in glass tubes. Serum was obtained and proteins were precipitated by addition of 3 volumes of precooled acetone with subsequent centrifugation. The supernatants were evaporated and the residues were resuspended in Tris-HCl buffer (5o mM, pH 7.4).

$PGF_2\alpha$ and cysteinyl-LT contents were analysed by means of sensitive radioimmunoassays (11,12). The anti-cysteinyl-LT antibodies used exhibit 1oo% cross-reaction with LTC_4 and 4o% cross-reaction with both LTD_4 and LTE_4. A standard curve was constructed using synthetic LTC_4. Reversed phase HPLC using a C_{18}-Nucleosil column (25o x 4 mm, particle size 5 μm) and the solvent system methanol:water:acetic acid (68:32:o.o1, v/v/v, pH 5.5) was performed as previously described (5).

RESULTS AND DISCUSSION

Incubation of human brain tissue slices from grey and white matter under basal conditions resulted in spontaneous release of LTC_4-like material (Fig. 1, Fig. 2). While the solvent DMSO did not significantly affect the release of cysteinyl-LT, ionophore A23187 (1o.o μM) induced release of large amounts of cysteinyl-LT from human grey (Fig. 1) and white matter (Fig. 2) tissue slices. In fact, cysteinyl-LT production by human brain tissue slices was approximately 25 (grey matter) to 4o (white matter)-fold higher than that from rat brain tissue slices incubated under similar conditions (1). Preincubation of human brain tissue in the presence of indomethacin did not affect cysteinyl-LT release from grey (Fig. 1) or white matter (Fig. 2) which is in contrast to rat brain tissue where cysteinyl-LT release was approximately doubled (1). The lipoxygenase inhibitor NDGA (1o.o μM) tended to decrease basal release of cysteinyl-LT from grey (Fig. 1) and white matter (Fig. 2) and abolished the ionophore A23187-induced increase in cysteinyl-LT production.

Release of $PGF_2\alpha$, which is considered to be the major prostanoid formed by human brain tissue (13), was not stimulated by ionophore A23187 (1o.o μM) (22.o + 4.5 ng/g vs. 17.8 + 2.6 ng/g, n.s. and 11.o + 2.3 ng/g vs. 9.2 + 1.9 ng/g, n.s., for human grey and white matter tissue slices, respectively, n=1o each) and was significantly inhibited by indomethacin (2.8 μM) (25.o + 4.6 ng/g vs. 5.1 + 1.6 ng/g, P < o.oo1, and 11.8+ 2.3 ng/g vs. 2.7 + o.7 ng/g, P < o.oo5, n=1o each). It seems remarkable that cysteinyl-LT formation exceeded that of $PGF_2\alpha$.

Cysteinyl-LT released from both grey and white matter tissue slices were shown to have biological activity in that the iso-

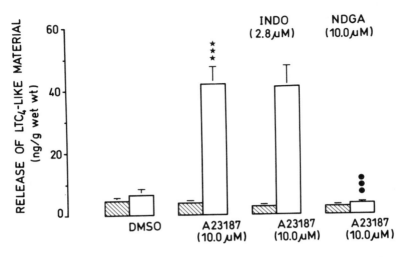

FIG. 1. Release of LTC4-like material from non-pathological human grey matter tissue slices during a 3o min preincubation period (hatched bars) and during a 3o min incubation in the presence of ionophore A23187 (1o.o µM) or its solvent DMSO (open bars) and the effects of indomethacin (2.8 µM) and NDGA (1o.o µM). Results are means + S.E.M. of 1o experiments. *** P < 0.oo1 compared to DMSO, ●●● P < 0.oo1 compared to iono- phore A23187 in the absence of NDGA.

lated guinea-pig ileum as bioassay tissue was contracted by incubation buffer of ionophore A23187-stimulated brain tissue slices (14). This contractile response was nearly completely antagonized by the slow-reacting substance of anaphylaxis (SRS-A) antagonist FPL-55712 (14,15).

Since the antibody used for cysteinyl-LT determination cross- reacts with LTC4, LTD4 and LTE4, cyteinyl-LT were further charac- terized by reversed phase HPLC. Material from human grey matter comigrated with authentic LTC4, LTD4 and LTE4 (14) which have also been described to be released from rat brain tissue incu- bated in vitro (2) as well as in gerbil brain tissue after seizures (6). In material from guinea-pig cortical slices main- ly LTC4 and smaller amounts of LTD4 have been found (16). Mate- rial obtained from human white matter coeluted with authentic LTD4 and smaller amounts with authentic LTE4 which indicates a higher activity for γ-glutamyl transpeptidase in human white matter as compared to human grey matter (14).

Despite extensive washing, long preincubation time and small tissue slices it may be assumed that some blood remained in our brain tissue preparations. Therefore, we investigated cys- teinyl-LT formation in whole blood. Spontaneous clotting for 3o min resulted in formation of LTC4-like material (o.38+o.1 ng/ml serum, n=6) which by reversed phase HPLC was shown to consist

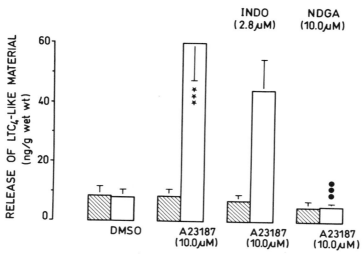

FIG. 2. Release of LTC4-like material from non-pathological human white matter tissue slices during a 3o min preincubation period (hatched bars) and during a 3o min incubation in the presence of ionophore A23187 (1o.o µM) or its solvent DMSO (open bars) and the effects of indomethacin (2.8 µM) and NDGA (1o.o µM). Results are means + S.E.M. of 1o experiments. *** P < o.oo1 compared to DMSO, ●●● P < o.oo1 compared to iono- phore A23187 in the absence of NDGA.

of LTC4, LTD4 and LTE4. Ionophore A23187 (1o.o µM) significantly stimulated cysteinyl-LT production (14.1 + 2.2 ng/ml serum, n=6, P < o.oo1) in whole human blood. Thus, if one would esti- mate the blood content of the tissue slices to be 1o% of the wet weight, then cysteinyl-LT formation by whole blood would account for less than 2% of the total cysteinyl-LT release by the tissue slices.

In conclusion our data demonstrate that human grey and white matter tissue slices possess the capacity to synthesize large amounts of cysteinyl-LT in vitro. The identity of cysteinyl-LT was verified using an antibody which recognizes not only the fatty acid moiety but also the presence of an aminoacid side- chain of the cysteinyl-LT-molecule (12), furthermore by the guinea-pig ileum bioassay employing FPL 55712 as SRS-A antago- nist (14) and finally by reversed phase HPLC (14).

ACKNOWLEDGEMENTS

We wish to thank Dr. J. Rokach, Merck Frosst Laboratories, Pointe-Claire, Dorval, Canada, for synthetic cysteinyl-LT and Prof. Dr. H. Breining, Department of Pathology, Bundesknapp- schaft, D-43oo Essen, for histopathological examination of the tissue samples. FPL 55712 was donated by Dr. P. Sheard,

Fisons Ltd., Loughborough, England. This work was supported by the Deutsche Forschungsgemeinschaft.

REFERENCES

1. Dembińska-Kieć A, Simmet Th, Peskar BA. Eur J Pharmacol 1984;99:57-62.

2. Lindgren JA, Hökfelt T, Dahlén SE, Patrono C, Samuelsson B. Proc Natl Acad Sci USA 1984;81:6212-6216

3. Moskowitz MA, Kiwak KJ, Hekimian K, Levine L. Science 1984; 224:886-889.

4. Kiwak KJ, Moskowitz MA, Levine L. J Neurosurg 1985;62:865-869.

5. Simmet Th, Seregi A, Hertting G. Neuropharmacology 1987; 26:1o7-11o.

6. Simmet Th, Seregi A, Hertting G. J Neurochem 1988;(in press).

7. Hulting AL, Lindgren JA, Hökfelt T et al. Proc Natl Acad Sci USA 1985;82:3834-3838.

8. Palmer MR, Mathews R, Murphy RC, Hoffer BJ. Neurosci Lett 198o;18:173-18o.

9. Palmer MR, Mathews WR, Hoffer BJ, Murphy RC. J Pharmacol Exp Ther 1981;219:91-96.

1o. Piomelli D, Volterra A, Dale N, Siegelbaum SA, Kandel ER, Schwartz JH, Belardetti F. Nature 1987;328:38-43.

11. Peskar BA, Hertting G. Naunyn-Schmiedeberg's Arch Pharmacol 1973;279:227-234.

12. Aehringhaus U, Wölbling RH, König W, Patrono C, Peskar BM, Peskar BA. FEBS Lett 1982;146:111-114.

13. Abdel-Halim SM, von Holst H, Meyerson B, Sachs C, Änggård E. J Neurochem 198o;34:1331-1333.

14. Simmet Th, Luck W, Delank WK, Peskar BA. Brain Res 1988; (in press).

15. Augstein J, Farmer JB, Lee TB, Sheard P, Tattersall M. Nature (New Biol) 1973;245:215-217.

16. Shimizu T, Takusagawa Y, Izumi T, Ohishi N, Seyama Y. J Neurochem 1987;48:1541-1546.

Advances in Prostaglandin, Thromboxane, and Leukotriene Research, Vol. 19, edited by B. Samuelsson, P. Y.-K. Wong, and F. F. Sun, Raven Press, Ltd., New York ©1989.

RAS ONCOGENES AND PHOSPHOLIPASE C

R.R. Gorman, A.H. Lin, P.L. Olinger and C.W. Benjamin

Department of Cell Biology,
The Upjohn Co., Kalamazoo, MI 49008

INTRODUCTION

The ras genes are a highly conserved gene family in eukaryotic cells. Ras genes encode proteins with molecular masses of 21 kDa (p21s). Point mutations in the cellular-ras genes (c-ras) at amino acids 12, 13, or 61 confer on p21 the ability to transform some cell types in culture (1-5). It is known that both mutated and normal p21 bind GTP with similar affinity and display GTPase activity.

Previous work from our laboratory showed that both the basal and hormone-stimulated adenylate cyclase activities were reduced in NIH-3T3 cells expressing the mutated ras gene from the human EJ bladder carcinoma (EJ-ras) (6). We also found a decrease in adenylate cyclase activity in cells expressing high levels of the normal c-ras gene. These data supported the concept that both normal and mutated p21 are related to mammalian G proteins. We now report that another vertebrate system thought to be regulated by G proteins, hormone-sensitive phospholipase C activity, is also inhibited in cells expressing high levels of the EJ-ras gene. Thus, platelet-derived growth factor (PDGF) stimulated prostaglandin E_2 (PGE$_2$) and arachidonate release from EJ-ras-transformed NIH-3T3 cells is markedly reduced compared to that in control cells.

RESULTS AND DISCUSSION

Control NIH-3T3 cells (transfected with only calf thymus DNA and pUCNeo DNA) release significant amounts of PGE$_2$ as determined by RIA, when exposed to PDGF at 2 units/ml (Fig. 1). PGE$_2$ is observed immediately, with maximal levels occurring at 2 hr. EJ-ras transformed cells release only low levels of PGE$_2$ in response to PDGF; after 2 hr these cells have released only 3% as much PGE$_2$ as controls.

407

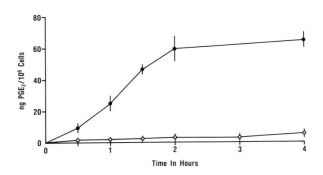

FIG 1.   PDGF-stimulated   PGE$_2$ release   in   control   and
EJ-ras-transformed cells.   NIH-3T3 cells (approximately 1.5
x $\overline{10^6}$ cells per 35-mm well) were stimulated with PDGF at 2.0
units/ml.   PGE$_2$ was quantitated by RIA at the indicated times.
●—●, control + PDGF; O—O, EJ-ras-transformed + PDGF.

This loss of PDGF-stimulated PGE$_2$ biosynthesis is not due
to a loss of cyclo-oxygenase or PGE$_2$ isomerase activity, since
control and EJ-ras cells synthesize equivalent amounts of
PGE$_2$ from arachidonate (7).   Direct HPLC measurements of
PDGF-stimulated phosphoinositide levels show that PDGF induces
a rapid accumulation of IP$_3$ levels in EJ-ras transformed cells
(Figure 2).   These data indicate that mutated ras uncouples
the PDGF receptor from phospholipase C.   Confirmation of this
is found in measurements of intracellular Ca^{2+} levels by fura-2
fluorescence and digital imaging techniques.   In control cells,
PDGF stimulates intracellular Ca^{2+} concentration over a time
course   that   parallels   IP$_3$ synthesis.   However,   EJ-ras
transformed cells show little or no PDGF-stimulated Ca^{2+}
accumulation.   In the few cells that do respond, both the
magnitude and duration of the response diminished when compared
to   the   control   response   (8).   A   normal   consequence   of
PDGF-stimulated phospholipase C activation, IP$_3$ synthesis,
and Ca^{2+} accumulation is the induction of the protooncogene
c-fos.   Figure 3 shows a Northern analysis of c-fos m-RNA
levels in control cells, but not in EJ-ras transformed cells.
Cholera toxin or 8-bromo-cyclic AMP enhance c-fos m-RNA levels
in both cell types.   Thus three measurements of PDGF-stimulated
phospholipase C activity (IP$_3$ generation, Ca^{2+} mobilization,
and c-fos induction) are all blunted in EJ-ras transformed
cells.

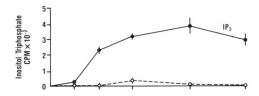

FIG 2. Time course of PDGF-stimulated IP$_3$ synthesis. NIH-3T3 cells were grown in media containing 10 μCi of myo-[^{3}H]inositol. After 24 hrs the cells were washed and challenged with 10 ng/ml PDGF, and [^{3}H]IP$_3$ synthesis quantitated by HPLC. ●—●, control cell IP$_3$ levels, O—O, EJ-<u>ras</u> transformed cell IP$_3$ levels.

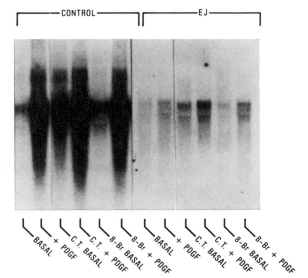

FIG. 3. PDGF-stimulated c-<u>fos</u> m-RNA levels. Control and EJ-<u>ras</u> transformed cells were stimulated with 10 ng/ml PDGF for 30 minutes and c-<u>fos</u> m-RNA quantitated by Northern analysis.

In summary, the transforming activity of mutated <u>ras</u> has now been associated with two vertebrate cellular systems thought to be regulated by G proteins, namely phospholipase and adenylate cyclase. In both cases the enzyme activity is reduced in cells expressing mutated <u>ras</u> at high levels. Since cells expressing c-<u>ras</u> at high levels also exhibited reduced phospholipase and adenylate cyclase activities, we believe that c-<u>ras</u> may normally help modulate systems that are regulated by G proteins and that <u>ras</u> transformation may result from a concerted aberration of guanine-nculeotide-regulated systems.

REFERENCES

1. Tabin CJ, Bradley SM, Bargmann CL, et al. <u>Nature (London)</u> 1982;300:143-149.

2. Reddy EP, Reynold RK, Santo E and Barbacid M. <u>Nature (London)</u> 1982;300:149-152.

3. Taparowski E, Suard Y, Fasano O, Shimizu K, Goldfarb M and Wigler M. <u>Nature (London)</u> 1982;300:762-765.

4. Yuasa Y, Srivastava SK, Dunn CY, Rhim JS, Reddy EP and Aaronson SA. <u>Nature (London)</u> 1983;303:775-779.

5. Bos JL, Toksoz D, Marshall CJ, et al. <u>Nature (London)</u> 1985;315:726-730.

6. Tarpley WG, Hopkins NK and Gorman RR. <u>Proc. Natl. Acad. Sci. USA</u> 1986;83:3703-3707.

7. Benjamin CW, Tarpley WG and Gorman RR. <u>Proc. Natl. Acad. Sci. USA</u> 1987;83:3703-3707.

8. Benjamin CW, Connor JA, Tarpley WG and Gorman RR. <u>Proc. Natl. Acad. Sci. USA</u> 1988;in press.

Advances in Prostaglandin, Thromboxane, and Leukotriene Research, Vol. 19, edited by B. Samuelsson, P. Y.-K. Wong, and F. F. Sun, Raven Press, Ltd., New York ©1989.

CYCLOPENTENONE PROSTAGLANDINS BLOCK CELL CYCLE PROGRESSION IN THE G_1 PHASE AND INDUCE THE G_1-SPECIFIC PROTEINS IN HELA S3 CELLS

Shuh Narumiya, Kouji Ohno, Masanori Fukushima* and Motohatsu Fujiwara

Department of Pharmacology, Kyoto University Faculty of Medicine, Yoshida, Sakyo-ku, Kyoto 606, Japan, and *Department of Internal Medicine, Aichi Cancer Center, Chikusa-ku, Nagoya 464, Japan

PGs of E, A and D series inhibit growth of cultured cells and in some cases induce differentiation (1,2). We showed that PGs of D and E undergo enzymatic dehydration in culture medium containing serum, and that growth inhibition by these PGs are actually caused by the dehydration products, PGJ and PGA, respectively (3,4). Unlike other PGs, cyclopentenone PGs such as PGs A and J do not act on a cell surface receptor. They are actively transported into cells by a specific carrier in the cell membrane and accumulate in cell nuclei (5,6). The cellular uptake and accumulation are well correlated with their growth inhibitory activities(5,7). Then, how does this accumulation of the PGs lead to growth inhibition ? Recently several groups have reported that the cyclopentenone PGs such as PGA_2 and Δ^{12}-PGJ_2 block cell progression from G_1 to S phase of cell cycle (8,9). Induction and suppression of specific proteins in cells treated with cyclopentenone PGs have also been reported (10,11). However, the cell cycle analysis reported so far used the exponentially growing cells, and it is difficult to relate a specific biochemical change with the PG-induced cell cycle arrest in randomly growing cell population. We, therefore, synchronized growth of HeLa S3 cells by serum starvation and analyzed effects of the PGs on cell cycle progression and protein synthesis in these cells (12,13).

INDUCTION OF G_1 BLOCK IN CELL CYCLE

HeLa S3 (CCL2.2) cells were enriched in G_1 phase by culture in the Ham's F-12 medium containing 0.5 % FCS for 84 h. Cells in G_1, S and G_2/M phase of cell cycle were 65, 20 and 15 % of the total cells, respectively. When these cells were supplemented with 10 % FCS, progression into the cell cycle was initiated. As shown in Fig. 1, cells enriched in G_1 phase progressed through the G_1 phase in the first 6 h, moved to the S phase from 6 to 12 h, and then accumulated in the G_2/M phase. To analyze PG effects on progression of G_1 phase cells, Δ^{12}-PGJ$_2$ (12 μM) was added to the culture at 0, 3, 6 and 9 h and cell cycle progression was analyzed at various time points until 24 h. As shown in Fig. 2, when the PG was added at 0 h, the proportion of G_1 phase cells decreased during the first 3 h to the extent as observed in the control cells (Fig. 1). However, no progression of G_1 phase cells was observed during the following incubation. S phase cells, on the other hand, slowly progressed into G_2/M phase and the proportion of S phase cells decreased to 10 % after 24 h. Inhibition of cell progression in G_1 phase was also observed when the PG was added at 3, 6 and 9 h. In each case, the inhibition became apparent about 6 h after the PG addition and the decrease in G_1 phase cells was completely inhibited. However, population of cells which had progressed into the S phase by this time proceeded through S phase and time-dependently accumulated in G_2/M. When 24 μM of PGA$_2$ was added to the cells instead of Δ^{12}-PGJ$_2$, it also inhibited the progression of G_1 phase cells with the time course similar to that observed with Δ^{12}-PGJ$_2$. However, the reversibility of this G_1-block is different between the two PGs. It was examined by exposing cells to the PGs for short time. Either 12 μM Δ^{12}-PGJ$_2$ or 24 μM PGA$_2$ was added at 0 time to G_1-enriched HeLa S3 cells and incubated for 3, 6, 9 or 12 h. The cells were washed and incubated without the PG until 24 h, and cell progression was analyzed. Cell cycle progression was arrested by more than 3 h exposure to Δ^{12}-PGJ$_2$ and scarcely resumed until 24 h. On the contrary, it was resumed in cells exposed to PGA$_2$ about 3 h after the cell wash, and the majority

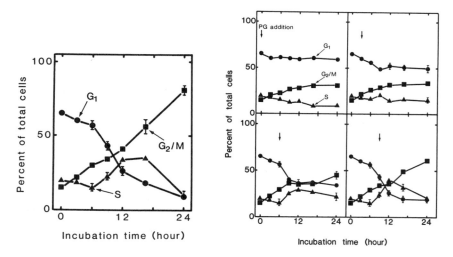

FIG. 1 (left)   Cell cycle progression of control HeLa S3 cells (From ref.12). FIG. 2 (right) Effect of Δ^{12}-PGJ$_2$ on cell cycle progression of HeLa cells. Δ^{12}-PGJ$_2$ (12 uM) was added to the culture at 0, 3, 6 and 9 h as indicated by arrows (From ref.12).

of cells accumulated in G_2/M phase at 24 h. Reversal of PGA_2 effect was also observed after 6 and 9 h treatment of cells with this PG. Thus, the G_1 block by Δ^{12}-PGJ_2 was irreversible, whereas that by PGA_2 was reversible. This difference in reversibility between the two PGs is consistent with that found in their pharmacodynamics in cells we reported previously (7). We have further found that this G_1 block by the PGs is exerted only when the PGs are added to G_1-phase cells and not to cells of other phases of cell cycle (12). In summary, these results suggest that cyclopentenone PGs act specifically in cells in the G_1 phase and induce the block of cell cycle progression at a point in the G_1 phase. From the kinetic analysis, this point appears to lie several hours before the G_1/S boundary.

INDUCTION OF THE G_1-SPECIFIC PROTEINS BY PGs

Since several groups reported induction of proteins by the cyclopentenone PGs (10,11) and protein synthesis inhibitors such as cycloheximide attenuate growth inhibition and cell cycle block by the PGs (12, 14), we analyzed change in protein synthesis in Hela S3 cells synchronized as above and investigated its relation with the PG-induced G_1 block. At various times of cell cycle, cells were washed with PBS and incubated at 37°C for 30 min with 10 µCi [^{35}S]methionine (1,200 Ci/mmol) in 1 ml of methionine-free MEM containing 10% dialyzed serum. After incubation cells were lyzed and labeled lyzates were analyzed by SDS-polyacrylamide gel electrophoresis. Fig. 3 compares the patterns of proteins synthesized in the control and Δ^{12}-PGJ_2-treated cells at various times during incubation. We found that proteins of 68-70 kDa were prominently synthesized in the control cells at 3 and 6 h incubation. The synthesis of these proteins was transient and

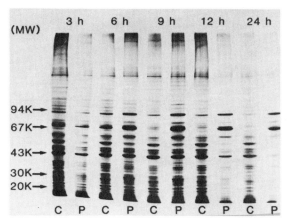

FIG. 3. SDS-polyacrylamide gel electrophoresis of proteins synthesized in control (C) and Δ^{12}-PGJ_2-treated (P) cells at various time of cell cycle.

rapidly decreased during further incubation. Since the majority of cells was in the G_1 phase at 3 and 6 h of incubation as shown in Fig. 1, these results suggest that they were the proteins specifically synthesized in cells at some point in the G_1 phase. Effect of Δ^{12}-PGJ_2 was then examined by adding the PG to cells at 0 h and incubating for 24 h. Under these conditions cell cycle progression was blocked in the G_1 phase. We found that synthesis of 68-70 kDa proteins was markedly elevated in these cells as shown in Fig. 3. This enhancement began at 3 h and continued until 24 h. When we compared these proteins with those transiently expressed in the G_1 phase of the control cells by two dimensional polyacrylamide gel electrophoresis, they overlaped each other, indicating that they were identical (13). Induction of these proteins by the cyclopentenone PGs was closely associated with the PG-induced G_1-block in terms of reversibility and sensitivity described above. In addition, when either cycloheximide or actinomycin D was added, they suppressed induction of these proteins and attenuated the G_1-block (13). Thus, these PG-induced proteins may play some functions in the PG-induced block in cell cycle progression. The causative relationship between the two phenomena will be investigated in future study.

REFERENCES

1. Honn KV, Bockman RS, Marnett LJ. Prostaglandins 1981;21:833-864.
2. Fukushima M, Kato T, Ueda R, Ota K, Narumiya S, Hayaishi O. Biochem Biophys Res Commun 1982;105:956-964.
3. Narumiya S, Fukushima M. Biochem Biophys Res Commun 1985;127:739-745.
4. Ohno K, Fujiwara M, Fukushima M, Narumiya S. Biochem Biophys Res Commun 1986;139:808-815.
5. Narumiya S, Fukushima M. J Pharmacol Exp Therap 1986;239:500-505.
6. Narumiya S, Ohno K, Fukushima M, Fujiwara M. J Pharmacol Exp Therap 1986;239:506-511.
7. Narumiya S, Ohno K, Fukushima M, Fujiwara M. J Pharmacol Exp Therap 1987;242:306-311.
8. Hughes-Fulford M, Wu J, Kato T, Fukushima M. In:Hayaishi O, Yamamoto S, eds. Adv. Prostaglandin Thromboxane and Leukotriene Res. vol 15. New York: Raven Press, 1985; 401-404.
9. Bhuyan BK, Adams EG, Badiner GT, Li LH, Barden K. Cancer Res 1986;46:1688-1693.
10. Santoro MG, Jaffe BM, Elia G, Benedetto A. Biochem Biophys Res Commun 1982;107:1179-1184.
11. Santoro MG, Crisari A, Benabente A, Amici C. Cancer Res 1986;46:6073-6077.
12. Ohno K, Sakai T, Fukushima M, Narumiya S, Fujiwara M. J Pharmacol Exp Therp 1988;245:in press
13. Ohno K, Fukushima M, Narumiya S, Fujiwara M. submitted
14. Shimizu Y, Todo S, Imashuku S. Prostaglandins 1986;32:517-525

Advances in Prostaglandin, Thromboxane, and Leukotriene Research, Vol. 19, edited by B. Samuelsson, P. Y.-K. Wong, and F. F. Sun, Raven Press, Ltd., New York ©1989.

PROSTAGLANDIN A AND J: ANTITUMOR AND ANTIVIRAL PROSTAGLANDINS

M. Fukushima[1], T. Kato[1], S. Narumiya[2], Y. Mizushima[3], H. Sasaki[4], Y. Terashima[4], Y. Nishiyama[5], and M.G. Santoro[6]

[1]Aichi Cancer Center, Nagoya 464, [2]Faculty of Med. Kyoto Univ., Kyoto 606, [3]St. Marianna Univ. School of Med., Kawasaki 213, [4]Jikei Univ. School of Med., Tokyo 105, [5]Nagoya Univ. School of Med., Nagoya 466, Japan, [6]Inst. Exp. Med., C.N.R., II Univ. of Rome, 00173 Rome, Italy

Summary

Prostaglandin(PG)s of the A and J series are categorized as antitumor, antiviral PGs. They have a reactive α, β -unsaturated carbonyl in the cyclopentenone ring, which could be the active moiety. They are actively incorporated into cells and in part transferred to the nuclei, and lead to cell cycle arrest at G1 or cell death depending on the dose.

Introduction

In the past, many investigators reported that PGE1,2 and PGD2 have antitumor activity, however, it is now believed that such activity is exclusively ascribed to their ultimate metabolites, PGA1,2 and Δ12-PGJ2, respectively. This paper overviews the research and describes new findings concerning actions of PGA and PGJ.

Chemistry and the mode of action of PGA and PGJ

In 1982, Fukushima and his collegues found that PGD2 is dehydrated to 9-deoxy-Δ9-PGD2 in aqueous solution (1). This new PG species was named PGJ2, since PGJ2 is a new cyclopentenon type PG. Following this discovery, they found that in serum or

Fig.1. Formation of PGJ2 and Δ12-PGJ2 from PGD2.

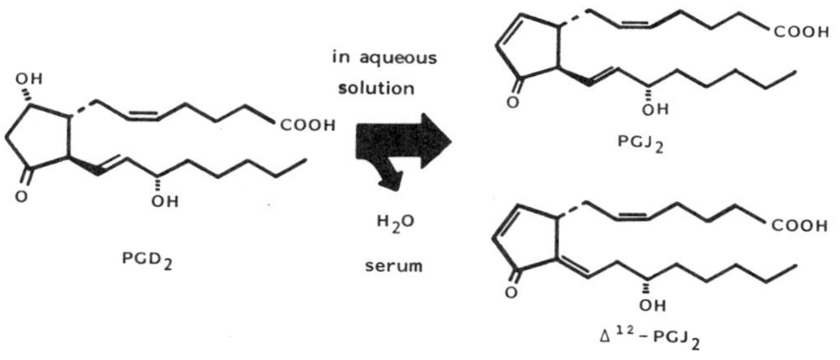

plasma, PGD2 is converted to Δ12-PGJ2 (2)(Fig. 1). Thus,
PGD2, as PGE2, undergoes dehydration in plasma or serum-con-
taining culture medium, and Δ12-PGJ2 and PGA2 are the active
ultimate compounds, respectively (3,4). PGA, PGJ, and Δ12-
PGJ have α, β-unsaturated carbonyl which is chemically very
reactive to form Michael adducts and could be related to their
unique pharmacodynamics and biochemical actions. As mentioned
above, Δ12-PGJ2 occurs in nature, whereas Δ7-PGA itself is
not reported to occur naturally, but acetoxy-derivatives of
Δ7-PGA1, 2 such as clavulone and punaglandin have been isolated from some octocorals (5).   Δ7-PGA1 and Δ12-PGJ2 have
an alkylidene-cyclopentenone which is more reactive than cyclopentenone, and they have potent antitumor(6) and antiviral activity (7) as mentioned later. Thus, the structure of 5-member
ring and adjacent double bonds in the α and ω chains appears
to be strictly related to the activity, while the -OH group in
C15 is not (6).   According to a comparative study using punaglandin and its analogues such as 10-Cl, 12-OH- Δ7-PGA1, 12-
OH- Δ7-PGA1 and 10-Cl- Δ7-PGA1, it was found that the cytotoxicity of Δ7-PGA1 is potentiated by introductions of -Cl and
-OH into C10 and C12, respectively (5)(Fig. 2).

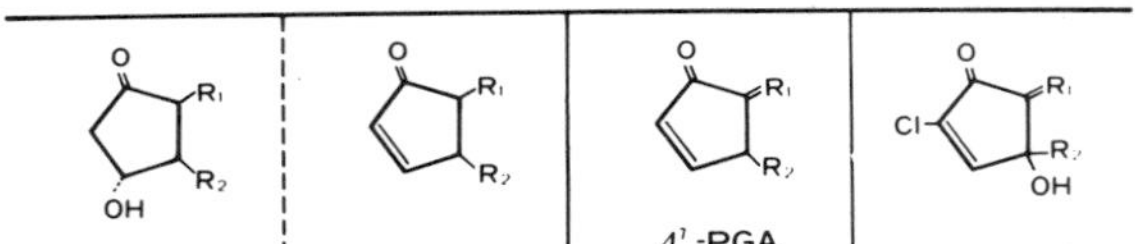

Fig.2.
Structure activity
relationship of
antitumor prosta-
glandins and
PG-derivatives.

	PGE, D	PGA, J	Δ^1-PGA, Δ^{12}-PGJ	Punaglandin
IC$_{50}$ (μg/ml)	2~5	0.7	0.3	0.03
Relative Cytotoxicity	1	5	10	100

    The prominent actions of PGA and J are cytotoxicity and cell
cycle arrest-inducing activity. Such PGs inhibit cell growth a
time and dose dependent manner. At a dose which induce 50% inhibition of cell growth, cells arrest in G1 phase (8). This
G1-arresting action also has the same structural requirements
as cytotoxicity. It should be emphasized that cyclopentenone
PGs and alkylidene-cyclopentenone PGs are quite different in
the reversibility of the action. When we looked at the action
of PGA2 and Δ12-PGJ2 on cell cycle, it was found that G1 arrest by PGA2 is reversed by washing, whereas that by Δ12-PGJ2
is not (9), indicating that the number of enones in the molecule is related to the reversibility of the action. In 1986,
we demonstrated that PGA2 and Δ12-PGJ2 are actively incorporated into cells (10): their uptake into cells reaches a peak
within few minutes and then declines due to the function of the
efflux system for PGs (11). Furthermore, strikingly they are
transferred to the nuclei, where particularly Δ12-PGJ2 binds
to nucleoproteins and is not released by washing, as PGA2 (12).

Antitumor activity

Although the pharmacological merit of PGs as antitumor agent is still unclear, the antitumor effect of PGD2 or J2 has been demonstrated using more than 40 human malignant cells including colonogenic assays in vitro and in vivo. Taking account of the pharmacodynamics and the higher sensitivity for such PGs, $\Delta 7$-PGA1 analogues which have more potent activity than PGA1 in vitro are now under preclinical investigation using nude mice, bearing human tumors such as ovarian cancer, neuroblastoma or melanoma. PGA1 effectively inhibited tumor growth of human melanoma inoculated subcutaneously into nude mice (13). Antitumor activity of PGs primarily depends on the structure of the 5-member ring; however, recently we have demonstrated that the lipophilic character of the side chains also contribute to cytotoxicity (14). Although the derivatives with larger log P value showed more potent cytotoxicity in vitro, a derivative with lower log P value showed greater antitumor activity in mouse P388 leukemia in vivo (14). We also studied the effect of lipid microsphere-integrated $\Delta 7$-PGA1 comparing with free $\Delta 7$-PGA1 and showed that in several tumor systems the former drug is more effective (15). Based on these results and from a view-point of drug delivery, sugar-conjugates are now under investigation.

Antiviral activity

Antiviral activity of PGA1,2 was first described by Santoro et al. in 1980 (16). Recently, again they demonstrated that PGJ2 also have potent antiviral activity on Sendai and herpes simplex Ⅱ viruses (HSV Ⅱ)(17,18). Following this study, antiviral activity of $\Delta 7$-PGA1 and $\Delta 12$-PGJ2 was studied in comparison with PGA1, PGJ2 and their parent molecule and we found that the above mentioned structure-activity relationship also exist for antiviral activity (7). Furthermore in experiments using HSV Ⅱ, it was found that such PGs inhibit primarily early synthesis of viral RNA (7). Topical use of PG resulted in marked suppression of viral production in HSV Ⅱ-infected mice. However, at the present, systemic use of this drug does not yield any selectivity.

Perspectives

Very recently Itoh et al. demonstrated $\Delta 12$-PGJ2 in human urine (Itoh S., personal communication). This fact suggest that $\Delta 12$-PGJ2 occurs in human body fluid physiologically. The hypothesis that PGA and J play a role in the regulation of cell cycle and defence mechanisms of cells against viral infections are of current interest.

References

1.   Fukushima M, Kato T, Ota K, Arai Y, Narumiya S, Hayaishi

0. Biochem Biophys Res Comm 1982;109:626-633.

2. Kikawa Y, Narumiya S, Fukushima M, Wakatsuka H, Hayaishi O. Proc Natl Acad Sci USA 1984;81:1317-1321.

3. Narumiya S, Fukushima M. Biochem Biophys Res Comm 1985; 127:739-745.

4. Ohno K, Fujiwara M, Fukushima M, Narumiya S. Biochem Biophys Res Comm 1986;139:808-815.

5. Fukushima M, Kato T. Adv Prostaglandin thromboxane and Leukotriene Res 1985;15:415-418.

6. Kato T, Fukushima M, Kurozumi S, Noyori R. Cancer Res 1986;46:3538-3542.

7. Yamamoto N, Fukushima M, Tsurumi T, Maeno K, Nishiyama Y. Biochem Biophys Res Comm 1987;146:1425-1431.

8. Hughes-Fulford M, Wu J, Kato T, Fukushima M. Adv Prostaglandin Thromboxane and Leukotriene Res 1985;15:401-404.

9. Ohno K, Sakai T, Fukushima M, Narumiya S, Fujiwara M. J Pharmacol Exp Ther 1988 (in press).

10. Narumiya S, Fukushima M. J Pharmacol Exp Ther 1986;239: 500-505.

11. Narumiya S, Ohno K, Fujiwara M, Fukushima M. J Pharmacol Exp Ther 1986;239:506-511.

12. Narumiya S, Ohno K, Fukushima M, Fujiwara M. J Pharmacol Exp Ther 1987;242:306-311.

13. Bregman MD, Funk C, Fukushima M. Cancer Res 1986;46: 2740-2744.

14. Fukushima M, Suzumura Y, Kato T, Hazato A, Kurozumi S. Proc Amer Assoc Cancer Res 29 abstract no.1307, 1988.

15. Mizushima Y, Shoji Y, Kato T, Fukushima M, Kurozumi S. J Pharm Pharmacol 1986;38:132-134.

16. Santoro MG, Benedetto A, Carruba G, Garaci E, Jaffe BM. Science 1980;209:1032-1034.

17. Santoro MG, Fukushima M, Benedetto A, Amici C. J Gen Virol 1987;68:1153-1158.

18. Santoro MG. In: Garaci E, Paoletti R, Santoro MG, eds. Prostaglandins in Cancer Res Heidelberg:Springer-Verlag, 1987;97-114.

Advances in Prostaglandin, Thromboxane, and Leukotriene Research, Vol. 19, edited by B. Samuelsson, P. Y.-K. Wong, and F. F. Sun, Raven Press, Ltd., New York ©1989.

EFFECTS OF PROSTAGLANDIN E_2 ON

PHENOTYPE OF OSTEOBLASTS-LIKE CELLS

I. Morita, K. Toriyama, and S. Murota

Department of Physiological Chemistry, Tokyo Medical and Dental University, Yushima, Tokyo-113, Japan

Bone metabolism is regulated by two kinds of cells, osteo-blasts and osteoclasts. These cells have been interacted on each other by coupling factors produced by both cells. The origin of osteoblasts has been recognized to be mesenchymal cells and osteo-blasts are further differentiated into osteocytes. The progeni-tors of osteoclasts may be thought CFU-GM (colony forming unit in granulocyte-macrophages) and pre-osteoclasts. Pre-osteoclasts are fused to osteoclasts, which are multi-nucleated cells. Pre-vious investigators have reported that PGE_2 stimulates bone resorp-tion both in vitro (1) and in vivo (2). It has been also reported bone resorption mediated by endogenous PGE_2 formation has been shown in response to several stimuli in organ culture (3).

In the present paper, we will determine the effects of PGE_2 on the proliferation and differentiation of osteoblasts and osteo-clasts. We will show the possible mechanisms for the effects of PGE_2.

PG production in osteoblasts

Osteoblast-like cells, MC 3T3-E_1, which was established by Kodama et al.(4), were cultured with 10% FBS containing α-MEM. Characteristics of the cells are follows ; growing in multi-layers, having high alkaline phosphatase, showing calcification in vitro, etc. Therefore, the cells have been used as a good model for studying differentiation processes with bone formation in vitro. First, we examined the synthesizing activity of PGs in cell-free system. The main product was PGE_2 and minor ones were PGI_2 and 12-HETE. The synthesizing activity of PGE_2 was gradually reduced with culture and at 40 days in culture (late stage) the synthesi-zing activity was about 1/10 of that at 10-day culture (early stage) (Fig. 1). To shorten the experimental time, we used α-glycerophosphate Ca salt. The cells cultured with α-glycerophos-phate Ca salt mineralized even at 14-day culture. The dose depen-dency of this drug was shown in Fig. 2. Therefore, following exper-

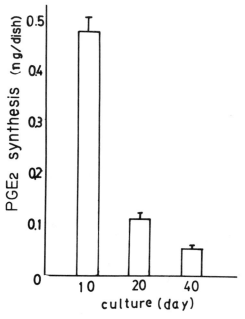

Fig. 1

Change of PGE$_2$ synthesizing activity in MC 3T3-E$_1$ with cultured period.

iments were carried out containing α-glycerophosphate. It was interesting that the PGE$_2$ synthesizing activity may be related to arachidonic acid content in phospholipids in cell membrane. That is, the ratio of arachidonic acid to all fatty acids in the phospholipids was very low in the early stage of culture and the ratio increased gradually as a mirror image of PGE$_2$ synthesis.

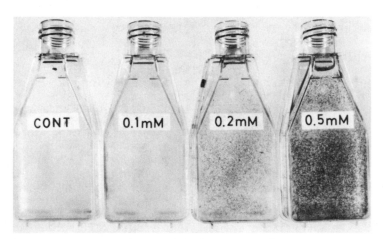

Fig. 2. Effect of α-glycerophosphate Ca salt on calcification in MC 3T3-E$_1$.

Effects of endogenous and exogenous
PGE_2 on the phenotype of osteoblasts

Since MC3T3-E_1 cells had high capacity for PGE_2 synthesis as above mentioned, we studied the effects of PGE_2 on the phenotype of osteoblasts. In the early stage of the culture, indomethacin suppressed the proliferation and addition of 3 μM of PGE_2-to the culture stimulated the proliferation of the cells. In the late stage of the culture, the cells differentiated to osteocytes and mineralized (calcification). In this stage, if the PGE_2 synthesis was blocked by indomethacin, the appearance of the mineral crystal was stimulated. On the contrary, the addition of 3 μM of PGE_2 suppressed the mineralization completely.

These data suggest that PGE_2 stimulates cell proliferation and inhibits cell differentiation in osteoblasts.

Mechanism of the stimulatory effect
of PGE_2 on the proliferation of osteoblasts

Next, we tried to evaluate the mechanism of the stimulatory effect of PGE_2 on the proliferation of osteoblasts. As cAMP could not mediate the proliferation, we measured cytosolic free Ca^{++} level. Elevation of cytosolic free Ca^{++} is considered to stimulate proliferation through the activation of calmodulin. Cytosolic free Ca^{++} was measured with fura-2. The level of cytosolic free Ca^{++} was about 10^{-7}M at resting cells. PGE_2-treatment induced dose-dependent increase in Ca^{++} and 6 μM of PGE_2 it reached 7×10^{-7}M. Next, the change in the effect of PGE_2 on the elevation of cytosolic free Ca^{++} was examined during culture (Fig. 3). The cells on 3 and 4 days after inoculation were the most sensitive to PGE_2.

At the early stage of culture cells produced much more PGE_2 and they were most sensitive to PGE_2. These results suggest endogenous PGE_2 regulating proliferation of osteoblasts.

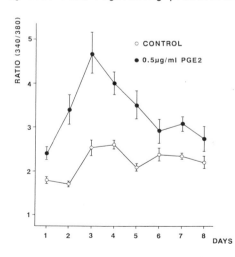

Fig. 3

Effect in the effect of PGE_2 on the elevation of cytosolic free Ca^{++} in MC3T3-E_1

Effect of PGE₂ on differentiation toward osteoclasts (5)

Effect of PGE₂ on differentiation of stem cells into osteoclasts was examined. We used mouse bone marrow cells and they
were cultured for 8 days with or without several PGs. The formation of multi-nucleated osteoclasts were found in this system,
and PGE₂ was the most strong promotor for differentiation among
PGs tested. At the same time, we measured cAMP level. The
potency of the PGs in inducing osteoclasts was highly correlated
with the cAMP inducing capacity of the PGs. Addition of dibutyryl
cAMP to the bone marrow culture also induced osteoclasts formation.
These data suggest that PGE₂ promotes osteoclasts formation
by a mechanism involving cAMP.

CONCLUSION

As shown in Fig. 4, several stimuli to bone metabolism will
act on osteoblasts and let them produce PGE₂. Released PGE₂, in
turn, will affect progenitor cells of osteoclasts and promote
their differentiation into osteoclasts.

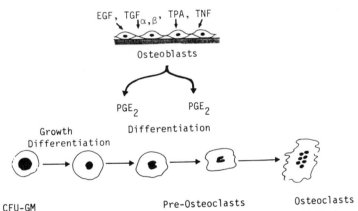

Fig. 4. Hypothetical scheme for the action of stimuli on bone

REFERENCES

1. Raisz LG, Vanderhoek JY, Simmons HA et al. Prostaglandins,1979;
   17:905-914.
2. Goodson JM, McClatchy K, Revell C. J.Dent.Res.1974,53:670-677.
3. Tashjian AH, Levine L. Biochem.Biophys.Res.Commun.1978;85:
   966-975.
4. Kodama H, Amagai H, Sudo S. et al., Jap.J.Oral.Biol. 1981,23:
   899-901.
5. Akatsu T, Takahashi N, Morita I. et al. to be submitted.

Advances in Prostaglandin, Thromboxane, and Leukotriene Research, Vol. 19, edited by B. Samuelsson, P. Y.-K. Wong, and F. F. Sun, Raven Press, Ltd., New York ©1989.

ROLE OF PROSTAGLANDINS IN DIFFERENTIATION
OF GROWTH PLATE CHONDROCYTES

Mary Lynn S. Kemick, Jia E. Chin* and Roy E. Wuthier
Department of Chemistry,
University of South Carolina, Columbia, SC 29208
*E.I. DuPont Co., Glenolden, PA 19036

While prostaglandins (PG) are known to inhibit synthesis of sulfated proteoglycans (1), to stimulate degeneration of the extracellular matrix in **articular** cartilage (2), and have been implicated in the development of lesions in inflammatory arthritis (3), little is known of their action on **growth plate** cartilage. That prostanoids may be involved in growth plate differentiation stems from early work demonstrating progressive increase in phospholipase A_2 activity down the growth plate (4). Subsequent isolation of PGB_1 from growth plate cartilage (5), and demonstration of high levels of PG synthetase and degradative activity by Wong (6) fueled further interest in this area. Later, Northington (7) showed that PGE_2, PGD_2 and $PGF_2\alpha$ were synthesized by growth plate cartilage microsomes. Chondrogenesis in embryonic tissues also has been associated with PGE_2 (8). Current studies were aimed at defining the role of PG in the development and differentiation of growth plate chondrocytes.

MATERIALS AND METHODS

Growth plate chondrocytes were isolated from the proliferative and hypertrophic region of the tibia of 8-10 week old broiler-type chickens and cultured as previously described (9). Cells were gradually changed to a serum-free medium after confluency. On day 21 of culture and thereafter, the cells were fed 100% serum-free DMEM. The serum-free medium had been previously shown to maintain viable chondrocytes under the defined conditions of culture (10). For administration to cultures, PG and arachidonate were dissolved in ethanol, added to sterile solution of bovine serum albumin (0.1 mg/ml), lyophilized, and redissolved in DMEM. Indomethacin was dissolved in DMEM and filter-sterilized. ECF was expressed from cartilage slices according to the method of Hubbard (11). Slices of growth plate cartilage were collected in ice-cold synthetic cartilage fluid (12) containing indomethacin (1 mM) to block further PG synthesis. PG levels in the ECF were assessed by RIA using assay kits from New England Nuclear (Boston, MA).

RESULTS

Expression of **AP** by hypertrophic chondrocytes was affected in a biphasic manner, each PG tested causing graded stimulation of AP activity (Fig. 1A). Maximal effect (191% and 266%) seen at 10^{-14}M with PGD_2 and PGE_1, and at 10^{-12}M with PGE_2, higher levels causing decreases in activity. Stimulation of AP could be blocked by cycloheximide, indicating protein synthesis was required. Differential effects on **cell division** were also seen with the various PG (Fig. 1B). PGE_2 and PGD_2 were both stimulatory to ^{3}H-thymidine incorporation, showing maximal effect at 10^{-12}M and 10^{-8}M, respectively; whereas PGE_1 was inhibitory with maximal effect at 10^{-14}M. While inhibition of cell division by PGE_1 was correlated with suppression of polyphosphoinositide synthesis, studies with Li^+ and neomycin indicate that inhibition of the phosphatidylinositol cycle stimulates cellular AP expression.

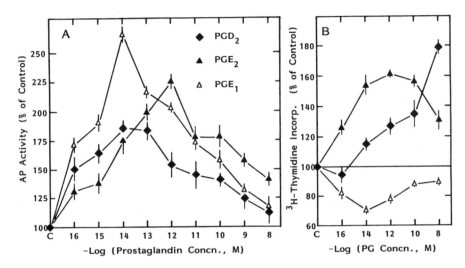

Fig. 1A. Effect of PG on cellular   Fig. 1B. Effect of PG on
AP Activity.   cell division.

Indomethacin, at levels inhibitory to cyclooxygenase activity, blocked AP stimulation produced by PGE_2 and PGE_1 (Fig. 2), indicating that further PG synthesis in response to PG administration must be involved.

Analyses of ECF from the proliferative and hypertrophic zones of growth plate cartilage revealed high levels of PGE, 6-keto $PGF_1\alpha$ and thromboxane B_2 (TXB_2) (Table I). Highest levels of the latter prostanoids were seen in ECF from the proliferative zone.

TABLE I
Levels of Prostanoids in Growth Plate Cartilage ECF

Prostanoid	Growth Plate Zone	
	Proliferative	Hypertrophic
	(nmol/L)	
PGE[a]	2.11 ± 0.68	1.71 ± 0.28
6-Keto $PGF_1\alpha$	7.66 ± 1.89	2.98 ± 0.56
TXB_2	12.00 ± 2.39	3.62 ± 0.58

[a] RIA cannot distinguish PGE_1 from PGE_2.

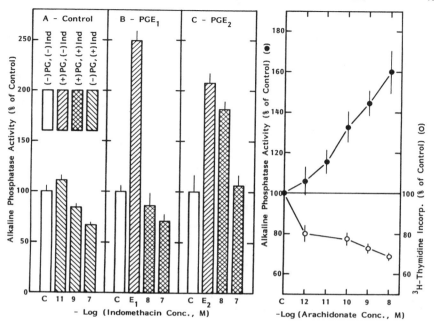

Fig. 2. Effect of indomethacin on PG-stimulation of AP expression.

Fig. 3. Effect of arachidonate on cell AP and cell division.

DISCUSSION

While past work had shown high levels of phospholipase A_2 (4) and PG synthetase activity (6) in growth plate tissue, the present studies demonstrate for the first time that **growth plate** chondrocytes are exquisitely sensitive to exogenous PG. Significant increases in cellular AP levels were seen at PG levels as low as 10^{-16}M. In fact, the various PG classes tested differentially affected both cell division (as measured by ^{3}H-thymidine incorporation) and differentiation (as indicated by AP activity and matrix vesicle formation), but had minimal effect on protein synthesis. Thus, the effects seen were highly selective.

The importance of using serum-free media in studies with growth plate chondrocytes is shown by the fact that <u>fmolar</u> levels of PGE_1 and PGD_2 strongly effected the cells. Thus, although serum contains very low levels of PGE_2 (10^{-13} M), maximal stimulation of AP activity was seen well below this level with both PGE_1 and PGD_2.

The biphasic response of the chondrocytes to the different PG classes (Fig. 1), with progressively lowered AP activity at the higher PG levels, suggests that PG desensitized the cells. Down-regulation of PG receptors has been seen in hepatocytes exposed to high levels of a PG analog (13). The marked differences in cellular response to the different PG classes suggest that separate receptors for PGE_1 and PGE_2 exist in growth plate cells, as has been observed in other cell types (14).

The high levels of 6-keto $PGF_1\alpha$, TXB_2, and PGE found in cartilage ECF also support a role for prostanoids in growth plate development. While these levels are over 1000-fold above that found to maximally stimulate chondrocyte activity (Fig. 1), trauma to the tissue during collection of the ECF must have raised levels well above normal values of PG, even though indomethacin was used to block synthesis. Surprisingly, careful analysis of the fatty acids of growth plate phospholipids has revealed little arachidonate or omega-6 eicosatrienoate precursors of PG. This and the discovery of the omega-9 eicosatrienoate as the dominant polyunsaturate, indicate that growth plate cartilage is deficient in PG precursor fatty acids. This finding may explain the extreme sensitivity of growth plate cells to added PG.

REFERENCES

1. Lipiello L, Yamamoto K, Robinson D, Mankin HJ Arth Rheum 1978; 21: 909-917.

2. Fulkerson JP, Ladenbauer-Bellis IM, Chrisman OD Arth Rheum 1979; 22: 1117-1126.

3. Robinson DR, Levine L. In: Robinson HJ, Vane JR, eds. Prostaglandin Synthetase Inhibitors, New York: Raven Press, 1974; 223-228.

4. Wuthier RE Clin Orthop 1973; 90: 191-200; Stillo, JV PhD Thesis, Univ. of S. Carolina, Columbia, 1980; 75-79.

5. Wong PYK, Wuthier RE Prostaglandins 1974; 8: 125-132.

6. Wong PYK, Majeska RJ, Wuthier RE Prostaglandins 1977; 14:839-851.

7. Northington FK, Oglesby TD, Ishikawa Y, Wuthier RE Calcif Tiss Res 1978; 26: 227-236.

8. Chepenik KP, Ho WC, Waite BM, Parker CL Calcif Tiss Int 1984; 36: 175-181; Parker CL, Biddulph DM, Ballard TA Calcif Tiss Int 1981; 33: 641-648.

9. Wuthier RE, Chin JE, Hale JE, Register TC, Hale LV, Ishikawa Y J Biol Chem 1985; 260: 15972-15979.

10. Hale LV, Hale JE, Kemick MLS, Ishikawa Y, Wuthier RE In Vitro 1986; 22: 597-603.

11. Hubbard HL PhD Thesis, Univ. of S. Carolina, Columbia, 1984; 8-10.

12. Majeska RJ, Wuthier RE Biochim Biophys Acta 1975; 391: 51-60.

13. Garrity MJ, Andreasen TJ, Storm DR, Robertson RP J Biol Chem 1983; 258: 8692-8697.

14. Kuehl FA, Humes JL, Tarnoff J, Cirillo VJ, Ham EA Science 169: 883-886.

Advances in Prostaglandin, Thromboxane, and Leukotriene Research, Vol. 19, edited by B. Samuelsson, P. Y.-K. Wong, and F. F. Sun, Raven Press, Ltd., New York ©1989.

CYCLO-OXYGENASE INHBITORS AND CELL KILLING BY CYTOTOXIC DRUGS

A. Bennett, J.D. Gaffen and E. Chambers

Dept Surgery, King's College School of Medicine and Dentistry, The Rayne Institute, 123 Coldharbour Lane, London, SE5 9NU, UK.

Our experiments on prostaglandins (PGs) and human mammary cancer (1) led us to study PG synthesis and the murine NC carcinoma. Flurbiprofen or indomethacin (INDO) prolonged the survival of the host mice and potentiated the anticancer effect of the cytotoxic drugs methotrexate (MTX) plus melphalan (2). This beneficial interaction with INDO also occurs when MTX is used without melphalan, both in vivo and in vitro, and INDO appears to increase the retention or uptake of MTX by NC isolated cancer cells (3).

The possibility that INDO potentiates MTX by inhibiting PG formation is in doubt since the cyclo-oxgenase inhibitor flurbiprofen did not potentiate MTX. Aims of the present experiments were to determine whether (a) another PG synthesis inhibitor, piroxicam, affects the response of NC cells to MTX, (b) PGE_2 counteracts the effect of INDO on MTX uptake, (c) INDO increases the response of NC cells to the unrelated cytotoxic drug melphalan, and (d) whether INDO alters the effect of MTX on human malignant cells.

MATERIALS AND METHODS

Cells and cell culture. All culture media contained penicillin and streptomycin each 50 units/mL. NC cancer cells, obtained from a mouse with peritoneal metastases (3), were maintained as a suspension in MEM containing 10% newborn bovine serum (NBS), L-glutamine 292mg/L, and 1% nonessential amino acids (Flow Laboratories). DU4475 human breast cancer cells were maintained as a suspension in RPMI 1640 containing 5% NBS and L-glutamine 300mg/L. T47D human breast cancer cells were grown as monolayers in DMEM containing 10% NBS and L-glutamine 584 mg/mL. LoVo human colon cancer cells were cultured as monolayers in Ham's F-12 medium plus 15% NBS and L-glutamine 146mg/mL. Monolayers of LS174T human colon cancer cells were grown in the type of medium used for the NC cells.

Drugs. These were dissolved as follows: indomethacin in water containing $NaHCO_3$ (final pH 7.8); piroxicam (Pfizer) and melphalan (Burroughs Wellcome) in 70% ethanol; methotrexate (Lederle) in 154 mM NaCl adjusted to pH 8.4 with 0.1M NaOH; PGE_2 in ethanol and diluted as necessary in phosphate buffered saline pH 7.4 (pbs). All water was double-distilled in glass, and the solutions were sterilised by filtration.

Determination of cell growth. For both NC and DU4475 cells, growth in suspension was determined by microturbidimetry (4). Cells were pelleted by centrifugation, resuspended in 1mL trypsin/ EDTA solution (0.05%: 0.02% w/v) and incubated for 30 s at 37°C. After rapidly adding 9 mL medium, the cells were gently disaggregated by repeated pipetting. The cell numbers were adjusted so that 100µl contained 25,000 NC cells or 100,000 DU4475 cells. 100 or 200µl of medium containing drugs at x2 or x1.5 the desired final concentration (NC cells and DU4475 cells respectively), or vehicle only were added to each of the 96 wells of a microtest plate, followed by 100µl of the cell suspension or medium alone. The plates were incubated at 37°C, 5% CO_2 in humidified air, and after 4 days the transmission of 600 nm light in each well was determined with a Dynatech microplate reader.

Growth of the T47D, LoVo and LS174T cells was determined by dye uptake (5). Each well of a 96-well plastic micro-test plate received 100µl growth medium + vehicle or drugs at twice the desired final concentration. The cell monolayers, were detached by treatment with trypsin/ EDTA solution (0.5: 0.02% w/v), counted (Coulter counter), and diluted in growth medium so that 100µl contained 12,000 T47D cells, 6000 LoVo cells or 10,000 LS174T cells. 100µl of cell suspension (or medium only for blanks) were added to each well, and the plates were incubated at 37°C, 5% CO_2 in humidified air. After 4 days (7 for the T47D cells) the medium was removed, leaving the cells attached to the plastic. After adding 100µl of 10% formol saline to each well for 15 min, the fixative was replaced with 100µl stain (crystal violet 0.5% in 154mM saline) which was removed after 15 min. The plates were washed twice with distilled water, dried in air, and the stain in the cells eluted with 100µl acidified methanol (5 drops 1M HCl to 100 mL methanol). The amount of dye, which depends on the number of cells, was estimated by measuring the absorbance through each well at 600 nm using a Dynatech microplate reader. Growth curves were obtained for each cell line with appropriate concentrations of MTX (see later) alone or with INDO 1µg/mL, and with melphalan ± INDO 1.2 µg/mL using NC cells.

Methotrexate accumulation studies. 'MTX accumulation' was studied with a method modified from Henderson et al (6). NC cells (2×10^6; 1.8mL medium in glass centrifuge tubes) were pre-incubated for 15 min at 37°C under the conditions described previously, with drugs or vehicle only. Radiolabelled MTX (0.2mL of 20µM [3',5',7' ^{3}H]-MTX sodium salt, 250mCi/mmol, Amersham, UK) in pbs was then added to each tube and the cells incubated at 37°C for 1hr with either INDO 1µg/mL, PGE_2 1µg/mL, both substances together or vehicle alone. Identical control samples were placed in an ice/water bath 5 min before and during incubation with the isotope. The cell suspensions were washed twice with ice-cold pbs (8 mL and then 10mL), and centrifuged at 700 x g and 1900 x g respectively for 5 min at 4°C. The cell pellets were suspended in

1mL distilled water, and transferred to glass counting vials using 2 aliquots of scintillation fluid (final volume 10mL). Active accumulation of label was taken as the difference in the radioactivity between the experimental and control samples. There were at least 5 experiments in each part of the study.

RESULTS

1. Piroxicam effect on MTX cytotoxicity in NC cancer cells. MTX 5-15 ng/mL concentration-relatedly reduced NC cell growth, as measured by microturbidimetry. Although the growth was somewhat further reduced with piroxicam 1µg/mL + MTX ($P<0.02$ for overall mean difference), this was probably because of an additive effect with piroxicam, and not a potentiation as seen with INDO. When used alone, piroxicam 1µg/mL reduced cell growth by 14% ($P<0.02$).

2. PGE_2 effect on MTX accumulation in NC cells. When NC cells were incubated with [3H]-MTX for 60 min, INDO 1µg/mL increased the mean accumulation of label by 50% compared to the control ($P<0.025$). With INDO + PGE_2 (both 1µg/mL) the mean increase was 55% higher than the control ($P<0.005$), but similar to that with INDO alone ($P<0.8$). PGE_2 1µg/mL alone had little or no effect on the [^{3}H] accumulation.

3. INDO effect on melphalan toxicity in NC cells. Melphalan 0.06-12.2µg/mL decreased NC cell growth in a concentration-related fashion. INDO 1.2µg/mL alone had little or no effect on cell growth, and it did not alter the cytotoxicity of melphalan.

4. MTX/INDO in human breast cancer cells. MTX concentration-relatedly reduced the growth of both human breast cancer cell lines (2.5-10ng/mL and 25-100 ng/mL repectively for the DU4475 and T47D cells). INDO 1µg/mL alone had little or no effect on the growth of either cell line, but it increased the cytotoxicity of MTX by 6.8-20.5% for the DU4475 cells and by 2-14% for the T47D cells ($P<0.001$ and $P<0.005$ respectively, overall mean difference).

5. MTX/INDO human colon cancer cells. INDO 1µg/mL alone had little or no effect on the growth of either cell line. The LoVo cells were refractory even to high concentrations of MTX (2.5-10µg/mL), and this was not altered by INDO. In contrast, MTX 5-20 ng/mL reduced the growth of LS174T cells in a concentration-related fashion, but as with the LoVo cells INDO 1µg/mL had little or no effect on the response.

DISCUSSION

These results confirm our previous finding (3) that the beneficial interaction between the cytotoxic drug combination MTX/melphalan and INDO on the survival of mice with NC tumours may be explained by the interaction between INDO and just the MTX component. Our previous work showed that INDO potentiated MTX when used without melphalan, and we have now shown that INDO does not interact with melphalan on NC cells in vitro.

When L1210 cells were incubated with $[^3H]$-MTX, PGE_2 inhibited the accumulation of label possibly by stimulating adenylate cyclase (6). It would therefore follow logically that INDO could increase MTX accumulation by inhibiting PGE_2 formation. However, it was not clear from our previous work that the interaction of INDO with MTX involves inhibition of PG synthesis; flurbiprofen had little or no effect on MTX cytotoxicity to NC cells (3), and exogenous PGE_2 at most partially counteracted the INDO-induced increase in accumulation of tritium when NC cells were incubated with $[^3H]$-MTX (7). Our present experiments clearly indicate that PGE_2 does not counteract the effect of INDO, and the unrelated cyclo-oxygenase inhibitor piroxicam is similarly ineffective. This strengthens the evidence that INDO does not potentiate MTX just by inhibiting PG synthesis; one or more of its other actions (including inhibition of protein kinases, calcium binding and phosphodiesterase) may be involved. However, we cannot rule out cyclo-oxygenase inhibition as at least part of the mechanism, since we studied only PGE_2 versus INDO, and the anti-inflammatory drugs may differ in their PG synthesis inhibition and diversion of substrate metabolism into lipoxygenase products.

INDO increased the cytotoxicity of MTX to the human breast cancer cell lines, but not to the colon cancer cell lines which in this respect resemble the normal epithelial cells from human intestine (3). INDO may therefore increase the MTX effect in breast cancer, without increasing the problem of damage to the gut epithelium.

We thank the King's Joint Research Committee, the CRC, MRC and AICR for support.

REFERENCES

1. Bennett A, Charlier EM, McDonald AM, Simpson JS, Stamford IF, Zebro T. Lancet 1977;ii:624-6

2. Bennett A, Berstock DA, Carroll MA. Br J Cancer 1982;45:762-8

3. Bennett A, Gaffen JD, Melhuish PB, Stamford IF. Br J Pharmacol 1987; 91:229-35

4. Gaffen JD, Bennett A, Barer MR. J Pharm Pharmacol 1985;37:261-3

5. Barer MR, Lyon H, Drasar BS. Histochem J 1987;18:122-8

6. Henderson GB, Zevely EM, Huennekens FM. Cancer Res 1987;38:859-61

7. Gaffen JD, Tsang R, Bennett A. Prog Lipid Res 1986;25:543-5

Advances in Prostaglandin, Thromboxane, and Leukotriene Research, Vol. 19, edited by B. Samuelsson, P. Y.-K. Wong, and F. F. Sun, Raven Press, Ltd., New York ©1989.

APPEARANCE OF METABOLIC ACTIVITIES FOR ARACHIDONATE DURING DEVELOPMENT OF MOUSE EMBRYOS

Yasuko Koshihara and *Mitsugu Fukuda

Department of Pharmacology and*Biochemistry, Tokyo Metropolitan Institute of Gerontology, 35-2 Sakaecho, Itabashi-ku, Tokyo-173, Japan

Arachidonic acid metabolites, especially prostaglandins (PG) and hydroperoxides are reported to be related with fertilization, adherence of eggs to the uterus and maturation. The role of arachidonic acid on fertilization of sea urchin was first examined by Perry and his workers (1,2). Rabbit blastocysts produce PG E-A-B and F (3). One of the earliest events after implantation is increased in capillary permeability at the site of blastocyst attachment. This reaction is triggered by production of PG by the blastocyst (3). Arachidonic acid induces maturation of starfish oocytes as 1-methyladenine dose (4), which is a metabolite produced by lipoxygenase, like 12-HETE and 15-HETE. Furthermore the hatching factor of barnacle eggs was shown to be 10,11,12-trihydroxy-5,8,14,17-eicosatetraenoic acid, which was probably formed by oxidation of eicosapentaenoic acid catalyzed by 12-lipoxygenase (5).

However, the appearance of activities for metabolism of arachidonic acid during development has not been investigated.

The first step in metabolism of arachidonic acid is its conversion to PG by PG endoperoxide synthetase and to HPETE by lipoxygenases, which are subsequently reduced into the corresponding HETEs by peroxidase. Therefore, we investigated the times of appearance of PG endoperoxide synthetase and lipoxygenase activities during development of mouse embryos using ^{14}C-arachidonic acid as substrate. In some experiments, we used enzyme-linked immunoassay method for measurement of PG endoperoxide synthetase. In general, PG endoperoxide synthetase is localized in membranous fractions, especially microsome, whereas lipoxygenase is the localized in soluble fractions of cells, but the localization of these enzymes in embryos are unknown. Therefore we fractionated the embryos into mitochondria (M) and high-speed supernatant (S) and precipitate (P) fractions, and examined the enzyme activities in each fraction.

First we used 15 day embryo for assays of PG endoperoxide synthetase and lipoxygenase. Each fraction was incubated with ^{14}C-arachidonic acid in the presence of hematin and tryptophan at 37°C for 20 min. The arachidonate metabolites produced were extracted with ethylacetate and analyzed by silica-gel thin layer chromatography. The activities of lipoxygenase or PG endoperoxide synthetase was expressed as the sum of the radioactivities due to HETEs or to PGs synthesized, respectively (6,7). Fig.1 shows radiochromatograms of the metabolites of arachidonic acid. Mainly 6-keto-PGF$_{1\alpha}$ and PGE$_2$, with small amounts of PGF$_{2\alpha}$, thromboxane B$_2$ and PGD$_2$ were obtained with the P-fraction, while mainly 6-keto-PGF$_{1\alpha}$ with some PGF$_{2\alpha}$ and PGE$_2$ were formed by the M-fraction. The S-fraction did not produce any PGs as reported by Ånggård et al. (8).

Low polar products which were presumably formed by the lipoxygenase were obtained with the P- and M-fractions. The production of low polar products were inhibited by indomethacin (4 x 10^{-5} M), but inhibited more than 90 % by caffeic acid methylester (4 x 10^{-5} M) which is a selective inhibitor of lipoxygenase. CaCl$_2$ (1mM) which is an activator of lipoxygenase increased their production. These findings support the conclusion that the low polar products (indicated as peak I and peak II in Fig. 1) are arachidonic acid metabolites formed by lipoxygenase.

Next we examined the appearance of activities for metabolism of arachidonic acid in mouse embryos during development. Mice are generally born after a gestation period of 20 days. As it is easy to distinguish embryos from day 9 of gestation, we used embryos obtained on days 9, 10, 11, 13 and 15 and eggs for the assay.

When measured per mg protein, lipoxygenase activity appeared in the membranous fractions on day 11, and in the soluble fraction on day 15. PG endoperoxide synthetase activity appeared in the M-fraction on day 11, in the P-fraction weakly on day 11 and distinctly on day 13. The proportion of 6-keto-

PGF$_{1\alpha}$ in the total PG produced increased during development (Fig. 2). When measured per embryo, lipoxygenase and PG endoperoxide synthetase activities were both clearly detected in the membranous fraction from day 13. In the S-fraction, only lipoxygenase activity was detected, appearing on day from 15. Neither activity was detected in fertilized

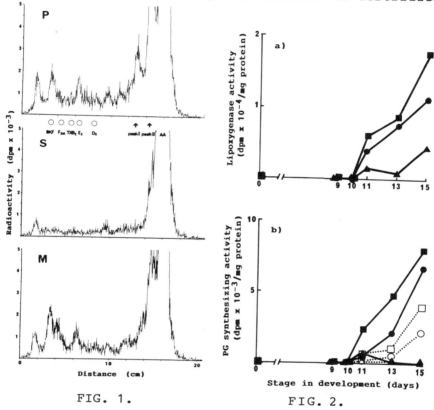

FIG. 1.   FIG. 2.

FIG. 1. Radiochromatogram of arachidonic acid into M-, P- and S- fractions, corresponding to mitochondria-rich, microsome-rich and soluble fractions, and metabolism of ^{14}C-arachidonic acid by the fractions was examined. AA:arachidonic acid.

FIG. 2. Activities of lipoxygenase (a) and PG endoperoxide synthetase (b) per mg protein of mouse embryos at various stages of development. Embryos were separated into M (■), P (●) and S (▲)fractions. 6-Keto-PGF$_{1\alpha}$ synthesis in the M (□), P (○) and S (△) fractions were also measured.

or unfertilized eggs.

Since the assays of enzyme activity as described above may not have been very sensitive, we next measured the amount of PG endoperoxide synthetase by enzyme-linked immunoassay. The purified PG endoperoxide synthetase from bovine seminal vesicles which gave a single band on SDS-polyacrylcmide gel electrophoresis, was used as a standard. The purified enzyme also use to prepare antiserum by injecting rabbit. The anti-serum against bovine PG endoperoxide synthetase cross-reacted with the mouse enzyme (9). By our method of peroxide-linked immunoassay of PG endoperoxide synthetase was used. By this method 6.8 ng to 102 ng of enzyme can be detected, but the sensitivity of PG endoperoxide synthetase activity using ^{14}C-arachidonic acid as substrate is more than 50 μg. Since PG endoperoxide synthetase is membrane-bound as mentioned above, it was solubilized with 1% Tween 20 before assay. Up to 350 μg of protein of crude fractions of embryos could be immobilized in a multi-well plastic plate and in practice we used samples of 200 μg protein of the P-fraction from embryos at various stages. No enzyme was detected in unfertilized eggs even when measured using 100 eggs, but the amounts appeared and increased during development, being 4.8, 7.7 and 8.7 ng per 100 μg protein on day 11, 13 and 15 respectively. Results obtained by enzyme linked immunoassay were consistent with those obtained by measurement of enzyme activity.

REFERENCES

1   Perry, G. Ph.D. Thesis. Univ. of California, San Diego. 1987.
2   Epel, D., Perry, G and Schmidt, T. In Gerish, G., Hoffman, J. eds. Membrane in Growth and Development New York: A.R. Liss, 1982; 171-183.
3   Dey, S.K., Chien, S.M., Cox, C.L. et al. Prostaglandins 1980; 19: 449-453.
4   Meijer, L., Guerrer, P. and Maclouf, J. Dev. Biol. 1984; 106: 368-378.
5   Holland, D.L. and East, J. Prostaglandins 1985; 29: 1021-1029.
6   Koshihara, Y., Senshu, T., Kawamura, M. et al. Biochim. Biophys. Acta 1980; 617: 536-539.
7   Koshihara, Y., Mizumura, M. and Murota, S. J. Biol. Chem. 1982; 257: 7302-7305.
8   Änggård, E., Bohman, S.O., Griffin, J.E. et al. Acta Physiol. Scand. 1972; 84: 231-246.
9   Kondo, M., Koshihara, Y., Kawamura, M. et al. Biochem. J. 1983; 212: 219-222.

Advances in Prostaglandin, Thromboxane, and Leukotriene Research, Vol. 19, edited by B. Samuelsson, P. Y.-K. Wong, and F. F. Sun, Raven Press, Ltd., New York ©1989.

THE ACTION OF PARATHYROID HORMONE ON BONE METABOLISM MAY BE REGULATED BY ENDOGENOUSLY SYNTHESIZED PROSTAGLANDIN E_2

,*C.Y. Yang,*W.A. Gonnerman, and *P.R. Polgar

*Department of Biochemistry, Boston University School of Medicine, Boston, MA; **Department of Dentistry, Tri-Service General Hospital, National Defense Medical Center, ; and ***Institute of Biomedical Sciences, Academia Sinica, Nankang, Taiwan, R.O.C.

INTRODUCTION

The physiological function of PTH is to maintain the balance of extracellular fluid calcium concentration. The action of PTH on bone resorption was proposed by stimulating the activity of osteoclasts (1). On the contrary, PTH may activate the production of cAMP in osteoblasts, which then stimulate osteoclastic bone resorption. Evidence for local prostaglandin stimulated bone resorption in vivo has been reported by Goodson et al. (2). Bone itself can synthesize prostaglandins and local production of PGE_2 leads to stimulation of bone resorption (3,4,5,6).

Cyclic AMP, calcium, and Na-Ca exchange mechanism have been proposed to be the intracellular mediator of PTH action (7,8,9). Prostaglandins may be a direct mediator in regulating several physiological and pathological functions in the body. The possibilities of prostaglandins to be the second messenger of the PTH act on bone metablism have been examined. Powles and his coworkers (10) proposed that PGE_1 may mediated the action of PTH, whereas Marcus and Orner (11) suggested that the cAMP response to PTH is not mediated by prostaglandins. We found that human parathyroid hormone N-terminal 1-34 fragment (hPTH 1-34) stimulates PGE_2 production in intact chick calvaria (12), and stimulates PGE_2 synthesis in osteoblast-like cells isolated from the same bone (13). In this report, we further examined the action of hPTH 1-34 on bone resorption and DNA synthesis in embryonic chick calvaria.

MATERIALS AND METHODS

Bone resorption stimulated by hPTH 1-34 was assessed by measuring the extent of release of [^{45}Ca] from prelabeled chick calvaria. Calvaria were dissected aseptically from 17-day chick embryos and divided along the midsaggital suture. The paired bones were incubated separately in 24-well tissue culture plates containing 2 ml of BGJ_b medium (Fitton-Jackson Modification) with ascorbic acid (50 ug/ml), penicillin (100 U/ml) and streptomycin (100 ug/ml) in a humidified atmosphere of 5% CO_2 / 95% air at 37°C. The calvaria were pulsed for 24 h with 0.25 uCi/ml of [^{45}Ca]. The pulse medium was replaced with identical medium without radioactive calcium and the bones were incubated for an additional 24 h. This chase period was designed to remove loose or unbound [^{45}Ca]. At the end of this chase period, the medium was removed from one half-calvariae and then replaced with fresh medium containing the materials to be tested; fresh medium without any additions was replaced on the other half-calvariae as a control group. The incubations were continued, aliquots of medium were removed at different time points, and the [^{45}Ca] radioactivity was measured as described (11).

DNA synthesis was examined by studying the uptake of [^{3}H]-thymidine and the total content. Incorporation of labeled thymidine into DNA was measured by incubating intact and dissected calvaria with [^{3}H]-thymidine (5 uCi/ml) for the last 60 min of the culture period. Labeled DNA was isolated according to a modification of the method of Dietrich et al. (14). Intact and dissected calvaria were extracted with 5% trichloroacetic acid (TCA) overnight. The tissues were homogenized in cold isotonic saline, the homogenated were treated with cold 5% TCA and centrifuged, and the amount of TCA-extractable radioactivity in the supernatant was determined. The TCA precipitate was resuspended in fresh 5% TCA, heated at 90°C for 15 min, cooled, and centrifuged; 80% of the label remained in the hot TCA-digestible DNA fraction. To determine total DNA content, calvaria were homogenized in 2 ml of H₂0. Aliquots of samples (0.5 ml) plus 0.5 ml of 5% perchloric acid (PCA) and 14 ul of 70% PCA were hydrolyzed at 70°C for 30 min and centrifuged. Equal amounts of the diphenylamine reagent (DPA) was added to the supernatant and incubated at 37°C overnight. DNA content was read at 600 nm in a spectrophotometer (Beckman Model 24).

RESULTS AND DISCUSSION

The time course of hPTH 1-34 on the release of pre-labeled [^{45}Ca] by chick calvaria is illustrated in figure 1. The effect of this hormone on calcium mobilization was relatively slow. Significant calcium mobilization developed 48 h after the bones were exposed to this hormone. The effect persisted up to 120 h and the response increased with time. The significant increase in [^{45}Ca] mobilization did not develop until 48 h after exposure to this hormone. This prolonged increase in bone resorption in vitro is in accordance with several studies (15,16). For example, Raisz found that the addition of 0.01 to 1.0 U per ml of parathyroid extract or purified parathyroid hormone to the medium was found to stimulate resorption in 72-h cultures of bone shafts from radius and ulna removed from 19-day rat embryos.

Table 1 illustrates that hPTH 1-34 stimulated [^{3}H]-thymidine incorporation in intact calvaria. When the periosteum was removed from the bone, this stimulatory effect was in the nonperiosteal central bone, not in the periosteum. There was no difference between 6 ug/ml and 0.6 ug/ml ug.ml of hPTH 1-34 concentrations.

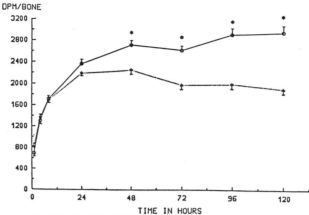

Fig. 1. The time course of hPTH 1-34 effect on mineral mobilization in chick calvaria.

All the bones were labeled with ^{45}Ca for 24 h and incubated with plain medium for an additional 24 h. On the third day, one half-calvariae was treated with hPTH 1-34 (0.6 ug/ml), while the other half-calvariae was incubated with plain medium without additions. Aliquots of samples were taken at different time points. Data are expressed as mean ± SE of 5 determinations.

* Significantly different from corresponding control using paired t-test, P   0.05.

Table 1. Effects of hPTH 1-34 on the incorporation of ^{3}H-thymidine and DNA content in intact and dissected calvaria.

Additions	^{3}H-thymidine incorporation (dpm/bone)	DNA content (ug/bone)
Intact calvariae		
control	29250 ± 2210	11.58 ± 0.68
hPTH (6 ug/ml)	51080 ± 3170 *	13.41 ± 0.86 NS
control	28000 ± 1230	12.58 ± 0.60
hPTH (0.6 ug/ml)	58340 ± 4080 *	13.98 ± 0.55 NS
Dissected calvariae		
Nonperiosteal bone		
control	5000 ± 430	8.42 ± 0.53
hPTH (6 ug/ml)	9440 ± 300 *	9.55 ± 0.93 NS
control	3360 ± 470	8.47 ± 0.51
hPTH (0.6 ug/ml)	10580 ± 1640 *	8.78 ± 0.51 NS
Periosteum		
control	860 ± 60	3.83 ± 0.48
hPTH (6 ug/ml)	1020 ± 130 NS	4.84 ± 0.13 NS
control	960 ± 50	4.38 ± 0.61
hPTH (0.6 ug/ml)	1100 ± 100 NS	4.37 ± 0.16 NS

Values are the mean ± SE for 5 calvaria cultured with or without hPTH 1-34 for 48 h. Periostea were removed by dissection after this incubation was completed in the dissected calvaria group. Bones and periostea were pulsed with ^{3}H-thymidine (5 uCi/ml) for 1 h. For details see Materials and Methods.

* Significantly different from corresponding control using paired t-test, P < 0.05.

NS: Not significant from corresponding control.

There were no differences between hPTH 1-34 treated and control bones in total DNA content either in intact or dissected calvaria. The ability of hPTH 1-34 to stimulate cell division appears to be cell or tissue speciffic since this hormone, stimulates cell division in the central bone which is rich in osteoblasts, but not in the periosteum which is rich in fibroblasts and progenitor cells. In addition, we have demonstrated that hPTH 1-34 did stimulate PGE_2 synthesis in intact chick calvaria and osteoblast-like cells isolated from the same bone (11,12). It is possible that hPTH 1-34 stimulated proliferation of osteoblasts which are the cells responsible for the endogenously synthesized PGE_2 and calcium mobilization. These results suggest that hPTH 1-34 regulate bone metabolism may related to the endogenously synthesized PGE_2 by osteoblasts.

REFERENCES

1. Holtrop, M.E., King, G.J., Cox, K.A. and Reit, B. (1979): Calcif. Tissue. Int., 27:129
2. Goodson, J.M., McClatchy, R., and Revell, C. (1974): J. Dent. Res., 53:670
3. Wong, P.Y.K., Majeska, R.J., and Wuthier, R.E. (1977): Prostaglandins, 14:839
4. Voelkel, E.F., Tashjian, A.H.Jr. and Levine, L. (1980): Biochim. Biophys. Acta., 620:418
5. Tashjian, A.H.Jr and Levine, L. (1978): Biochem. Biophys. Res. Commun., 85:966
6. Katz, J.M., Wilson, T., Skinner, S.J.M. and Gray, D.H. (1981): Prostaglandins, 22:537
7. Chase, L.R. and Aurbach, G.D. (1967): Proc. Natl. Acad. Sce. U.S.A., 58:518
8. Marcus, R. and Orner, F.B. (1980): Calcif. Tissue. Int., 32:207
9. Krieger, N.S. and Tashjian, Jr.A.H. (1980): Nature, 287:843
10. Powles, T.J., Easty, D.M., Easty, G.C., Bondy, P.K. and Munro-Neville, A. (1973): Nature [New Biol], 245:83
11. Marcus, R. and Orner, F.B. (1977): Endocrinology, 101:1570
12. Yang, C.Y., Gonnerman, W.A., Taylor, L., Nimberg, R.B. and Polgar, P.R. (1978): Endocrinology, 120:63
13. Yang, C.Y., Gonnerman, W.A. Menconi, M., Taylor, L. and Polgar, P.R. (1988): Endocrinology (Submitted for publication)
14. Dietrich, J.W. and Paddock, D.N. (1979): Endocrinology, 104:493
15. Raisz, L.G. (1965): J. Clin. Invest., 44:103
16. Klein, D.C. and Raisz, L.G. (1970): Endocrinology, 86:1436

Advances in Prostaglandin, Thromboxane, and Leukotriene Research, Vol. 19, edited by B. Samuelsson, P. Y.-K. Wong, and F. F. Sun, Raven Press, Ltd., New York ©1989.

Lipoxygenase Regulation of Membrane Expression of Tumor Cell Glycoproteins and Subsequent Metastasis

K. V. Honn, I. M. Grossi, B. W. Steinert, H. Chopra, J. Onoda, K.K. Nelson, and J. D. Taylor

Department of Radiation Oncology and Biological Sciences, Wayne State University, Detroit, MI 48202, USA, and Gershenson Radiation Oncology Center, Harper/Grace Hospitals, Detroit, MI 48201, USA

The metastatic cascade is a multifactorial process, the successful completion of which requires distinct, but coordinated responses by tumor cells to both their own internal stimuli and external stimuli presented by the host (1). The hematogenous phase of the metastatic cascade involves multiple cell-cell (i.e., tumor cell-platelet, tumor cell-endothelial cell, etc.) and cell-matrix (i.e., tumor cell-subendothelial matrix) interactions (1). These interactions are mediated by receptors on the surface of tumor cells, normal cells, and by adhesion proteins which comprise the subendothelial matrix. We recently reported immunological evidence for a glycoprotein complex (IRGpIIb/IIIa) related to the platelet IIb/IIIa complex on the surface of human and rodent tumor cells (2-6). In addition, we recently performed Northern blot analysis of mRNA isolated from a variety of human and rodent tumor cells using GpIIb and GpIIIa cDNA probes and demonstrated that these tumor cells expressed specific transcripts which hybridize to the GpIIb cDNA probe and to the GpIIIa cDNA probe (4,7).

Honn et al (8,9) first proposed the hypothesis that eicosanoids produced by the platelet, the tumor cell and the vessel wall were key determinents in the interaction of those three cell types. They proposed that prostacyclin (PGI_2) or PGI_2 stimulating agents may limit tumor cell metastasis, whereas thromboxane A_2 (TXA_2) would promote tumor cell metastasis (8,9). In addition, Honn et al (10) proposed that lipoxygenase (LOX) products of arachidonic acid, produced by the tumor cell, platelet and endothelial cell affect their interactions, possibly by altering vessel wall prostacyclin (PGI_2) biosynthesis (11). Recently, we demonstrated that products of the 12-lipoxygenase (i.e., 12-HETE) stimulate tumor cell adhesion to endothelial cells (EC), subendothelial matrix (SEM) and fibronectin (FN) (5,12). Therefore, we investigated the role of other eicosanoids (e.g., PGI_2) on 12-HETE mediated tumor cell adhesion and determined the role of IRGpIIb/IIIa in 12-HETE mediated adhesion and metastasis.

MATERIAL AND METHODS

The Lewis lung carcinoma (3LL) and B16 amelanotic melanoma (B16a) were propagated in vivo, enzymatically dispersed, and tumor cells separated from host cells by centrifugal elutriation as described previously (3). Tumor cell LOX metabolism was measured (13,14) and 12-HETE was found to be the major product (14). IRGpIIb/IIIa was identified with specific polyclonal (i.e., pAbIIb/IIIa) and monoclonal (i.e., mAb10E5, mAb7E3, mAbAP-2) antibodies and tumor cell surface expression quantitated by flow cytometric analysis as described previously (2-5). Rat endothelial cells were isolated from the dorsal aorta, cloned, characterized, removed, and the underlying SEM characterized as described previously (15). Tumor cell adhesion to EC, SEM, FN, etc., and lung colony formation were evaluated (2-6,8,15) and compared to expression of IRGpIIb/IIIa and 12-HETE biosynthesis. Eicosanoids were purchased from Cayman Chemical (Ann Arbor, MI) except 13-hydroxyoctadecadienoic acid (13-HODE) which was generously supplied by Dr. Lawrence Marnett (Wayne State University, Detroit, MI).

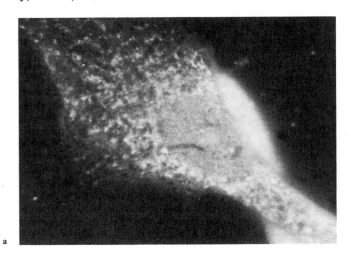

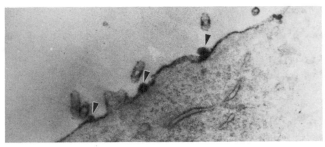

FIG 1. Immunohistochemical identification (a, mAb10E5) and localization (b, arrows) of IRGpIIb/IIIa on B16a cells

RESULTS AND DISCUSSION

Both B16a (Fig 1a) and 3LL (not shown) cells demonstrated positive immunofluorescence when stained with pAb's and mAb's specific for platelet GpIIb/IIIa (2-6). As a result of the immunological relatedness and specific Northern blot analyses (4,7), we designated this glycoprotein IRGpIIb/IIIa. Immunocytochemical localization at the ultrastructural level reveals a punctate distribution of reaction product (Fig 1b) which suggests areas of high receptor concentration and possibly prefered sites for attachment of platelets to the tumor cell plasma membrane (4) and attachment of tumor cells to EC and SEM (2-4).

In the platelet GpIIb/IIIa is a multifunctional receptor which interacts with several adhesion proteins (i.e., FN, fibrinogen, vonWillebrand factor, vitronectin, etc.) (16, 17). Therefore, IRGpIIb/IIIa may be important in metastasis as tumor cell adhesion to EC and SEM are critical events in the metastatic cascade (1). We observed a high degree of correlation (r=0.90) between B16a tumor cell expression of IRGpIIb/IIIa and formation of pulmonary colonies in the experimental metastasis assay (Fig 2 and ref 3). We demonstrated

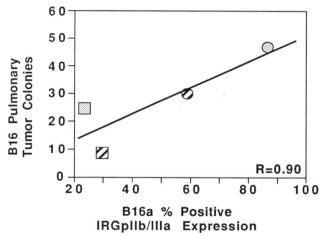

FIG 2. Correlation between IRGpIIb/IIIa expression on B16a cells and tumor colony formation

previously that 12-HETE and the phorbol ester, TPA, enhance surface expression of IRGpIIb/IIIa by human cervical carcinoma cells (6). Similarly IRGpIIb/IIIa expression in 3LL cells (Fig 3a) and B16 cells (not shown) is enhanced by 12-HETE and TPA. The 12-HETE effect is specific for the (S) isomer (Fig 3a). The LOX product of linoleic acid, 13-HODE, decreases 12-HETE and TPA expression of IRGpIIb/IIIa, an effect which was enhanced by PGI$_2$ (Fig 3a). Adhesion of 3LL cells to EC monolayers was enhanced by 12(S,R)-HETE and TPA (Fig 3b). This enhanced adhesion is specific for the (S) isomer (not shown) and is inhibited by PGI$_2$ and 13-HODE (Fig 3b). In order to demonstrate that 12-HETE and TPA enhanced adhesion to EC was mediated, in part, by the IRGpIIb/IIIa receptor, we treated 3LL tumor cells with specific antibodies against

GpIIb/IIIa which crossreact with IRGpIIb/IIIa (2-6). Both pAbIIb/IIIa and mAb10E5 reduced 12-HETE and TPA stimulated 3LL adhesion to EC (Fig 3c). Finally, we determined whether the TPA response was mediated via a LOX metabolite by pretreating 3LL cells with LOX inhibitors (BW755C and NDGA) or the cyclooxygenase (COX) inhibitor, indomethcin. Inhibition of the LOX pathway reduced 3LL cell adhesion to SEM while the COX inhibitor was ineffective (Fig 3d). TPA and 12-HETE enhanced adhesion to SEM is mediated, in part, by IRGpIIb/IIIa as, pAbIIb/IIIa (Fig 3d) and mAb10E5, mAb7E3, (not shown) reduce tumor cell adhesion to that substrata. A 5-LOX (i.e., 5-HETE) or a 15-LOX (i.e., 15-HETE) metabolite did not enhance tumor cell adhesion to EC, SEM or FN (not shown). Finally, tumor cell (i.e., B16a) metabolism of arachidonic acid to 12-HETE correlates with metastatic potential (6).

Our results suggest that a 12-LOX (i.e., 12-HETE) metabolite regulates tumor cell surface expression of a multifunctional receptor (i.e., IRGpIIb/IIIa) which may be a critical determinant in tumor cell adhesion to EC, SEM, and subsequent metastasis. In addition, we propose a bidirectional control of IRGpIIb/IIIa expression and possibly metastasis by LOX metabolites of arachidonic acid (i.e., 12-HETE; stimulation) and LOX metabolites of linoleic acid (i.e., 13-HODE; inhibition).

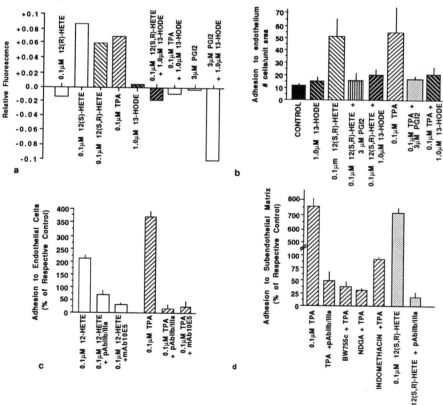

FIG 3. Role of 12-HETE in adhesion of 3LL cells to EC and SEM

ACKNOWLEDGEMENT

This work supported by grants CA29997 and CA47715 awarded to K.V. Honn and a grant from Harper/Grace Hospitals. I.M. Grossi is a fellow on NIH training grant CA-09531-03.

REFERENCES

1. Weiss L, Orr FW, Honn KV. FASEB J 1988;2:12-21.

2. Grossi IM, Hatfield JS, Fitzgerald LA, et al. FASEB J (in press).

3. Honn KV, Grossi IM, Nelson KK, et al. Cancer Res (in press).

4. Chopra H, Hatfield JS, Chang YS, et al. Cancer Res (in press).

5. Honn KV, Grossi IM, Fitzgerald LA, et al. Biochem Biophys Res Commun (in press).

6. Honn KV, Grossi IM, Chopra H, et al. In: Nigam S, McBrien DCH, Slater TG, eds. Eicosanoids, lipid peroxidation and cancer, Berlin: Springer-Verlag, 1988; (in press).

7. Chang YS, Fitzgerald LA, Grossi IM, et al. FASEB J 1988; 2:A1406

8. Honn KV, Cicone B, Skoff A. Science 1981; 212: 1270-1272

9. Honn KV, Busse WD, Sloane BF. Biochem Pharmacol 1983; 32: 1-11.

10. Honn KV, Menter DG, Onoda JM, et al. In: Nicolson GL, Milas L, eds. Cancer invasion and metastasis: biologic and therapeutic aspects, New York: Raven Press, 1984;361-388.

11. Honn KV, Onoda JM, Menter DG, et al. In: Honn KV, Sloane, BF, eds. Hemostatic mechanisms and metastasis Boston, Martinus-Nijhoff, 1984; 207-231.

12. Grossi IM, Nelson KK, Hatfield JS, et al. FASEB J 1988;2:A1406.

13. Honn KV, Dunn JR. FEBS Lett 1982; 139:65-68.

14. Dunn JD, Ohannesian DW, Tefend S, et al. In: Garaci E, Paoletti R, Santoro MG, eds. Prostaglandins in cancer research, Berlin, Springer-Verlag 1987;257-260.

15. Menter DG, Steinert BW, Sloane BF, et al. Cancer Res 1987; 47:6751-6762.

16. Charo IF, Bekeart LS, Phillips DR. J Biol Chem 1987;262:9935-9938.

17. Ruoslahti E, Pierschbacher MD. Science 1987; 238:491-497.

Advances in Prostaglandin, Thromboxane, and Leukotriene Research, Vol. 19, edited by B. Samuelsson, P. Y.-K. Wong, and F. F. Sun, Raven Press, Ltd., New York ©1989.

MOLECULAR MECHANISM OF CYCLOOXYGENASE REGULATION

IN CLONED MOUSE OSTEOBLASTIC CELL (MC3T3-E1)

Shozo Yamamoto[1], Takeo Oshima[1], Masami Kusaka[1], Kazushige Yokota[1], Tanihiro Yoshimoto[1], Koji Sumitani[2], Terushige Kawata[2], and Masayoshi Kumegawa[3]

[1]Department of Biochemistry, School of Medicine,
[2]Department of Orthodontics, School of Dentistry, Tokushima University, Kuramoto-cho, Tokushima, and
[3]Department of Oral Anatomy, Meikai Dental University, Sakado, Saitama 350-02, Japan

MC3T3-E1 cell was cloned from newborn mouse calvaria by Kodama and his associates (1). The cell line differentiates into an osteoblast in the cell culture, and is characteristic of its calcification in vitro. Parameters of bone formation change in response to various hormones and growth factors (2). With this unique and useful cell line we have investigated the biosynthesis of PGE_2 and its regulatory mechanism. The PGE_2 is well known as a bone resorption factor (3), and is produced as a major arachidonate metabolite by this cell line. Earlier we reported that the PGE_2 synthesis by MC3T3-E1 cells was markedly stimulated by the addition of epidermal growth factor (EGF) to the culture medium (4). First, we found that the cyclooxygenase step was stimulated. The cyclooxygenase reaction was initiated with a lag phase of 1-2 h after the addition of EGF. Even if the cells were pretreated with aspirin or indomethacin to irreversibly inhibit the cyclooxygenase, the PGE_2 synthesis was stimulated by the addition of EGF indicating that the role of EGF was not to activate an inactive constitutive enzyme. The EGF-dependent stimulation of PGE_2 synthesis was inhibited by actinomycin D or cycloheximide. These experimental results suggested that the cyclooxygenase protein was induced or synthesized de novo in the presence of EGF.

By our further studies on the regulatory mechanism of PGE_2 synthesis in this osteoblast cell line, we found that epinephrine also stimulated the PGE_2 synthesis. The PGE_2 release in the culture medium started 1-2 h after the addition of epinephrine. Fig. 1 shows effect of epinephrine concentration on the PGE_2 synthesis. About 0.1 µM epinephrine gave a maximal stimulation.

444

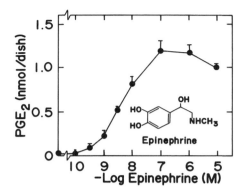

Fig. 1.   Effect of epinephrine concentration on PGE$_2$ synthesis.

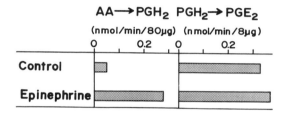

Fig. 2.   Effect of epinephrine on cyclooxygenase and PGE synthase reactions.

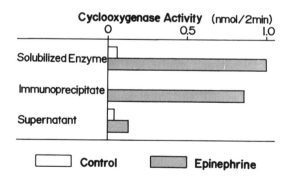

Fig. 3.   Effect of epinephrine to increase immunoprecipitable cyclooxygenase activity.

The PGE$_2$ synthesis from arachidonic acid involves three enzymatic steps (5). Arachidonic acid is transformed to PGG$_2$ by the reaction of fatty acid cyclooxygenase, followed by the PG hydroperoxidase reaction from PGG$_2$ to PGH$_2$, and then the PGH$_2$ is isomerized to PGE_2 by PGE synthase. As shown in Fig. 2, we examined which of the three steps was affected by epinephrine. Microsomes were prepared from the epinephrine-treated cells and the control cells. The conversion of arachidonic acid to PGH_2 occurred at a higher rate in the epinephrine-treated cells. In contrast, the conversion of PGH_2 to PGE_2 was not significantly affected by the presence of epinephrine in the cell culture. These observations indicated that the overall synthesis of PGE_2 was stimulated by epinephrine at the step of cyclooxygenase. Fig. 3 presents the result of an experiment using an anti-cyclooxoygenase antibody. Cyclooxygenase contained in the epinephrine-treated cells and control cells was solubilized by the use of Tween 20, and the solubilized enzyme was incubated with a monoclonal anti-cyclo-oxygenase antibody. Most of the cyclooxygenase activity of the solubilized enzyme was recovered in the immunoprecipitate, and the epinephrine-treated cells showed a markedly increased acti-vity of immunoprecipitable cyclooxygenase.

Such a stimulatory effect of epinephrine on the cyclooxygenase led us to examine a possible involvement of adrenergic receptors. First, we tested whether α-agonist or β-agonist could replace epinephrine and stimulate the production of PGE_2. Isoproterenol as a β-agonist was as active as epinephrine giving a maximal stimulation at a concentration of 0.1 µM. In contrast, phenyl-ephrine as an α-agonist was much less effective. Propranolol as a β-antagonist at 1 µM abolished the stimulatory effect of 1 µM epinephrine. These results suggested a role of β-adrenergic receptor in the stimulation of PGE_2 production by MC3T3-E1 cells.

The next subject we must investigate was a possible involve-ment of cAMP. After 5-min incubation of the cells with various concentrations of epinephrine, we found a marked accumulation of cAMP within the cells depending on the epinephrine concentration.

The time courses of cAMP and PGE_2 production were compared (Fig. 4). The intracellular cAMP level reached a maximum almost

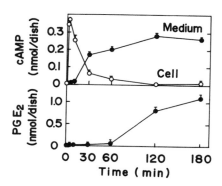

Fig. 4.   Time courses of epinephrine-dependent production of cAMP and PGE_2.

immediately when epinephrine was added to the cell culture, while there was no PGE_2 synthesis for at least 1 h and the PGE_2 level reached a maximum after 2-3 h. We applied another method to increase the intracellular cAMP level. Cholera toxin was given to MC3T3-El cells. Both the cAMP level and the PGE_2 release were increased depending on the concentration of cholera toxin. Forskolin which also increased the intracellular cAMP, stimulated the PGE_2 synthesis. Both 8-bromo-cAMP and dibutyryl cAMP added to the cell culture, also stimulated the PGE_2 production. All these data supported a view that the stimulation of PGE_2 synthesis by epinephrine is mediated by cAMP.

The stimulation of cyclooxygenase by cAMP may be discussed in terms of two possible mechanisms. First, constitutive inactive cyclooxygenase may be activated by the addition of cAMP. Alternatively, cAMP may cause a de novo synthesis of the cyclooxy-

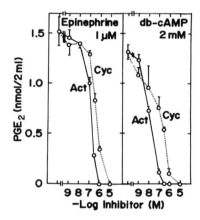

Fig. 5. Inhibition of epinephrine- and dibutyryl cAMP-dependent PGE_2 synthesis by actinomycin D (Act) and cycloheximide (Cyc).

genase protein. We used well-known inhibitors of transcription and translation. The left panel of Fig. 5 demonstrates that the epinephrine-stimulated PGE_2 synthesis was inhibited in a dose-dependent manner by actinomycin D, a transcription inhibitor, and by cycloheximide, a translation inhibitor. These inhibitors did not affect the cAMP production. Similar results were obtained with α-amanitin and puromycin. As presented in the right panel, the PGE_2 production stimulated by dibutyryl cAMP was also inhibited by actinomycin D and cycloheximide. These findings suggested that cyclooxygenase was induced for 1-2 h after the addition of either epinephrine or dibutyryl cAMP.

In summary, when epinephrine was added to the cell culture, PGE_2 synthesis started after a lag phase of 1-2 h. Among the enzymes involved in the PGE$_2$ synthesis, the activity of cyclo-oxygenase was enhanced. This was shown more specifically by the use of anti-cyclooxygenase antibody. The study with various agonists and antagonists suggested that the stimulatory effect of epinephrin was mediated by a β-receptor. Intracellular cAMP level was rapidly increased by the addition of epinephrine, and the cAMP increase was followed by the PGE$_2$ synthesis. The addition of dibutyryl cAMP also increased the PGE$_2$ production. The PGE$_2$ synthesis thus stimulated by epinephrine or dibutyryl cAMP was blocked by the transcription and translation inhibitors. cAMP is known as an intracellular messenger and activates protein kinases resulting in phosphorylation of various enzymes and proteins. An alternative function of cAMP is a transcriptional role which was earlier found in bacterial cells (6). Recently the biosynthesis of various mammalian enzymes and proteins has been found to be controlled by cAMP at the gene level; phospho-enolpyruvate carboxykinase of rat liver cytosol (7), bovine and human vasoactive intestinal polypeptide (8), rat somatostatin (9), human chorionic gonadotropin (10), and proenkephalin (11). The use of deletion mutants clarified the region of the gene regulated by cAMP, and the homology in these polypeptides was demonstrated (9,12,13). As I have discussed, the PGE$_2$ synthesis in MC3T3-E1 cells was enhanced by cAMP presumably by induction of cyclooxygenase. However, such a mechanism of cyclooxygenase induction mediated by cAMP must be confirmed by our further investigations at the gene level, and the PGE$_2$ synthesis system in MC3T3-E1 cells will provide a unique subject for the study to elucidate the molecular mechanism of the arachidonate cascade regulation.

ACKNOWLEDGEMENTS

This work was supported by grants-in-aid for scientific research from the Ministry of Education, Science and Culture and the Ministry of Health and Welfare of Japan, and grants from the Japanese Foundation of Metabolism and Diseases, Takeda Science Foundation, Mochida Memorial Foundation, Tokyo Biochemical Research Foundation, and Pfeizer Central Research (Nagoya).

REFERENCES

1 Sudo, H., Kodama, H., Amagai, Y., Yamamoto, S., and Kasai, S. (1983) J. Cell Biol. 96, 191-198

2 Kumegawa, M., Hiramatsu, M., Hatakeyama, K., Yajima, T., Kodama, H., Osaki, T., and Kurisu, K. (1983) Calcif. Tissue Int. 35, 542-548

3 Raisz, L.G., and Kream, B.E. (1983) New Engl. J. Med. 309, 29-34

4 Yokota, K., Kusaka, M., Ohshima, T., Yamamoto, S., Kurihara, N., Yoshino, T., and Kumegawa, M. (1986) J. Biol. Chem. 261, 15410-15415

5 Miyamoto, T., Ogino, N., Yamamoto, S., and Hayaishi, O. (1976) J. Biol. Chem. 251, 2629-2636

6 Watson, J.D., Hopkins, N.H., Roberts, J.W., Steitz, J.A., and Weiner, A.M. (1987) Molecular Biology of the Gene 4th edition, pp.478-479, Benjamin/Cummings Publishing Company, Menlo Park

7 Lamers, W.H., Hanson, R.W., and Meisner, H.M. (1982) Proc. Natl. Acad. Sci. USA 79, 5137-5141

8 Hayakawa, Y., Obata, K., Itoh, N., Yanaihara, N., and Okamoto, H. (1984) J. Biol. Chem. 259, 9207-9211

9 Montminy, M.R., Sevarino, K.A., Wagner, J.A., Mandel, G., and Goodman, R.H. (1986) Proc. Natl. Acad. Sci. USA 83, 6682-6686

10 Burnside, J., Nagelberg, S.B., Lippman, S.S., and Weintraub, B.D. (1985) J. Biol. Chem. 260, 12705-12709

11 Eiden, L.E., Giraud, P., Affolter, H.-U., Herbert, E., and Hotchkiss, A.J. (1984) Proc. Natl. Acad. Sci. USA 81, 3949-3953

12 Short, J.M., Wynshaw-Boris, A., Short, H.P., and Hanson, R.W. (1986) J. Biol. Chem. 261, 9721-9726

13 Tsukada, T., Fink, J.S., Mandel, G., and Goodmann, R.H. (1987) J. Biol. Chem. 262, 8743-8747

Advances in Prostaglandin, Thromboxane, and Leukotriene Research, Vol. 19, edited by B. Samuelsson, P. Y.-K. Wong, and F. F. Sun, Raven Press, Ltd., New York ©1989.

REGULATION OF CYCLOOXYGENASE

SYNTHESIS BY EGF AND CORTICOSTEROIDS

J. Martyn Bailey

The George Washington University
School of Medicine and Health Science, Washington, D.C. U.S.A.

In this chapter we describe the use of cultured vascular smooth muscle cells, in which cyclooxygenase has been inactivated by prior treatment with aspirin, as a model to study regulation of cyclooxygenase expression. The interaction of corticosteroids and lipomodulin with this EGF-dependent recovery process provides a new mechanism for the suppression of prostaglandin synthesis by corticosteroids.

Recovery of cyclooxygenase activity in aspirin inactivated cells was assayed by incubating the cells with [^{14}C]-arachidonic acid for 10 minutes and measuring prostacyclin

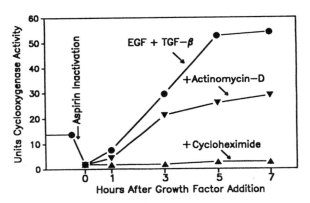

Figure 1. TIME COURSE OF EGF-DEPENDENT CYCLOOXYGENASE RECOVERY AFTER ASPIRIN INACTIVATION. *Influence of cycloheximide and actinomycin-D. Cultures were inactivated with 300 μM aspirin and then incubated with 10 ng/mL EGF and 1 ng/mL TGF-ß for 1, 3, 5 and 7 hours ± 2 μg/mL cycloheximide or 2 μg/mL actinomycin-D and cyclooxygenase assayed.*

synthesis. There was essentially no recovery in chemically-defined serum-free medium. Addition of EGF (10 ng/mL) to the serum-free medium resulted in a marked stimulation of enzyme recovery(Figure 1). Addition of TGF-β (1 ng/mL), while only moderately active on its own synergized with EGF to give a recovery of activity which fully reproduced that of medium containing 10 % fresh fetal bovine serum. The time-course for recovery of enzyme activity and the influence of cycloheximide and actinomycin-D on inhibition of protein and mRNA synthesis was investigated.

Rapid induction of cyclooxygenase occurred during the first 5 hours, to levels which were several fold greater than the baseline levels prior to aspirin treatment. Addition of 2 μg/mL cycloheximide totally blocked recovery of activity. Addition of 2 μg/mL actinomycin-D to the incubation had essentially no effect on recovery for the first 3 hours. Incubation of cultures with dexamethasone (2 μM) prior to inactivation by aspirin completely blocked the recovery of cyclooxygenase induced by EGF and TGF-β or fresh serum (Fig.2). Incubation of cultures with pure bovine lipocortin

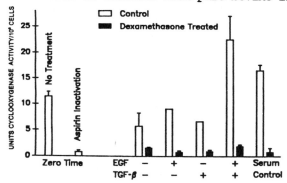

Figure 2. SUPPRESSION OF EGF-INDUCED CYCLOOXYGENASE ENZYME RECOVERY BY DEXAMETHASONE. *Confluent rat smooth muscle cell cultures were incubated with fresh serum-medium for 9 hours either with or without 2 μM dexamethasone, followed by inactivation for 30 minutes with 300 μM aspirin. The cells were washed and incubated in Hams F-12 medium containing 1 mg/mL BSA and 0.1 mM uric acid ± dexamethasone (2 μM) plus the indicated additions (10 ng/mL EGF; 1 ng/mL TGF-ß; or 10 ng/mL EGF plus 1 ng/mL TGF-ß; 10% fetal bovine serum). After 3 hours the media were removed and cyclooxygenase activity assayed.*

(2-4 μg/mL) prior to aspirin inactivation duplicated the effects of dexamethasone and gave a dose-dependent inhibition of stimulation by EGF.

Total protein synthesis as measured by incorporation of

[^{35}S]-methionine into TCA precipitable protein was not significantly different in control and EGF/TGF-β-treated cells, under conditions in which cyclooxygenase synthesis was completely suppressed. Binding of [^{125}I]-radiolabeled EGF to the cells was also unaffected by dexamethasone treatment indicating that the corticosteroid effects were not due to suppression of EGF receptors. Pre-labeled smooth muscle cell cultures were incubated with 10 ng/mL EGF and 1 ng/mL TGF-β. Maximal stimulation of prostacyclin release by EGF and TGF-β occurred between 1 and 2 hours. Addition of cycloheximide (2 μg/mL) to the recovery medium completely prevented the activation of prostacyclin synthesis by EGF and TGF-β, whereas actinomycin D (2 μg/ml) had no effect. Release of arachidonic acid was measured in the same incubations and was not significantly affected by EGF and   TGF-β nor by cycloheximide or actinomycin-D. Thus activation of endogenous prostacyclin synthesis by EGF and TGF-β was related to increased cyclooxygenase and not phospholipase activity.

The ability of EGF to induce phosphorylation of endogenous cell proteins was studied by incubating smooth muscle cell membranes at 4°C for 10 minutes with either EGF or EGF plus TGF-β after which [γ-^{32}P]-ATP was added for an additional 5 minutes. Acrylamide gel electrophoresis revealed an additional, heavily radioactive band in EGF-treated cultures which comigrated with authentic lipocortin and had an apparent molecular weight of 35 kDa.

Previous reports that EGF stimulates prostaglandin synthesis were usually attributed to increased release of the arachidonic acid substrate (2). That this is not the case in the present experiments is clearly evident since the increased levels of cyclooxygenase are assayed directly using [^{14}C]-arachidonic acid as substrate. In addition, stimulation of prostacyclin synthesis directly by EGF and TGF-β without enhancing arachidonic acid release from cellular lipids was also demonstrated. Furthermore, cycloheximide reduced prostacyclin synthesis to basal levels without affecting arachidonic acid release in either control or growth-factor stimulated cultures. These results demonstrate that the enhancement by EGF of prostacyclin synthesis from both exogenous and endogenous substrate is related to an increase in the level of cyclooxygenase enzyme.

The antiinflammatory activity of the corticosteroids has traditionally been attributed in part to their demonstrated ability to inhibit prostaglandin synthesis. The proposed mechanism implied that lipocortin, the synthesis of which is induced by corticosteroids, was an inhibitory subunit of phospholipase A$_2$ (3). Recent reports have questioned this interpretation since it has been shown that inhibition of phospholipase by lipocortin is an artifact due to binding of phospholipid substrate by lipocortin in the assay systems used (4-6). Our finding that EGF-dependent cyclooxygenase synthesis is blocked by dexamethasone thus offers a new explanation for the mechanism whereby the corticosteroids inhibit prostaglandin synthesis.

Recent work by Pepinsky and Sinclair (7) and by Haigler suggests the nature of a possible link between the two systems. The primary target of the EGF-receptor tyrosine kinase in several cell lines was shown to be lipocortin. As shown here membrane extracts of cells treated with EGF under the conditions used to activate cyclooxygenase synthesis, selectively phosphorylated a 35 kDa protein which comigrated with authentic lipocortin.

The results described in this paper suggest that stimulation of cyclooxygenase synthesis in vascular smooth muscle cells utilizes preexisting mRNA and is accompanied by EGF-induced phosphorylation of lipocortin.

SCHEME FOR REGULATION OF CYCLOOXYGENASE EXPRESSION
BY EGF AND CORTICOSTEROIDS

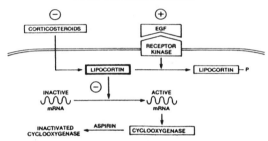

The previously accepted role of lipocortin as a regulatory subunit of phospholipase A_2 is being questioned. Our findings of a direct suppression of EGF-dependent cyclooxygenase synthesis by corticosteroids together with the recently established link between EGF and lipocortin thus offer an alternative explanation for the prostaglandin inhibiting and anti-inflammatory activity of these compounds (8).

References

1. Bailey, J.M.; et al. *J. Lipid Res.* 26: 54-61; 1985.
2. Levine, L.; Hassid, A. *Biochem. Biophys. Res. Comm.* 76: 1181-1187; 1977.
3. Hirata, F.; et al. *Proc. Natl. Acad. Sci. (USA).* 77: 2533-2536; 1980.
4. Davidson, F.F.; et al, *J. Biol. Chem.* 262: 1698-1705; 1987.
5. Schlaepfer, D.D.; Haigler, H.T. *J. Biol. Chem.* 262: 6931-6937; 1987.
6. Aarsman, A.J.; et al. *FEBS Lett.* 219: 176-180; 1987.
7. Pepinsky, R.B.; Sinclair, L.K. *Nature.* 321: 81-84; 1986.
8. Pash, J.; Bailey, J.M. *FASEB J.* 2: 10; 1988 in press.

*Advances in Prostaglandin, Thromboxane, and
Leukotriene Research*, Vol. 19, edited by
B. Samuelsson, P. Y.-K. Wong, and F. F. Sun,
Raven Press, Ltd., New York ©1989.

MOLECULAR CLONING OF PROSTAGLANDIN G/H SYNTHASE

David L. DeWitt, E.A. El-Harith and William L. Smith

Department of Biochemistry, Michigan State University,
East Lansing, Michigan, 48824, U.S.A.

Prostaglandin G/H (PGG/H) synthase catalyzes the rate-limiting, committed step in the formation of prostaglandins and thromboxanes from precursor fatty acids. This enzyme exhibits both dioxygenase (cyclooxygenase) and hydroperoxidase activities (1,2). The cyclooxygenase activity, but not the hydroperoxidase activity, is inhibited by non-steroidal anti-inflammatory drugs (3). There is evidence from studies with mouse 3T3 cells (4), rat Graafian follicles (5), smooth muscle cells (6), and sheep uterus (7) that PGG/H synthase protein levels can fluctuate during growth and differentiation in response to agents such as steroids, peptide hormones, growth factors and tumor promoters. The goal of the work summarized in this report was to prepare a cDNA coding for the sheep vesicular gland enzyme in order (a) to determine the primary structure of PGG/H synthase and (b) to investigate the biochemical mechanisms underlying changes in PGG/H synthase levels.

RESULTS AND DISCUSSION

PGG/H synthase from sheep vesicular gland microsomes was purified by immunoaffinity chromatography using a monoclonal antibody, (IgG_{2b}(cyo-7)) prepared previously (2). The reduced, alkylated enzyme was proteolyzed with trypsin. Tryptic peptides were isolated by reverse phase HPLC on a Varian Protein-C18 column. The sequences of peptides 1-4 and the sequence of the first 16 residues at the N-terminus were determined (see Fig. 1). Two ^{32}P-labeled oligonucleotide probes modeled from portions of the N-terminus and peptide 2 (amino acid residues 34-40 and 232-238; Fig. 1) were used to screen a λgt10 cDNA library prepared from sheep vesicular gland poly (A)$^+$ RNA. Phage which hybridized strongly with both probes were plaque purified, amplified, and the DNA isolated from each. The DNA inserts of three clones each yielded five Eco-R1 fragments (1609, 490, 285, 189, 129 bp). The sum of the sizes of the fragments (2.7 kb) was about the

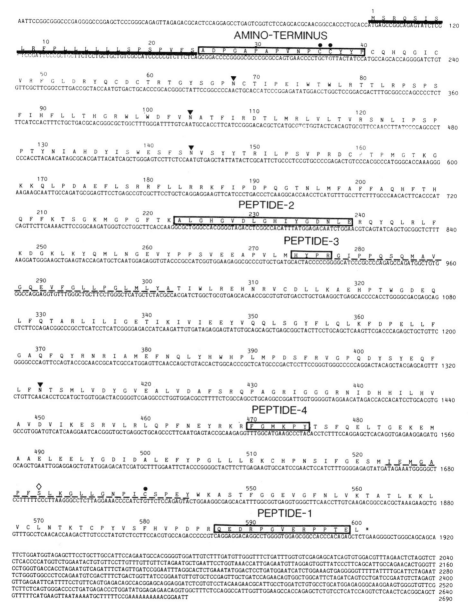

FIG. 1. Nucleotide sequence and deduced amino acid sequence of PGHS$_{ov}$, a cDNA for PGG/H synthase from sheep vesicular gland (8).

size of the sheep vesicular gland mRNA species which hybridized with the two oligonucleotide probes on Northern blots (2.75 kb; Fig. 2). Reasoning that the cDNA inserts we obtained were near full-length cDNAs, we determined the nucleotide sequence of one of the inserts, $PGHS_{ov}$ (8). The full-length cDNA encodes a protein of 600 amino acids, including a signal sequence (Fig. 1). Identification of the cDNA as coding for PGG/H synthase is based on comparison of amino acid sequences of seven peptides comprising 103 amino acids with the amino acid sequence deduced from the nucleotide sequence. PGG/H synthase is a glycoprotein (3) and there are four potential sites for N-glycosylation (residues 68, 104, 144, and 410). The serine reported to be acetylated by aspirin (9) is at position 530 near the C-terminus.

The 1.6 kb Eco-R1 fragment prepared from the cDNA for the sheep vesicular gland PGG/H synthase was radiolabeled with ^{32}P and hybridized with mRNA species prepared from sheep vesicular gland, bovine endothelial cells, human umbilical cord endothelial cells, and mouse 3T3 cells. As shown in Fig. 2, cross-hybridization of the sheep cDNA was observed with mRNA species of approximately 2.75 kb derived from bovine, human, and sheep cells; the mouse mRNA was slightly larger (3.1 kb). These results suggest that the cDNA sequences of PGG/H synthase from various species are closely related, consistent with known immunological similarities among mammalian PGG/H synthases.

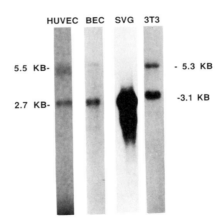

FIG. 2 Cross-species reactivity of the ovine PGG/H synthase cDNA. The 1.6 kb Eco-R1 fragment of the $PGHS_{ov}$ cDNA was radiolabeled and hybridized to northern blots of poly-(A+) mRNA from: sheep vesicular glands (SVG, 10 µg); bovine endothelial cells (BEC, 10 µg); mouse 3T3 fibroblasts (3T3, 10 µg); and human umbilical vein endothelial cells (HUVEC, 5 µg). The ovine cDNA hybridized with a major mRNA band of 2.75 kb from all species except mouse, which exhibited a major hybridizing band of 3.1 kb. Minor hybridizing bands were also observed at 5.3-5.5 kb, which may represent the unspliced mRNA for PGG/H synthase.

The availability of a cDNA probe for PGG/H synthase should now permit quantitation of changes in PGG/H synthase mRNA levels (i.e. PGG/H synthase gene expression) and examination of the factors responsible for changes in gene expression. In addition, the availability of a full-length cDNA should permit us to use in vitro mutagenesis to determine what features of the primary structure of PGG/H synthase underlie the unique catalytic and pharmacological activities of this enzyme.

ACKNOWLEDGMENTS

This work was supported in part by U. S. Public Health Service Grant DK 22042.

REFERENCES

1. Ohki S, Ogino N, Yamamoto S, Hayaishi O. J Biol Chem 1979; 254:829-836.

2. Pagels WR, Sachs RJ, Marnett LJ, DeWitt DL, Day JS, Smith WL. J Biol Chem 1983;258:6517-6523.

3. Van der Ouderaa FJ, Buytenhek M, Nugteren DH, Van Dorp DA. Eur J Biochem 1980;109:1-8.

4. Goerig M, Habenicht AJR, Heitz R, et al. J Clin Invest 1987;79:903-911.

5. Hedin L, Gaddy-Kurten D, DeWitt DL, Smith WL, Richards JS. Endocrinology 1987;121:722-731.

6. Bailey JM, Muza B, Hla T, Salata K. J Lipid Res 1985;26:54-61.

7. Huslig RL, Fogwell RL, Smith WL. Biol Reprod 1979;21:589-597.

8. DeWitt DL, Smith WL. Proc Natl Acad Sci USA 1988;85:1412-1416.

9. Roth GJ, Machuga ET, Ozols J. Biochemistry 1983;22:4672-4675.

Advances in Prostaglandin, Thromboxane, and Leukotriene Research, Vol. 19, edited by B. Samuelsson, P. Y.-K. Wong, and F. F. Sun, Raven Press, Ltd., New York ©1989.

LOCALIZATION OF THE PEROXIDASE ACTIVE SITE OF PGH SYNTHASE

Lawrence J. Marnett, Ying-Nan Pan Chen, Krishna Rao Maddipati, Regine Labeque and Patrick Ple

Department of Chemistry
Wayne State University
Detroit, MI 48202
USA

Prostaglandin H (PGH) synthase catalyzes the first two reactions of prostaglandin and thromboxane biosynthesis - bis-dioxygenation of arachidonic acid to the hydroperoxy endoperoxide PGG_2 and reduction of PGG_2 to the hydroxy endoperoxide PGH_2 (1-3). The cyclooxygenase and peroxidase activities are not separable by physical methods (1). Purified PGH synthase is a homodimer of 70 kDa subunits (4-6) and the prosthetic group is $Fe^{3+}PPIX$ (7). There is some disagreement on the stoichiometry of heme binding but both cyclooxygenase and peroxidase activities are fully reconstituted at no more than one heme per subunit (8,9). Spectroscopic studies indicate the fifth ligand to iron is an imidazole nitrogen from histidine and EPR experiments implicate histidine or tyrosine as the sixth ligand (9-11). The amino acid sequence of PGH synthase was recently deduced by recombinant DNA methods but no potential heme binding sites were apparent (12,13).

RESULTS AND DISCUSSION

Fully reconstituted PGH synthase is resistant to cleavage by trypsin whereas the apoprotein is rapidly cleaved (14). Trypsin appears to cause a single scission of the polypeptide backbone generating two protein fragments - a 33 kDa fragment containing the N-terminus of the protein and a 38 kDa fragment containing the aspirin-labeling site. Figure 1 displays the time courses for PGH synthase cleavage, loss of cyclooxygenase activity, and loss of guaiacol peroxidase activity following addition of trypsin to apo-PGH synthase. After 30 min of trypsin treatment, 90% of the apoprotein was cleaved. Addition of a saturating amount of hematin reconstituted 60% of the cyclooxygenase activity but only 10% of the peroxidase activity of an undigested control. Similar results were obtained when tetramethylphenylenediamine or epinephrine oxidation was used instead of guaiacol oxidation to assay peroxidase activity.

10-OOH-18:2 is a useful diagnostic probe for the mechanism of hydroperoxide cleavage by the metal center of peroxidases (15). Heterolytic cleavage produces 10-OH-18:2 as the exclusive product whereas homolytic cleavage generates an alkoxyl radical that undergoes ß-scission to 10-oxo-10:1 or is oxidized to 10-oxo-18:2. Intact PGH synthase is a typical heme peroxidase that cleaves the hydroperoxide bond heterolytically (15,16). It reduces 10-OOH-18:2 to 10-OH-18:2 in 95% yield. Incubation of trypsin-treated PGH synthase with 10-OOH-18:2 in the presence of phenol (as reducing substrate) generated two products, in addition to 10-OH-18:2 (39%), that were identified as 10-oxo-10:1 (32%) and 10-oxo-18:2 (28%). This indicates that trypsin treatment alters the mechanism of reaction of fatty acid hydroperoxide substrates with the peroxidase of PGH synthase.

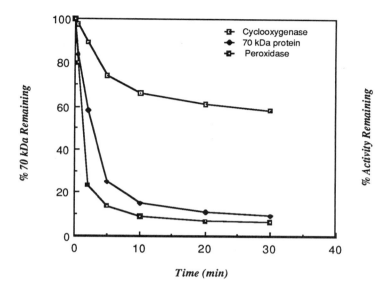

Figure 1. Time courses for protein cleavage, loss of cyclooxygenase activity, and loss of guaiacol peroxidase activity following treatment of apo-PGH synthase with trypsin.

Figure 2 displays the results of heme reconstitution experiments performed with apo-PGH synthase, trypsin-treated apo-PGH synthase, and boiled apo-PGH synthase. Trypsin treatment of apo-PGH synthase decreased the ability of the protein to bind heme by approximately 50% (assuming that the hemes bound at all sites of the protein have similar molar absorptivities). The extent of heme binding to trypsin-cleaved apo-PGH synthase was approximately the same as the extent of heme binding to boiled apo-PGH synthase. In a subsequent experiment, we found that similar titration curves were exhibited by trypsin-treated apo-PGH synthase and boiled, trypsin-treated apo-PGH synthase.

Tryptic cleavage of apoprotein occurs at the peptide bond between the Arg residue at position 253 and the Gly residue at position 254 (12,13). The four amino acids immediately preceding the cleavage site are His-Tyr-Pro-Arg. The presence of His and Arg residues in the sequence is provocative because these amino acids are present at the active sites of several other heme peroxidases in which they appear to facilitate heterolytic peroxide bond cleavage (17-19). In addition, Karthein *et al* recently detected a tyrosine radical cation in PGH synthase formed by intramolecular electron transfer to the first spectrally detectable peroxidase higher oxidation state (20). Estimates from EPR measurements place the Tyr 7-12 Å from the metal center of the peroxidase heme (20).

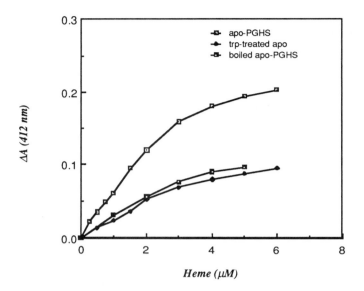

Figure 2. Spectrophotometric titration of apo-PGH synthase, boiled apo-PGH synthase, and trypsin-treated apo-PGH synthase with hematin.

We propose that the sequence His[250]-Arg[253] is at the active site of the peroxidase of PGH synthase. Most likely His[250] is the sixth ligand to the heme iron. This would explain the observations that (1) binding of heme at this position reduces the sensitivity of the peptide bond between Arg[253] and Gly[254] to cleavage by trypsin, (2) trypsin cleavage alters the mechanism of reaction between hydroperoxides and enzyme-bound heme, (3) trypsin cleavage substantially reduces peroxidase activity, and (4) trypsin cleavage abolishes one specific heme binding site on the protein. A corollary to this hypothesis is that the heme-binding site exists in a cleft located between the 33 and 38 kDa domains of the intact protein.

ACKNOWLEDGMENTS

This work was supported by a research grant from the National Institutes of Health (GM23642).

REFERENCES

1. Ohki S, Ogino N, Yamamoto S and Hayaishi O. *J Biol Chem* (1979);**254**:829-836.
2. Hamberg M and Samuelsson B. *Proc Natl Acad Sci USA* (1973);**70**:899-903.
3. Nugteren, D. H. and Hazelhof, E. *Biochim Biophys Acta* (1973);**326**:448-461.
4. Miyamoto.T, Ogino N, Yamamoto S and Hayaishi O. *J Biol Chem* (1976);**251**:2629-2636.
5. Hemler M, Lands WEM, and Smith WL. *J Biol Chem* (1976);**251**:5575-5579.
6. Van der Ouderaa FJ, Buytenhek M, Nugteren DH and Van Dorp DA *Biochim Biophys Acta.* (1977);**487**:315-331.
7. Ogino N, Ohki S, Yamamoto S and Hayaishi O. *J Biol Chem* (1978);**253**:5061-5068.
8. Kulmacz RJ and Lands WEM. *J Biol Chem* (1984);**259**:6358-6363.
9. Karthein R, Nastainczyk W and Ruf HH. *Eur J Biochem* (1987);**166**:173-180.
10. Lambeir AM, Markey CM, Dunford HB and Marnett LJ. *J Biol Chem* (1985);**260**:14894-14896.
11. Kulmacz RJ, Tsai A-L and Palmer G. *J Biol Chem* (1987);**262**:10524-10531.
12. DeWitt DL and Smith WL. *Proc Natl Acad Sci USA* (1988);**85**:1412-1416.
13. Merlie JP, Fagan D, Mudd J and Needleman P. *J Biol Chem* (1988);**263**:3550-3553.
14. Kulmacz RJ and Lands WEM. *Biochem Biophys Res Comm* (1982);**104**:758-764.
15. Labeque R and Marnett LJ. *J Am Chem Soc* (1987);**109**:2828-2829.
16. Markey CM, Alward A, Weller PE and Marnett LJ. *J Biol Chem* (1987);**262**:6266-6279.
17. Poulos TL and Kraut J. *J Biol Chem* (1980);**255**:8199-8205.
18. Welinder KG. *FEBS Letts* (1976);**72**:19-23.
19. Welinder KG and Mazza G. *Eur J Biochem* (1977);**73**:353-358.
20. Karthein R, Dietz R, Nastainczyk W and Ruf HH. *Eur J Biochem* (1988);**171**:313-320.

Advances in Prostaglandin, Thromboxane, and Leukotriene Research, Vol. 19, edited by B. Samuelsson, P. Y.-K. Wong, and F. F. Sun, Raven Press, Ltd., New York ©1989.

CLONING, NUCLEOTIDE SEQUENCE AND GENE EXPRESSION OF BOVINE LUNG PROSTAGLANDIN F SYNTHETASE

[*]K. Watanabe, [*]Y. Fujii, [†]K. Nakayama, [†]H. Ohkubo, [Ψ]S. Kuramitsu, [*]H. Hayashi, [Ψ]H. Kagamiyama, [†]S. Nakanishi, and [*]O. Hayaishi

[*]Hayaishi Bioinformation Transfer Project, Kyoto Laboratory, Research Development Corporation of Japan, Nishioji-Hachijo, Minami-ku, Kyoto 601, Japan. [†]Institute for Immunology, Kyoto University Faculty of Medicine, Kyoto 606, Japan. [Ψ]Department of Medical Chemistry, Osaka Medical College, Takatsuki 569, Japan.

Prostaglandin (PG) F synthetase purified from bovine lung catalyzed the reduction of PGH_2 to $PGF_2\alpha$ and that of PGD_2 to $9\alpha,11\beta-PGF_2$ at different active sites on the same molecule (1,2). To study the primary structure and molecular mechanism of the enzyme, we isolated cloned cDNA sequences specific for PGF synthetase from a cDNA library of bovine lung mRNA sequences and determined the cDNA sequence encoding the entire bovine lung PGF synthetase and the deduced amino acid sequence (3). Moreover, we compared the amino acid sequence of PGF synthetase with those of aldo-keto reductases and with the National Biomedical Research Foundation (NBRF) protein data base (3). To characterize PGF synthetase at the molar level, we tried to express the PGF synthetase gene in E. coli.

Fig. 1 shows the complete nucleotide sequence and the deduced amino acid sequence. The insert contained 1220 nucleotides(nt). The length of the poly (A) tail was not included in this determination. The cDNA inserts contained 6 nt in the 5' noncoding region, 969 nt in the coding region that were followed by the termination codon UAA, and 245 nt in the 3' untranslated region preceding the poly (A) tail. PGF synthetase contains 323 amino aicds, and the calculated Mr. of 36,666. The Mr. of the mature protein is 36,517 excluding the initiation methionine. As shown in Fig. 1, nine tryptic peptides (amino acid residues, 2-4, 8-35, 48-66, 67-76, 137-153, 217-236, 259-263,

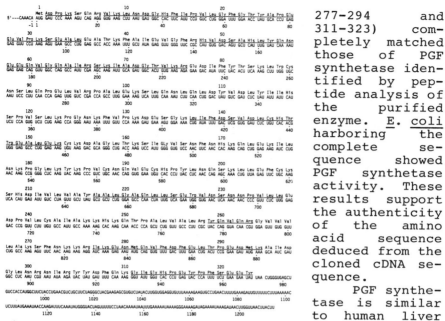

Fig. 1. Primary structure of bovine lung PGF synthetase mRNA

277-294 and 311-323) completely matched those of PGF synthetase identified by peptide analysis of the purified enzyme. E. coli harboring the complete sequence showed PGF synthetase activity. These results support the authenticity of the amino acid sequence deduced from the cloned cDNA sequence.

PGF synthetase is similar to human liver aldehyde reductase and rat lens aldose reductase in terms of Mr. and substrate specificity. These three enzymes belong to a group of aldo-keto reductases in terms of substrate specificity. Wermuth et al. (4) and Carper et al. (5) recently reported the amino acid sequences of human liver aldehyde reductase and rat lens aldose reductase, respectively. The amino acid sequence of PGF synthetase showed about 65% similarity with deletions/additions to those of human liver aldehyde reductase and to rat lens aldose reductase (Fig. 2). Possibly the amino acid sequences for the active sites of these enzymes show similarity. These findings may be helpful in elucidating the two active sites in PGF synthetase, and a group of aldo-keto reductases may form a gene family.

On the other hand, comparison of the amino acid sequence of PGF synthetase with the NBRF protein database reveals that the sequences of 225 amino acids from the C termini of ρ-crystallin of the European frog lens and of PGF synthetase show 77% similarity (Fig. 2). The Mr. of European common frog ρ-crystallin is about 35 KDa. The N-terminal region of the amino acid sequence of ρ-crystallin may also be similar to that of PGF synthetase, and ρ-crystallin of

```
        10          20          30          40          50          60          70
AASC L HT QKM LI L  WKS PGQVKA V--- Y LS  Y  I C AI G  PEI E L---- EDV      ALD
    ASHLE  N TKM T  L  WKSPPGQVT V--- V  DM Y  I C QV   KE  V LQEKL EQV      AR
DPKSQR K  D HFI V  F  YAP EVPKS  LEAT F  E F  V S HL    EQ  Q I--RS IAD      PGFS

      80          90         100         110         120         130         140
PGKA P  EL V    NTKHH  D E   R T AD   E L   LM W YAFER DNPF  NAD T- CY       ALD
----    Q L IV   TFHDQSM KGACQ T SD    L  L W TGF  PDYF L A  NV PS T         AR
---T    I Y     NSLQ  L R    S QN    V  I  S       NKFV   E  KL -P           PGFS
                            RS RDVGM  L  FLM W     SGASD S KDKPF -Y N        RHO

        150         160         170         180         190         200         210
THYKE  K  ALVAK  VQAL L    SR IDD  SVASVR-- AVL     A NE IAH QARGL           ALD
- FVD  T M QLV E  V A      PL I R        AV I      T E  I Y HCKG             AR
     H    KC    T        HK  K                    S  L F   H                 PGFS
     A    AR    VR       RR  R               V    N HSY    K                 RHO

        220         230         240         250         260         270         280
EVT  -P  SS-DRA RDPDE    E  VL L E YGRS  QIL  W   K ICIP  ITPS  LQ I         ALD
VT  SP  SP-DRP AKPED S   RIKE  A YNK T Q LI FPI  NL IP  VTPA   A  F          AR
    AA  AQLLSE  NSNN       C   K HKQ   L  Y        NKK      M                PGFS
T SV  SHRDRN  DLSL    D  I NKV A YNR S EI M FIL   I       TPA   Q L          RHO

    290         300         310         320
K    TFS  E  QLNA  K W  IVPMLTVDGKRVPRDA   L   NDP                          ALD
K    SN    ATLLSY  W VC-ALMSC--------AK KD   HA V                          AR
Q    T     AIDG    I  Y-D QKG--------I        SE                           PGFS
G  E  K    SLES D  LH G-P REV--------KQ       HD                           RHO
```

Fig. 2. Comparison of PGF synthetase (PGFS) with human liver aldehyde reductase (ALD), rat lens aldose reductase (AR) and European common frog lens -crystallin (RHO). Dark grey and light grey between sequences indicate exact matches and conservative substitutions (3), respectively.

European frog lens may be identical to PGF synthetase. Crystallins have been regarded simply as soluble, structural proteins. The strong similarity of the amino acid sequences of PGF synthetase and ρ-crystallin suggests that the enzyme protein is related to the structural protein.

To characterize PGF synthetase at the molar level, we tried to express this enzyme in E. coli. The full length bovine lung PGF synthetase cDNA clone

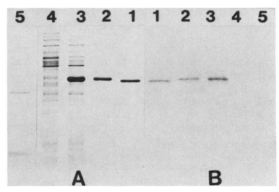

Fig. 3. SDS-PAGE and immunoblotting of the expressed protein in E. coli and of bovine lung PGF synthetase. lane 1, marker; lane 2, E. coli cells harboring pUC8; lane 3, E. coli cells harboring the full length sequence; lane 4, purified expressed protein; lane 5; bovine lung PGF synthetase.

was constructed from restriction fragments of the two partial cDNA clones and inserted into the plasmid pUC8. The extracts of E. coli cells harboring the full length sequence were electrophoresed on SDS-PAGE gels (Fig. 3A). Coomassie brilliant blue staining of the gel indicated that an approximately 35-KDa protein is produced in cells containing the expression plasmid (Fig. 3A). Western blot analysis revealed that the 35-KDa protein is recognized by the PGF synthetase-specific antibody (Fig. 3B). No protein from E. coli cells harboring pUC8 only interacted with the antibody. This expressed protein was purified to apparent homogeneity. The expressed protein represents that 9 amino acids contributed by the lac Z gene of pUC8, the noncoding region and the initiation codon of PGF synthetase are fused to N-terminus to native enzyme. The purified expressed protein reduced not only PGD_2 and carbonyl compounds (eg. phenanthrenequinone) but also PGH_2. The Km values for PGD_2 and H_2 were 100 μM and 10 μM, respectively. These values and the Km values for other substrates are almost equivalent to those for substrates of bovine lung PGF synthetase. PGD_2 reductase activity is inhibited competitively by phenanthrenequinone, but the PGH_2 reductase activity is not inhibited by phenanthrenequinone. The expressed protein catalyzed the reduction of PGD_2 to $9\alpha,11\beta$-PGF_2 and that of PGH_2 to $PGF_2\alpha$ at different active sites. These results suggest that the properties of the expressed protein in E. coli are essentially identical to those of the bovine lung PGF synthetase. Therefore, PGF synthetase is a dual function enzyme catalyzing the reduction of PGH_2 and that of PGD_2 on a single protein.

REFERENCES

1. Watanabe K, Yoshida R, Shimizu T, and Hayaishi O. J Biol Chem 1985;260:7035-7041.
2. Watanabe K, Iguchi Y, Iguchi S, Arai Y, Hayaishi O, and Roberts II, LJ. Proc Natl Acad Sci USA 1986;83:1583-1587.
3. Watanabe K, Fujii Y, Nakayama K, et al. Proc Natl Acad Sci USA 1988;85:11-15.
4. Wermuth B, Omar A, Forster A, et al. In: Weiner H, Flynn TG, eds. Enzymology and Molecular Biology of Carbonyl Metabolism: Aldehyde Dehydrogenase, Aldo-keto Reductase, and Alcohol Dehydrogenase, New York: Alan R. Liss, Inc, 1987;297-307.
5. Carper D, Nishimura C, Shinohara T, et al. FEBS Lett 1987;220:209-213.

Advances in Prostaglandin, Thromboxane, and Leukotriene Research, Vol. 19, edited by
B. Samuelsson, P. Y.-K. Wong, and F. F. Sun,
Raven Press, Ltd., New York ©1989.

MOLECULAR CLONING AND AMINO ACID SEQUENCE OF HUMAN 5-LIPOXYGENASE

Takashi Matsumoto*, Colin D Funk, Olof Rådmark, Jan-Olov Höög,
Hans Jörnvall and Bengt Samuelsson

Department of Physiological Chemistry,
Karolinska Institutet, S-104 01 Stockholm, Sweden

*Permanent address: Life Science Research Laboratory,
Japan Tobacco Inc., 6-2, Umegaoka, Midori-ku, Kanagawa 227 Japan

INTRODUCTION

The leukotrienes constitute a group of arachidonic acid derived
metabolites with biological activities suggesting important roles
in inflammation and immediate hypersensitivity (1). The enzyme, 5-
lipoxygenase (arachidonate:oxygen 5-oxidoreductase, EC 1.13.11.34)
catalyzes the formation of 5-hydroperoxy-6,8,11,14-icosatetraenoic
acid (5-HPETE) from arachidonic acid, as well as the subsequent
conversion of 5-HPETE to 5,6-oxido-7,9,11,14-icosatetraenoic acid
(leukotriene A_4)(2-5). It is also involved in the formation of lipoxins, a group of biologically active compounds derived from arachidonic acid (6).

The 5-lipoxygenase has been isolated from human and porcine
leukocytes, murine mast cells, and rat basophilic leukemia cells
(3,5,7). The enzyme is dependent on Ca^{2+} and ATP. The human leukocyte enzyme displays even greater complexity by the requirement
for three cellular components for maximal activity.

In this study we describe the isolation of cDNA clones for
human lung and placenta 5-lipoxygenase and deduce the complete
amino acid sequence of the enzyme.

METHODS

A cDNA clone corresponding to human leukocyte 5-lipoxygenase
was isolated from a human lung λgt11 expression library by immuno
screening with a polyclonal antibody. Additional clones from a
human placenta λgt11 cDNA library were obtained by plaque hybridization with the ^{32}P-labeled lung cDNA clone. DNA sequencing was
carried out by the dideoxy chain-termination method. 5-Lipoxyge-
nase and its proteolytic fragments were analyzed directly. The
details of these procedures have been published elswhere (8).

RESULTS AND DISCUSSION

Antibody Screening of a Lung λ gt11 cDNA Library.

In order to clone the cDNA for 5-lipoxygenase, we prepared a specific antiserum against purified human leukocyte 5-lipoxygenase for immunoscreening a λ gt11 library. The specificity of the purified IgG fraction was tested by immunoblot analysis of 100,000 x g human leukocyte sonicate supernatant that had been electrophoresed in a NaDodSO₄/10% polyacrylamide gel. A distinct single band was observed at ~80 KDa.

A human lung λ gt11 cDNA library was screened with the IgG fraction. The insert from the positive cDNA clone (λ luS1) was isolated and sequenced. λ luS1 had a 397-bp insert and was found to contain a coding sequence for a segment that was known for 17 amino acids from the peptide analyses of the lipoxygenase fragments. This finding identifies λ luS1 as part of the 5-lipoxygenase cDNA.

Screening for Additional 5-Lipoxygenase Clones.

The insert from λ luS1 was nick-translated and used as a probe for finding clones with longer inserts from a λ gt11 human placenta cDNA library. Four strongly positive clones were obtained after screening ~8 x 10⁵ cDNA clones. These clones were purified and the sizes of the EcoRI inserts were determined to be 1.3, 1.6, 2.2 and 2.6 kbp.

Nucleotide Sequence of cDNA and Deduced Amino Acid Sequence for 5-Lipoxygenase.

The insert of the clone containing the 2.6-kbp insert (λ p15BS) was sequenced. λ p15BS contains a 2552-bp insert, excluding EcoRI linkers, with 2073 bp from the initiator codon ATG to the stop codon TGA in a continuous open reading frame. Within this insert there are two adjacent exact 51-bp repeating units (Fig. 1 legend). The presence of this repeat suggested the possibility of a cloning artifact. Therefore, two additional clones, λ p19AS (1.6-kbp insert) and λ p16S (2.2-kbp insert) were sequenced. Only one copy of the 51-bp unit was present in each of these inserts. All other sequenced nucleotides were identical to the insert of λ p15BS. Consequently, the true 5-lipoxygenase is concluded also to lack the repeat, and the open reading frame would encode a mature protein of 673 amino acids (the initiator methionine is not present in the mature protein: direct sequence analysis revealed the subsequent proline residue to constitute the amino terminus) with a calculated molecular weight of 77,856 (Fig. 1). The 5' noncoding region is 34 bp long. The 3' noncoding region is 442 bp long and contains an AATAAA polyadenylylation signal 11 bases upstream from the poly(A) tail. The deduced amino acid sequence of the first 17 amino acids is identical to the sequence determined by Edman degradation of the purified protein. In addition, the deduced sequence agrees with the sequences of internal peptides generated by proteolytic

```
                                                                                                      -34                              -1
                                                                                                     GGGC CCGGCGCTCGCTGCTCCCGCGGCCCGCGCC
                             30                              60                              90                             120                             150
ATGCCCTCCTACACGGTCACCGTGGCCACT GGCAGCCAGTGGTTCGCCGGCACTGACGAC TACATCTACCTCAGCCTCGTGGGCTCGGCG GGCTGCAGCGAGAAGCACCTGCTGGACAAG CCCTTCTACAACGACTTCGAGCGTGGCGCG
MetProSerTyrThrValThrValAlaThr GlySerGlnTrpPheAlaGlyThrAspAsp TyrIleTyrLeuSerLeuValGlySerAla GlyCysSerGluLysHisLeuLeuAspLys ProPheTyrAsnAspPheGluArgGlyAla
                            180                             210                             240                             270                             300
GTGGATTCATACGACGTGACTGTGGACGAG GAACTGGGCGAGATCCAGCTGGTCAGAATC GAGAAGCGCAAGTACTGGCTGAATGACGAC TGGTACCTGAAGTACATCACGCTGAAGACG CCCCACGGGGACTACATCGAGTTCCCCTGC
ValAspSerTyrAspValThrValAspGlu GluLeuGlyGluIleGlnLeuValArgIle GluLysArgLysTyrTrpLeuAsnAspAsp TrpTyrLeuLysTyrIleThrLeuLysThr ProHisGlyAspTyrIleGluPheProCys
                            330                             360                             390                             420                             450
TACCGCTGGATCACCGGCGATGTCGAGGTT GTCCTGAGGGATGGACGCGCAAAGTTGGCC CGAGATGACCAAATTCACATTCTCAAGCAA CACCGACGTAAAGAACTGGAAACACGGCAA AAACAATATCGATGGATGGAGTGGAACCCT
TyrArgTrpIleThrGlyAspValGluVal ValLeuArgAspGlyArgAlaLysLeuAla ArgAspAspGlnIleHisIleLeuLysGln HisArgArgLysGluLeuGluThrArgGln LysGlnTyrArgTrpMetGluTrpAsnPro
                            480                             510                             540                             570                             600
GGCTTCCCCTTGAGCATCGATGCCAAATGC CACAAGGATTTACCCCGTGATATCCAGTTT GATAGTGAAAAAGGAGTGGACTTTGTTCTG AATTACTCCAAAGCGATGGAGAACCTGTTC ATCAACCGCTTCATGCACATGTTCCAGTCT
GlyPheProLeuSerIleAspAlaLysCys HisLysAspLeuProArgAspIleGlnPhe AspSerGluLysGlyValAspPheValLeu AsnTyrSerLysAlaMetGluAsnLeuPhe IleAsnArgPheMetHisMetPheGlnSer
                            630                             660                             690                             720                             750
TCTTGGAATGACTTCGCCGACTTTGAGAAA ATCTTTGTCAAGATCAGCAACACTATTTCT GAGCGGGTCATGAATCACTGGCAGGAAGAC CTGATGTTTGGCTACCAGTTCCTGAATGGC TGCAACCCTGTGTTGATCCGGCGCTGCACA
SerTrpAsnAspPheAlaAspPheGluLys IlePheValLysIleSerAsnThrIleSer GluArgValMetAsnHisTrpGlnGluAsp LeuMetPheGlyTyrGlnPheLeuAsnGly CysAsnProValLeuIleArgArgCysThr
                            780                             810                             840                             870                             900
GAGCTGCCCGAGAAGCTCCCGGTGACCACG GAGATGGTAGAGTGCAGCCTGGAGCGGCAG CTCAGCTTGGAGCAGGAGGTCCAGCAAGGG AACATTTTCATCGTGGACTTTGAGCTGCTG GATGGCATCGATGCCAACAAAACAGACCCC
GluLeuProGluLysLeuProValThrThr GluMetValGluCysSerLeuGluArgGln LeuSerLeuGluGlnGluValGlnGlnGly AsnIlePheIleValAspPheGluLeuLeu AspGlyIleAspAlaAsnLysThrAspPro
                            930                             960                             990                            1020                            1050
TGCACACTCCAGTTCCTGGCCGCTCCCATC TGCTTGCTGTATAAGAACCTGGCCAACAAG ATTGTCCCCATTGCCATCCAGCTCAACCAA ATCCCGGGAGATGAGAACCCTATTTTCCTC CCTTCGGATGCAAAATACGACTGGCTTTTG
CysThrLeuGlnPheLeuAlaAlaProIle CysLeuLeuTyrLysAsnLeuAlaAsnLys IleValProIleAlaIleGlnLeuAsnGln IleProGlyAspGluAsnProIlePheLeu ProSerAspAlaLysTyrAspTrpLeuLeu
                           1080                            1110                            1140                            1170                            1200
GCCAAAATCTGGGTGCGTTCCAGTGACTTC CACGTCCACCAGACCATCACCCACCTTCTG CGAACACATCTGGTGTCTGAGGTTTTTGGC ATTGCAATGTACCGCCAGCTGCCTGCTGTG CACCCCATTTTCAAGCTGCTGGTGGCACAC
AlaLysIleTrpValArgSerSerAspPhe HisValHisGlnThrIleThrHisLeuLeu ArgThrHisLeuValSerGluValPheGly IleAlaMetTyrArgGlnLeuProAlaVal HisProIlePheLysLeuLeuValAlaHis
                           1230                            1260                            1290                            1320                            1350
GTGAGATTCACCATTGCAATCAACACCAAG GCCCGTGAGCAGCTCATCTGCGAGTGTGGC CTCTTTGACAAGGCCAACGCCACAGGGGGC GGTGGGCACGTGCAGATGGTGCAGAGGGCC ATGAAGGACCTGACCTATGCCTCCCTGTGC
ValArgPheThrIleAlaIleAsnThrLys AlaArgGluGlnLeuIleCysGluCysGly LeuPheAspLysAlaAsnAlaThrGlyGly GlyGlyHisValGlnMetValGlnArgAla MetLysAspLeuThrTyrAlaSerLeuCys
                           1380                            1410                            1440                            1470                            1500
TTTCCCGAGGCCATCAAGGCCCGGGGCATG GAGAGCAAAGAAGACATCCCCTACTACTTC TACCGGGACGACGGGCTCCTGGTGTGGGAA GCCATCAGGACGTTCACGGCCGAGGTGGTA GACATCTACTACGAGGGCGACCAGGTGGTG
PheProGluAlaIleLysAlaArgGlyMet GluSerLysGluAspIleProTyrTyrPhe TyrArgAspAspGlyLeuLeuValTrpGlu AlaIleArgThrPheThrAlaGluValVal AspIleTyrTyrGluGlyAspGlnValVal
                           1530                            1560                            1590                            1620                            1650
GAGGAGGACCCGGAGCTGCAGGACTTCGTG AACGATGTCTACGTGTACGGCATGCGGGGC CGCAAGTCCTCAGGCTTCCCCAAGTCGGTC AAGAGCCGGGAGCAGCTGTCGGAGTACCTG ACCGTGGTGATCTTCACCGCCTCCGCCCAG
GluGluAspProGluLeuGlnAspPheVal AsnAspValTyrValTyrGlyMetArgGly ArgLysSerSerGlyPheProLysSerVal LysSerArgGluGlnLeuSerGluTyrLeu ThrValValIlePheThrAlaSerAlaGln
                           1680                            1710                            1740                            1770                            1800
CACGCCGCGGTCAACTTCGGCCAGTACGAC TGGTGCTCCTGGATCCCCAATGCGCCCCCA ACCATGCGAGCCCCGCCACCGACTGCCAAG GGCGTGGTGACCATTGAGCAGATCGTGGAC ACGCTGCCCGACCGCGGCCGCTCCTGCTGG
HisAlaAlaValAsnPheGlyGlnTyrAsp TrpCysSerTrpIleProAsnAlaProPro ThrMetArgAlaProProProThrAlaLys GlyValValThrIleGluGlnIleValAsp ThrLeuProAspArgGlyArgSerCysTrp
                           1830                            1860                            1890                            1920                            1950
CATCTGGGTGCAGTGTGGGCGCTGAGCCAG TTCCAGGAAAACGAGCTGTTCCTGGGCATG TACCCAGAAGAGCATTTTATCGAGAAGCCT GTGAAGGAAGCCATGGCCCGATTCCGCAAG AACCTCGAGGCCATTGTCAGCGTGATTGCT
HisLeuGlyAlaValTrpAlaLeuSerGln PheGlnGluAsnGluLeuPheLeuGlyMet TyrProGluGluHisPheIleGluLysPro ValLysGluAlaMetAlaArgPheArgLys AsnLeuGluAlaIleValSerValIleAla
                           1980                            2010                            2040                            2070                            2100
GAGCGCAACAAGAAGAAGCAGCTGCCATAT TACTACTTGTCCCCAGACCGGATTCCGAAC AGTGTGGCCATCTGAGCACACTGCCAGTCT CACTGTGGGAAGGCCAGCTGCCCCAGCCAG ATGGACTCCAGCCTGCCTGGCAGGCTGTCT
GluArgAsnLysLysLysGlnLeuProTyr TyrTyrLeuSerProAspArgIleProAsn SerValAlaIle---
                           2130                            2160                            2190                            2220                            2250
GGCCAGGCCTCTTGGCAGTCACATCTCTTC CTCCGAGGCCAGTACCTTTCCATTTATTCT TTGATCTTCAGGGAACTGCATAGATTGATC AAAGTGTAAACACCATAGGGACCCATTCTA CACAGAGCAGGACTGCACAGCGTCCTGTCC
                           2280                            2310                            2340                            2370                            2400
ACACCCAGCTCAGCATTTCCACACCAAGCA GCAACAGCAAATCACGACCACTGATAGATG TCTATTCTTGTTGGAGACATGGGATGATTA TTTTCTGTTCTATTTGTGCTTAGTCCAATT CCTTGCACATAGTAGGTACCCAATTCAATT
                           2430                            2460
ACTATTGAATGAATTAAGAATTGGTTGCCA TAAAAATAAATCAGTTCATTTAAAAAAAAA AAAAAAA
```

FIG. 1. Nucleotide sequence of 5-lipoxygenase cDNAs and the predicted amino acid sequence. Nucleotides are numbered beginning with the first base of the ATG initiator codon. Nucleotides to the 5' side are designated by negative numbers. Amino acids are numbered from the amino-terminal proline residue of the mature protein. Solid underlining represents regions determined also by direct peptide analysis (broken underlines indicate amino acids incompletely identified in the peptide analyses but with analytical data compatible with the deduced amino acid sequence). The polyadenylylation signal is wavy-underlined. The double-underlined region is repeated in λp15BS and would be inserted between nucleotides 1228 and 1229.

cleavages of purified leukocyte 5-lipoxygenase (Fig. 1).
As 5-lipoxygenase requires Ca^{2+} and ATP for maximal activity, the amino acid sequence was examined for the presence of consensus binding sites for these cofactors. A search for typical "E-F hand" Ca^{2+}-binding domain associated with Ca^{2+}-binding proteins revealed no such sites in 5-lipoxygenase. No strong homology was observed in the sequence to any ATP binding sites. Recent studies (9) indicate the possibility that Ca^{2+} may effect a translocation of the normally soluble enzyme to a membrane site, which may be related to the activation of the enzyme.

RNA Blot Analysis.

Poly(A)$^+$ RNA obtained from human lung, placenta and peripheral leukocytes was subjected to blot analysis using the insert of λ-luS1 as a hybridization probe. Hybridization to a discrete mRNA of ~2700 nucleotides occurred in all three tissues. The hybridization intensity was greatest for leukocyte poly(A)$^+$RNA, followed by the preparations from placenta and lung tissue.

Acknowledgements

We thank Lena Eliasson, Carina Palmberg, Anne Peters and Gunilla Lundquist for excellent assistance. This study was supported by fellowships from Japan Tobacco Inc. (to T.M.) and Fonds de la Recherche en Santé du Québec (to C.D.F.) and by grants from the Swedish Medical Research Council(03X-217, 03X-7467, and 03X-3532), the Konung Gustav V 80-års fond, the Magnus Bergwall foundation, and the Swedish Cancer Society (1806).

REFERENCES

1. Samuelsson B. Science 1983; 220: 568-575.
2. Rouzer CA, Matsumoto T, Samuelsson B. Proc. Natl. Acad. Sci. USA 1986; 83: 857-861.
3. Shimizu T, Izumi T, Seyama Y, Samuelsson B. Proc. Natl. Acad. Sci. USA 1986; 83: 4175-4179.
4. Ueda N, Kaneko S, Yoshimoto T, Yamamoto S. J. Biol. Chem. 1986; 261: 7982-7988.
5. Hogaboom GK, Cook M, Newton JF, et al. Mol. Pharmacol. 1986; 30: 510-519.
6. Serhan CN, Nicolaou KC, Webber SE, et al. J. Biol. Chem. 1986; 261: 16340-16345.
7. Rouzer CA, Samuelsson B. Proc. Natl. Acad. Sci. USA 1985; 82: 6040-6044.
8. Matsumoto T, Funk CD, Rådmark O, Höög JO, Jörnvall H, Samuelsson B. Proc. Natl. Acad. Sci. USA 1988; 85: 26-30.
9. Rouzer CA, Samuelsson B. Proc. Natl. Acad. Sci. USA 1987; 84: 7393-7397

Advances in Prostaglandin, Thromboxane, and
Leukotriene Research, Vol. 19, edited by
B. Samuelsson, P. Y.-K. Wong, and F. F. Sun,
Raven Press, Ltd., New York ©1989.

CHARACTERIZATION OF THE HUMAN 5-LIPOXYGENASE GENE

Colin D. Funk, Takashi Matsumoto, Shigeru Hoshiko,
Olof Rådmark and Bengt Samuelsson

Department of Physiological Chemistry
Karolinska Institutet
S-104 01 Stockholm, Sweden

The cDNA for 5-lipoxygenase has recently been cloned
from human placenta (1) and differentiated HL-60 cell
(2) cDNA libraries. However, little is known about
the mechanisms controlling 5-lipoxygenase expression
in various tissues. In this study we have begun characterization of the 5-lipoxygenase gene. Clones
spanning the gene have been isolated and characterized.

METHODS

Three genomic DNA libraries were screened in these
studies and are as follows: (i) an EMBL-3 human
leukocyte library (Clontech); (ii) an EMBL-4 human
leukemia cell library (gift from Dr. J. Sumegi) and ;
(iii) an AluI/HaeIII human fetal liver library in the
cloning vector λCharon 4A (constructed by T. Maniatis
and obtained from the American Type Culture Collection). Screening was carried out with various 5-li-
poxygenase cDNA probes (1).
Standard DNA techniques (3) were employed.

RESULTS

Isolation and characterization of 5-lipoxygenase
genomic clones.

Three different genomic libraries were screened in
multiple screenings with several different 5-lipoxy-
genase cDNA probes. Clones 1x3A, 1x9A, 1x12A, 1x15A
and 1x17A were isolated from the EMBL-3 human leukocyte library. Clones 1x22A and 1x27A were isolated
from the EMBL-4 leukemia cell library and 1x43A was
isolated from the λCharon4A human fetal liver library
(Fig.1).
Twelve complete exons were sequenced. They ranged
in size from 87 bp (exon 8) to 611 bp (exon 13). A

genomic segment containing putative exon 3 has not yet been cloned. All introns conform to the GT-AG rule (4) and surrounding sequences are closely related to the consensus sequences surrounding splice junctions (5). Introns ranged in size from 192 bp (intron J) to 10.5 kb (intron F). The total length of the human 5-lipoxygenase gene is at least 45 kb.

5' Flanking region of the human 5-lipoxygenase gene

The nucleotide sequence of a 270 bp region upstream from the ATG start codon was determined. The region is very GC rich (80 %) and contains several interesting features. There are six tandem repeats of the sequence CGGGGG and two repeats of CCCGCCC or socalled "GC- boxes". There are four copies of the sequence CCGGG, as well as an 11-bp inverted repeat sequence GCCGGGAGCCT. The region contains neither a "TATA-box" nor a "CAAT-box".

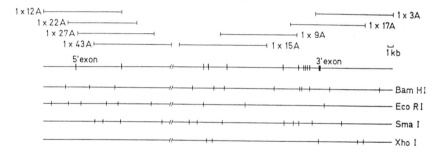

Fig. 1 The human 5-lipoxygenase gene. Top; genomic clones. Middle; exon-intron map. Bottom; restriction sites for selected enzymes.

DISCUSSION

Gene organization and putative protein domains

The structure and organization of the human 5-lipoxygenase gene has been investigated in the present study. The gene consists of 13 exons divided by 12 introns and is relatively long (at least 45 kb) considering the length of the coding sequence. There are three introns with lengths greater than 8 kb. Exons 1-6, encoding the amino-terminal half of 5-lipoxygenase are spread out over more than 30 kb of DNA, whereas the carboxyl-terminal encoding exons, 7-13 are clustered in a 6 kb segment of DNA. At present it is difficult to say if certain exons correspond to structural or functional domains of 5-lipoxygenase. Very little information is known about the structure of 5-lipoxygenase and putative Ca^{2+}- and ATP-binding sites could not be easily predicted from the cDNA sequence (1,2). However, exon 6, which encodes amino acids 278-326 corresponds exactly to one of the most hydrophobic segments of 5-lipoxygenase (1) (Fig.2). Thus, this segment could represent a catalytic domain

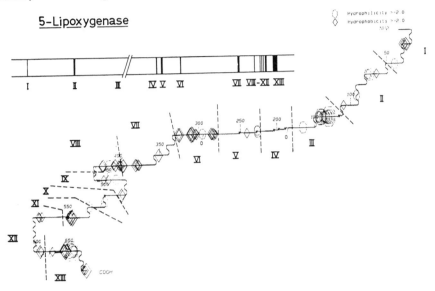

Fig.2   5-Lipoxygenase gene-protein relationship.
         Exons corresponding to various regions of
         5-lipoxygenase are displayed on a predicted
         secondary structure/hydropathy plot.

involved in arachidonic acid binding and conversion to 5-HPETE. In vitro mutagenesis analysis could substantiate this possibility.

The 5-lipoxygenase gene is likely represented by a single copy in the human haploid genome. Total genomic DNA hybridization analysis (data not shown) and the fact that phage clones from three different genomic libraries exhibited identical restriction maps tend to confirm this hypothesis.

5' Flanking region of the 5-lipoxygenase gene

The putative promoter region of the 5-lipoxygenase gene is lacking typical TATA and CAAT boxes, sequences purportedly involved in ensuring accurate transcription initiation and in controlling transcriptional rate. However, this region exhibits features common to the promoter regions of the housekeeping genes. These common characteristics include high GC content upstream of the cap site, the existence of potential binding sites for the transcription factor Sp1, as well as, the absence of TATA and CAAT boxes. The 5' flanking region of the 5-lipoxygenase gene contains 8 potential sites for Sp1 binding (GGGCGG or CCGCCC) in addition to similar short GC repeating units. The presence of two 11-bp inverted repeat units could also have some relevance to transcription factor binding and thus to transcriptional regulation.

The 5' flanking sequence shows some sequence similarity (65%) to a region of intron 2 of the human zeta-globin pseudogene (6). The latter sequence contains multiple copies of the sequence CGGGG, similar to the repeating CGGGGG units in the 5-lipoxygenase gene. The 177-bp intron 2 sequence of the bovine arginine vasopressin-neurophysin II gene (7) displays similar homology.

If, in fact, the human 5-lipoxygenase gene is constitutively expressed like the other housekeeping genes, this raises questions about the importance of 5-lipoxygenase in normal cellular biochemical processes and to 5-lipoxygenase enzyme turnover.

REFERENCES

1. Matsumoto, T., Funk, C.D., Rådmark, O., Höög, J-O, Jörnvall, H. and Samuelsson, B. (1988) Proc. Natl. Acad. Sci. USA 85, 26-30.

2. Dixon, R.A.F., Jones, R.E., Diehl, R.E., Bennett, C.D., Kargman, S. and Rouzer, C.A. (1988) Proc. Natl. Acad. Sci. USA 85, 416-420.

3. Maniatis, T., Fritsch, E.F., and Sambrook, J. (1982) Molecular Cloning: A Laboratory Manual (Cold Spring Harbor Laboratory, Cold Spring Harbor, NY).

4. Breathnach, R. and Chambon, P. (1981) Annu. Rev. Biochem. 50, 349-383.

5. Mount, S.M. (1982) Nucleic Acids Res. 10, 459-472.

6. Proudfoot, N.J., Gil, A. and Maniatis, T. (1982) Cell 31, 553-563.

7. Ruppert, S., Scherer, G. and Schutz, G. (1984) Nature 308, 554-557.

Advances in Prostaglandin, Thromboxane, and Leukotriene Research, Vol. 19, edited by B. Samuelsson, P. Y.-K. Wong, and F. F. Sun, Raven Press, Ltd., New York ©1989.

CLONING AND EXPRESSION OF HUMAN LEUKOCYTE 5-LIPOXYGENASE

*Carol A. Rouzer, +Carl D. Bennett, + Ronald E. Diehl,
+Raymond E. Jones, *Stacia Kargman, + Elaine Rands, and
+Richard A.F. Dixon

*Department of Pharmacology, Merck Frosst Canada, Inc.,
Pointe Claire-Dorval, Québec, Canada, H9R 4P8

and

+Department of Molecular Biology,
Merck Sharp and Dohme Research Laboratories,
West Point, Pennsylvania 19486

INTRODUCTION

The enzyme, 5-lipoxygenase (5-LO), catalyzes the first two steps in the biosynthesis of leukotrienes (LT) from arachidonic acid (20:4) (1-4). Therefore, an understanding of the regulation of this enzyme is of considerable importance to the delineation of the regulation of LT biosynthesis. Recent progress in the biochemistry of 5-LO has included the purification of the enzyme from human and other mammalian sources and the discovery of the stimulation of its activity by Ca^{2+}, ATP, and several other cellular components (1-5). However, very little is known concerning the regulation of 5-LO at the level of gene expression. Consequently, we have cloned the cDNA for human 5-LO from the promyelocytic leukemic cell line HL-60, obtained the complete nucleotide sequence of this cDNA, and achieved expression of 5-LO activity in an osteosarcoma cell line transfected with the cDNA. We summarize here the results of these studies (6-7).

RESULTS

Sequence of 5-LO Peptides

5-LO was purified from human leukocytes as previously described (8). The protein was subjected to cyanogen bromide cleavage, and three peptides were isolated by reverse phase, high pressure liquid chromatography. The N-terminal sequences of these peptides, and the intact protein were as follows:

N-terminus: PSYTVTVATGSQWFAGTDDYIYLSLVGSA
Peptide 8: VQRA
Peptide 18: YPEEHFIEKPVKEA
Peptide 27: ARFRKNLEAIVSVIAERNKKKOLPYYYLSPDRIPNS

Corresponding to the sequences of the N-terminus and peptide 27, two overlapping complementary oligonucleotides were constructed, based on preferred codon usage. From peptide 18 (amino acids 3-10) a pool of oligonucleotides was synthesized that corresponded to all possible codon choices (6).

cDNA Cloning

Although 5-LO was purified from human peripheral blood leukocytes, these cells proved to be a poor source of mRNA for cDNA cloning. We therefore utilized the human promyelocytic HL-60 cell line. These cells had previously been shown to differentiate in culture upon exposure to 1.3% dimethyl sulfoxide/10 μM dexamethasone (DMSO/dex) to yield cells that closely resemble mature neutrophils (9). During differentiation, the cells acquire the capacity to synthesize LT (10), and we have shown that from 1 to 7 days of exposure to DMSO/dex there is a linear increase in 5-LO activity in supernatants prepared from the cells, suggesting that 5-LO is being actively synthesized. Consequently poly (A)$^+$ RNA was isolated from HL60 cells cultured for 5 days in DMSO/dex, and used to construct a cDNA library in λgt10.

Recombinants (2 x 10^6) from the HL60 cDNA library were screened with the oligonucleotide probes described above. A total of 35 clones were isolated that hybridized to oligonucleotides corresponding to peptides 18 and 27, whereas no clones hybridized to oligonucleotides corresponding to the N-terminus. Sequence analysis of the inserts from the three longest positive clones (1.3 kilobases) indicated that all contained identical overlapping sequences which included a stretch of poly (A) residues 428 bases 3' of the open reading frame. Thus we could conclude that these clones encoded for the C-terminal region of 5-LO.

In order to obtain a full length cDNA clone for 5-LO, a second library was constructed using poly (A) from DMSO/dex differentiated HL60 cells. In this case, the cDNAs had been size selected to include only cDNAs > 2.2 kilobases prior to ligation. For screening the 500,000 recombinants of this library, a restriction fragment (310 bases) from one of the 5-LO cDNA clones described above was used along with oligonucleotide probes based on the N-terminus of 5-LO. A total of 8 clones were isolated that hybridized to both probes. All of these contained inserts that were 2.4 to 2.6 kilobases in length and had restriction maps that overlapped those of the clones that corresponded to the 3' end of the 5-LO mRNA.

DNA sequencing of two of the clones revealed that both contained identical open reading frames encoding for 674 amino acids which would yield a 78,000 dalton polypeptide. The corresponding amino acid sequence contained all known peptide sequences from the 5-LO. There were no signal sequences or membrane spanning regions. Although the central region was moderately hydrophobic, the sequence was hydrophilic overall, consistent with the fact that 5-LO is a soluble, cytosolic protein.

Closer examination of the amino acid sequence of 5-LO revealed a region (amino acids 368-382) that is related to the interface-binding domains of human lipoprotein lipase and rat hepatic lipase. This region may be involved in an interaction of 5-LO with membrane phospholipid that would explain the stimulation of enzymatic activity by phosphatidylcholine and leukocyte membranes (1,3-5). In addition, two regions of the enzyme (amino acids 16-28 and 488-512) exhibited weak homology to the Ca^{2+} binding sites from lipocortin and calmodulin respectively. Possibly one or both of these regions is responsible for the stimulatory effects of Ca^{2+} on 5-LO activity. In addition, significant homology was noted between regions of human 5-LO and both the soybean Lox 1 and rabbit reticulocyte 15-LO gene products. Of particular interest was a region (amino acids 547 through 559) in which 12 of 13 amino acids were identical to amino acids 685 through 697 of the Lox 1 protein. This degree of homology suggests that this region may play an important role in enzyme function.

Expression of 5-LO Activity in Transfected Cell Lines

In order to confirm that the cDNA isolated from the HL-60 cell library did, in fact, encode 5-LO, we sought to express the enzyme activity in cells that do not constitutively contain 5-LO. For this purpose we chose the human osteosarcoma cell line 143.98.2, because it exhibits high efficiency transfection with the $CaPO_4$ procedure (7,11). The 5-LO cDNA was cloned into the expression vector pR135 in both the forward and reverse orientation. Cells were transfected with the plasmids pR135, pLOX1 (pR135 containing 5-LO cDNA in the correct orientation) or pLOX2 (pR135 containing 5-LO cDNA in the reverse orientation). The 10,000 xg supernatants from hygromycin resistant clones were assayed for 5-LO activity. No activity was detected in control 143.98.2 cells, or cells transfected with pR135 or pLOX2. In contrast, supernatants from 2 of 5 clones containing pLOX1 contained significant 5-LO activity. One of these, clone 4, was selected for further study. The specific activity of clone 4 cell 10,000 xg supernatants varied from 0.72 to 41 units 5-LO/mg protein. This variability was presumably due to the fact that the expression plasmid was episomal, and therefore, its copy number varied from cell to cell. The variability was minimized by utilizing cultures at low passage number, and did not interfere with experiments performed to characterize the expressed protein (7).

Immuno-blot analysis of 10,000 xg supernatants from clone 4 cells utilizing a polyclonal antiserum to purified human leukocyte 5-LO revealed a specifically labelled 80,000 dalton polypeptide that was immunologically related to the 5-LO in human leukocyte supernatants. The relative quantities of immunoreactive protein in leukocyte and clone 4 supernatants correlated with the relative 5-LO specific activities of the supernatants. The expressed enzyme possessed both 5-LO activity and LTA_4-synthase activity at the same ratio as that observed for the enzyme from human leukocytes. The enzyme activity in clone 4 cell supernatants was stimulated by Ca^{2+}, ATP, and two leukocyte stimulatory factors, behavior that was also observed in the 5-LO activity of human leukocyte supernatants. These data indicated that, in terms of molecular weight, immunogenicity, products synthesized, and response to stimulatory factors, the expressed protein was indistinguishable from the human leukocyte 5-LO (7).

Interestingly, intact clone 4 cells challenged with ionophore A23187 synthesized no 5-LO products under conditions in which leukocytes synthesized LTB_4, and its polar metabolites, and minor quantities of the nonenzymatic hydrolysis products of LTA_4. If 20:4 (50 μM) was added with the ionophore, clone 4 cells produced 5-hydroxyeicosatetraenoic acid and nonenzymatic hydrolysis products of LTA_4. Clearly it is possible to activate the 5-LO in the intact clone 4 cells, however one must also provide the enzyme with exogenous substrate to observe product formation, and normal LT synthesis does not occur. This is not surprising since the osteosarcoma cells probably lack most if not all of the components of the LT synthetic pathway (7).

SUMMARY

In conclusion, we have cloned a full-length cDNA for human leukocyte 5-LO from differentiating HL-60 cells. The complete amino acid sequence of 5-LO has been determined from the nucleotide sequence of the cDNA. Some interesting features of the sequence include potential lipid and Ca^{2+} binding sites and sequence homologies with other lipoxygenases. Human osteosarcoma cells transfected with the 5-LO cDNA expressed 5-LO and LTA_4 synthase activities that were indistinguishable from those of the human leukocyte enzyme confirming that the cloned cDNA was the correct gene.

REFERENCES

1. Rouzer CA, Matsumoto T, Samuelsson B. Proc Natl Acad Sci USA 1986; 83:857–861.

2. Ueda N, Kaneko S, Yoshimoto T, Yamamoto S. J Biol Chem 1986; 261:7982–7988.

3. Shimizu T, Izumi T, Seyama Y, Tadokoro K, Radmark O, Samuelsson B. Proc Natl Acad Sci USA 1986; 83:4175–4179.

4. Hogaboom GK, Cook M, Newton JF, et al. Mol Pharmacol 1986; 30:510–519.

5. Goetze AM, Fayer L, Bouska J, Bornemeier D, Carter GW. Prostaglandins 1985; 29:689–701.

6. Dixon RAF, Jones RE, Diehl RE, Bennett CD, Kargman S, Rouzer CA. Proc Natl Acad Sci USA 1988; 85:415–420.

7. Rouzer CA, Rands E, Kargman S, Jones RE, Register RB, Dixon RAF. submitted manuscript.

8. Rouzer CA, Samuelsson B. Proc Natl Acad Sci USA 1985; 82:6040–6044.

9. Collins JJ, Ruscetti FW, Gallagher RE, Gallo RC. Proc Natl Acad Sci USA 1978; 75:2458–2462.

10. Bonser RW, Siegel MI, McConnell RT, Cuatrecasas P. Biochem Biophys Res Commun 1981; 102:1269–1275.

11. Yates JL, Warren N, Sugden B. Nature (London) 1985; 313:812–815.

Advances in Prostaglandin, Thromboxane, and Leukotriene Research, Vol. 19, edited by
B. Samuelsson, P. Y.-K. Wong, and F. F. Sun,
Raven Press, Ltd., New York ©1989.

MOLECULAR CLONING AND EXPRESSION OF HUMAN LEUKOTRIENE A4

HYDROLASE cDNA

Michiko Minami, Yasufumi Minami[1], Sigeo Ohno[1], Koichi Suzuki[1],
Nobuya Ohishi, Takao Shimizu, and Yousuke Seyama

Department of Physiological Chemistry and Nutrition, Faculty of
Medicine, University of Tokyo, Hongo, Bunkyo-ku, Tokyo 113
[1]Department of Molecular Biology, Tokyo Metropolitan Institute of
Medical Science, Honkomagome, Bunkyo-ku, Tokyo 113, Japan

SUMMARY

We have isolated a near full-length cDNA encoding human leukotriene A4 (LTA4) hydrolase from a human spleen cDNA library. The
mature form of the enzyme consists of 610 amino acid residues and
its molecular weight is calculated to be 69,153. The cDNA was
inserted into an expression vector (pUC 9) and expressed in
Escherichia coli. The fusion protein (EX85) possessed the LTA4
hydrolase activity with kinetic properties similar to the native
enzyme.

MOLECULAR CLONING OF LTA4 HYDROLASE cDNA

A human spleen λgt10 cDNA library was constructed according to
the method of Ohno et al. (1). Double-stranded cDNA was prepared
from the human spleen poly(A)$^+$ RNA by the procedure of Gubler and
Hoffman (2) with slight modifications. The double-stranded cDNA
larger than 2 kb was purified and then inserted into the vector
λgt10 (3). An oligonucleotide probe corresponding to the partial
amino acid sequence of human leukocyte LTA4 hydrolase was designed based on mammalian codon usage frequencies as described (4)
and synthesized with a DNA synthesizer. From 5 x 10^4 plaques of
the cDNA library, five positive clones were selected, whose cDNA
inserts were practically identical (2.1 kb) in size. Then, a
phage clone designated as LTA85 was chosen for further analyses.

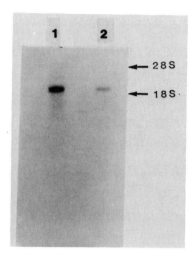

FIG. 1. Northern hybridization analysis (9). One μg each of poly(A)⁺ RNA from human leukocyte and spleen was electrophoresed and transferred to a nitrocellulose membrane, and then hybridized with a nick-translated cDNA fragment. Positions of ribosomal marker RNA are shown by arrows.

Northern blotting analysis revealed that the size of human LTA₄ hydrolase mRNA is 2.2 kb (FIG. 1). The content of the mRNA was larger in leukocytes than in the spleen, which is consistent with the observation that the enzyme activity in the former is higher than in the latter. Assuming that the mRNA is 2.2 kb in size and contains 100-200 bp of poly(A)⁺ sequence, the cDNA insert of LTA85 comprised a near full-length sequence of the mRNA for LTA₄ hydrolase. Accordingly, the nucleotide sequence of LTA85 was determined by the dideoxy chain termination method (5).

Nucleotide and deduced amino acid sequences of LTA85 are shown in FIG. 2. The nucleotide sequence of the cDNA (2,060 bp) had an open reading frame of 1,833 bp, which contained all the sequences of peptides determined with the leukocyte enzyme. Since the in-phase TGA termination codon exists at the nucleotide position -15, as shown in FIG. 2, ATG preceding the N-terminal proline was identified as the initiation codon. Consequently the mature form of this enzyme consists of 610 amino acid residues and its molecular weight is calculated to be 69,153, which agrees with the value estimated by SDS-polyacrylamide gel electrophoresis (68,000-70,000) (6-8). The amino acid composition obtained from the deduced sequence was in good accordance with those for the purified enzymes (6, 8). All these results lead to the conclusion that the cDNA is derived from the mRNA for the LTA₄ hydrolase.

A relatively short 3'-untranslated sequence significantly AT-rich suggests that LTA₄ hydrolase may have a short half-life,

```
                                                                          -11
CTCTATCGACGAGTCTGGTAGCTGAGCGTTGGGCTGTAGGTCGCTGTGCTGTGTGATCCCCCAGAGCCATGCCCGAGATAGTGGATACCTGTTCGTTGGCCTCTCCGGCTTCCGTCTGC
                                                                   ***      MetProGluIleValAspThrCysSerLeuAlaSerProAlaSerValCys
                                                                             1
                100
CGGACCAAGCACCTGCACCTGCGCTGCAGCGTCGACTTTACTCGCCGGACGCTGACCGGGACTGCTGCTCTCACGGTCCAGTCTCAGGAGGACAATCTGCGCAGCCTGGTTTTGGATACA
ArgThrLysHisLeuHisLeuArgCysSerValAspPheThrArgArgThrLeuThrGlyThrAlaAlaLeuThrValGlnSerGlnGluAspAsnLeuArgSerLeuValLeuAspThr
                200
AAGGACCTTACAATAGAAAAAGTAGTGATCAATGGACAAGAAGTCAAATATGCTCTTGGAGAAAGACAAAGTTACAAGGGATCGCCAATGGAAATCTCTCTTCCTATCGCTTTGAGCAAA
LysAspLeuThrIleGluLysValValIleAsnGlyGlnGluValLysTyrAlaLeuGlyGluArgGlnSerTyrLysGlySerProMetGluIleSerLeuProIleAlaLeuSerLys
      300                                                            400
AATCAAGAAATTGTTATAGAAATTTCTTTTGAGACCTCTCCAAAATCTTCTGCTCTCCAGTGGCTCACTCCTGAACAGACTTCTGGGAAGGAACACCCATATCTCTTTAGTCAGTGCCAG
AsnGlnGluIleValIleGluIleSerPheGluThrSerProLysSerSerAlaLeuGlnTrpLeuThrProGluGlnThrSerGlyLysGluHisProTyrLeuPheSerGlnCysGln
          100
                                                                   500
GCCATCCACTGCAGAGCAATCCTTCCTTGTCAGGACACTCCTTCTGTGAAATTAACCTATACTGCAGAGGTGTCTGTCCCTAAAGAACTGGTGGCACTTATGAGTGCTATTCGTGATGGA
AlaIleHisCysArgAlaIleLeuProCysGlnAspThrProSerValLysLeuThrTyrThrAlaGluValSerValProLysGluLeuValAlaLeuMetSerAlaIleArgAspGly
                                                                   600
GAAACACCTGACCCAGAAGACCCAAGCAGGAAAATATACAAATTCATCCAAAAAGTTCCAATACCCTGCTACCTGATTGCTTTAGTTGTTGGAGCTTTAGAAAAGCAGGCAAATTGGCCCA
GluThrProAspProGluAspProSerArgLysIleTyrLysPheIleGlnLysValProIleProCysTyrLeuIleAlaLeuValValGlyAlaLeuGluGluLysGlnAlaAsnTrpPro
          700                                                        200
AGAACTTTGGTGTGGTCTGAGAAAGAGCAGGTGGAAAAGTCTGCTTATGAGTTTTCTGAGACTGAATCTATGCTTAAAATAGCAGAAGATCTGGGAGGACCGTATGTATGGGGACAGTAT
ArgThrLeuValTrpSerGluLysGluGlnValGluLysSerAlaTyrGluPheSerGluThrGluSerMetLeuLysIleAlaGluAspLeuGlyGlyProTyrValTrpGlyGlnTyr
              800
GACCTATTGGTCCTGCCACCATCCTTCCCTTATGGTGGCATGGAGAATCCTTGCCTTACTTTTGTAACTCCTACTCTACTGGCAGGCGACAAGTCACTCTCCAATGTCATTGCACATGAA
AspLeuLeuValLeuProProSerPheProTyrGlyGlyMetGluAsnProCysLeuThrPheValThrProThrLeuLeuAlaGlyAspLysSerLeuSerAsnValIleAlaHisGlu
          900                                                        1000
ATATCTCATAGCTGGACAGGGAATCTAGTGACCAACAAAACTTGGGATCACTTTTGGTTAAATGAGGGACATACTGTGTACTTGGAACGCCACATTTGCGGACGATTGTTTGGTGAAAAG
IleSerHisSerTrpThrGlyAsnLeuValThrAsnLysThrTrpAspHisPheTrpLeuAsnGluGlyHisThrValTyrLeuGluArgHisIleCysGlyArgLeuPheGlyGluLys
              300
                                                                   1100
TTCAGACATTTTAATGCTCTGGGAGGATGGGGAGAACTACAGAATTCGGTAAAGACATTTGGGGAGACACATCCTTTCACCAAACTTGTGGTTGATCTGACAGATATAGACCCTGATGTA
PheArgHisPheAsnAlaLeuGlyGlyTrpGlyGlyTrpGlyGluLeuGlnAsnSerValLysThrPheGlyGluThrHisProPheThrLysLeuValValAspLeuThrAspIleAspProAspVal
                                  1200                              400
GCTTATTCTTCAGTTCCCTATGAGAAGGGCTTTGCTTTACTTTTTTACCTTGAACAACTGCTTGGAGGACCAGAGATTTTCCTAGGATTCTTAAAAGCTTATGTTGAGAAGTTTTCCTAT
AlaTyrSerSerValProTyrGluLysGlyPheAlaLeuLeuPheTyrLeuGlyIleGlnIleLeuGlyGlyProGluIlePheLeuGlyPheLeuLysAlaTyrValGluLysPheSerTyr
                                      1300
AAGAGCATAACTACTGATGACTGGAAGGATTTCCTGTATTCCTATTTTAAAGATAAGGTTGATGTTCTCAATCAAGTTGATTGGAATGCCTGGCTCTACTCTCCTGGACTGCCTCCCATA
LysSerIleThrThrAspAspTrpLysAspPheLeuTyrSerTyrPheLysAspLysValAspValLeuAsnGlnValAspTrpLeuTyrSerProGlyLeuProProIle
                              1400
AAGCCCAATTATGATATGACTCTGACAAATGCTTGTATTGCCTTAAGTCAAAGATGGATTACTGCCAAAGAAGATGATTTAAATTTCAATGCCACAGACCTGAAGGATCTCTCTTCCT
LysProAsnTyrAspMetThrLeuThrAsnAlaCysIleAlaLeuSerGlnArgTrpIleThrAlaLysGluAspAspLeuAsnSerPheAsnAlaThrAspLeuLysAspLeuSerSer
          1500                                                      1600
CATCAATTGAATGAGTTTTTAGCACAGACGCTCCAGAGGGCACCTCTTCCATTGGGGCACATAAAGCGAATGCAAGAGGTGTACAACTTCAATGCCATTAACAATTCTGAAATACGATTC
HisGlnLeuAsnGluPheLeuAlaGlnThrLeuGlnArgAlaProLeuProLeuGlyHisIleLysArgMetGlnGluValTyrAsnPheAsnAlaIleAsnAsnSerGluIleArgPhe
          500
                                                                   1700
AGATGGCTGCGGCTCTGCATTCAATCCAAGTGGGAGGACGCAATTCCTTGGCGCTAAAGATGGCAACTGAACAAGGAAGAATGAAGTTTACCCGGCCCTTATTCAAGGATCTTGCTGCC
ArgTrpLeuArgLeuCysIleGlnSerLysTrpGluAspAlaIleProLeuAlaLeuLysMetAlaThrGluGlnGlyArgMetLysPheThrArgProLeuPheLysAspLeuAlaAla
                                      1800
TTTGACAAATCCCATGATCAAGCTGTCCGAACCTACCAAGAGCACAAAGCAAGCATGCATCCCGTGACTGCAATGCTGGTGGGGAAAGACTTAAAAGTGGATTAAAGACCTGCGTATTGA
PheAspLysSerHisAspGlnAlaValArgThrTyrGlnGluHisLysAlaSerMetHisProValThrAlaMetLeuValGlyLysAspLeuLysValAsp***
                                                    600
TGATTTTAGAGATTTCTCTTTTTTAAATGGAATTCGTAAAGAAATATAAAACTTCAGCTCACAATTAAAACTGTCTTTTTAGTTTTGGCTTTTTATTGTTTTGTTGGTGATTTTACTGAA
AATAAAGATGAGCTACTTCTTC
```

FIG. 2.   Nucleotide and deduced amino acid sequences of the cDNA clone LTA85 (10).   Amino acid sequences of peptides determined at the protein level are indicated by thin underlines, and the polyadenylation signal sequence (AATAAA) is shown by a thick underline. ***, termination codons.

as proposed by Clemens (9). A region of amino acid residues 196–210 is the only hydrophobic portion of this enzyme, which is supposed to be involved in the interaction with the hydrophobic substrate, LTA₄. In addition, it is known that this enzyme is inactivated by SH-modifying reagents. In this respect, it should be emphasized that there exists a cysteine residue within this hydrophobic region (position 200).

EXPRESSION OF LTA₄ HYDROLASE cDNA

The cDNA fragment encoding human LTA₄ hydrolase was inserted into the expression vector pUC9 and the resultant expression plasmid was used to transform Escherichia coli YA21. After IPTG-induced overproduction of the fusion protein (EX85) with the first 10 amino acid residues derived from the vector, cell suspension was sonicated (FIG. 3, lanes 1 and 2). Since the LTA₄ hydrolase activity was recovered in the soluble fraction, it was further purified according to the methods described below. The amount of EX85 in the soluble fraction increased up to 2 h after IPTG induction, but thereafter remained constant, while EX85 in the inclusion bodies of bacteria increased time-dependently (data not shown). To the soluble fraction obtained by centrifugation of the sonicated bacterial suspension, ammonium sulfate was added and the precipitate formed between 40 and 70 % saturation was collected. The obtained protein preparation was applied to Mono-Q and then Mono-P column chromatographies to purify EX85 (FIG. 3). A 3 l culture yielded 9 mg of EX85 which has a similar electrophoretic mobility to the native enzyme from human lung (FIG. 3, lane 5).

Human LTA₄ hydrolase has been purified from neutrophils and lung (6, 8) by 4 steps of column chromatographies with yields lower than from the bacterial system. Therefore, the transfor-

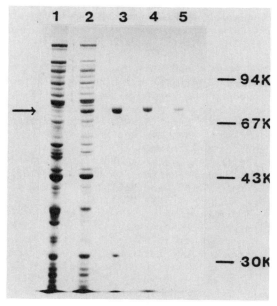

FIG. 3. SDS-polyacrylamide gel electrophoresis of protein preparations (11). Crude extracts from transformants with pUC9 alone (lane 1) or expression plasmid (lane 2); preparations from Mono-Q column chromatography (lane 3); Mono-P column chromatography (lane 4); and the human lung LTA₄ hydrolase (lane 5). The arrow indicates the position of EX85.

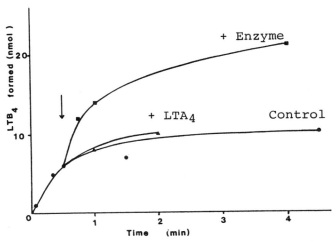

FIG. 4. The time course of the LTB$_4$ synthesis by EX85 (11). EX85 (2 μg/10 μl) was incubated with LTA$_4$ (20 μM) in 50 μl of 0.1 M Tris-HCl (pH 7.8) containing 2 mg/ml bovine serum albumin at 37° C for 5 min (circles). After the 30-s incubation (indicated by the arrow), EX85 (squares) or LTA$_4$ (triangles) were further added to the reaction mixture.

mant is a good source for LTA$_4$ hydrolase. The N-terminal sequence of EX85 revealed that it contained 10 amino acids (TMIT-PSLAAG), followed by the N-termial sequence (PEIVDT) determined for human neutrophil and lung enzymes (6, 8).

The Km value of EX85 for LTA$_4$ was 27 μM and the Vmax value was 4.3 μmol LTB$_4$/min·mg. These values are comparable with those of human (6, 8) and rat (7) enzymes.

As noted for the native LTA$_4$ hydrolase purified from human lung (8), SH-modifying reagents, NEM (N-ethylmaleimide), PCMB (p-chloromercuribenzoic acid), and HgCl$_2$, inhibited the activity of EX85. The IC$_{50}$ values of NEM, PCMB, and HgCl$_2$ were 1 mM, 0.02 μM, and 0.026 μM, respectively.

The reaction of LTB$_4$ synthesis by EX85 almost reached a plateau in 1 min as shown in FIG. 4. The rapid deceleration of the enzyme reaction was due to the suicide-type inactivation of LTA$_4$ hydrolase caused by its substrate, LTA$_4$ (8, 12), and not due to the depletion of the substrate. Therefore, the initial velocity of the reaction was recovered by the addition of the enzyme but not of the substrate.

Accordingly, it is concluded that EX85 possesses a full enzyme activity with all the properties reported for LTA$_4$ hydrolase. The acquisition of the expression system makes it feasible to elucidate the reaction mechanism of the enzyme and to synthesize substantial amount of LTB$_4$, thereby leading a clarification of its physiological significances.

REFERENCES

1. Ohno, S., Emori, Y., Sugihara, H., Imajoh, S., and Suzuki, K. Methods in Enzymology, 1987; 139, 363-379

2. Gubler, U., and Hoffman, B.J. Gene, 1983; 25, 263-269

3. Huynh, T.V., Young, R.A., and Davis, R.W. in DNA Cloning (Glover, D.M., ed) Vol 1, IRL Press, Wash. D.C. 1985; 49-78

4. Lathe, R. J. Mol. Biol., 1985; 183, 1-12

5. Hattori, M., and Sakaki, Y. Anal. Biochem., 1986; 152, 232-238

6. Rådmark, O., Shimizu, T., Jörnvall, H., and Samuelsson, B. J. Biol. Chem., 1984; 259, 12339-12345

7. Evans, J.F., Dupuis, P., and Ford-Hutchison, A.W. Biochim. Biophys. Acta, 1985; 840, 43-50

8. Ohishi, N., Izumi, T., Minami, M., Kitamura, S., Seyama, Y., Ohkawa, S., Terao, S., Yotsumoto, H., Takaku, F., and Shimizu, T. J. Biol. Chem., 1987; 262, 10200-10205

9. Clemens, M. Cell, 1987; 49, 157-158

10. Minami, M., Ohno, S., Kawasaki, H., Rådmark, O., Samuelsson, B., Jörnvall, H., Shimizu, T., Seyama, Y., and Suzuki, K. J. Biol. Chem. 1987; 262, 13873-13876

11. Minami, M., Minami, Y., Emori, Y., Kawasaki, H., Ohno, S., Suzuki, K., Ohishi, N., Shimizu, T., and Seyama, Y. FEBS Lett. 1988; 229, 279-282

12. McGee, J., and Fitzpatrick, F.A. J. Biol. Chem., 1985; 260, 12832-12837

Advances in Prostaglandin, Thromboxane, and Leukotriene Research, Vol. 19, edited by B. Samuelsson, P. Y.-K. Wong, and F. F. Sun, Raven Press, Ltd., New York ©1989.

Leukotriene A_4-hydrolase, cloning of the human enzyme and tissue distribution in the rat.

Rådmark, O., Funk, C.D., Ji Yi Fu, Matsumoto, T., Jörnvall, H., Shimizu, T., Medina, J.F., Haeggström, J., Kumlin, M., and Samuelsson, B.

Department of Physiological Chemistry
Karolinska Institutet
S-104 01 Stockholm, Sweden

Leukotriene A_4-hydrolase catalyzes the conversion of leukotriene A_4 (LTA$_4$) into the chemotactic agent leukotriene B_4 (LTB$_4$). This enzyme has been purified primarily from human tissues [1-4] and has been found to have several features distinguishing it from other epoxide hydrolases, both soluble and microsomal. The kinetics of LTA$_4$ hydrolase were studied by several groups, and regardless of the enzyme source, it has been characterized by a quick initial burst of product formation together with self-inactivation of the enzyme.

In this report the cloning of a cDNA corresponding to LTA$_4$-hydrolase, and a study of the tissue-distribution of enzymes metabolizing LTA$_4$ in the rat, are briefly described.

Methods

These are described in the corresponding original papers (5,6).

Results and Discussion

1. Cloning of LTA$_4$-hydrolase. A λGT11 cDNA library derived from human lung was screened with a polyclonal antiserum for human leukocyte LTA$_4$-hydrolase. A short clone (λlu H6-1a) was picked up (fig 1) and found to contain a known peptide sequence. The identity was confirmed also by antibody selection. This clone was subsequently used in screening of a human placenta cDNA library by plaque hybridization. A clone (λpl 16a) containing the entire protein coding region (1830 bp) was sequenced, and identified by the complete match with N-terminal, internal and near C-terminal peptide sequences.

Predictions of secondary structure (7) and calculations of hydropathy (8) indicated some interesting features of a region centering around position 200 of the protein (fig 2). Thus the segment 170-185 was the most hydrophilic of the entire protein, closely followed by the segment 190-205 which was the most hydrophobic part. These were separated by a strongly predicted reverse turn, and a long α-helix was also found in close proximity (220-240).

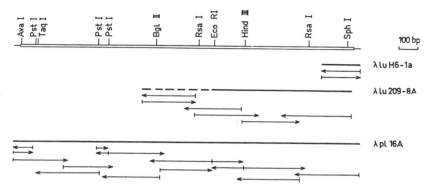

Fig 1. Partial restriction map and sequencing strategy of cDNAs encoding LTA$_4$-hydrolase. The protein coding region is shown by the open bar.

It was previously demonstrated that the hydrophobic substrate LTA$_4$ could be covalently bound to the enzyme, possibly of significance for the selfinactivation of LTA$_4$-hydrolase (3). The thiol group of cys 199, within the hydrophobic region, is a possible candidate for such an interaction. LTA$_4$-hydrolase was also cloned from a human spleen cDNA-library (9), the protein coding sequence was identical.

LTA$_4$ hydrolase

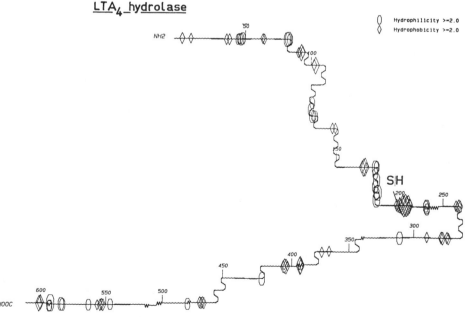

Fig 2. Prediction of secondary structure and hydropathy of LTA$_4$-hydrolase.

2. Metabolism of LTA₄ in rat tissues. After careful perfusion, homogenates were prepared from nine rat tissues. Aliquots were incubated with LTA₄ (35μM, 37°C, 15min) after supplementation with glutathione (10mM)⁴ and albumin (10 mg/ml). Samples were extracted with chloroform and fractionated on a silicic acid column, giving one fraction containing dihydroxyacids (yield 70-85%), and another containing peptido-leukotrienes (yield 55-70%). The respective fractions were finally analyzed by reverse phase HPLC.

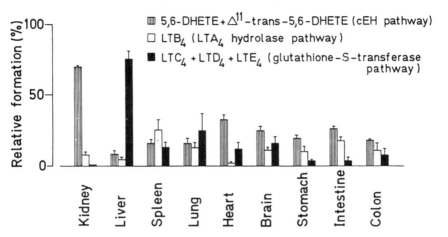

Fig 3. Metabolism of LTA₄ in rat homogenates. Bars represent the yields of metabolites expressed as percentages of the total products (mean ± S.D., n=4).

Fig 3 summarizes the relationships between the different metabolic pathways of LTA₄ in the respective homogenates. Note that nonenzymatic hydrolysis of LTA₄ was considerable in several cases, thus the sum of bars (fig 3) did not add up to 100%. Formation of 5(S),6(R)-dihydroxy-7,9-trans-11,14-cis-eicosatetraenoic acid (5,6-DHETE), catalysed by cytosolic epoxide hydrolse (10), was detectable in all cases. This was the major metabolite in kidney, heart and brain, in agreement with a previous report regarding tissue distribution of cEH in rat (11). The 11-trans isomer of 5,6-DHETE was found in the incubations of kidney homogenate. It was indicated that this isomerization was primarily enzymatic.

Conversion to LTC₄ was demonstrated in all homogenates, however very small amounts were formed in kidney. Both soluble and particulate enzymes should have contributed to these levels of LTC₄. Since glutathione was added, further metabolism to LTD₄ was inhibited.

LTB₄-formation was also almost ubiquituous (very low in heart), however this was the predominant pathway only in spleen. The apparent wide distribution of LTA₄-hydrolase is in agreement with a previous study of the conversion of LTA₄ to LTB₄ in different organs of the guinea pig (12). The cellular origin of LTA₄ hydrolase in various tissues merits further study.

Acknowledgements

This project was supported by grants from the Swedish medical research council (03X-217, 03X-07467, 03X-3532).

References

1. Rådmark, O., Shimizu, T., Jörnvall, A. and Samuelsson, B.: (1984) J. Biol. Chem., 259, 12339-12345.

2. Mcgee, J and Fitzpatrick, F.: (1985) J. Biol. Chem., 260, 12832-12837.

3. Evans, J.F., Nathaniel, D.J., Zamboni, R.J. and Ford-Hutchinson, A.W.: (1985) J. Biol. Chem., 260, 10966-10970.

4. Ohishi, N., Izumi, T., Minami, M., Kitamura, S., Seyama, Y., Ohkawa, S., Terao, S., Yotsumoto, H., Takaku, F. and Shimizu, T.: (1987) J. Biol. Chem., 262, 10200-10205.

5. Funk, C.D., Rådmark, O., Fu, Ji Yi, Matsumoto, T., Jörnvall, H., Shimizu, T., and Samuelsson, B.: (1987) Proc. Natl. Acad. Sci. USA 84, 6677-6681.

6. Medina, J.F., Haeggström, J., Kumlin, M. and Rådmark, O.: (1988) Biochim. Biophys. Acta, in press.

7. Chou, P.Y. and Fasman, G.D.: (1974) Biochemistry, 13, 211-221.

8. Hopp, T.P. and Woods, K.R.: (1981) Proc. Natl. Acad Sci. USA, 78, 3824-3828.

9. Minami, M., Ohno, S., Kawasaki, H., Rådmark, O., Samuelsson, B., Jörnvall, H., Shimizu, T., Seyama, Y. and Suzuki, K.: (1987) J. Biol. Chem. 262, 13873-13876.

10. Haeggström, J., Meijer, J. and Rådmark, O.: (1986) J. Biol. Chem. 261, 6332-6327.

11. Schladt, L., Wörner, W., Setiabudi, F. and Oesch, F.: (1986) Biochem. Pharmacol., 35, 3309-3316.

12. Izumi, T., Shimizu, T., Seyama, Y., Ohishi, N. and Takaku, F. (1986) Biochem. Biophys. Res. Commun., 135, 139-145.

Advances in Prostaglandin, Thromboxane, and Leukotriene Research, Vol. 19, edited by
B. Samuelsson, P. Y.-K. Wong, and F. F. Sun,
Raven Press, Ltd., New York ©1989.

LEUKOTRIENES AND HUMAN AIRWAYS

P.J. Piper, M.N. Samhoun, D.M. Conroy,
*N.C. Barnes, **J. Evans and **J.F. Costello

Dept.of Pharmacology, Royal College of Surgeons, Lincoln's Inn
Fields, London WC2A 3PN, *London Chest Hospital, Bonner Road,
London E2 9JX and **King's College School of Medicine and
Dentistry, Denmark Hill, London SE5 8RX

Leukotrienes (LTs) are a family of biologically-active compounds produced from fatty acids, incorporated into the phospholipids of the cell membrane by the action of 5-lipoxygenase (1).
In this paper, we shall consider only LTs derived from arachidonic
acid. For many years, the mediator, slow-reacting substance of
anaphylaxis (SRS-A) (2) has been thought to play an important role
in asthma. It is now known that the cysteinyl-containing LTs,
LTC_4, LTD_4 and LTE_4, account for the biological activity of SRS-A
(3,4). These LTs have potent actions on airway smooth muscle in
vitro and in vivo, which suggests that these phospholipid-derived
substances may be involved in respiratory disease.

GENERATION OF LEUKOTRIENES

Leukotrienes are released by both immunological and non-immuno-
logical challenge of human lung in vitro but the exact cellular
origin of LTs is unclear. The LTs generated from lung vary both
with the stimulus used and between the parenchyma (small airways
and blood vessels) and bronchi. Dahlén et al (5) showed the
formation of LTs C_4, D_4 and E_4 during antigen challenge of
asthmatic lung tissue but did not detect LTB_4. In our studies,
when chopped parenchyma from normal human lung was stimulated with
anti-IgE, generation of LTB_4 and LTD_4 was detected (Table 1).
Challenge of parenchyma with the calcium ionophore A23187 results
in formation of larger quantities of both LTB_4 and LTD_4, LTB_4
being the predominant LT formed. In this study, levels of LTE_4
were not determined. When human chopped bronchial tissue was
challenged with A23187, LTB_4 was generated but no cysteinyl-
containing LTs were detected (6).
A 5-lipoxygenase system is also present in vascular tissue (7).
Intralobar pulmonary arteries were dissected from human lung and
challenged with anti-IgE or A23187. Radioimmunoassay was used to

TABLE 1. Generation of leukotrienes from human lung parenchyma stimulated with A23187 or anti-IgE

Stimulus:	A23187 5 ug ml^{-1} (n = 5)		Anti-IgE 1:160 (n = 4)	
	LTB_4	LTD_4	LTB_4	LTD_4 pmol g^{-1}
Normal	664	472	20	16
	976	441	12	20
	764	250	10	64
	429	233	–	–
	310	27	11	N.D.
Mean ± sem	629±119	285±81	13±2	25±14
asthmatic	130	205	9	32
asthmatic	220	1308	N.D.	N.D.

N.D. = None detected

show that anti-IgE caused release of LTB_4 6.71+1.55, LTC_4 7.37+ 2.43 and LTD_4 11.98+5.49 pmol g^{-1} (n=5). In a similar study, chopped pulmonary arteries were stimulated with A23187 and LT-like material quantitated by bioassay on guinea-pig ileum smooth muscle. The amount of LTD_4-like material generated was 90+32.21 pmol g^{-1} (n=7), again suggesting that larger quantities of LTs are generated following stimulation with A23187 with A23187 than by immunological challenge. Since lung parenchyma contains a large amount of micro-vessels in addition to small airways, vascular tissue may be an important source of LTs released from lung tissue.

ACTIONS OF LEUKOTRIENES ON
RESPIRATORY SMOOTH MUSCLE IN VITRO

The fact that cysteinyl-containing LTs have very potent actions on airway smooth muscle has been well documented (see 5,8,9,10). On the other hand, LTB_4 has little direct smooth muscle stimulating activity on human bronchus (HBr) and any initial contraction rapidly develops tachyphylaxis. There are specific receptors for LTs on airway smooth muscle. In guinea-pig trachea, there are distinct receptors for LTC_4 and LTD_4; LTE_4 appears to occupy the LTD_4 receptor (11). However, in HBr, there seems to be one receptor which is acted on by LTs C_4, D_4 and E_4 (12). LTC_4 and LTD_4 contract isolated Hbr at the picomolar level and are more potent than LTE_4. However, whilst being less active than LTs C_4 or D_4, LTE_4 causes contractions of HBr which are longer lasting than those induced by its parent metabolites (13).

Leukotriene E_4 is a metabolite of LTC_4 and is itself further degraded. In rodents, LTE_4 undergoes N-acetylation (14). The N-acetyl derivative of LTE_4 ($N-AcLTE_4$) retains considerable biological activity and is about equiactive with LTE_4 in contracting guinea-pig trachea (GPT) and lung parenchymal strip (GPP) (15).

N-AcLTE$_4$ contracts isolated HBr, is less active than LTD$_4$ but, like LTE$_4$, causes protracted responses.

Strips of HBr and lung parenchyma (HP) from an asthmatic patient were superfused in series with Tyrode's solution containing mepyramine, hyoscine, propranolol, phenoxybenzamine and methysergide. Challenge of the tissues with anti-IgE (0.3:160–1:160 dilution) caused long-lasting contractions of HBr and HP which closely resembled those induced by LTE$_4$. The LT antagonist FPL 55712 (1.9 uM) inhibited the immunologically-induced contractions, strongly suggesting that LTs were generated within the bronchial strip. Similar findings have been described by Dahlen et al (9,16). In another experiment, isolated bronchus from an asthmatic subject was superfused as described, and challenged with anti-IgE. The effluent was collected during the initial part of the protracted contraction (>40 min). Radioimmunoassay was used to quantitate LTs present in the effluent. LTB$_4$, LTC$_4$ and LTD$_4$ were present in the effluent but in low levels of less than a picomole per ml.

LEUKOTRIENES IN THE AIRWAYS

Leukotrienes C$_4$ and D$_4$ have been detected in bronchoalveolar lavage (BAL) fluid from asthmatics (17). In addition LTs B$_4$, C$_4$ and D$_4$ have been shown to be present in sputum from patients with asthma, chronic bronchitis and cystic fibrosis (18,19). The major LT found in sputum was LTB$_4$, which may reflect the inflammatory component of these conditions. The detection of LTs in sputum and BAL fluid shows that LTs can be present in the airways for some length of time where they may act on airway smooth muscle, mucous secreting cells (20) or, in the case of LTB$_4$, act as a chemotactic agent for inflammatory cells (21).

EFFECTS OF INHALED LEUKOTRIENES IN HUMANS

Leukotrienes are active in causing narrowing of both large and small airways in normal man when given by inhalation. As predicted by studies on isolated HBr in vitro, LTs C$_4$ and D$_4$ are more active than histamine by about 3 orders of magnitude (22). Although less active than LTC$_4$ or LTD$_4$, LTE$_4$ is still 2 orders of magnitude more active than histamine. As previously shown in studies in vitro (21), bronchoconstriction induced by LTE$_4$ is also longer lasting than that of the other LTs (23). Leukotrienes given by inhalation cause wheezing in normal subjects (22) but were reported to induce cough in only one study (24).

Asthmatic subjects also bronchoconstrict to inhaled LTC$_4$ or LTD$_4$ and show hyperreactivity to these agonists (see 23). However, the sensitivity to LTs is increased 4-fold whereas the sensitivity to histamine is increased by a factor of 11. There is some evidence that cysteinyl-containing LTs may induce hyperreactivity of the airways. A non-bronchoconstrictor dose of LTD$_4$ increased the sensitivity of normals to inhaled prostaglandin (PG) F$_{2\alpha}$ (see 23), and inhaled LTE_4 increased the sensitivity of asthmatics to methacholine (25).

Leukotriene B_4 is present in sputum of patients with inflammatory diseases of the airways (18,19) and might be expected to contribute to hyperreactivity of the respiratory tract. However, LTB_4 inhaled alone or in conjunction with PGD_2 failed to increase bronchial reactivity to histamine in normal subjects (26).

STUDIES WITH LEUKOTRIENE ANTAGONISTS

In order to investigate whether LTs play a significant role in asthma, it will be necessary to find whether a potent LT antagonist substantially improves the condition of asthmatics. However, before such drugs can be tested against asthma, basic studies against inhaled LTs in normal man are required.

FPL 55712 (27) was prepared as an antagonist of SRS-A before it was known that SRS-A comprised LTs C_4, D_4 and E_4. Recently, a number of antagonists of cysteinyl-containing LTs, which are most active against LTD_4, have been synthesised and shown to be potent antagonists of LTs in various animal models in vitro and in vivo. The structures of some of these antagonists are based on that of FPL 55712. Only limited studies of FPL 55712 have been carried out in man because it has a short half-life and poor oral absorption. However, inhaled FPL 55712 or a related compound, FPL 59257, partially inhibited bronchoconstriction to inhaled LTC_4 or LTD_4 in normal subjects (24) and improved FEV_1 of asthmatic patients (28).

Some of the new LT antagonists have been investigated in man. L-649,923 is structurally related to FPL 55712 but is active by the oral route (29). L-649,923 (1.0g, p.o.) was investigated against bronchoconstriction induced by inhaled histamine or LTD_4 in normal man (30). L-649,923 had no action against histamine but shifted the LTD_4 dose-response curve to the right in all subjects. The geometric mean shift was 3.8-fold in all subjects for both PC_{35} sGaw and PC_{30} $\dot{V}max_{30}$. The side effects of colicky abdominal pain and watery diarrhoea prevented higher doses of the compound being administered. The same dose of L-649,923 had a small protective effect against the early response of asthmatic patients to antigen challenge but had no effect against the late phase (31).

LY 171883 is also structurally related to FPL 55712 (32) and has been shown in normals to shift the dose-response to inhaled LTD_4 to the right (33). The shift for FEV_1 was 4.6-fold and that for $\dot{V}max_{30}$ 6.3-fold. In a long-term study in asthmatics, LY 171883 was shown to produce a significant reduction in symptom score, a decrease in usage of $ß_2$ agonists and an increase in FEV_1 (34).

Another LTD_4 antagonist based on the structure of FPL 55712, L-648,051, has been given by inhalation to normal subjects against inhaled LTD_4. In a dose of 1.6 mg, L-648,051 partially inhibited the bronchoconstriction induced by LTD_4 and shortened its duration. L-648,051 did not have any unwanted side effects (35).

CONCLUSIONS

The potent actions of cysteinyl-containing LTs in human airways in vitro and in vivo suggest that these mediators may be involved in respiratory diseases such as asthma. In addition, both LTB_4 and cysteinyl LTs may contribute to inflammation of the airways.

Studies with LT antagonists in man have shown that it is possible to antagonise LTD_4-induced bronchoconstriction with drugs given orally or by inhalation. So far, however, the antagonists used, although reported to be potent in animal models, have been only weakly active in man. Recently, two LT antagonists, SK+F 104,353 (36) and ICI 198,615 (37) have been shown to have higher pA_2 values against LTD_4 than previously reported for any other antagonist: 8.6 and 10.1 respectively. It will be of great interest to find whether these antagonists are more active against inhaled LTD_4 in man than those previously described. If such extremely potent compounds do not improve lung function in asthmatics, it will suggest that LTs are not important mediators of asthma. In addition, it would show that good results with such compounds in animals do not accurately predict their efficacy in man.

REFERENCES

1. Samuelsson B. In: Piper PJ, ed. SRS-A and Leukotrienes. Chichester, New York, Brisbane, Toronto: Research Studies Press, Wiley, 1981;45-64

2. Brocklehurst WE. J Physiol 1960;150:416-435.

3. Morris HR, Taylor GW, Rokach J, Girard Y, Piper PJ, Tippins JR, Samhoun MN. Prostaglandins 1980;20:601-607.

4. Lewis RA, Austen KF, Drazen JM, Clark DA, Corey EJ. Proc Natl Acad Sci 1980;77:3710-4

5. Dahlén S-E, Hansson G, Hedqvist P, Bjorck T, Granstrom E, Dahlén B. Proc Natl Acad Sci 1983;80:1712-1716.

6. Barnett K, Piper PJ. Br J Pharmac, 1985;86:642P.

7. Piper PJ, Letts LG, Galton SA. Prostaglandins 1983;25:591-599

8. Dahlén S-E, Hedqvist P, Hammarström S, Samuelsson B. Nature (London) 1980;288:484-486.

9. Piper PJ. Br Med Bull 1983;39:255-259.

10. Piper PJ, Samhoun MN. Br. Med. Bull., 1987;43(2);297-311.

11. Krell RD, Tsai BS, Berdoulay A, Barone M, Giles RE. Prostaglandins 1983;25:171-178.

12. Buckner CK, Krell RD, Laravuso RB, Coursin DB, Bernstein PR, Will JA. J Pharm exp Ther 1986;237:558-562.

13. Samhoun MN, Piper PJ. Prostaglandins, Leukotrienes and Medicine 1984;13:79-87.

14. Bernstrom K, Hammarstrom S. Arch Biochem Biophys 1986;244:485-490.

15. Conroy DM, Piper PJ, Samhoun MN. Br J Pharmac 1987;91:365P.

16. Bjork, J, Dahlen S-E. Acta Physiol Scand 1988;132(2)Abs.23.

17. Diaz P, Galleguilos FR, Gonzalez MC, Pantin C, Kay AB. J Allergy Clin Immunol 1984;74:41-48.

18. O'Driscoll BR, Cromwell O, Kay AB. Clin exp Immunol 1984;55:397-404.

19. Zakrzewski JT, Barnes NC, Piper PJ, Costello JF. Br J clin Pharmac 1987;23:19-27

20. Marom Z, Shelhamer JK, Bach MK, Morton DR, Kalmer M. Am Rev Respir Dis 1982;126:449-451

21. Ford-Hutchinson AW, Bray MA, Doig MV, Shipley ME, Smith MJH. Nature 1980;286:264-265.

22. Barnes NC, Piper PJ, Costello JF. Thorax 1984;39:500-504.

23. Barnes NC, Piper PJ. In: The Leukotrienes: their biological significance. Piper PJ, ed. New York: Raven Press 1986;199-211.

24. Holroyde MC, Altounyan REC, Cole AH, Dixon M, Elliott EV. Lancet 1981;II:17-18.

25. Arm JP, Spur BW, Lee TH. Thorax 1987;42:220(Abs).

26. Black PN, Fuller RW, Taylor GW, Barnes PJ, Dollery CT. Br J Pharmac 1988; in press

27. Augstein J, Farmer JB, Lee TB, Sheard P, Tattersall ML. Nature New Biol 1973;245:215-217.

28. Lee TH, Walport MJ, Wilkinson AH, Turner-Warwick M, Kay AB Lancet 1981;2:304-305.

29. Jones TR, Guindon Y, Young R et al. Can J Physiol Pharmacol 1986;64:1532-1542.

30. Barnes NC, Piper PJ and Costello JF. In: <u>Advances in Prostaglandin, Thromboxane and Leukotriene Research</u> 1987;17:1000-1002.

31. Britton JR, Hanley SP, Tattersfield AE. <u>J Allergy Clin Immunol</u> 1987;79:811.

32. Fleisch JH, Rinkema LE, Haisch KD et al. <u>J Pharm exp ther</u> 1985;233:148-157.

33. Phillips GD, Rafferty P, Holgate ST. <u>Thorax</u> 1987;42:723.

34. Fleisch JH, Cloud ML, Marshall WS. <u>Ann NY Acad Sci</u> (in press).

35. Barnes NC, Evans JM, Zakrzewski JT, Piper PJ, Costello JF. Proc. Xth IUPHAR 1987;Abs.034 (in press).

36. Hay DWP, Muccitelli RM, Tucker SS et al. <u>J Pharm Exp Ther</u> 1987;243:474-481.

37. Snyder DW, Giles RE, Keith RA, Yee YK, Krell RD. <u>J Pharm Exp Ther</u> 1987;243:548-556.

Advances in Prostaglandin, Thromboxane, and Leukotriene Research, Vol. 19, edited by
B. Samuelsson, P. Y.-K. Wong, and F. F. Sun,
Raven Press, Ltd., New York ©1989.

REGULATED GENERATION OF LEUKOTRIENES IN MONONUCLEAR CELLS

Robert A. Lewis, *John A. Rankin, Anthony C. Allison,
and **Julian L. Ambrus, Jr.

Syntex Research, 3401 Hillview Ave., Palo Alto, CA 94304;
*Research Service, West Haven Veterans' Hospital, Yale
University School of Medicine Pulmonary Disease Section,
New Haven, CT 06510; and **Laboratory of Immunoregulation,
National Institute of Allergy and Infectious Diseases,
National Institutes of Health, Bethesda, MD 20892, USA

Among human mononuclear cells, macrophages and monocytes have
been documented to produce 5-lipoxygenase products in response
to a limited set of cellular activators, whereas lymphocytes are
generally believed to produce little or none of these arachidonic acid metabolites. This manuscript addresses mechanisms by
which leukotriene generation in monocytes and macrophages may be
regulated and introduces the possibility that under certain conditions, even lymphocyte subsets may be capable of producing
such products. Additionally, in contrast to previous demonstra-
tions that LTB_4 provides a sufficient stimulus for the differentiation of CD8+ suppressor lymphocytes (1,2), the action of
LTD_4 in opposing the differentiation of promonocytes to monocytes is suggested.

MONOCYTES AND MACROPHAGES

The calcium ionophore A23187 is a highly effective in vitro
activator of human monocytes and pulmonary alveolar macrophages
for the generation of leukotrienes. LTB_4 is thus produced in
both cell types (3-5); LTC_4 has been measured from A23187-
activated monocytes and LTD_4 from activated macrophages (5,6).
Zymosan is a non-ionophoric, and, thus, presumably more physio-
logically-relevant, activator of each of these cells (4,5), especially since it activates via a naturally-occurring (B-glucan)
receptor; the same assessment can be made of the relevance of
activation by N-formylated peptides, e.g. fMLP, which elicits
production of LTB_4 and LTC_4 from monocytes that have been
pretreated with cytochalasin B (7). Aggregates of IgG, IgA, or
IgE – but not of IgM – also activate human monocytes to generate
LTB_4 and LTC_4 (8) by receptor-mediated mechanisms.
We have recently assessed the effectiveness of heat-

aggregated IgG as an activator of human pulmonary alveolar
macrophages for generation of leukotrienes (9 and Manuscript
Submitted). Although there was little generation of LTB_4 from
cells of various healthy donors in response to this ligand,
despite ample numbers of the IgG1 receptor (averaging 1–2 x
10^5/cell), the response could be greatly augmented to produce
LTB_4 in tens of nanograms/10^6 cells by preincubation of the
cells with γ-interferon for 24 hours prior to challenge with the
aggregated IgG. Concentrations of γ-interferon as low as 10U/ml
were effective, and higher concentrations, to 1000U/ml, yielded
additional dose-dependent increases in LTB_4 generation in
response to the activating stimulus. By itself, γ-interferon
effected no production of LTB_4, although incubation of the
cells with 1000U/ml for 24 hours effectively doubled the number
of IgG1 Fc receptors. Incubation of the human pulmonary alveolar macrophages with α- or β-interferons (1000U/ml each) elicited no increases in IgG receptors and did not augment the capacity of aggregated IgG to activate the cells for LTB_4 generation. In the context of a 24-hour preincubation with γ-inter-
feron, the leukotriene-generating response was dependent on the
dose of heat-aggregated IgG from 250ng/ml to 25g/ml and upon
time, with a notable effect at, or even before, 2.5 minutes.

The bone marrow precursor of the macrophage and monocyte,
which is termed a "promonocyte," is presumed to proliferate in
response to the interaction of certain colony-stimulating factors (e.g., CSF-1) with surface receptors (e.g., the c-fms
protooncogene product [10]). The human promonocytic cell line
U-937 spontaneously proliferates in culture, but can be induced
to cease proliferation and differentiate by incubation with
inhibitors of the 5-lipoxygenase or antagonists of the LTD_4
receptor (R.V. Waters and A.C. Allison, unpublished data). The
differentiation markers, which are increasingly expressed in
response to compounds with 5-lipoxygenase inhibitory activities
(AA-861, NDGA, BW-755c, R-830, WY-47,288) or receptor antagonists (LY-171883, FPL 55712), included IgG Fc receptors, C3b
receptors, Mo1 surface antigen, and lysozyme. That LTD_4 could
overcome the differentiating effects of 5-lipoxygenase inhibition suggests that endogenously generated LTD_4 might provide a
proliferative signal and even act as a post-receptor regulator
in normal promonocytes for effecting the proliferative response
to an appropriate colony-stimulating factor.

LYMPHOCYTES

Of all the leukocyte types that exist in the human, only the
lymphocytes cannot be demonstrated to produce 5-lipoxygenase
products in vitro. Among the likely explanations for this is
that critical regulatory molecules for 5-lipoxygenase gene
expression are not produced in these cells or that a repressor
is uniquely generated during the differentiation of lymphocytes
from the pluripotential leukocyte precursor. In either case,

the lack of stability of the phenotype in transformed cells — with the demonstrated activity of the 5-lipoxygenase pathway in certain naturally-occurring lymphocytic neoplasias suggests the possibility that such phenotypic expression could also arise during an <u>in vivo</u> inflammatory event.

Recent work using normal human T-lymphocytes as fusion partners with a CD4+ lymphoma (CEM-6) has provided an additional demonstration along these lines, in that 3 of 180 tested hybridomas produced LTC_4 constitutively (11). Because of the novelty of this observation, several independent criteria were used to define the identity of the LTC_4. It was shown to elute from reverse phase-high performance liquid chromatography (HPLC) at the retention time of authentic LTC_4 in two mobile phase solvent systems. It was double-labeled in one hybridoma clone, using $[^{14}C]$-arachidonic acid and $[^3H]$-glutathione, and resolved at the appropriate retention time on HPLC; and, when the hybridoma supernatant was preabsorbed on an anti-LTC_4-Sepharose affinity column, the labeled peak was removed, as assessed by HPLC. Finally, it was recognized as immunoreactive LTC_4 by a specific radioimmunoassay.

Of the 5-lipoxygenase products, LTB_4 has been shown to suppress immunoglobulin production in pokeweed mitogen-stimulated human lymphocytes (1) via induction of CD8+ suppressor T cells (1,2); at much higher concentrations, the cysteinyl-leukotrienes LTC_4 and LTD_4 also are inhibitory (1). That LTC_4 could be produced by some, but not all of the T cell hybridomas created by fusing normal T cells with CEM-6, as described above (11), was then shown to correlate with the capacities of the supernatants to suppress Ig synthesis. Hybridoma supernatants containing 0.5 to 10 ng LTC_4/ml could suppress 50 to 70% of Ig production from unfractionated human mononuclear cells stimulated with pokeweed mitogen; from normal human B cells stimulated with Staphylococcus aureus Cowan I and cultured with concanavalin A-stimulated mixed lymphocyte supernatants as a source of B cell differentiation factors; and from the EBV-transformed human B cell line SDK.6 in the presence of B cell differentiation factors. Chemically-synthesized LTC_4 in the same concentration range as the hybridoma supernatants suppressed Ig production from each of these cell preparations equally with the biological material. Hybridoma supernatants which lacked suppressor activity, and which were tested for the presence of immunoreactive LTC_4, also lacked this arachidonic acid metabolite. The best-characterized supernatant of an active suppressor hybridoma clone did not contain additional suppressor eicosanoids, including LTB_4 and PGE_2. Protein suppressors produced by T cells, such as the soluble immune response suppressor (12) did not make a significant contribution to the observed suppressive activity, since the activity was largely removed by the anti-LTC_4-Sepharose column.

CONCLUDING REMARKS

It is thus suggested that the capacity for leukotriene biosynthesis in various mononuclear cells may be regulated both in terms of the expression of critical anabolic enzyme function and of the capacity of the cell to heighten its response to marginal agonists, and that the maturation of monocytes as well as of lymphocyte subsets may be regulated by 5-lipoxygenase products. In the cooperative and sequential processes by which complicated cell-cell signalling among monocyte/macrophages, T lymphocyte subsets, and B cells ultimately determine the level of Ig synthesis effected in the humoral immune response, the regulation of 5-lipoxygenase product generation may be critical at several stages.

REFERENCES

1. Atluru D, Goodwin JS. J Clin Invest 1984;74:1444-50.

2. Rola-Pleszczynski M. J Immunol 1984;135:1357-60.

3. Fels AO, Pawlowski NA, Cramer EB, King TKC, Cohn ZA, Scott WA. Proc Natl Acad Sci USA 1982;79:7866-70.

4. Martin TR, Altman LC, Albert RK, Henderson WR. Am Rev Respir Dis 1983;129:106-11.

5. Williams JD, Czop JK, Austen KF. J Immunol 1984;132:3034-40.

6. Damon M, Chavis C, Godard P, Michel FB, Crastes de Paulet A. Biochem Biophys Res Commun 1983;111:518-24.

7. Williams JD, Robin JL, Lewis RA, Lee TH, Austen KF. J Immunol 1986;136:642-48.

8. Ferreri NR, Howland WC, Spiegelberg HL. J Immunol 1986;136:4186-93.

9. Rankin JA, Schrader CE, Lewis RA. Fed Proc 1986;45:212

10. Sherr CJ, Rettenmier CW, Sacca R, Roussel MF, Look AT, Stanley ER. Cell 1985;41:665-76.

11. Ambrus JL Jr, Jurgensen CH, Witzel NL, Lewis RA, Butler JL, Fauci AS. J Immunol 1988;140:2382-8.

12. Schnaper HW, Pierce CW, Aune TM. J Immunol 1984;132:2429-35.

Advances in Prostaglandin, Thromboxane, and Leukotriene Research, Vol. 19, edited by B. Samuelsson, P. Y.-K. Wong, and F. F. Sun, Raven Press, Ltd., New York ©1989.

Transformation of Prostaglandin D_2 to Isomeric Prostaglandin F_2 Compounds by Human Eosinophils: A Potential Mast Cell-Eosinophil Interaction

Willis G. Parsons, III and L. Jackson Roberts, II

Departments of Pharmacology and Medicine
Vanderbilt University
Nashville, Tennessee 37232

PGD_2 is produced in large quantities by immunologically activated human mast cells (1). PGD_2 exerts a number of potent biological actions which may be relevant in immediate hypersensitivity reactions (2-4).

PGD_2 is metabolized stereoselectively <u>in vivo</u> by 11-ketoreductase to $9_\alpha,11_\beta$-PGF_2, which is biologically active (5,6). More recently PGD_2 has been shown to undergo extensive isomerization <u>in vivo</u> to a number of PGD_2 isomers which are reduced by 11-ketoreductase yielding a family of isomeric PGF_2 compounds (7).

Since eosinophils accumulate around mast cells at sites of immediate hypersensitivity reactions, and because PGF_2 compounds can exert biological actions which differ from PGD_2, we examined whether human eosinophils have the capacity to transform PGD_2 to PGF_2.

Methods

Human peripheral blood eosinophils were purified to 88-100% purity as described (8). The presence of 11-ketoreductase activity was assessed by monitoring the conversion of PGD_2 to PGF_2. Reaction mixtures contained 0 to 2×10^{-4}M PGD_2 and 5×10^5 eosinophils in PBS in a total volume of 500 μl. Incubations were carried out for 2 hours except for time-course experiments. The formation of PGF_2 compounds was detected and quantified by GC/MS as described (7).

Production of cyclooxygenase products by human eosinophils was quantified by GC/MS following incubation of 1×10^6 eosinophils in 1 ml Tyrode's buffer with 2μM A23187 for 30 minutes at 37° C.

Results

Formation of PGF_2 compounds was determined using eosinophils from four different donors. Following incubation of eosinophils in the absence of added PGD_2, formation of PGF_2 compounds was not detected. However, in the presence of PGD_2, formation of PGF_2 compounds was detected with eosinophils from all four donors. Eosinophils from each donor transformed PGD_2 not only to $9_\alpha,11_\beta$-PGF_2, but also to 12-epi-$9_\alpha,11_\beta$-PGF_2. In the presence of 2×10^{-4}M PGD_2, the amount of $9_\alpha,11_\beta$-PGF_2 and 12-epi-$9_\alpha,11_\beta$-PGF_2 formed by eosinophils from the four donors ranged from 1.7-17.6 ng/10^6 eosinophils and 0.39 to 0.98 ng/10^6 eosinophils, respectively. In experiments examining the time-course of formation of PGF_2 compounds, formation occurred rapidly during the first 30 minutes of incubation and tended to plateau by 2 hours.

Experiments were then carried out examining the effect of varying substrate (PGD_2) concentration over the range of 2×10^{-6} to 2×10^{-4}M on the formation of $9_\alpha,11_\beta$-PGF_2 and its 12-epi isomer. In each donor, the formation of $9_\alpha,11_\beta$-PGF_2 increased with increasing substrate concentration over the range of concentrations tested. However, for reasons which are unclear, in three of four donors, the formation of 12-epi-$9_\alpha,11_\beta$-PGF_2 decreased substantially at the highest concentration of PGD_2 used (2×10^{-4}M).

An interesting observation emerged during the studies. One donor's eosinophils were obtained on four separate occasion for various experiments. On three of the occasions, incubation of the eosinophils with PGD_2 resulted in the formation of $9_\alpha,11_\beta$-PGF_2 and its 12-epi isomer as expected. However, on the fourth occasion, two additional compounds were also present and these were formed in greater amounts than $9_\alpha,11_\beta$-PGF_2 and its 12-epi isomer. These compounds were not detected in the absence of added PGD_2 indicating they arose from PGD_2 metabolism. Analysis of the compounds as a deuterated trimethylsilyl ether derivative indicated the presence of three hydroxyl groups. These data provided considerable evidence that these compounds were additional PGF_2 isomers. Insufficient material was present to permit further structural characterization. Why these two additional compounds were only formed on this one occasion is not known but it is provocative that this person is atopic and at the time that these eosinophils were obtained, the donor was experiencing a marked exacerbation of allergic rhinitis and conjunctivitis.

Because the above data established that eosinophils contain 11-ketoreductase activity, we examined whether eosinophils produced substantial quantities of PGD_2 following incubation with the ionophore A23187. Consistent with previous data using human peritoneal eosinophils (9), Tx was the major cyclooxygenase product produced (2247 pg/106 eosinophils) (mean of results from 3 experiments). Levels of PGE_2, $PGF_{2\alpha}$, PGD_2, and 6-keto-$PGF_{1\alpha}$ produced were 483, 265, 50, and 6 pg/10^6 eosinophils, respectively. The amount of PGD_2 was calculated from the sum of PGD_2 and its PGF_2 metabolites produced. Thus, PGD_2 is a relatively minor cyclooxygenase product and is produced in only small quantities by the eosinophil.

Discussion

These studies establish the presence of 11-ketoreductase in human circulating eosinophils. Eosinophils not only reduce PGD_2 to $9_\alpha,11_\beta$-PGF_2 but also catalyze isomerization of PGD_2, leading to the formation of additional PGF_2 isomeric compounds. It is attractive to speculate that the eosinophil major basic protein may catalyze isomerization of PGD_2 since albumin also catalyzes isomerization of PGD_2, which is thought to be due to the alkaline microenvironment of albumin binding sites (7).

Eosinophils were found to produce only very small quantities of PGD_2. The absence of production of large quantities of PGD_2 by the eosinophil would likely enhance the availability of the eosinophil 11-ketoreductase to metabolize PGD_2 from exogenous sources, such as from adjacent mast cells.

The potential relevance of these findings to the pathophysiology of disorders of mastocyte activation, such as immediate hypersensitivity, relates to differences in biological actions of PGD_2 and its isomeric PGF_2 metabolites. One example is that PGD_2 is a vasodilator, whereas $9_\alpha,11_\beta$-PGF_2 is a vasoconstrictor (5). Preliminary studies indicate that 12-epi-$9_\alpha,11_\beta$-PGF_2 is also biologically active. However, because the complete spectrum of the biological activity of PGF_2 metabolites of PGD_2 is not known, it is not possible to predict at this time all of the potential biological ramifications of transformation of PGD_2 to PGF_2 compounds. Because these biochemical transformations of PGD_2 by eosinophils could alter the local biological consequences of PGD_2 released from adjacent mast cells, this may represent a physiologically relevant mast cell-eosinophil interaction.

References

1. Lewis, RA, Soter NA, Diamond PT, Austen KF, Oates JA, Roberts LJII. *J. Immol* 1982;129:1627-1631.

2. Hardy CC, Robinson C, Tattersfield AE, Holgate ST. *N. Engl. J. Med.* 1984;311:209-213.

3. Fuller RW, Dixon CMS, Dollerty CT, Barnes PJ. <u>Am. Rev. Resp.</u> <u>Dis.</u> 1986;133:252.

4. Goetzl EJ, Weller PF, Valone FH. In: Weissman B, Samuelsson, Paoletti R, eds. <u>Advances in inflammation research</u>, vol 1. New York: Raven Press, 1979;157-167.

5. Liston TE, Roberts LJII. <u>Proc. Natl. Acad. Sci. USA</u> 1985;82:6030-6034.

6. Seibert K, Sheller JR, Roberts LJII. <u>Proc. Natl. Acad. Sci. USA</u> 1987;84:256-260.

7. Wendelborn DF, Seibert K, Roberts LJ II. <u>Proc. Natl. Acad. Sci. USA</u> 1988;85:304-308.

8. Vadas MA, David JR, Butterworth A, Pisani HJ, Siongok TA. <u>J. Immol.</u> 1979;122:1228-1236.

9. Foegh ML, Maddox YT, Ramwell PW. <u>Scand. J. Immunol.</u> 1986;23:599-603.

Acknowledgements

Supported by Grant GM 15431 from the National Institutes of Health. L. Jackson Roberts, II, is a Burroughs Wellcome Scholar in Clinical Pharmacology.

Advances in Prostaglandin, Thromboxane, and Leukotriene Research, Vol. 19, edited by B. Samuelsson, P. Y.-K. Wong, and F. F. Sun, Raven Press, Ltd., New York ©1989.

INVOLVEMENT OF LEUKOTRIENES IN IMMEDIATE HYPERSENSIVITY REACTIONS IN THE RAT

B.A. Jakschik and W. Leng

Department of Pharmacology, Washington University School of Medicine St. Louis, Missouri 63110

Peptidoleukotrienes, when applied exogenously, have been shown to cause vasoconstriction and plasma exudation (1-3). The effect of intravenously administered leukotrienes (LT) on blood pressure has been variable (3,4). We used anaphylaxis in the rat as a model of endogenously generated LT, and followed changes in vascular permeability in the mesentery by intravital fluorescence microscopy (FITC-BSA) and in systemic pressure (5). Anaphylaxis in the rat peritoneal cavity has been used to generate slow reacting substance of anaphylaxis (6), a mixture of LTC_4, D_4 and E_4. We have shown that not only peptido-LT but also LTB_4, prostaglandins and thromboxane are released (7). The exogenous application of LTD_4 to the mesenteric microvasculature resulted in a dose dependent extravasation of macromolecules (5).

CARDIOVASCULAR CHANGES DURING SYSTEMIC ANAPHYLAXIS

Rats were passively sensitized (I.V.) with monoclonal anti-DNP IgE, and two days later anaphylaxis was induced by injecting DNP-BSA I.V. (5). Antigen challenge was followed by a marked increase in peristaltic movement of the intestine, plasma exudation (Fig. 1) and vasospasms in the mesenteric vasculature and a biphasic fall in systemic pressure. The first phase was immediate and lasted approximately two minutes. The second phase was prolonged. All of the cardiovascular changes observed increased in severity with the dose of antigen (0.125 - 0.5 mg/kg).

EFFECT OF INHIBITORS ON SYSTEMIC ANAPHYLAXIS

Various mediators are released during anaphylaxis in the rat, including leukotrienes, histamine and serotonin. Therefore, leukotriene inhibitors were tested alone and in combination with the antihistamine, pyrilamine, and/or the serotonin antagonist, methysergide. The leukotriene inhibitors used were the 5-lipoxygenase inhibitor, ONO-LP-049, and the LTD_4 receptor antagonist, L-649,923. ONO-LP-049 caused a partial inhibition of the second phase and the duration of the hypotension and of the plasma exudation in the mesentery (Fig. 2). The dose dependent effects (1 - 10 mg/kg) corresponded to the inhibiton of leukotriene formation during anaphylaxis in the peritoneal cavity (5).

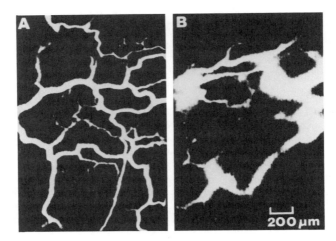

Figure 1. EXTRAVASATION IN THE MESENTERY AFTER ANTIGEN CHALLENGE. A passively sensitized rat was challenged with DNP-BSA, 0.5 mg/kg, I.V. Plasma exudation in the mesentery was followed by intravital fluorescence microscopy (FITC-BSA). A. Control (before DNP-BSA). C. After DNP-BSA (same rat as A).

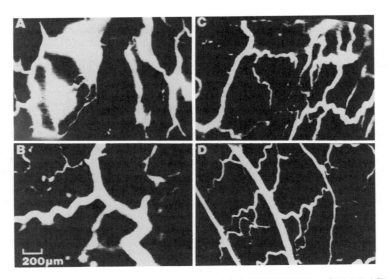

Figure 2. EFFECT OF A 5-LIPOXYGENASE INHIBITOR ON PLASMA EXUDATION IN THE MESENTERY AFTER ANTIGEN. Passively sensitized rats were challenged with DNP-BSA, 0.5 mg/kg, I.V. A. No pretreatment. B. Pretreatment with ONO-LP-049, 10 mg/kg. C. Pretreated with pyrilamine, 2 mg/kg. D. Pretreatment with ONO-LP-049 and pyrilamine.

L-649,923 decreased the plasma exudation to a lesser extent than ONO-LP-049 and did not significantly alter the hypotension. Pyrilamine extensively inhibited the first phase of the hypotension and partially its second phase and duration, as well as the plasma exudation in the mesentery (Fig. 2) in a dose dependent manner. Methysergide partially blocked the vascular leakage in the mesentery, and the second phase and the duration of the hypotension. When ONO-LP-049 or L-649,923 where used in combination with pyrilamine and/or methysergide the plasma exudation in the mesentery was almost complety prevented (Fig.2). This combination of antagonists also caused a high degree of blockade of the hypotension. The vasospasms were inhibited by methysergide, but not by the leukotriene antagonists. The cyclooxygenase inhibitor, indomethacin, did not alter the hypotension and caused a further marked increase in the peristaltic movement so that it was difficult to evaluate the effect on the microvasculature. The data from the inhibitor studies are summarized in Fig. 3. The increase in the intestinal peristalsis due to antigen was partially inhibited by each type of inhibitor. When these inhibitors were used in combination, peristalis was similar to control conditions. These findings indicate that leukotrienes play an important role in the microvascular changes and in the second phase of the hypotension caused by systemic anaphylaxis. The first phase of the hypotension seems to be mainly due to histamine. Cyclooxygenase products did not appear to significantly contribute to the cardiovascular changes studied.

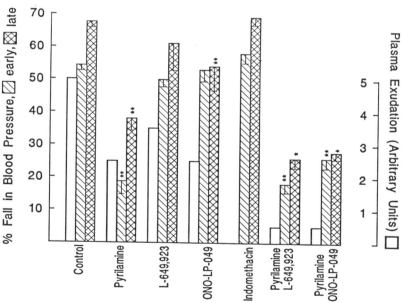

Figure 3. EFFECT OF INHIBITORS ON CARDIOVASCULAR CHANGES IN ANAPHYLAXIS. Passively sensitized rats were challenged with DNP-BSA, 0.5 mg/kg, I.V. Plasma exudation was evaluated on a scale of 1 to 5 (5 most extensive). Inhibitor pretreatment (I.V.): pyrilamine, 2 mg/kg; L-649,923, 3 mg/kg; ONO-LP-049, 10 mg/kg; indomethacin, 10 mg/kg. Mean ± SEM, n=3-7.

PASSIVE CUTANEOUS ANAPHYLAXIS AND LEUKOTRIENES

Passive cutaneous anaphylaxis (PCA) in rats caused plasma exudation which was not affected by ONO-LP-049 or L-649,923, when used either alone or in combination with an antihistamine or antiserotonergic agent. The extravasation was partially blocked by pyrilamine and methysergide when used alone and almost completely when used in combination (5). These data indicate that, in contrast to the mesentery, leukotrienes do not seem to play a role in PCA. This may be due to differential sensitivity of the microvasculature to peptidoleukotrienes and/or due to the types of mast cells present in the tissues. LTC_4 and LTD_4 have been shown to cause plasma exudation in rat skin (3). However, we found that LTD_4, up to 1 nmol, did not consistently initiate extravasation in rat skin, while in the mesentery 0.12 nmol caused extensive plasma exudation. With regard to mast cells, only the conncetive tissue type is present in the skin, while in the peritoneal cavity both, connective tissue and mucosal mast cells are found. The latter contain less histamine and have a higher capacity to synthesize leukotrienes.

CONCLUSION

The inhibitor studies in immediate hypersensitivity reactions indicate that leukotrienes play an important role in systemic anaphylaxis but not in PCA. They contribute to the hypotension and the plasma exudation in the mesentery but not to the increased vascular permeability in PCA. Our findings are in agreement with the observation that antihistamines are not efficacious in the treatment of cardiovascular or pulmonary manifestaions of immediate hypersensitivity reactions, but are very effective in cutaneous allergy.

Acknowledgements: We thank Dr. J. Rokach of Merck Frosst Laboratories, Canada, for the gift of LTD_4, LTC_4 and L-649,923, and Ono Pharmaceutical Co., Japan, for ONO-LP-049. The work was supported by NIH grant HL 31922.

REFERENCES

1. Dahlen SE, Bjork J, Hedqvist, P. Arfors KE, Hammarstrom S, Lindgren JA, Samuelsson B. Proc Nat Acad Sci USA 1981; 78:3887-3891.

2. Drazen JM, Austen KF, Lewis RA, Clark DA, Goto G, Marfat A., Corey EJ. Proc Nat Acad Sci USA 1980;77:4354-4358.

3. Ueno A, Tanaka K, Katori M, Hayashi M, Arai Y. Prostaglandins 1981;21:637-648.

4. Zukowska-Grojec Z, Bayorh MA, Kopin IJ, Feuerstein G. J Pharmacol Exp Therap 1982; 223:183-189.

5. Leng W, Kuo CG, Qureshi R, Jakschik BA. J Immunol 1988; 140, in press.

6. Orange RP, Vallentine MD, Austen KF. J Exp Med 1968;127:767-782.

7. Wei Y, Heghinian K, Bell RL, Jakschik AB. J Immunol 1986;137:1993-2000.

Advances in Prostaglandin, Thromboxane, and Leukotriene Research, Vol. 19, edited by
B. Samuelsson, P. Y.-K. Wong, and F. F. Sun,
Raven Press, Ltd., New York ©1989.

THE USE OF LEUKOTRIENE D$_4$ RECEPTOR ANTAGONISTS AND 5-LIPOXYGENASE INHIBITORS TO DEFINE A ROLE FOR LEUKOTRIENES IN ALLERGIC REACTIONS

A.W. Ford-Hutchinson

Merck Frosst Canada Inc., P.O. Box 1005,
Pointe Claire-Dorval, Québec, H9R 4P8, Canada

The peptidolipid leukotrienes, leukotrienes C$_4$, D$_4$ and E$_4$, have been proposed as important mediators of allergic conditions (1). Leukotriene D$_4$ has structurally specific, high affinity receptor sites on a number of smooth muscle preparations, interaction with which results in smooth muscle contraction (vasoconstriction or bronchoconstriction). In addition, leukotriene D$_4$ and other peptidolipid leukotrienes may have other important actions suggestive of a role in allergic reactions including mediation of changes in vascular permeability, mucous production, decreases in mucocilliary clearance and induction of nonspecific bronchial hyperreactivity. The role of peptidolipid leukotrienes in animal models of immediate hypersensitivity has been demonstrated through the use of specific 5-lipoxygenase inhibitors, such as L-656,224 (7-chloro-2-[(4-methoxyphenyl)methyl]-3-methyl-5-propyl-benzofuranyl) (2), and selective leukotriene D$_4$ receptor antagonists such as L-660,711 (3-(((3-(2-(7-chloro-2-quinolinyl)ethenyl)phenyl) ((3-(dimethyl amino-3-oxo-propyl)thio)methyl)thio)propanoic acid (3).

L-660,711 is an example of a new class of potent and selective leukotriene D$_4$ receptor antagonists (3). _In vitro_ the compound is a selective and competitive inhibitor of the binding of [^{3}H]-leukotriene D$_4$ binding to both guinea-pig (IC$_{50}$ value 0.9 nM) and human (IC$_{50}$ value 8.5 nM) lung homogenates. In contrast the compound is virtually inactive at inhibiting the binding of [^{3}H]-leukotriene C$_4$ in the same homogenates (IC$_{50}$ values > 20 μM). The compound is a functional and competitive antagonist of contractions of both the guinea-pig trachea and ileum induced by leukotriene D$_4$ (pA$_2$ values respectively of 9.4 and 10.5) and leukotriene E$_4$ (pA$_2$ values of 9.1 and 10.4 respectively). The compound also competitively inhibits contractions of human trachea induced by leukotriene D$_4$ (pA$_2$ value 8.5). The selectivity of L-660,711 on these tissues was indicated by the failure to block contractions induced by other agonists such as histamine, acetylcholine, 5-hydroxytryptamine, prostaglandin $F_{2\alpha}$, U-44069 and prostaglandin D_2. Leukotriene D_4 receptor antagonism was also observed in vivo where L-660,711 (i.v. or i.d.) inhibited bronchoconstriction induced in anesthetized guinea pigs by intravenous administration of leukotrienes C_4 or D_4 but failed to block bronchoconstriction induced by arachidonic acid, U-44069, histamine, acetylcholine or 5-hydroxytryptamine.

Compounds such as L-656,224 and L-660,711 have been tested in a variety of animal models of allergic bronchoconstriction and have been used to indicate a major role for leukotriene D_4 in allergen-induced bronchoconstriction in hyperreactive rats (2,4), ascaris-induced immediate and late phase bronchoconstriction in squirrel monkeys (2,5,6) and ascaris-induced late phase responses in sheep (7,8). In the hyperreactive rat model bronchoconstriction is assessed by monitoring the duration of dyspnea following administration of an aerosol of antigen to sensitized rats. A major mediator of the bronchoconstriction in this model is serotonin, a principal release product of rat mast cells. The activity of 5-lipoxygenase inhibitors or leukotriene D_4 receptor antagonists can only be revealed following inhibition of the serotonin component by pretreatment with methysergide (4). Under these conditions dose-related inhibition of duration of dyspnea has been observed with both 5-lipoxygenase inhibitors such as L-656,224 (3) (ED_{50} 0.7 mg/kg) and L-660,711 (3) (ED_{50} 0.068 mg/kg, both compounds administered p.o. 4 h prior to the induction of dyspnea). Further evidence for the role of leukotrienes in this model has been the demonstration of large increases in the production of peptidolipid leukotrienes as assessed by the excretion of biliary metabolites following induction of bronchoconstriction by intratracheal administration of allergen (9). Evidence for a role for peptidolipid leukotrienes in immediate bronchoconstriction induced by aerosols of ascaris to sensitize squirrel monkeys has been obtained through inhibition of the response by 5-lipoxygenase inhibitors such as L-656,224 (2) and L-651,392 (5) as well as leukotriene D_4 receptor antagonists, including L-660,711 (3). In addition, certain of these squirrel monkeys have been shown to produce a late phase bronchoconstriction primarily reflected in a decrease in dyanamic compliance (10). This response was also abolished by pretreatment with the 5-lipoxygenase inhibitor, L-651,392 (5). In a sheep model of immediate and late phase bronchoconstriction, continuous infusion of L-660,711 (0.025 mg/kg/min) attenuated the immediate bronchoconstriction and completely abolished the late phase bronchoconstriction (Abraham, unpublished results). In contrast, to the effects of these leukotriene D_4 receptor antagonists and 5-lipoxygenase inhibitors in the rat, squirrel monkey and sheep model, compounds such as L-660,711 had only a minor effect on antigen-induced anaphylaxis in sensitized guinea pigs, even in the presence of other blockers such as atropine, mepyramine and indomethacin.

Evidence that man may more closely relate to the squirrel monkey or the sheep rather than the guinea pig has been obtained with in vitro studies using isolated trachea. Following challenge of human trachea in vitro with goat anti-human IgE a contraction was elicited which could be largely blocked by pretreatment or reversed by addition of L-660,711 (Jones, unpublished results). In contrast, on guinea-pig trachea in vitro, L-660,711 produced only a minor attenuation of the antigen-induced response both in the presence or absence of blockers such as atropine, mepyramine and indomethacin.

Allergen-induced permeability changes may also be mediated by leukotriene D_4. Evidence for this has been obtained in a guinea-pig model of allergic conjunctivitis where the inhibitory effects of leukotriene D_4 receptor antagonists on the antigen response were correlated with inhibitory effects on the leukotriene D_4 response and the inhibitory effects of topical 5-lipoxygenase inhibitors with inhibition of leukotriene B_4 production in the conjunctiva following ex vivo challenge with ionophore A23187 (11,12). In this model both leukotriene D_4 receptor antagonists and 5-lipoxygenase inhibitors produced inhibition of the response when applied in conjunction with antihistamines following a second application of antigen (11,12). L-660,711 also inhibits leukotriene D_4-induced permeability changes and has been shown to partially inhibit responses in the guinea-pig skin following intradermal administration of either enterotoxin to normal animals or antigen to sensitized animals (Chan and Hamel, unpublished results).

Clinical trials with leukotriene D_4 receptor antagonists have tested such agents first against leukotriene D_4-induced bronchoconstriction in normal volunteers and secondly against antigen challenge of mild asthmatics. Some data has been obtained with first generation compounds such as L-649,923, L-648,051 and LY-171883 (13,14,15). All three of the compounds have produced only small shifts in the leukotriene D_4 response curve in man at their maximum tolerated doses. Under these conditions minor effects on antigen challenge have been observed with L-649,923 and in a six week study with LY-171883 small effects on FEV_1, symptom score and a more dramatic reduction in β-agonist usage were observed. Because of the relative lack of activity of these compounds against the leukotriene D_4 response in man in vivo it is difficult to determine if the results indicate a minor role for leukotrienes in immediate antigen responses in man or whether the results simply reflect lack of potency of the compounds. L-660,711 is a much more potent compound which should produce at least 50-fold shifts in the leukotriene D_4 dose response curve in man which would then allow for a more definitive evaluation of the role of leukotrienes in allergic diseases including bronchial asthma.

REFERENCES

1. Piper PJ. *Physiol Rev* 1984;64:744-761.

2. Bélanger P, Maycock A, Guindon Y, Back T, Dallob AL, Dufresne C, Ford-Hutchinson AW, Gale PH, Hopple S, Lau CK, Letts LG, Luell S, McFarlane CS, MacIntyre E, Meurer R, Miller DK, Piechuta H, Riendeau D, Rokach J, Rouzer C, Scheigetz J. Can J Physiol Pharmacol 1987;65:2441-2448.

3. Jones TR, Zamboni R, Belley M, Champion E, Charette L, DeHaven RN, Ford-Hutchinson AW, Frenette R, Gauthier JY, Leger S, Masson P, McFarlane CS, Piechuta H, Pong SS, Rokach J, Williams H, Young RN. Can J Physiol Pharmacol (submitted for publication).

4. Piechuta H, Ford-Hutchinson AW, Letts GL. Agents Actions 1987;22:69-74.

5. McFarlane CS, Hamel R, Ford-Hutchinson AW. Agents Actions 1987; 22:63-68.

6. Letts LG, McFarlane C, Piechuta H, Ford-Hutchinson AW. In: Samuelsson B, Paoletti PW, eds. Advances in Prostaglandin, Thromboxane and Leukotriene Research, vol 17. New York: Raven Press, 1987;1007-1011.

7. Abraham WM, Wanner A, Stevenson JS, Chapman GA. Prostaglandins 1986;31:457-467.

8. Lanes S, Stevenson JS, Codias E, Hernandez A, Sielczak MW, Wanner A, Abraham WM. J Appl Physiol 1986;61:864-872.

9. Foster A, Letts G, Charleson S, Fitzsimmons B, Blacklock B, Rokach J. J Immunol (submitted for publication).

10. Hamel R, McFarlane CS, Ford-Hutchinson AW. J Appl Physiol 1986;61:2081-2087.

11. Garceau D, Ford-Hutchinson AW. Eur J Pharmacol 1987;134:285-292.

12. Garceau D, Ford-Hutchinson AW, Charleson S. Eur J Pharmacol 1987;143:1-7.

13. Barnes N, Piper PJ, Costello J. J Allergy Clin Immunol 1987;79:816-821.

14. Britton JR, Hanley SP, Tattersfield AE. J Allergy Clin Immunol 1987;79:811-816.

15. Mathur PN, Callaghan JT, Farid MA, Sylvester AJ. Clin Res 1986;34:580A.

Advances in Prostaglandin, Thromboxane, and Leukotriene Research, Vol. 19, edited by B. Samuelsson, P. Y.-K. Wong, and F. F. Sun, Raven Press, Ltd., New York ©1989.

STUDIES OF SYNERGISM BETWEEN INHIBITORS OF THE 5-LIPOXYGENASE PATHWAY

Michael K. Bach and John R. Brashler

Hypersensitivity Diseases Research, The Upjohn Company, Kalamazoo, MI 49001, USA

We have studied the cumulative effects on leukotriene (LT) synthesis in suspensions of rat basophil leukemia (RBL) cells (1) of combinations of inhibitors which are selective for each of the three known enzymes (2) which are involved in LT synthesis. To assess the manifestation of synergism between a given pair of inhibitors, the experiments were set up so that cells were exposed to a series of increasing concentrations of one inhibitor in the presence of increasing concentrations of the other inhibitor, and LT production was estimated by selective radioimmunoassay for LTC_4 (3). The average LT production in duplicate incubations was expressed relative to production in uninhibited control incubations. The expected relative LT production in the presence of any given combination of two inhibitors was calculated from the relative LT production in the presence of each inhibitor taken singly using the equation,

$$\text{Predicted Activity}_{combination} = \text{Activity}_A \times \text{Activity}_B$$

where "activity" stands for the relative production of LT. If the ratio of the observed relative LT production to the expected relative LT production for any given combination was smaller than unity, synergism was observed and, the smaller the ratio, the greater the synergism.

The following inhibitors have been studied: 1. **Para bromophenacyl bromide (PBPB)**, an irreversible inhibitor of phospholipase A2, having an EC_{50} of 87 ± 20 μM (average of 10 experiments). 2. **Piriprost (U-60,257)**, a presumed inhibitor of the 5-lipoxygenase (5-LO), EC_{50} 10.5 ± 2.3 μM (17 experiments). 3. **AA861**, 2-(12-hydroxy-5,10-dodecadinyl)-3,5,6-trimethyl-2,5-cyclohexadiene-1,4-dione, a 5-LO inhibitor, EC_{50} 22.2 ± 4.9 nM (15 experiments). 4. **Itazigrel**, [4,5-bis (p-methoxyphenyl)-2-(trifluoromethyl)]-thiazole, a known inhibitor of cyclooxygenase (4) which also has 5-LO inhibitory activity; (E_{50} 12.4 ± 3.1 μM (4 experiments). 5. **4-Phenoxybutyl, phenyldisulfide**, a presumed 5-LO inhibitor of the phenyldisulfide type (5), EC_{50} 3.6 ± 1.9 μM (2 experiments). 6. **U-74,006F**, 21-[4-(2,6-di-1-pyrrolidinyl-4-pyrimidinyl)-1-piperazinyl]-16-methyl-16-α-pregna-1,4,9(11)-triene-3,20-dione monomethane sulfonate, a "Lazaroid" (6), EC$_{50}$ 7.5 ± 3.3 μM (3 experiments).   7. **Sulfasalazine** (SFZ) , an inhibitor of LTC synthase, competitive with glutathione (1), EC$_{50}$ 54 ± 16 μM, (4 experiments).   8. **Diethylcarbamazine** (DEC), an inhibitor of LTC synthase, competitive with LTA$_4$ (7), EC$_{50}$ 27.4 ± 2.0 mM (9 experiments).

The following combinations of inhibitors showed essentially additive inhibition and no synergism: 1. DEC and SFZ, the two inhibitors of the LTC synthase.   2. PBPB with either piriprost or AA861.   3. AA861 with U-74,006F, Itazigrel, or 4-phenoxybutyl, phenyl-disulfide.   4. SFZ with either AA861 or piriprost. On the other hand, there was profound synergism between DEC and either AA861 or piriprost as well as between the latter two inhibitors of the 5-LO themselves.

Interpretation of these results is complicated by the fact that not all of these inhibitors are completeley selective and, furthermore, their modes of action are not always known. PBPB is an alkylating agent and, while it is an inhibitor of phospholipase A$_2$, it is known to have numerous other activities outside the 5-LO pathway. The specificities of several of the 5-LO inhibitors are not defined, and there are a number of publi-cations suggesting that both DEC and SFZ are inhibitors of the 5-lipoxygenase. While this cannot be ruled out in the present studies, dose-response studies with the isolated LTC synthase suggest that the inhibition of this enzyme by itself is sufficient to account for the activities of the last two compounds in our system. Thus, in interpreting our results, there remains the caveat that lack of inhibitor specificity may be at the basis of other possible explanations of the observed effects.

One might expect, a priori, that two inhibitors which inhibit the same enzyme in two different manners should synergize each other. We therefore expected so see synergism between DEC and SFZ since we had already demonstrated that both these compounds inhibited the same enzyme at the concentrations which were being used and, furthermore, that their mechanisms of inhibition were different kinetically. We expected that any combination of inhibitors which act at different steps in the pathway, such as a phospholipase inhibitor and a lipoxygenase inhibitor or a lipoxygenase inhibitor and an LTC synthase inhibitor, should act synergistically. Again, with but one exception, these combinations did not display significant synergism. On further reflection, however, we believe that our observations all point to a single conclusion which is that in order for there to be synergism between two inhibitors acting on a single pathway, both inhibitors must limit the formation of a product whose concentration is rate-limiting to the final reaction. It follows that no synergism would be expected between an inhibitor which interferes with the utilization of glutathione (ie using SFZ) and any other inhibitor of LT synthesis since the concentration of glutathione in the cells is not likely to be limiting. Similarly in a reaction which is initiated by the calcium ionophore, the mobilization of arachidonate must far exceed the needs of the 5-LO in the cells. This could explain our failure to observe synergism between an inhibitor of the phospholipase and a 5-LO inhibitor. On the other hand, both the inhibitors of the 5-LO which were tested showed marked synergism with DEC. This further supports our conclusion that the primary site of action of DEC is by competing with LTA_4 in the LTC synthase reaction rather than acting as an inhibitor of the 5-LO. It seems very likely that the concentration of LTA_4 is rate limiting since the apparent K_m of the LTC synthase for LTA_4 in the presence serum albumin was 0.1 mM (7) while in the absence of a stabilizing protein the half-life of this intermediate would be too short to permit the accumulation of a significant pool size.

It is axiomatic that inhibitors having an identical mode of action cannot display synergism. Thus, the failure to find synergism between several presumed inhibitors of the 5-LO is consistent with the interpretation that, as far as the kinetics of the reaction are concerned, these compounds have a similar mechanism of action. On the other hand, this makes the observation that there was profound synergism between AA861 and piriprost particularly interesting. In contrast to AA861 which is a potent inhibitor of the solubilized 5-LO (8), we and others have repeatedly failed in atempts to demonstrate the inhibition of this enzyme in cell-free incubations with piriprost. The observation of profound synergism between these two inhibitors thus adds another dimension to the argument that the mechanisms of action of these two compounds are different. It is possible that piriprost may act by interfering with the regulation of the 5-LO by one of its cofactors (9) rather than affecting the "constitutive" enzyme itself.

These studies are consistent with our general understanding of the biosynthesis of the LTs. While they suggest some new insights into the mechanisms of action of inhibitors of this pathway, the generalizations which have been offered will require extension of these studies to many more examples of interactions between specific inhibitors of each step in the pathway and further careful analysis of the biochemical basis of the actions of these inhibitors.

REFERENCES

1. Bach MK, Brashler JR, Johnson MA. <u>Biochem. Pharmacol.</u> 1985;34:2695-2704.

2. Bach MK. In: Chakrin LW, Bailey DM, eds. <u>The Leukotrienes. Chemistry and Biology</u>, New York: Academic Press, 1984;163-194.

3. Bach MK, Brashler JR, White GJ, Galli SJ. <u>Biochem. Pharmacol.</u> 1987;36:1461-1466.

4. Nishizawa EE, Mendoza AR, Honohan T, Annis KA. <u>Thromb. Haemostasis</u> 1982;47:173-176.

5. Egan RW Gale PH. <u>J. Biol. Chem.</u> 1985;260:11554-11559.

6. Braughler JM, Pregenzer JF, Chase RL, Duncan LA, Jacobsen EJ, McCall JM. <u>J. Biol. Chem.</u> 1987;262:10438-10440.

7. Bach MK Brashler JR. <u>Biochem. Pharmacol.</u> 1986;35:425-433.

8. Yamamoto S, Yoshimoto T, Furukawa M, Horie T, Watanabe-Kohno S. <u>J. Allergy Clin. Immunol.</u> 1984;74:349-352.

9. Rouzer CA, Matsumoto T, Shimizu T, Samuelsson B. <u>Adv. Prostaglandin, Thromboxane, Leukotriene Res.</u> 1986;16:2-16.

Advances in Prostaglandin, Thromboxane, and Leukotriene Research, Vol. 19, edited by B. Samuelsson, P. Y.-K. Wong, and F. F. Sun, Raven Press, Ltd., New York ©1989.

ANALYSIS OF THE EFFECTS OF CYCLOOXYGENASE AND LIPOXYGENASE INHIBITORS ON LEUKOCYTE ACCUMULATION IN THE INFLAMMATORY SITE

Susumu Tsurufuji, Noriyasu Hirasawa and Izumi Kamo

Department of Biochemistry, Faculty of Pharmaceutical Sciences, Tohoku University, Aoba, Aramaki, Sendai 980, JAPAN.

We have developed an experimental model of allergic inflammation of air pouch type in rats using azobenzenearsonate-conjugated acetyl bovine serum albumin (ABA-AcBSA) as an antigen (1). In brief, 9 days after the immunization, animals are injected with 8ml of air subcutaneously to make an air pouch on the back. Twenty-four hours later, the antigen dissolved in 2% sodium carboxymethylcellulose (CMC) solution is injected into the pouch to provoke an allergic inflammation. Immediately after the challenge injection, a strong response of plasma exudation into the pouch fluid from the surrounding tissues occurs, reaching maximum within 30 minutes, and then it decreases quickly down to about half of the maximum within 1.5 hour after the challenge injection.(2). Thereafter, a moderate response of the plasma exudation is maintained over the period of 48 hours. Migration of leukocytes is very active during the period of 3-15 hours. The number of leukocytes in the pouch fluid reaches maximum about 24 hours after the challenge injection and then it decreases gradually (1, 3).

Time course study of histamine levels disclosed that histamine in the pouch fluid shows bi-phasic increase. Namely, the sudden and rapid increase in the anaphylactic phase, reaching maximum coincidently with the time course of the immediate response of plasma exudation, is followed by quick fall to a very low level by 1.5 hour (4). Thereafter, it again increases gradually toward the second time maximum which is reached about 24 hours after the challenge injection, and then it decreases gradually. The first phase increase of histamine has been shown to be responsible for the anaphylactic increase of the vascular permeability. Then we investigated into the role of histamine increase of the second phase (post-anaphylactic phase) and disclosed that histamine in the post-anaphylactic phase exerts an inhibitory effect on leukocyte migration toward inflammatory sites. The inhibitory effect of histamine on the leukocyte migration is mediated by the histamine H_2 mechanism, because the inhibitory effect is unaffected by the treatment with pyrilamine, an H_1 blocker, but blocked by cimetidine, an H_2 blocker (4, 5).

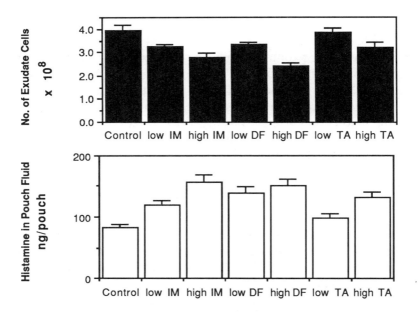

Fig. 1. CYCLOOXYGENASE INHIBITORS ADMINISTERED LOCALLY IN THE INFLAMMATORY POUCH SUPPRESS LEUKOCYTE ACCUMULATION THROUGH RAISING HISTMAINE LEVEL IN THE SITE OF INFLAMMATION.
low IM: 1μg/ml of indomethacin, high IM: 10μg/ml, low DF: 1μg/ml of diclofenac, high DF: 10μg/ml, low TA: 1μg of tiaprofenic acid, high TA: 10μg/ml.

Prostaglandin E_2 in the pouch fluid begins to rise about 1 hour after the antigenic challenge and reaches maximum at 8 hour. Then the maximum level is maintained up to 48 hour after the challenge (5), and then it declines toward a very low level by day 5 (6). The role of PGE2 in the vascular permeability reaction in the site of inflammation is not so simple as generally thought. In the anaphylactic stage, PGE2 level is not high enough to rise the vascular permeability (2). In the early post-anaphylactic stage, i.e. about 4 hour after the challenge, PGE2 plays no significant role in rising the vascular permeability, though the level has been already elevated close to the maximum. In contrast, PGE2 in more later phase, when examined at 8 and 24 hour after the antigenic challenge, augments plasma exudation (5, 7).

PGE2 plays also a significant role in augmenting neutrophil accumulation in inflammatory site through inhibiting histamine-generating system in the inflammatory tissues (7), since histamine in the late phase of acute inflammation, i.e. in the period of 4-48 hour after the onset of the inflammation, exerts a downward regulatory effect on the accumulation of neutrophils (4). Cyclooxygenase inhibitors such as indomethacin, diclofenac and tiaprofenic acid, when applied locally into the pouch together with the challenging antigen, inhibit PGE2 production. Thus they exert significant inhibitory effects on the accumulation of neutrophils, as illustrated in Fig. 1, by raising histamine levels in the inflammatory site (7).

Peptide leukotrienes begin to rise immediately after the antigenic challenge, reach maximum about 1 hour later and then decline gradually. However, they play no significant role in the vascular permeability reaction in the anaphylactic phase (2), probably because their local levels are not so high enough to cause a significant reaction. Leukotriene B4 also occurs in the inflammatory site to reach maximum about 4 hours after the challenge, and then it declines and almost disappears by 8 hour. Lipoxygenase inhibitors administered locally in the pouch are highly effective in inhibiting the generation of LTB4, but ineffective in inhibiting either leukocyte emigration into the pouch or occurrence of chemotactic activity in the pouch fluid. In other words, some chemotactic factors other than LTB4 seem to play more significant role in inducing the leukocyte emigration. An antiinflammatory steroid dexamethasone is not only capable of inhibiting the generation of LTB4 and leukocyte accumulation but also effectively suppresses the generation of the chemotactic activity in the pouch fluid. Therefore, mechanisms other than the inhibition of the generation of LTB4 should be responsible for the inhibitory effect of dexamethasone on leukocyte accumulation in the inflammatory site.

References.

(1) Tsurufuji S, Yoshino S, Ohuchi K. Int Arch Allerg Appl Imm 1982;69:189-198.

(2) Ohuchi K, Hirasawa N, Watanabe M, Tsurufuji S. Europ J Pharmac 1985;117:337-345.

(3) Kurihara A, Ohuchi K, Tsurufuji S. Int Arch Allerg Appl Imm 1983;71:368-370.

(4) Hirasawa N, Ohuchi K, Watanabe M, Tsurufuji S. J Pharmac Exp Therap 1987;241:967-973.

(5) Hirasawa N, Ohuchi K, Sugio K, Tsurufuji S, Watanabe M, Yoshino S. Brit J Pharmac 1986;87:751-756.

(6) Watanabe M, Ohuchi K, Tsurufuji S. Int Arch Allerg Appl Imm 1987;83:390-397.

(7) Hirasawa N, Ohuchi K, Watanabe M, Tsurufuji S. Europ J Pharmac 1987;144:267-275.

Advances in Prostaglandin, Thromboxane, and Leukotriene Research, Vol. 19, edited by B. Samuelsson, P. Y.-K. Wong, and F. F. Sun, Raven Press, Ltd., New York ©1989.

GLUCOCORTICOID INHIBITION OF Ca^{2+} AND

PHOSPHOLIPID-DEPENDENT ENZYMES REGULATING

LEUKOTRIENE C_4 FORMATION AND ACTION

IN ALLERGIC AND INFLAMMATORY RESPONSES.

U. Zor, E. Her, I. Ostfeld, J. Talmon and *Y. Lahav

Departments of Hormone Research and
*Polymer Research, The Weizmann Institute of Science,
Rehovot, 76100, Israel.

Activation of allergic and inflammatory cells by various stimulants require prior elevation of cytosolic Ca^{2+} concentration ($[Ca^{2+}]_i$), this being an essential cofactor for some of the key enzymes for this process (for review see ref. 1). Another probable prerequisite for cellular activation is availability (by unmasking) of certain phospholipids (PL; Fig. 1). These include phosphatidylserine (PS) and phosphatidyl-inositol (PI), which are located in and on the surface of the plasma membrane.

Allergic and Inflammatory Cells

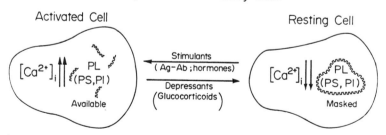

Fig. 1. Transformation of cell from resting to activated state by various stimulants (immune response; Ag-Ab etc.) and its reversal by HC.

Hydrocortisone (HC) induces a spectrum of proteins (including lipocortins) which mediate its multiple actions. These proteins can prevent the development of the allergic reaction or can "defuse" activated allergic cells returning them to the resting state. Some of the lipocortins bind PL in such a way as to mask their site of action from the enzymes which use PL either as a substrate or as a cofactor (see Fig. 1). Recently, we showed for the first time that HC could prevent the elevation of $[Ca^{2+}]_i$ induced by Ag-Ab complex (1) and consequently leukotriene C_4 (LTC_4) formation.

In the presence of high $[Ca^{2+}]_i$, 5-lipoxygenase (5-LOX) is gradually recruited from the cytosol and bound tightly to the membrane. The translocation induces activation of the enzyme (2). Some enzymes require PL in addition to high Ca^{2+} con-centration, for example, phospholipase A_2 (PLA_2), phospholipase C (PLC) and protein kinase C (PKC).

In this paper we will demonstrate that one of the main actions of the natural hormone HC in rat basophilic leukemia cells (RBL) is to reduce $[Ca^{2+}]_i$ and consequently inhibit PLA_2, PLC and 5-LOX activity. Secondly, by using antibodies recognizing PL located on the outer plasma membrane (3), we examine the role of membrane PL, specifically PI, in collagen-induced platelet adhesion and aggregation.

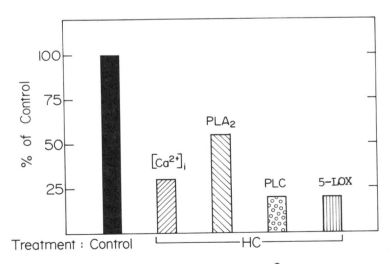

Fig. 2. Inhibitory effect of HC on $[Ca^{2+}]_i$, PLA_2, PLC and 5-LOX. HC (3×10^{-6}M) was incubated for 6 hr with RBL cells and then the cells challenged with IgE-DNP.

RESULTS

Pretreatment with HC markedly reduced $[Ca^{2+}]_i$ (70%) following antigen-antibody (IgE-DNP) challenge to RBL cells (ref. 1 and Fig. 2). The inhibitory effect became apparent only after 2 hrs preincubation and was maximal at 5 hrs. It could be totally suppressed by addition of a steroid receptor antagonist or cycloheximide (4). The effect was specific to glucocorticoids, dexamethasone, for example, being active, whereas estradiol and aldosterone were not (for review see 4).

The enzymes PLA_2, 5-LOX and PLC which are all involved in LTC_4 production and/or action, were activated by IgG-DNP in RBL cells. Activities of PLC and 5-LOX were almost abolished by HC, while that of PLA_2 was reduced only 45% (Fig. 2 and refs 1 and 4). When Ca^{2+} was omitted from the medium (in the absence of HC) PLA_2 and 5-LOX activities following stimulation by IgE-DNP or by Ca^{2+} ionophore were totally suppressed (refs. 1 and 4). Thus low Ca^{2+} produced effects similar to those resulting from addition of HC.

The effect of antibodies (Ab) against PL (mainly PI and, to a lesser extent, PS) was examined on adhesion and aggregation of purified human platelets. Collagen-induced platelet adhesion was inhibited by about 50% by prior addition of anti-PL Ab. When the Ab were preincubated with PI, they did not display any inhibitory effect and adhesion was normal (Fig. 3A). Collagen-induced platelet aggregation at submaximal concentrations was markedly reduced (80%) by prior addition of Ab. The Ab however, were almost inactive, if they were first preincubated with cardiolipin (Fig 3B).

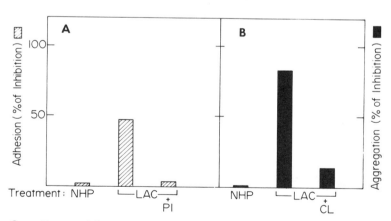

<u>Fig. 3.</u>   Prevention by anti-PL Ab of collagen-induced platelet adhesion (A) and aggregation (B). NHP: normal human plasma; LAC: anti-PL Ab (Lupus anticoagulant); CL: cardiolipin.

DISCUSSION

Reduction of $[Ca^{2+}]_i$ elevated by various stimulants should cause abatement of cellular activity. This may be achieved by regulation of the following biochemical pathways: a) inhibition of Ca^{2+} influx; b) enhancement of Ca^{2+} efflux (Ca^{2+}-Mg^{2+} ATPase); c) prevention of mobilization of internal bound calcium from organelles. Ca^{2+} influx serves as the main source for elevation of $[Ca^{2+}]_i$ in RBL cells, but we have no indication whatsoever whether HC has any inhibitory effect on it. With regard to Ca^{2+} efflux, our preliminary data indicates that HC magnifies plasma membrane Ca^{2+}-pump activity. Reinforcement of this pathway could certainly account for the large reduction in $[Ca^{2+}]_i$ seen after HC treatment. Finally, HC (and other glucocorticoids) were found to be very potent inhibitors of PLC activity Fig. 2), which means that less inositol 1,4,5-triphosphate is available to mobilize calcium from the organelles.

High $[Ca^{2+}]_i$ enhances binding of 5-LOX to the membrane and activates the enzyme (1,2). Since HC reduces $[Ca^{2+}]_i$, Ca^{2+} becomes a rate-limiting factor for activation of 5-LOX, PLA_2 and PLC. This, we contend, is one of the main mechanisms by which HC suppresses allergy and inflammation.

Phospholipids (PC, PE and PI) serve as substrates for receptor-mediated PLA_2 and PLC. PS, however, is a cofactor for the binding of PKC to the plasma membrane, binds to lipocortin in a Ca^{2+}-dependent manner and is involved in platelet activation. Recently, we showed that antibodies against PL (mainly PI but also PS) prevent cellular activation induced by various stimulants or by exogenous PLA_2 or PLC (3). We interpret the data in Fig. 3 to mean that the anti-PL Ab bind and neutralize PS and PI located on the outer plasma membrane. Thus platelet adhesion cannot be fully induced by collagen, nor can platelet aggregation, which may be PLC-dependent. It is possible that PL Ab act in the same way as the lipocortins, namely bind to PL thereby preventing the interaction between PLC and PLA_2 and their respective PL.

We conclude, therefore, that high $[Ca^{2+}]_i$ and PL availability are among the agents that control cellular activation during allergy and inflammation. The therapeutic action of HC is probably related to its ability to reduce $[Ca^{2+}]_i$ and to induce "depletion" of essential membrane PL. The regulation by HC is thus due to limiting cofactors and substrate availability, rather than directly inhibiting key enzymes which induce the mediators of the allergic and inflammatory response.

Acknowledgement: This study is supported by Institut Henri Beaufour, France. We are grateful to Mrs. Malka Kopelowitz for typing of this manuscript, and to Dr. Sandra Moshonov for valuable editing. U. Zor is an incumbent of the W.B. Graham Professorial Chair in Pharmacology.

REFERENCES

1. Zor U, Her E, Talmon J, et al. <u>Prostaglandins</u> 1987;34:29-40.

2. Rouzer CA, Samuelsson B. <u>Proc</u> <u>Natl</u> <u>Acad</u> <u>Sci</u> <u>USA</u> 1987;84:7393-7397.

3. Sömjen D, Zor U, Kaye AM, et al. <u>Biochim</u> <u>Biophys</u> <u>Acta</u> 1987;931:215-223.

4. Her E, Weizzman A, Zor U. <u>J</u> <u>Biol</u> <u>Chem</u> (submitted).

Advances in Prostaglandin, Thromboxane, and Leukotriene Research, Vol. 19, edited by B. Samuelsson, P. Y.-K. Wong, and F. F. Sun, Raven Press, Ltd., New York ©1989.

BETA ADRENOCEPTOR DESENSITIZATION IN LUNG:
A ROLE FOR PROSTAGLANDINS.

Claudio Omini, Luisa Daffonchio, Maria Pia Abbracchio, Flaminio Cattabeni and Ferruccio Berti;

Institute of Pharmacological Sciences and Biological Sciences, University of Milan and Pisa, Italy.

INTRODUCTION

One of the important side effects of beta agonist therapy is a decrease in their efficacy after prolonged use of these drugs attributed to beta-receptor desensitization (1). We have already demonstrated an involvement of prostaglandins (PGs) in this phenomenon, in fact PGE_2 release by guinea-pig trachea during beta-receptor induced relaxation is increased after the homologous desensitization procedure (2). Moreover the inhibition of cyclo- and lipo-oxygenase prevents the development of beta-receptor down-regulation in guinea-pig and rat lung (2,3). In addition the possible site of action of PGs in beta-receptor desensitization seems to be located at the coupling between adenylate cyclase and beta-receptor (3,4).
In this regard it has been proposed that an impairment of beta-adrenergic function might be a cause of asthma. Therefore we investigated the possible occurrence of beta-adrenoceptor desensitization after antigen challenge in ovalbumin (OA) sensitized guinea-pigs and the possible involvement of PGs in this phenomenon.

MATERIALS AND METHODS

Male guinea-pigs (300-350 g) were actively sensitized to OA by s.c. and i.p. injection of the antigen (OA, Sigma grade V, 100 mg/kg) 18-28 days before the experiments. The tracheas were removed after sacrifice, cut into zig-zag strips and placed in an organ bath. After 1h equilibration the tracheas were challenged with the specific antigen (OA 50 µg/ml) or saline and 1h later washed with Krebs solution containing pilocarpine (2×10^{-5}M). Cumulative epinephrine (EPI) concentration response curves were performed. INDO (1.5×10^{-5}M) and hydrocortisone (HYDRO 6.2×10^{-5}M) were added 1h before challenge and throughout all the experiment.

RESULTS

Fig 1. Effect of antigen challenge on EPI induced relaxation
in guinea-pig trachea.

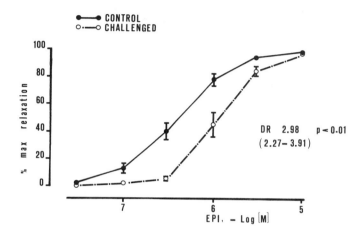

Each point represent the mean+SE of 5 replications.
DR= dose ratio

The in vitro challenge with OA in tracheas obtained from
actively sensitized guinea-pigs resulted in an impairment of
beta-receptor activity. In fact EPI concentration response
curves were significantly ($p < 0.01$) shifted to the right in
OA challenged tracheas as compared to controls (fig. 1). A
preliminary binding study using $\pm$ 125 iodocyanopindolol showed
a parallel decrease in the number of beta-receptors after antigen challenge; the B_{max} calculated were 149 and 50 fmol/mg
prot in control and challenged tracheas respectively. The pretreatment of the tissue with INDO completely prevented the
decrease in beta-receptor function due to the antigen challenge
(fig. 2). Similar results were obtained with HYDRO pretreatment.

Fig 2. Effect of INDO on beta-receptor desensitization induced by antigen challenge in guinea-pig trachea.

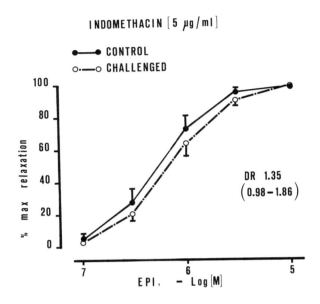

Each point represent the mean±SE of 5 replications.
DR= dose ratio

DISCUSSION

Homologous desensitization of pulmonary beta-adrenoceptors and the involvement of PGs in this phenomenon have been already established (5). However the role of adrenergic system in the genesis of asthma may be also important, since a decrease in beta-adrenergic function was observed in asthmatic patients (6). Our data, obtained in OA actively sensitized guinea-pig, speak in favour of an involvement of adrenergic beta receptors in asthma. It has been questioned that the decrease in adrenergic function in asthmatic may be a consequence rather than a cause of asthma (6); our results seem to avvalorate this hypothesis in fact the beta adrenoceptor reactivity seems to be not modified by the active sensitization (unpublished observation) and only the antigen challenge induces the impairment of adrenergic relaxation. However asthmatic patients have several antigen challenges in their life and the subsequent decrease in adrenergic function may exacerbate their disease. In this regard our data, showing that PGs are involved in the desensitization of beta-receptor after antigen challenge, may have a pathological explanation. In fact it is well known that asthma is often associated to airway inflammation (7), therefore a consequence of eicosanoid release during inflammation may be a decrease in pulmonary adrenergic inhibitory control, which in turn may contribute to the genesis of airway hyperreactivity present in asthmatic subjects.

REFERENCES

1. Plummer AL. Chest 1987;73:949-957.

2. Berti F, Daffonchio L, Folco GC, Omini C, Vigano' T. J Autonom Pharmacol 1982;2:247-253.

3. Omini C, Abbracchio MP, Coen E, Daffonchio L, Fano M, Cattabeni F. Eur J Pharmacol 1984;106:601-606.

4. Fano M, Abbracchio MP, Cattabeni F, Daffonchio L, Hernandez A, Omini C. J Autonom Pharmacol 1986;6:47-51.

5. Abbracchio MP, Daffonchio L, Omini C. Pharmac Res Comm 1986; 18:93-110.

6. Barnes PJ. In:Bianco S, Pasargiklian M, Grassi C, eds. Respiration, vol 50 Basel: Karger, 1986;9-16.

7. Nadel JA, Holtzman MJ. In:Kay AB, Austen KF, Lichtenstein LM, eds. Asthma; physiology, immunopharmacology and treatment, vol 9 Academic Press Inc, 1984;129-155.

Advances in Prostaglandin, Thromboxane, and Leukotriene Research, Vol. 19, edited by
B. Samuelsson, P. Y.-K. Wong, and F. F. Sun,
Raven Press, Ltd., New York ©1989.

EFFECT OF AN ORAL THROMBOXANE SYNTHETASE INHIBITOR (OKY-046)

ON ANTIGEN - INDUCED BRONCHOCONSTRICTION IN GUINEA PIGS

F. Nambu, T. Shiraji, M. Motoishi, M. Sawada, N. Omawari,
H. Terashima, T. Okegawa, A. Kawasaki, and S. Ikeda*

Minase Research Institute, Ono Pharmaceutical Co., Ltd.,
Shimamoto, Mishima, Osaka 618, Japan and
*Central Research Laboratories, Kissei Pharmaceutical Co., Ltd.,
Matsumoto 399, Japan

OKY-046, (E)-3-$[p$-$(1H$-imidazol-1-ylmethyl)phenyl]-2-propenoic acid is a potent and selective inhibitor of thromboxane synthetase in various species(1). We examined the effect of OKY-046 on airway hyperresponsiveness induced by antigen and various spasmogens such as platelet activating factor(PAF) and peptide leukotrienes(LTs) in anesthetized guinea pigs. Further, the spectrum of inhibiting activities of OKY-046 was investigated by measuring the release of cyclooxygenase products in bronchoalveolar lavage fluid (BALF) and plasma.

MATERIALS AND METHODS

Normal or ovalbumin(OVA)-sensitized guinea pigs were anesthetized with pentobarbital sodium(75 mg/kg, i.p.) and artificially ventilated at 70 strokes per minute(2). The change in lung resistance was measured using a pressure transducer. Changes in respiratory overflow were expressed as a percentage of maximal bronchoconstriction obtained by clamping down the trachea completely. Airway hyperresponses were induced by OVA and various spasmogens such as LTC_4, STA_2(a stable thromboxane A_2 analog), prostaglandin D_2(PGD$_2$), serotonin(5-HT), histamine(His), acetylcholine(ACh) and PAF. Increases of thromboxane B_2(TXB$_2$) and 6-keto-PGF$_{1\alpha}$ induced by antigen challenge were measured both in BALF samples and plasma samples. OKY-046 was administered orally 1 hr before spasmogen treatments.

RESULTS AND DISCUSSION

Antigen-induced bronchoconstriction showed a biphasic pattern under the treatment of mepyramine. The systemic blood pressure showed a biphasic pattern to OVA challenge: an initial hypertension and a delayed hypotension.

OKY-046 significantly inhibited antigen-induced bronchoconstriction at an oral dose of 300 mg/kg. OKY-046 also inhibited the
initial hypertensive phase but not the delayed hypotensive phase
(Fig. 1). The combination of oral OKY-046 and intravenous ONO-

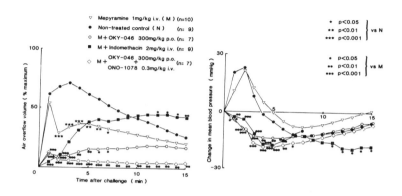

Fig. 1. Effect of OKY-046 and indomethacin on antigen-induced
bronchoconstriction and change in blood pressure in actively
sensitized guinea pigs under treatment of mepyramine.

Table 1. Antigen-induced generation of TXB_2 in plasma and BALF
in actively sensitized guinea pigs

Compound	Dose (mg/kg)	Concentration (ng/ml) Time after OVA challenge (min)		
		0	1	15
BALF				
Control		0.02+0.03	0.73+0.15	0.47+0.08
OKY-046	100 p.o.	0.15+0.02	0.24+0.02**	0.22+0.06*
	300 p.o.	0.11+0.01**	0.19+0.02**	0.09+0.01***
Indomethacin	2 i.v.	0.16+0.03	0.12+0.02***	0.13+0.02***
Plasma				
Control		0.35+0.1	5.20+1.39	1.37+0.22
OKY-046	100 p.o.	0.40+0.13	1.88+0.39*	0.50+0.13**
	300 p.o.	0.35+0.17	0.93+0.22**	0.19+0.03***
Indomethacin	2 i.v.	0.12+0.02	0.18+0.03**	0.16+0.04***

*: $P<0.05$, **: $P<0.01$, ***: $P<0.001$.

1078(an antagonist of LTs) inhibited both the initial and late phases of bronchoconstriction. Antigen-challenge significantly increased TXB_2 but had no effect on 6-keto-$PGF_1\alpha$ in both BALF and plasma. OKY-046 (100 and 300 mg/kg, p.o.) and indomethacin (2 mg/kg, i.v.) inhibited significantly the increases of TXB_2 after antigen challenge in both BALF and plasma(Table 1). OKY-046 inhibited both the bronchoconstriction and the hypertension induced by PAF and LTs. OKY-046 did not inhibit bronchoconstrictions induced by His, ACh, 5-HT, PGD_2 and STA_2 (Table 2).

Table 2. Effect of OKY-046 on spasmogens-induced bronchoconstriction in guinea pigs in vivo

Spasmogen	Dose (μg/kg i.v.)	OKY-046 Dose (mg/kg)	Route	Effect
PAF	0.3	3 - 10	i.v.	+
		30 - 300	p.o.	+
LTC_4	2	0.1 - 1.0	i.v.	+
		3 - 30	p.o.	+
LTD_4	2	0.1 - 1.0	i.v.	+
LTE_4	5	0.3 - 1.0	i.v.	+
STA_2	3	30	i.v.	−
PGD_2	100	30	i.v.	−
His	10	30	i.v.	−
ACh	30	30	i.v.	−
5-HT	10	30	i.v.	−

These results suggested that PAF and LTs may be involved in TXA_2 release from lung parenchyma in antigen-induced bronchoconstriction and that OKY-046 suppressed this response through the inhibition of TXA_2 generation.

REFERENCES

1. Hiraku S, Taniguchi K, Wakitani K, et al. Japan J Pharmacol 1986;41:393.

2. Obata T, Katsube N, Miyamoto T, et al. Adv Prostaglandin Thromboxane Leukotriene Res 1985;15:229.

Advances in Prostaglandin, Thromboxane, and
Leukotriene Research, Vol. 19, edited by
B. Samuelsson, P. Y.-K. Wong, and F. F. Sun,
Raven Press, Ltd., New York ©1989.

DETERMINATION OF THE EFFECTS OF INHIBITION OF PULMONARY
THROMBOXANE A_2 SYNTHASE ACTIVITY, IN VIVO AND IN VITRO

D.B. McNamara, M.D. Kerstein, J.K Harrington, J.A. Bellan, G.B.
Graybar, A.L. Hyman, and P.J. Kadowitz

Department of Pharmacology, Surgery and Anesthesiology, Tulane
University School of Medicine, New Orleans, Louisiana 70112 USA

INTRODUCTION

The enzymatic conversion of arachidonic acid (AA) to
biologically active metabolites, prostaglandins (PG) and
thromboxanes (TX), is thought to mediate airway and vascular
responses in the lung (1,2). PGI_2 has bronchodilator and
vasodilator actions, whereas TXA_2, $PGF_{2\alpha}$, and PGD_2, produce
bronchoconstriction and vasoconstriction (1,3,4). The present
study was undertaken to investigate the effects of CGS 13080, a
TXA_2 synthase inhibitor, on airway responses to AA. The effects
of CGS 13080 on pulmonary PGI_2 and TXA_2 synthase activities were
also determined.

METHODS

Thirty mongrel cats unselected as to sex (mean weight 2.1 kg)
were sedated with ketamine hydrochloride (15 mg/kg i.m.) and
were anesthetized with pentobarbital sodium (15 mg/kg i.p.). the
animals were catheterized for recording pressure in the aorta
(P_{Ao}), and for i.v. administration of drugs. The cats were
mechanically ventilated with room air. Transpulmonary pressure
(P_{TP}) and tidal airflow ($\dot{V}_T$) were measured. Tidal volume (V_T),
lung resistance (R_L), and dynamic compliance (C_{DYN}) were
calculated on a breath-to-breath basis from P_{TP} and $\dot{V}_T$
signals by a Hewlettt-Packard model 8816A respiratory analyzer.
R_L was computed at early (passive) expiration by dividing
calculated instantaneous resistant pressure by instantaneous
airflow. C_{DYN} was computed at points of zero flow by dividing
V_T by the change in P_{TP}. All procedures were as previously
published (1,4). In all experiments, control responses to AA
and U 46619 were obtained prior to injection of CGS 13080 (10
mg/kg i.v.), which was administered over a period of 1 to 2 min.

The test agents were again administered 10-20 min after injection of CGS 13080. After responses were obtained, sodium meclofenamate (2.5 mg/kg i.v.) was administered and responses to U 46619 and AA were determined in order to assess the effects of cyclooxygenase blockade.

Microsomal fractions were isolated by differential centrifugation. The reaction mixture for AA metabolism contained 200 μg of microsomal protein in 100 μl of 0.1 M potassium phosphate buffer, pH 8, 5 mM tryptophan, and 20 μM (1-^{14}C) AA. The reaction mixture for PGH_2 metabolism contained 200 μg of microsomal protein in 100 μl of 0.1 M potassium phosphate buffer, pH 7.4, and 10 μM PGH_2. The reactions were initiated by the addition of the microsomal suspension to a cold (0° C) 1.5 ml Brinkman centrifuge tube containing either AA or PGH_2 (previously blown dry under a stream of nitrogen) and incubated at 37°C for 1 hr (AA metabolism) or 2 min (PGH_2 metabolism). Product formation was maximal after incubations with AA or PGH_2, for 1 hr and 2 min, respectively, and as such, represent the profile of products formed during end-point incubations. The reaction was stopped and the products extracted, separated, and quantified as previously described (2). PGI_2 and TXA_2 synthesis was determined by formation of the hydrolysis products 6 keto $PGF_{1\alpha}$ and TXB_2 respectively.

RESULTS AND DISCUSSION

CGS 13080 does not affect baseline bronchopulmonary parameters or aortic pressure at a dose of 10 mg/kg, i.v., which significantly affects responses to AA suggesting that neither is under the influence of tonic formation of TxA_2. CGS 13080 did not affect either bronchopulmonary parameters or aortic pressure responses to U 46619, an analog of PGH_2 and mimic of TXA_2, suggesting that it does not have receptor antagonist propertities. However, increases in P_{TP} and R_1 and decreases in C_{DYN} in response to AA are reduced by CGS 13080. These data support the hypothesis that bronchoconstrictor responses to AA are mediated in part by formation of TXA_2. Airway responses to AA were reduced to an even greater extent after meclofenamate (2.5 mg/kg, i.v.) than after CGS 13080 in the same animal indicating that the responses to AA are mediated by formation of other cyclooxygenase bronchoconstrictor products in addition to TXA_2. The preceeding data are not shown.

TABLE 1. Effect of In Vitro Administration of CGS 13080 On PGH_2 Metabolism by Cat Lung Micrsomes

Picomoles of Product Formed

CGS 13080	6-keto-$PGF_{1\alpha}$		TxB_2		PGE_2	
	−GSH	+2 mM GSH	−GSH	+2 mM GSH	−GSH	+2mM GSH
10^{-9}M	211+64	252+68	65+13	26+5	157+46	283+76
10^{-8}M	218+57	269+79	65+17	22+3	126+26	282+65
10^{-7}M	191+41	276+75	46+14	17+4	162+31	306+62
10^{-6}M	172+49	256+83	23+11*	12+5	172+33	305+70
10^{-6}M	213+70	250+83	11+4*	11+5	182+52	308+63

Data are expressed as mean + SEM of duplicate incubations. *Indicated value is significantly different from control (p < 0.05); n=4 animals

The data presented in Table 1 indicate that CGS 13080 inhibits TXA_2 synthase activity in the cat lung microsomal fractions but it did not significantly affect the formation of 6-keto-$PGF_{1\alpha}$, suggesting that inhibition of TXA_2 synthase activity did not produce a shunting of PGH_2 to PGI_2 formation and that CGS 13080 does not directly affect PGI_2 synthase activity. The total amount of cat lung cyclooxygenase product formation was not altered significantly, it therefore is unlikely that CGS 13080 inhibited cyclooxygenase activity (data not shown). Addition of GSH to the reaction mixture produced an increase in PGE_2 formation indicating the presence of an active GSH-dependent PGH_2 to PGE_2 isomerase in these fractions. The decrease in TXB_2 formation upon the addition of GSH most probably represents a shunting of available substrate to PGE_2 formation. GSH did not significantly alter 6-keto-$PGF_{1\alpha}$ formation. Addition of CGS 13080 did not alter GSH-dependent PGE_2 formation, indicating that this substance does not affect GSH-dependent PGE_2 isomerase activity.

TABLE 2: Effect of In Vivo Administration of CGS13080 on Cat Lung Microsomal AA and PGH_2 Metabolism

Picomoles of Product Formed

Substrate	6-keto-$PGF_{1\alpha}$		TXB_2		PGE_2	
	−GSH	+2 mM GSH	−GSH	+2 mM GSH	−GSH	+2 mM GSH
PGH_2	414+64	441+73	18+5	(4+1)	67+27	245+59

Data are expressed as mean + SEM of duplicate incubations; () indicates value is equal to or below the limits of detection; n=4 animals; meclotenamate was not administered to these animals.

Microsomal fractions isolated from lungs of animals which had received CGS 13080 (10 mg/kg i.v.) exhibited decreased TXB_2 and a two-fold increase in $6-keto-PGF_{1\alpha}$ formation (Table 2). Direct addition of CGS 13080 to the reaction mixture containing microsomes isolated from CGS 13080 naive animals did not augment $6-keto-PGF_{1\alpha}$ formation (Table 1). These data suggest that there may be differences in the effect of CGS 13080 on the formation of $6-keto-PGF_{1\alpha}$ based on route of administration; they further suggest that in vivo administration of CGS 13080 may have a stimulatory effect on PGI_2 synthase in addition to an inhibitory effect on TXA_2 synthase activity.

In conclusion, the present data indicate that CGS 13080 is a potent and selective inhibitor of TXA_2 synthase activity and suggest that it may be useful in defining the biologic role of TXA_2 in physiologic and pathophysiologic states in which TXA_2 formation is enhanced.

ACKNOWLEDGEMENTS

The authors wish to thank Ms. Laura P. Pope for her editorial assistance in preparing the manuscript. This work was supported by grants-in-aid from the National Heart, Lung and Blood Institute, HL18070, HL15580, HL29456, the American Heart Association-Louisiana Inc. and the American Heart Association.

REFERENCES

1. Spannhake EW, Colombo JL, Craigo PA, McNamara DB, Hyman AL, Kadowitz PJ. J Appl Physiol 1983;54:191-198.

2. She HS, McNamara DB, Spannhake EW, Hyman AL, Kadowitz PJ. Prostaglandins 1982;24:586-606.

3. Wasserman MA, DuCharme DW, Griffin RL, DeGraff GL, Robinson FG. Prostaglandins 1977;13:255-265.

4. Graybar GB, Harrington JK, Cowen KH, Spannhake EW, Hyman AL, and McNamara DB. Prostaglandins 1986; 31:167-177.

Advances in Prostaglandin, Thromboxane, and Leukotriene Research, Vol. 19, edited by B. Samuelsson, P. Y.-K. Wong, and F. F. Sun, Raven Press, Ltd., New York ©1989.

INHIBITION OF THROMBOXANE RESPONSES IN THE AIRWAY

OF THE CAT BY SQ29,548 AND OKY 1581

P.J. Kadowitz, D.B. McNamara, S.J. Tilden,
A.L. Hyman, and D.C. Underwood

Department of Pharmacology
Tulane University School of Medicine
New Orleans, Louisiana 70112

INTRODUCTION

Arachidonic acid (AA) is released from cell membranes by stimuli which activate phospholipase A_2 (1,2). After release, the AA is converted into PGH_2 by the membrane-bound cyclooxygenase (1,2). PGH_2 is then converted into classical PG's, TXA_2, or PGI_2 by terminal enzymes (1,2). $PGF_{2\alpha}$ and PGD_2 have bronchoconstrictor and pulmonary vasoconstrictor activity, whereas PGI_2 has bronchodilator and pulmonary vasodilator activity. The endoperoxide analog, U46619, has marked smooth muscle stimulating and platelet aggregating properties and has been reported to mimic the actions of TXA_2 on isolated smooth muscle (3). Although U46619 has marked bronchomotor and vasomotor activity in the lung, it is uncertain whether this chemically and biologically stable substance actually mimics the biologic properties of TXA_2 in the lung, since this substance has a short physiologic half-life of 32 sec at body temperature and pH (3,4). AA injections cause cyclooxygenase-dependent bronchoconstriction in the dog and cat (5-7). Although studies with thromboxane synthesis inhibitors suggest that a component of the bronchomotor response to AA is due to formation of TXA_2, the absolute contribution of TXA_2 cannot be ascertained by synthesis blockade, since more PGH_2 can be redirected into the other terminal enzyme pathways (5-7). The present study was undertaken to determine the selectivity and blocking effects of SQ29,548, a novel TXA_2 receptor blocking agent, in the airways of the cat and to determine the relative contribution of TXA_2 to the bronchoconstrictor response to exogenous AA (8).

535

RESULTS

Intravenous injections of AA, U46619, and $PGF_{2\alpha}$ elicited dose-related increases in P_{TP} and R_L and dose-dependent decreases in C_{dyn} in the cat. AA injections caused dose-dependent decreases in P_{Ao}, whereas iv injections of U46619 and $PGF_{2\alpha}$ caused only small inconsistent changes in aortic pressure. After administration of SQ29,548 (5 mg/kg iv), the increases in P_{TP} and R_L and the decreases in C_{dyn} in response to AA and U46619 were reduced significantly. The changes in lung mechanics elicited by AA were reduced 50-60% by treatment with SQ29,548, whereas responses to U46619 were almost completely abolished. In the same animals in which bronchomotor responses to AA and U46619 were decreased significantly by SQ29,548, airway responses to $PGF_{2\alpha}$ were not modified. SQ29,548 had little, if any, effect on baseline bronchopulmonary parameters.

Responses to AA were compared before and after treatment with SQ29,548 and again after cyclooxygenase blockade with sodium meclofenamate (2.5 mg/kg iv) in the cat. In these experiments SQ29,548 reduced airway responses to AA by 50-60%, whereas sodium meclofenamate almost abolished airway responses to the prostaglandin precursor. The decrease in aortic pressure in response to AA was blocked by meclofenamate.

The specificity of the blocking effects of SQ29,548 was further characterized in another group of cats. In these experiments, iv injections of PGD_2, serotonin (5-HT), and U46619 increased P_{TP} and R_L and decreased C_{dyn}. The increase in P_{TP} and R_L and decreases in C_{dyn} in response to PGD_2 and 5-HT were not altered by SQ29,548 (5 mg/kg iv). However, SQ29,548 reduced significantly bronchomotor responses to U46619 by approximately the same extent as observed in the previous set of experiments. In eight animals bronchomotor responses to midrange doses of methacholine and histamine were compared before and after administration of SQ29,548 (5 mg/kg iv). The TXA_2 receptor blocking agent did not alter significantly responses to these bronchoconstrictor agents.

Although interpretation of results of experiments with thromboxane synthesis inhibitors are theoretically more complicated than results with the TXA_2 receptor antagonist, the effect of OKY 1581 on airway responses to AA, the classical prostaglandins, and U46619 were investigated in the cat. The administration of OKY 1581 (5-10 mg/kg iv) had no significant effect on baseline bronchopulmonary parameters. However, the increases in P_{TP} and R_L and the decreases in C_{dyn} and C_{st} in response to AA were diminished significantly after treatment with OKY 1581. The decreases in P_{Ao} in response to AA were not changed significantly after administration of OKY 1581. Airway responses to PGD_2 and $PGF_{2\alpha}$ were not altered significantly by OKY 1581. The thromboxane synthesis inhibitor had no significant effect on the increases in P_{TP} and R_L and the decreases in C_{dyn} in response to U46619. There was a small reduction in the decrease in C_{st} in response to 0.1 μg dose of U46619. This effect was not seen with the other doses of U4b619. OKY 1581 produced no significant effect on changes in P_{TP}, R_L, or C_{dyn} in response to U46619.

Administration of sodium meclofenamate (2.5 mg/kg iv) to the same animals that had received OKY 1581 had no significant effect on baseline P_{TP}, R_L, C_{dyn}, C_{st}, or P_{Ao}. After administration of the cyclooxygenase inhibitor (meclofenamate), the increases in P_{TP} and R_L and decreases in C_{dyn} in response to AA were reduced significantly when compared with control values. For the highest dose of AA studied, changes in P_{TP}, R_L, C_{dyn}, and C_{st} were reduced significantly after administration of sodium meclofenamate when compared to responses obtained after administration of OKY 1581. The fall in P_{Ao} in response to the high dose of AA was reduced significantly after administration of sodium meclofenamate. Changes in P_{TP}, R_L, C_{dyn}, and C_{st} in response to PGD_2, $PGF_{2\alpha}$, and U46619 were not changed significantly by the administration of sodium meclofenamate. The inhibitory effects of OKY 1581 and of SQ29,548 on airway responses to AA suggest that bronchoconstrictor responses to the essential fatty acid precursor are mediated in part by the formation of TXA_2.

DISCUSSION

Results of the present investigation show that bronchoconstrictor responses to U46619 in the closed-chest cat are reduced by SQ29,548, a TXA_2 receptor blocking agent (8). The stable prostaglandin endoperoxide analog, U46619, has been shown to mimic the actions of TXA_2 and neither cyclooxygenase blockade nor thromboxane synthase inhibition affects the potent bronchoconstrictor activity in U46619 in the cat (3). The present results with SQ29,548 support the hypothesis that U46619 acts by directly stimulating TXA_2 receptors in the airways, since responses to U46619 are blocked by SQ29,548 (3). This interpretation is dependent on the specificity of the blocking effects of SQ29,548 in the cat. Since SQ29,548 reduced airway responses to U46619 but did not block bronchoconstrictor responses to $PGF_{2\alpha}$ and PGD_2, these data suggest that SQ29,548 in the dose studied does not block airway "prostaglandin receptors," and that PG receptors and the TXA_2 receptor are different in the feline airway in vivo, a finding that does not agree with studies in isolated airways (8). In the present study, bronchomotor responses to 5-HT, methacholine, and histamine were also shown to be unaffected by SQ29,548. These results, therefore, suggest that SQ 29,548, in a dose of 5 mg/kg iv can act as a highly selective TXA_2 receptor antagonist in the airways of the closed-chest cat.

In the present study, the duration of thromboxane receptor blockade by SQ29,548 (5 mg/kg iv) was approximately 1 to 2 hr, after which time airway responses to the 100-300 ng doses of U46619 returned toward control value. After TXA_2 receptor blockade with SQ29,548, large doses (1-3 μg) of U46619, which could not be administered in untreated animals, produced only small bronchoconstrictor responses in the blocked animals.

Thromboxane receptor blockade with SQ29,548 reduced AA-induced bronchoconstrictor responses approximately 50%, and this is in agreement with experiments employing thromboxane synthesis inhibitors. In the present as well as previous studies, cyclooxygenase inhibition with meclofenamate reduced significantly the remaining component of the airway response to AA after TXA$_2$ synthesis or receptor blockade (6,7). These data support the hypothesis that airway responses to AA are mediated by formation of cyclooxygenase products and, in large part, by the formation of TXA$_2$.

In conclusion, the results of the present studies suggest that the TXA$_2$ receptor antagonist, SQ29,548, may be useful as a pharmacological probe for studying the role of thromboxane in physiologic and pathophysiologic processes in the airways of the close-chest cat.

ACKNOWLEDGMENTS

The authors wish to thank Ms. Jan Ignarro for help in the preparation of the manuscript. This work was supported by NIH grants HL18070, HL15580, and HL11802.

REFERENCES

1. Spannhake EW, Hyman AL, Kadowitz PJ. Prostaglandins 1981;22: 1013-1026.
2. Hyman AL, Mathe AA, Lippton HL, Kadowitz PJ. Med Clinic N Am 1981;65:789-808.
3. Coleman RA, Humphrey PPA, Kennedy I, Levy GP, Lumley P. Br J Pharmacol 1981;73:773-778.
4. Hamberg M, Samuelsson B. Proc Natl Acad Sci USA 1973;70: 899-903.
5. Spannhake EW, Lemen RJ, Wegman MJ, Hyman AL, Kadowitz PJ. J Appl Physiol 1978;44:307-405.
6. Tilden SJ, Underwood DC, Cowen KH, Wegman MJ, Graybar GB, Hyman AL, McNamara DB, Kadowitz PJ. J Appl Physiol 1987;62: 2066-2074.
7. Underwood DC, Kriseman T, McNamara DB, Hyman AL, Kadowitz PJ. J Appl Physiol 1987;62:2193-2200.
8. Ogletree ML, Harris DH, Greenberg R, Haslanger MF, Nakane M. J Pharmacol Exp Ther 1985;234(2):435-441.

Advances in Prostaglandin, Thromboxane, and Leukotriene Research, Vol. 19, edited by B. Samuelsson, P. Y.-K. Wong, and F. F. Sun, Raven Press, Ltd., New York ©1989.

DUAL ACTION OF PROSTAGLANDIN E_2 IN ALLERGIC INFLAMMATION

Per Hedqvist, Johan Raud and Sven-Erik Dahlén

Department of Physiology, and Institute of Environmental Medicine, Karolinska Institutet, S-10401 Stockholm, Sweden.

The antiphlogistic effect of nonsteroidal anti-inflammatory drugs (NSAID:s) is well established and apparently correlates with inhibition of prostaglandin (PG) formation, in particular PGE_2 and PGI_2. In harmony with this view are observations that PGE_2 is released at sites of inflammation and that it potentiates the action of a number of inflammatory mediators in vivo. However, in vitro PGE_2 may inhibit the function of inflammatory cells, and there are instances when NSAID:s enhance inflammatory reactions in vivo.

We have recently explored these seemingly discordant findings by means of intravital microscopy of the terminal vascular bed of the hamster cheek pouch. Actively sensitized hamsters were used to characterize the influence by PGE_2 and the prototype of NSAID:s, indomethacin, on the sequence of microvascular reactions that ensue challenge with allergen. Our experiments indicate that PGE_2 may be both anti- and pro-inflammatory in one and the same tissue, with local factors determining the balance between the two actions.

SYNERGISM BETWEEN PGE_2 AND INFLAMMATORY MEDIATORS

The hamster cheek pouch has been extensively used to characterize microvascular reactions evoked by inflammatory mediators, such as histamine and leukotrienes (1,2). The microvascular responses to these substances, plasma leakage from postcapillary venules by histamine and leukotriene C_4, and accumulation and diapedesis of leukocytes plus secondary plasma leakage by leukotriene B_4, are all substantially enhanced by topical application of PGE_2 in low concentration (3). It should be pointed out, however, that PGE_2 per se produced no increase of microvascular permeability or leukocyte accumulation. Thus, the potentiation is rather a consequence of PGE_2 causing increased local blood flow. In that sense PGE_2 may be considered proinflammatory.

INHIBITION OF MAST CELL-DEPENDENT ALLERGIC INFLAMMATION BY PGE2

The hamster cheek pouch is known to have a rich supply of perivascular mast cells. Recently we have documented that hamsters can be immunized so as to give rise to functional expression of mast cell-fixed antibodies, probably of the IgE type, in the cheek pouch (3,4). The sequence of microvascular reactions induced by topical antigen challenge was shown to involve transient vasoconstriction followed by dilation, extravasation of plasma, and accumulation of leukocytes.

Pretreatment with indomethacin, in order to block prostaglandin biosynthesis, markedly increased and prolonged leakage of plasma induced by antigen challenge (Fig. 1). Accumulation of leukocytes was enhanced even more. In fact, the number of emigrated cells increased by approximately 1500 %. By itself indomethacin had virtually no effect on measured parameters.

Prostaglandin E2, which per se caused marked vasodilation, completely reversed indomethacin-induced potentiation of plasma extravasation (Fig. 1) as well as the enhanced number of endothelial and emigrated leukocytes. Furthermore, PGE2 markedly inhibited plasma leakage also in the absence of indomethacin treatment. In contrast, a nonprostaglandin vasodilator, nitroprusside, caused but enhancement of this reaction.

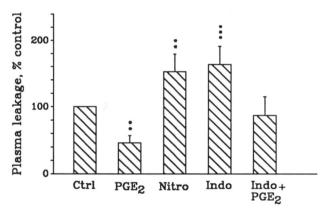

FIG. 1. Plasma extravasation in vivo in cheek pouches of actively immunized hamsters. Leakage induced by topical challenge with antigen alone (Ctrl) and in the presence of prostaglandin E2 (PGE2 30 nM topically), nitroprusside (Nitro 300 nM topically), indomethacin (Indo 5 mg/kg i.v. and 6 μM topically), or Indo + PGE2. Note inhibition by PGE2 but enhancement by Nitro (which caused vasodilation equal to PGE2), and reversal of potentiating effect of Indo by PGE2. Mean values ± SD, n=5-10, ** and *** indicate difference from control at 1.0 and 0.1 percent level (Mann-Whitney).

It thus seemed clear that the inhibitory effect of PGE$_2$ on antigen-induced reactions was not a consequence of vasodilation or influence on the target action of mediators. Rather, the results provided indirect evidence for PGE$_2$ interacting at the level of mediator release. Moreover, using the same protocol as above, and measuring in vivo release of histamine which is responsible for a major part of plasma leakage after antigen challenge, we obtained substantial support for this interpretation. Thus, PGE$_2$ inhibited antigen-evoked release of histamine by almost 60 %. Furthermore, indomethacin pretreatment markedly enhanced the release of histamine. Finally, PGE$_2$ effectively suppressed this potentiation. It is reasonable to suggest that PGE$_2$ inhibits also the release of mast cell-derived chemotactic mediator(s).

MAST CELL DISTRIBUTION

In the course of our investigation of mast cell-dependent allergic inflammation in the hamster cheek pouch, it was noted that mast cells, while generally having a perivascular location, were preferentially found along arterioles. Analysis of this observation (5) revealed a relative mast cell distribution of approximately 5:1 between arterioles and venules (Fig. 2). Moreover, after challenge with antigen, or the mast cell secretagogue compound 48/80, diapedesis and further migration of leukocytes from the venules consistently occurred with strong preference

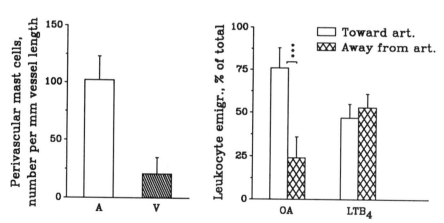

FIG. 2. **Left panel:** Distribution of perivascular mast cells between arterioles (A) and venules (V) in hamster cheek pouch. Mean values ± SD based on cell counting within 40 μm of 8-15 vascular segments in each of 4 pouches.
Right panel: Diapedesis and migration of leukocytes in hamster cheek pouch occur with strong preference towards arterioles after antigen challenge (OA 10 μg/ml topically) but is undirected after challenge with leukotriene B$_4$ (LTB$_4$ 20 nM topically). Mean values ± SD from 11 expts. ***= p < 0.001.

towards arterioles. In contrast, leukocyte diapedesis and subsequent tissue migration showed no preferential orientation when induced by the chemoattractant leukotriene B_4 (Fig. 2). Since diapedesis of leukocytes occurs exclusively from venules, it is concluded that release of leukotactic agents from periarteriolar mast cells may create a chemical gradient that optimizes leukocyte migration in the tissue.

SUMMARY

The findings reported here demonstrate that PGE_2 can exert both anti- and pro-inflammatory activities in one and the same tissue, as exemplified by inhibition of mediator release and enhancement of mediator action. Furthermore, the complete reversal of indomethacin potentiation of allergic inflammation by addition of PGE_2 in low concentration advocates a regulatory function of the endogenous and locally formed PGE_2. In the present in vivo model for mast cell-dependent inflammation the influence of PGE_2 was mainly on the release of mediators. However, factors such as the degree of local blood flow, or the state of the tissue and the site of prostaglandin production, may in other instances shift the Yin-Yang balance in favour of PGE_2 action at the target level for released mediators. Finally, it was noted that the cheek pouch mast cells, in addition to their pivotal role in the initiation of inflammatory reactions, have a predominant periarteriolar distribution that promotes oriented and, in terms of covered area, efficient migration of recruited leukocytes. Whether this previously unrecognized organization is specific for the hamster cheek pouch or exemplifies a more general phenomenon is presently not known.

ACKNOWLEDGEMENTS

Supported by grants from the Swedish Medical Research Council (project 14X-4342), National Institute of Environmental Medicine, National Environment Protection Board (5324067-7), Swedish Society for Medical Research, and Karolinska Institutet.

REFERENCES

1. Persson CGA, Svensjö E. In: Bonta IL, Bray MA, Parnham MJ, eds. Handbook of inflammation, vol 5.   Elsevier, 1985;61-82.

2. Dahlén SE, Björk J, Hedqvist P, et al. Proc Natl Acad Sci USA 1981;78:3887-3891.

3. Raud J, Dahlén SE, Sydbom A, Lindbom L, Hedqvist P. Proc Natl Acad Sci USA 1988;85:2315-2319.

4. Raud J, Dahlén SE, Smedegård G, Hedqvist P. Acta Physiol Scand (in press).

5. Raud J, Lindbom L, Dahlén SE, Hedqvist P. (submitted).

Advances in Prostaglandin, Thromboxane, and Leukotriene Research, Vol. 19, edited by B. Samuelsson, P. Y.-K. Wong, and F. F. Sun, Raven Press, Ltd., New York ©1989.

ON THE MECHANISM OF ASPIRIN ASTHMA

T. Viganò, M.T. Crivellari, A. Sala, C. Ortolani*, G. Galli and G.C. Folco**

Inst. of Pharmacological Sciences, School of Pharmacy, Univ. of Milan, 20133 Milan, *Pad. Bizzozzero, Ospedale Maggiore di Niguarda, 20162 Milan, **Inst. of Pharmacology and Pharmacognosy, Univ. of Parma, 43100 Parma, Italy.

Aspirin (ASA) is a widely used drug with well recognized gastrointestinal side-effects; adverse aspirin reactions such as urticaria, angioedema and shock have also been reported.

An altered respiratory tract reactivity following non-steroidal antiinflammatory drugs has prompted several investigators to propose the so called "prostaglandins synthetase inhibition hypothesis" which postulates a shunt of arachidonic acid (AA) from the cyclooxygenase (CO) to the 5-lipoxygenase pathway (5-LO). This diversion would be expected to augment the synthesis of leukotrienes (LTs) and thereby increase the amplitude of their component of bronchospasm (1,2).

In this report we provide evidence that in anti-IgE challenged human airways, cyclo-oxygenase blockade is not accompanied by a similar redistribution of AA metabolism towards any lipoxygenase.

Moreover nasal provocation (NP) with a lysine acetyl-salicylate solution in ASA-intolerant patients causes a release profile of immunoreactive LTC_4 that is not consistent with a primary triggering role of LTs in inducing the symptoms that characterize ASA intolerance.

METHODS

Macroscopically normal human lung parenchyma was challenged with anti-human IgE antibody as described (3). Aliquots of the incubating media were collected and analyzed for LTs, hydroxyacids and PGD_2 as reported (4).

Seven aspirin-intolerant subjects were selected for the study and 0.2 ml of a 10 mg/ml solution of lysine acetylsalycilate were sprayed into each nostril following the procedure reported by Naclerio et al. (5). Nasal lavages were then performed at different time intervals and mediator content assayed as described (6).

RESULTS AND DISCUSSION

Eicosanoids from CO as well as from different LO are released from immunologically challenged human lung; PGD_2 is by far the most abundant metabolite and, among sulfidopeptide LTs, LTE_4 is the one present in larger amount. 5-, 12-and 15-HETE are also detected in the incubation media. (Tab. 1)

Indomethacin (1.5×10^{-5} M) inhibits PGD_2 formation by appr. 90% without a redistribution of precursor metabolism among LTs. An increase in 5- and 12-HETE takes place without reaching statistical significance (N=6). Similar results were also found using a lower indomethacin concentration (3 μM).

In these experiments it was of interest to note that the bioassay of SRS-A activity, which was carried out on longitudinal strips of guinea-pig ileum at the end of the 15' incubation with the anti-IgE, almost invariably indicated presence of larger amounts of SRS-A like activity in the indomethacin treated samples compared to controls.

These results do not support the commonly accepted thesis on arachidonate diversion to LTs as a direct consequence of CO blockade in human airways. Other findings in agreement with our results have also been published (7). However recent findings by Undem et al. (8) have shown increased release of LTs, following antigen challenge, in indomethacin treated bronchial tissue but not in parenchymal specimen. These data suggest a difference in

TABLE 1. EFFECT OF INDOMETHACIN ON THE IMMUNOLOGICAL RELEASE OF SULFIDOPEPTIDE LEUKOTRIENES, 5-, 12-, 15-HETE AND PGD_2 FROM HUMAN LUNG.

	LTC_4	LTD_4	LTE_4	LTB_4	5-HETE	12-HETE	15-HETE	PGD_2
ANTI IgE N= 6	0.04 ± 0.02	0.43 ± 0.10	0.72 ± 0.27	0.14 ± 0.05	0.05 ± 0.02	0.08 ± 0.02	0.12 ± 0.04	1.56 ± 0.49
ANTI IgE +INDOMETHACIN 1.5×10^{-5}M N= 6	0.02 ± 0.02	0.48 ± 0.10	0.90 ± 0.12	0.19 ± 0.04	0.12 ± 0.02	0.19 ± 0.06	0.12 ± 0.02	0.13 *± 0.05

THE VALUES (X ± S.E.) ARE EXPRESSED IN NMOLES/G FRESH TISSUE.   *$P < 0.05$

bronchial and parenchymal mast cells with respect to CO blockade.

This available evidence, however, comes from studies performed in tissue from normal patients treated with aspirin or indomethacin.

It is plausible however that these patients possess a metabolic profile of arachidonates that is unique as indicated by the findings of Edenius et al. (9). We have therefore decided to investigate the release of LTs in nasal wash fluids of ASA-intolerant patients after provocation with a lysine acetylsalicilate solution. This approach has been developed recently as a new method of assessing release of inflammatory mediators in allergic reactions.

The results of the nasal provocations show that a significant increase of $i-LTC_4$ in relation to control values, takes place 60' only after aspirin exposure in the ASA-intolerant subjects. This increase was also different in relation to the levels of $i-LTC_4$ detected at 60' in nasal lavages from ASA-tolerant subjects and did not correlate with the onset of symptoms as well as with their type (LTs should cause primarily nasal obstruction).

The profile of assayable SRS-A activity parallelled that of $i-LTC_4$ as only the ASA-intolerant subjects presented a delayed increase of this activity, while in the controls no change was observed. In six ASA-intolerant subjects and in four controls PGD_2 levels in nasal washes after ASA nasal provocation were evaluated and no significant change in both groups observed.

As far as ASA intolerance is concerned, the experimental model utilized is not strictly adherent to the clinical reality since the provocation test was performed through the nasal route while normally ASA is taken orally. More work is therefore in progress in order to elucidate the mediators' release profile from nasal mucosa after oral ingestion of ASA.

Another consideration to be taken into account is the fact that release of mast cell mediators does not seem to constitute the fundamental mechanism of ASA intolerance. Only in a few ASA intolerant patients did Histamine increase in the nasal lavages without a clear relationship with the appearance of nasal symptoms. ASA could act on intolerant subjects triggering a release of mediators different from Histamine, LTs or PGD_2 which would successively imply a mast cell reaction; such a cellular activation could constitute a secondary amplification factor of an early unknown reaction.

The clinical data as well as the in vitro experiments using

human lung parenchyma do not confirm the importance of cyclo-oxygenase block in the induced reactions to ASA intolerance. Intrinsic errors in assaying LTs by guinea-pig ileum, the existence of different phospholipid pools of AA as precursor of CO- and LO- products, the abolition of negative feed-back mechanisms on mediator release following CO inhibition, are some of the proposed hypothesis to explain aspirin asthma and ASA idiosyncratic reactions in general (10). It is our opinion that only studies carried out using cells or tissue fragments from ASA intolerant subjects will help to solve this problem.

REFERENCES

1. Weissman G,

   N Engl J Med 1983;308:454-455.

2. Editorial Article. Arachidonic Acid, Analgesics and Asthma,

   The Lancet. 1981;1266-1267.

3. Viganò T, Sautebin L, Magni F, et al.

   Prostag Leukotr Med 1986;23:109-115.

4. Sautebin L, Viganò T, Grassi E, et al.

   J Pharmacol Exp Therap 1985;234:217-221.

5. Naclerio RB, Meier HL, Kagey-Sobotka A, et al.

   Am Rev Resp Dis 1983;128:597-603.

6. Miadonna A, Tedeschi A, Leggieri E, et al.

   Am Rev Resp Dis 1987;136:357-362.

7. Salari H, Borgeat P, Fournier M, et al.

   J Exp Med 1985;162:1904-1915.

8. Undem BJ, Pickett WC, Lichtenstein LM and Kenneth Adams III G

   Am Rev Resp Dis 1987;136:1183-1187.

9. Edenius C, Dahlen B, Zetterstrom O, et al. VI Intern Conf on Prostaglandins, Florence, June 1986;Abstract Book:195.

10. Humes JL, Sadowski S, Galavage M, et al. J Biol Chem 1982;257:1591–1594.

Advances in Prostaglandin, Thromboxane, and Leukotriene Research, Vol. 19, edited by B. Samuelsson, P. Y.-K. Wong, and F. F. Sun, Raven Press, Ltd., New York ©1989.

ENHANCED PRODUCTION OF LTC_4 IN LEUKOCYTES FROM ALLERGIC

ASTHMATIC SUBJECTS

Soo Ray Wang, Lilly Liang, Sharon SM Wang, Chia Li Yu, Benjamin N Chiang, Shou Hwa Han.

Section of Allergy, Immunology & Rheumatology, Department of Medicne, Veterans General Hospital; and Institute of Microbiology & Immunology, Yang-Ming Medical College, Taipei, Taiwan, ROC.

INTRODUCTION

Slow-reaction substance (SRS) is a major mediator in causing bronchospasm(1-3). We have previously reported that the A23187-induced production of SRS was enhanced in leukocytes from patients with asthma (4). The degree of enhancement is related to the degree of atopy.

SRS is known to include leukotriene(LT) C_4, D_4, and E_4. Among them, LTD_4 and LTE_4 are degrading products of LTC_4(5). The A23187-induced LTC_4 production in peripheral leukocytes, neutrophils, and eosinophils was compared in the normal subjects and asthmatic patients with intrinsic, mixed, and extrinsic types.

MATERIALS AND METHODS

Blood donors were selected from patients with asthma by physicians in the allergy clinic. Donors consisted of normal subjects (NL), and asthmatic patients with intrinsic (INT), mixed (MIX), and extrinsic (EXT) types.

Leukocytes in heparinized blood were separated by dextran sedimentation (2%, MW 500,000). Metrizamide discontinuous gradient centrifugation(6) was used to separate neutrophils (at metrizamide 20-22%) from eosinophils (at metrizamide 23-25%). Cells were reacted with A23187 (4 µg/ml) at 37°C for 10 min. Both intracellular and extracellular LTC_4 were extracted with methanol, lyophilized, and analyzed by a C_{18}-reverse phase HPLC. The retention time was 4 min. This peak was collected for radioimmunoassay (LTC_4 kit from New England Nuclear Co).

The data were analyzed by Kruskal-Wallis Test of nonparametric analysis.

RESULTS

As shown in Fig. 1, the amounts of LTC_4 produced in 1×10^7 leukocytes were 71 ± 12 ng (mean $\pm$ S.E.) for NL (N=18), 73 ± 19 ng for INT (n=17), 84 ± 26 ng for MIX (n=8), and 108 ± 17 ng for EXT (n=13). The LTC_4 produced in total leukocytes seemed to increase with the degree of atopy.

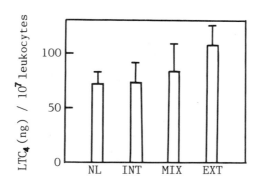

FIG. 1. LTC_4 production in leukocytes from normal subjects (NL), and asthmatic with intrinsic (INT), mixed (MIX), and extrinsic (EXT) types.

As shown in Fig 2, the amounts of LTC_4 produced in 1×10^7 neutrophils were 65 ± 12 ng (mean $\pm$ S.E.) for NL (N=18), 65 ± 15 ng for INT (n=17), 72 ± 26 ng for MIX (n=8), and 113 ± 20 ng for EXT (N=13). The LTC_4 prodcution was much increased in EXT.

As shown in Fig. 3, the amount of LTC_4 produced in 1×10^7 eosinophils were 127 ± 26 ng (mean $\pm$ S.E.) for NL (N=8), 175 ± 56 ng for INT (n=18), 91 ± 28 ng for MIX (n=8), and 194 ± 49 ng for EXT (n=12). LTC_4 produced in EXT is higher than the normal group, but is not impressively different from other asthmatic groups.

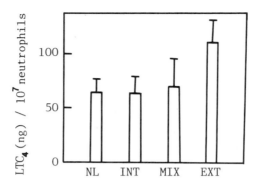

FIG. 2. LTC$_4$ production in neutrophils.

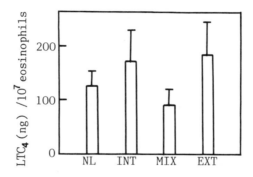

FIG. 3. LTC$_4$ production in eosinophils.

DISCUSSION

The A23187-induced biological activity of SRS measured by guinea pig ileum contraction, is higher in leukocytes from extrinsic asthma patients than those from the normal subjects (4). Probably the increased contractivity in extrinsic asthmatic cells is due to the total spasmotic leukotrienes produced. Present experiment was carefully performed. The cells separated by metrizamide discontinuous gradient (6) were rather clean with less than 10% contamination, in the average, for neutrophils, and less than 30% contamination for eosinophils. The contamination in the later was mainly neutrophils. The LTC$_4$ produced was separated and collected by C_{18}-reverse phase HPLC prior to radioimmunoassay. Thus the reproducibility of LTC_4 assay was excellent.

In this study, the individual variation of LTC_4 production is big. Although the LTC_4 production is constantly greater in cells from extrinsic asthmatics, the difference is not statistically significant ($p > 0.05$). These results are not compatible with the results of SRS study(4) in which SRS production was significantly enhanced in cells from extrinsic asthma patients. In that study, SRS activity was measured by guinea pig ileum contraction in the presence of atropine, propranolol, diphenhydramine and indomethacin. Probably, there are certain spasmotic substances still existing in the SRS preparation not suppressed by above inhibitors. These spasmotic substances, such as platelet activating factor, thromboxane, or other eicosanoid products, may represent part of spasmotic activity in the SRS preparation. This possibility deserves further study.

In conclusion, there was a trend to have a higher LTC_4 production in neutrophils and eosinophils from allergic asthmatics. These results imply the blood cells from these allergic subjects have a higher response to calcium ionophore stimulation which is certainly not an immune mechanism.

ACKNOWLEDGMENT

This work was partly supported by a grant NSC 76-0412-B010-40 from National Science Council of the republic of China, and partly supported by a grant from the Academia Sinica.

REFERENCES

1. Austen KF, Orange RP: Rev Respir Dis 1975;112:423.

2. Patterson R, Pruzansky JJ, Harris KE: J Allergy Clin Immunol 1981;67:444.

3. Wang SR, Yang CM, Wang SSM: Chinese J Microbiol Immunol 1984;17:48.

4. Wang SR, Yang CM, Wang SSM, Han SH, Chiang BN. J Allergy Clin Immunol 1986;77:465.

5. Hammarström S, Bernström K, Orning L, Dahlen SE, Hedqvist P. Biochem Biophysic Res Communic 1981;101:109.

6. Vadas MA, David JR, Butterworth A, Pisani NT, Siongok TA: J Immunology 1979;122:1228.

Advances in Prostaglandin, Thromboxane, and
Leukotriene Research, Vol. 19, edited by
B. Samuelsson, P. Y.-K. Wong, and F. F. Sun,
Raven Press, Ltd., New York ©1989.

ROLE OF CYSTEINYL LEUKOTRIENES

IN GASTRIC MUCOSAL DAMAGE IN RATS

B. M. Peskar

Department of Experimental Clinical Medicine
Ruhr-University of Bochum
D-4630 Bochum, FRG

INTRODUCTION

It has been demonstrated previously that in rats oral instillation of ethanol induces a dose-dependent increase in the ex vivo release of leukotriene (LT)C_4 from gastric mucosal fragments parallel to the production of gastric injury (1). LTC_4 is a potent constrictor of gastric submucosal vessels (2). Exogenous LTC_4 and LTD_4 have been shown to potentiate gastric mucosal lesions caused by a variety of noxious agents including ethanol (3,4). The lipoxygenase inhibitor nordihydroguaiaretic acid (NDGA) (1) and the dual lipoxygenase and cyclooxygenase inhibitor BW755C (5,6) inhibit rat gastric mucosal LTC_4 formation and simultaneously protect against gastric damage caused by ethanol. Both the sulfhydryl-containing agent cysteamine and the sulfhydryl-depleting compound diethylmaleate prevent the stimulatory action of ethanol on rat gastric mucosal LTC_4 formation parallel to their protective actions (7). Sodium salicylate is a non-steroidal anti-inflammatory drug (NSAID) which protects against the necrotizing effect of ethanol (8) and simultaneously inhibits the increase in LTC_4 release elicited by ethanol exposure (9). Finally, a number of chemically different LT receptor antagonists which preferentially bind to the LTD_4 receptor have been reported to protect against NSAID-induced gastric damage in mice (10) and ethanol-induced injury in rats (5,11). We have now further investigated the profile of cysteinyl-LT generated by the rat stomach and the interrelationship between inhibition of gastric LT synthesis and drug-induced gastroprotection.

METHODS

The stomach of anaesthetized male Wistar rats was perfused in situ under constant pressure with oxygenated Krebs-Henseleit buffer via the aorta and the perfusate was collected from the portal vein. Ionophore

A23187 (1µg/ml)-stimulated release of cysteinyl-LT into the perfusate was determined radioimmunologically and further characterized by reversed phase high pressure liquid chromatography (HPLC) as described (1). In 4 experiments each LTC4 and LTD4 (gift of Dr. A. Ford-Hutchinson, Merck-Frosst Laboratories, Pointe Claire/Dorval, Canada) were infused and the effects on gastric flow were determined. In further experiments groups of 6 rats were treated orally with graded doses of various sulfhydryl-containing or -blocking agents and metals. After 30 min the rats received 1.5 ml ethanol and were killed 5 min later. After evaluation of mucosal damage using a scoring system (1) fragments of gastric corpus mucosa were incubated in oxygenated Tyrode solution and release of LTC4 was determined radioimmunologically.

RESULTS AND DISCUSSION

In the isolated vascularly perfused rat stomach spontaneous release of cysteinyl-LT into the perfusate is close to or below the detection limit of the assay (5 ng/20 min). Ionophore A23187 (1µg/ml) increased release of cysteinyl-LT to 68 ± 16 ng/20 min, n=6. HPLC analysis revealed that the cysteinyl-LT found in the perfusate collected from the portal vein consisted of a mixture of LTC4, LTD4 and LTE4 (Fig. 1). Furthermore, exogenous LTC4 perfused through the gastric vascular bed was rapidly converted to LTD4 and LTE4. These findings are in contrast to results obtained with chopped rat gastric mucosa incubated in vitro which releases almost exclusively LTC4 (1). The discrepancy could possibly be due to different

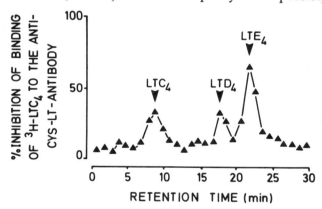

FIG. 1
Profile of cysteinyl-LT released from the isolated vascularly perfused rat stomach. Each point represents the inhibition of binding of 3H-LTC4 to an anti-plasma recognizing LTC4, LTD4 and LTE4 by 1 min HPLC eluate fractions of material extracted from gastric perfusates. Arrows indicate the retention times of standard cysteinyl-LT.

cellular sources of LT synthesis in both preparations. Alternatively, processing of LTC4 to LTD4 may be prevented in the chopped tissue by the high concentration of glutathione present in rat gastric mucosa (12) and probably released in large amounts during preparation of tissue fragments.

Infusion of exogenous LTC4 and LTD4 decreased vascular flow by 43±6% and 47±8%, respectively. Thus, in contrast to the lack of effect on the rat gastric submucosal microvasculature (2), LTD4 is as potent as LTC4 in reducing flow in the isolated perfused rat stomach. The potent vasoactive effects of LTD4 could explain that this LT potentiates gastric mucosal damage caused by noxious agents such as ethanol comparable to LTC4 (3,4). Whether the protection afforded by certain LT receptor antagonists (5,10,11) involves, indeed, blockade of LTD_4 effects or relies on other mechanisms remains to be elucidated.

Pretreatment of rats with thiols, sulfhydryl-blocking or -depleting agents and metals dose-dependently protected against gastric mucosal injury caused by ethanol confirming previous reports (13,14,15). All drugs studied simultaneously inhibited gastric mucosal LTC_4 formation. As shown in Table 1 the ID_{50} values for gastroprotection closely paralleled those for inhibition of LTC_4 release. These results together with the protective action of lipoxygenase inhibitors such as NDGA (1) and BW755C (5,6) have suggested that inhibition of gastric LT formation is an important mechanism of gastroprotection. However, it has recently been shown that in rats certain selective 5-lipoxygenase inhibitors which significantly reduced gastric mucosal LTC_4 formation did not prevent gastric damage caused by ethanol (5,16). Thus, although numerous examples demonstrate a close interrelationship between gastroprotection and inhibition of mucosal cysteinyl-LT formation, the lack of protective action of selective 5-lipoxygenase inhibitors indicates that this interrelationship is not absolute. This conclusion is further supported by the finding that ulcerogenic NSAID such as indomethacin or aspirin given orally inhibit the ex vivo release of LTC_4 from rat gastric mucosal fragments, although less potently than formation of cyclooxygenase-derived arachidonate metabolites (9).

TABLE 1.   Effect of sulfhydryl-modulating agents and metals on gastric lesion production and LTC_4 formation in ethanol-challenged rats.

Treatment		Protection ID_{50} (mg/kg)	LTC_4 formation ID_{50} (mg/kg)
Thiols	Cysteamine	20	26
	L-cysteine	180	130
	N-acetylcysteine	290	290
	Dimercaprol	15	5
Sulfhydryl blockers	Diethylmaleate	5	9
	N-ethylmaleimide	0.4	2
	Iodoacetamide	0.3	10
Metals	$CdSO_4$	8	25
	$ZnCl_2$	7	11
	LiCl	4	5
	$TeCl_4$	9	23

Rats were treated orally with graded doses of compounds 30 min prior to intragastric instillation of ethanol. Gastric mucosal damage and LTC_4 formation was determined as described in Methods.

Thus, in addition to cysteinyl-LT other mediators may play a role in ethanol-induced gastric damage and may be of particular importance when formation of cysteinyl-LT is suppressed. It remains to be investigated whether selective inhibition of the 5-lipoxygenase pathway of arachidonate metabolism increases formation of other lipoxygenase products which may contribute to mucosal damage. Formation of various hydroxy fatty acids has been demonstrated in human colonic mucosa (17). The 15S-

and 12S-hydroperoxides of arachidonic acid were found to be potent constrictors of cat coronary arteries (18). Furthermore, 15-hydroperoxy arachidonic acid and 13-hydroperoxy linoleic acid caused a marked enhancement of histamine and other anaphylactic mediators from guinea pig isolated perfused lungs (19). In view of these considerations it will be of interest to investigate the effect of combinations of inhibitors and/or antagonists of mediators in various types of gastric damage.

REFERENCES

1. Peskar BM, Lange K, Hoppe U, Peskar BA. Prostaglandins 1986;31:283-293.

2. Whittle BJR, Oren-Wolman N, Guth PH. Am J Physiol 1985;248:G580-G586.

3. Konturek SJ, Brzozowski T, Drozdowicz D, Becka G, Jendralla H. Gastroenterology 1987;92:1477.

4. Pihan G, Szabo S. Dig Dis Sci 1986;31:57S.

5. Wallace JL, Beck PL, Morris GP. Am J Physiol 1988;254:G117-G123.

6. Wallace JL, Whittle BJR. Eur J Pharmacol 1985;115:45-52.

7. Lange K, Peskar BA, Peskar BM. Adv Prostaglandin, Thromboxane, and Leukotriene Res 1987;17:299-302.

8. Robert A. Prostaglandins 1981;21,Suppl:139-146.

9. Peskar BM, Hoppe U, Lange K, Peskar BA. Br J Pharmacol 1988;93:937-943.

10. Rainsford KD. Agents Actions 1987;21:316-319.

11. Peskar BM. Gastroenterology 1988; Cysteinyl-leukotriene receptor antangonists protect against ethanol- and indomethacin-induced gastric mucosal damage in rats. (in press).

12. Boyd SC, Sasame HA, Boyd MR. Science 1979;205:1010-1012.

13. Dupuy D, Szabo S. Gastroenterology 1986;91:966-974.

14. Robert A, Eberle D, Kaplowitz N. Am J Physiol 1984;247:G296-304.

15. Szabo S, Trier JS, Frankel PW. Science 1981;214:200-202.

16. Boughton-Smith NK, Deakin MA, Whittle BJR. Proceedings of the Br. Pharmacological Society, January 1988, abstr. C146.

17. Boughton-Smith NK, Hawkey CJ, Whittle BJR. Gut 1983;24:1176-1182.

18. Trachte GJ, Lefer AM, Aharony D, Smith JB. Prostaglandins 1979;18:909-914.

19. Adcock JJ, Garland LG, Moncada S, Salmon JA. Prostaglandins 1978;16:163-177.

Advances in Prostaglandin, Thromboxane, and Leukotriene Research, Vol. 19, edited by B. Samuelsson, P. Y.-K. Wong, and F. F. Sun, Raven Press, Ltd., New York ©1989.

PROFILE AND SITES OF EICOSANOID RELEASE
IN EXPERIMENTAL NECROTIZING ENTEROCOLITIS

Mark J.S. Miller* and David A. Clark

Departments of Pharmacology and Pediatrics, New York Medical
College, Valhalla, N.Y.   10595 and *Research Department,
CIBA-GEIGY Corporation, 556 Morris Avenue, Summit, N.J.   07901

INTRODUCTION

Agents which attenuate eicosanoid formation alleviate the symptoms of inflammatory bowel disease and limit tissue injury (1). This suggests that eicosanoids play an important role in the underlying disease process. We have demonstrated that acute intestinal damage in a model of necrotizing enterocolitis (NEC) can be prevented by concomitant administration of superoxide dismutase (SOD, 2). The purpose of the present study was to determine if SOD therapy also attenuated eicosanoid releasing mechanisms in the gut. In addition, we developed an in vitro intestinal perfusion system to evaluate the vascular responsiveness of damaged versus salvaged intestine and the localization of eicosanoid release. In particular, it was hypothesized that eicosanoid relase would be contiguous with the intestinal vasculature and thereby, potentially influencing vascular tone and the activity of blood-borne elements.

MATERIAL AND METHODS

Induction of NEC in Rabbits

The model of NEC has been described previously(2). Briefly, weanling New Zealand white male rabbits were fasted for 8 hours prior to anesthesia induction with ketamine (50 mg/kg) and xylazine (10 mg/kg) I.M. After laparotomy, the intestine was ligated into a series of loops of approximately 10 cm in length, with care to preserve blood supply. Loops were then injected transmurally with saline (control) or a solution of bovine casein in saline (10 mg/ml) acidified with proprionic acid to pH 4.0 (treated). The peritoneum was closed and the animals sacrificed 3 hours later for ex vivo perfusion of the treated loop. A group of animals was sacrified 16 hours after NEC induction and eicosanoid release and intestinal motility determined in a superfusion bioassay cascade. In those animals treated with SOD (3 hr group only), an intravenous infusion (4mg/kg/hr) was commenced 15 min after NEC induction and continued until sacrifice. Prevention of intestinal damage by SOD treatment was confirmed by light microscopy.

Isolated Perfused Intestinal Loop

A branch of the mesenteric artery supplying the treated loop was cannulated and the loop flushed free of blood elements with Krebs-Henseleit solution. Collateral vessels were cut and tied to ensure adequate perfusion of the bowel. Silastic tubing was placed in both ends of the treated loop and intestinal contents displaced with Krebs-Henseleit solution. The loop was then transferred to a perfusion chamber and perfused through both arterial and intestinal cannulae at equal flow rates (10 ml/min). The venous and mucosal effluents were directed over separate but parallel banks of bioassay tissues for the detection of prostaglandins and leukotrienes. Effluents were also collected for radioimmunoassay of PGE_2, 6-keto $PGF_1\alpha$, TxB_2 and LTB_4.

Eicosanoid release was induced by intra-arterial injections of fMLP (100 ng) and PAF (100 ng, C18). Changes in perfusion pressure and bioassayable eicosanoid release were monitored continuously on a Soltec pen recorder. Indomethacin was infused into the arterial cannules at 1 µg/ml to determine the contribution of prostanoids to the vascular responses to fMLP and PAF challenges. Results in NEC and NEC + SOD were compared by a Students t-test for unpaired samples and by ANOVA. Significance was determined by a P value of less than 0.05.

RESULTS

Basal vascular resistance was significantly lower in NEC perfused loops ($p<0.02$). In addition, NEC loops displayed a dramatic shift in perfusate from the vascular to the mucosal side not evident in SOD-salvaged loops ($p<0.05$), suggesting enhanced vascular permeability in damaged loops. However, vascular responses to fMLP and PAF were comparable in the two groups. PAF administration caused a marked decrease in vascular resistance and fMLP produced an increase in vascular resistance. The vasoconstrictor response to fMLP was potentiated by indomethacin (Fig. 1), whereas PAF-induced vasodilation was still evident, although of shorter duration.

Both agents promoted the release of bioassayable and immunoreactive eicosanoids, primarily from the venous effluent. From the bioassay profile, fMLP released similar amounts of prostaglandins and peptido-leukotrienes (Fig. 1), whereas PAF greatly favored the release of prostaglandins. This was supported by radioimmunoassay, where PAF was a poor agonist for LTB_4 release.

Basal efflux of PGE_2, 6-keto $PGF_1\alpha$ and TxB_2 was significantly reduced in SOD-salvaged loops ($p<0.05$), although LTB_4 release was unaffected. Efflux of PGE_2, 6-keto $PGF_1\alpha$ and LTB_4 in response to fMLP was greatly reduced by SOD treatment. A notable exception

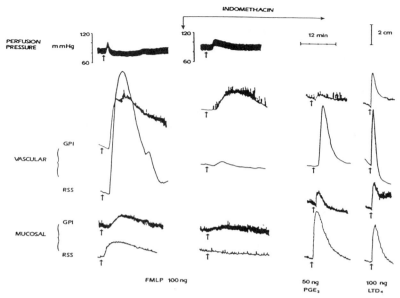

Fig. 1   Representative experiment of intestinal perfusion pressure and bioassay responses of an intestinal loop with NEC, following challenge with intra-arterial injection with fMLP (100 ng). Contractions of bioassay tissues perfused by vascular and mucosal effluents to PGE_2 and LTD_4 standards are depicted on the right. Indomethacin (1 μM) eliminated the contractile response on the rat stomach strip (RSS, PGE_2 bioassay) but guinea-pig ileum contractile substances (GPI, LTD_4 bioassay) were still evident. Note that in the presence of indomethacin, fMLP caused a prolonged vasoconstriction, as opposed to the biphasic response in the absence of indomethacin.

was TxB_2, with considerable release despite prevention of intestinal damage by SOD. Similarly with PAF administration, TxB_2 efflux was comparable in NEC and SOD-treated loops, whereas 6-keto $PGF_1\alpha$ efflux was dramatically attenuated. Release of PGE_2 was also reduced although this did not achieve significance. Furthermore, following SOD treatment, PAF failed to release LTB_4.

Loops removed from rabbits 10 hrs after NEC induction continued to display exaggerated fMLP-induced eicosanoid release (LTD_4 and PGE_2). Furthermore, treated loops failed to demonstrate contractile responses to a variety of agents (fMLP, acetylcholine, bradykinin) suggesting that intestinal motility was dramatically impaired in this region. Inter-loops, regions of normal tissue adjacent to the damaged treated loop elicited contractile responses to fMLP and acetylcholine. However, inter-loops released considerable quantities of LTD_4-like material and PGE_2, equivalent to the adjacent, damaged loops.

DISCUSSION

This model of NEC is based on the luminal contents of afflicted neonates; by mimicking these conditions in a rabbit intestinal loop preparation we can induce intestinal necrosis. The reduction in eicosanoid efflux with SOD treatment would suggest that arachidonic acid metabolism was enhanced by free radical-mediated cellular damage and that eicosanoids play a secondary role in the inflammatory process.

An important finding of this study was that PAF did not cause leukotriene-mediated vasoconstriction as has been reported in the rat intestine (3). The eicosanoid profile released by PAF from ex vivo perfused intestine greatly favored vasodilatory prostaglandins, with minimal release of thromboxane and leukotrienes. Further, PAF administration resulted in a profound vasodilatation which was partly attenuated by indomethacin administration whereas the vasconstrictor response to fMLP was potentiated. The vascular response to fMLP appears to reflect an interplay of vasoconstrictor leukotrienes and vasodilator prostaglandins. The finding that the release of peptido-leukotrienes was greatest at the border of normal and damaged tissue may suggest that leukotrienes contribute to the extension of tissue necrosis.

In summary, in this model of NEC, intestinal injury is initiated by free radical generation, and as a consequence, local release of PGE_2, 6-keto $PGF_1\alpha$ and LTB_4 is exaggerated. Eicosanoid release is contiguous with the vascular space and may contribute to the recruitment of inflammatory cells and the extension of tissue damage.

REFERENCES

(1) Zipser RD, Nast CC, Lee M, Kao HW and Duke R. Gastroenterology 1987;92:33-39.

(2) Clark DA, Fornabaio DM, McNeill H, Mullane KM, Caravella SS and Miller MJS. Amer. J. Pathol. 1988;130:537-542.

(3) Hseuh W, Gonzalez-Crussi F and Arroyave JL. Gastroenterology 1988;94:1412-1418.

Advances in Prostaglandin, Thromboxane, and
Leukotriene Research, Vol. 19, edited by
B. Samuelsson, P. Y.-K. Wong, and F. F. Sun,
Raven Press, Ltd., New York ©1989.

DEPLETION OF RESIDENT GLOMERULAR MACROPHAGES BY
ESSENTIAL FATTY ACID DEFICIENCY PROTECTS
AGAINST GLOMERULONEPHRITIS

J.B. Lefkowith[*o], B. Rovin[*], and G. F. Schreiner[*+]

Depts. of Medicine[*], Pharmacology[o], and Pathology[+], Washington
University School of Medicine, St. Louis, Mo. 63110 U.S.A.

Modulation of dietary fatty acids has been shown to prolong survival in
several animal models of the human disease systemic lupus erythematosus.
Hurd and colleagues demonstrated that essential fatty acid (EFA) deficiency
dramatically prolonged survival in NZB x NZW mice (1). Other investigators
have shown a similar strikingly beneficial effect for diets enriched for (n-3)
fatty acids in MRL lpr (2) and NZB x NZW mice (3) as well. Manipulation of
fatty acid intake appears to be especially effective in ameliorating the
glomerulonephritis associated with the development of autoimmunity in these
animals, reducing both the incidence of proteinuria and the severity of the
histologic changes that occur in the glomerulus (1-3). Because renal failure is
the predominant cause of death in murine lupus (4), the mechanism of the
beneficial effect of dietary fatty acid manipulation has been thought to be due
to its effects on the development of the glomerulonephritis. The mechanisms
by which modulation of fatty acid intake prevent the development of immune-
mediated glomerulonephritis, however, have hithertofore been ill-defined.

Suppression of autoimmunity has been proposed as a possible mechanism of
the protective effect (2). Available data, however, would seem to negate this
possibility. No unequivocal effect of EFA deficiency has been established
with respect to humoral or cellular immunity (5). Moreoever, dietary fatty
acid manipulation has been shown to exert a salutary effect despite the fact
that anti-dsDNA autoantibodies are not suppressed (2). Additionally,
institution of dietary fatty acid manipulation has been shown to be protective
even when started after the inception of renal disease (6).

Recent studies by our group suggest an entirely different possible
explanation for the protective effect of dietary fatty acid modification: that
modulation of the glomerular microenvironment, in terms of glomerular
resident macrophage number and eicosanoid production, may contribute to the
renal-sparing effects of dietary fatty acid restriction in lupus
glomerulonephritis (7). In a series of experiments we observed that EFA
deficiency led to a substantial reduction in the number of resident glomerular
macrophages (Fig. 1). This phenomenon was not strain-specific, was not due
to a decrease in circulating monocytes, was not a function of changes in cell
surface labeling characteristics, and was not restricted to a specific subset of
glomeruli.

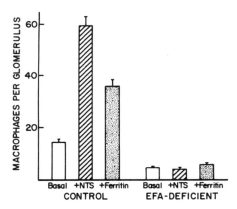

Fig. 1. Effects of EFA deficiency on glomerular macrophage number in basal (uninflamed) and inflamed glomeruli.   Nephrotoxic antiserum (NTS) and aggregated ferritin were used as inflammatory agents.   Macrophages were detected and enumerated using a double antibody fluorescence labeling technique (7).

   In conjunction with the decrease in glomerular macrophages seen with the deficiency state, a marked decrease in both basal and angiotensin II-stimulated glomerular prostaglandin E_2 and thromboxane B_2 production was noted (7).   These changes in glomerular eicosanoid production could not be attributed to changes in glomerular cyclooxygenase or reacylation capacity. Glomerular cyclooxygenase activity was actually enhanced several-fold by EFA deficiency.
   Interestingly, linoleic (18:2(n–6)) fatty acid supplementation, but not linolenic (18:3(n–3)) fatty acid supplementation, reversed both the decrease in glomerular macrophages and the diminished basal and agonist-stimulated eicosanoid metabolism seen with the deficiency state.   The fact that these changes are reversed concomitantly with (n–6) fatty acid supplementation suggests that these phenomena may be causally interrelated.   Available data would tend to support this conjecture.   Macrophages have been shown to enhance the arachidonate metabolism of a variety of mesenchymal cells (8), including mesangial cells (9).   This interaction occurs via the elaboration of soluble cytokines, most notably interleukin 1 (8).   The absence of macrophages from EFA-deficient glomeruli thus may explain the decrease in angiotensin II-stimulated eicosanoid production since mesangial cells are the only glomerular cell to express receptors for angiotensin II (10).   This hypothesis is further supported by experiments that demonstrate that leukocyte depletion prevents the influx of macrophages, as well as the enhanced agonist-stimulated eicosanoid production, seen in a model of experimental renal inflammation, hydonephrosis (11).
   In subsequent investigations, we have focused on the synthesis of leukotriene(LT)B_4 synthesis by glomeruli since this eicosanoid may play an important role in inflammatory phenomena, particularly as a chemotactic agent

(12). We found that glomeruli were able to synthesize LTB_4 when provided both with exogenous substrate and calcium ionophore A23187 (13). The identity of LTB_4 was confirmed in our studies by specific radioimmunoassay, high pressure liquid chromatography and gas chromatography/mass spectrometry. The synthesis of LTB_4 was also inhibited by BW755C (a dual lipoxygenase/cyclooxygenase inhibitor) but not indomethacin.

EFA deficiency was subsequently found to attenuate markedly the ability of glomeruli to synthesize LTB_4 from exogenous substrate (13). Because of our prior studies showing that EFA deficiency depletes glomeruli of their resident macrophages (7) and because macrophages are known to synthesize LTB_4 (14), we hypothesized that the lack of macrophages in EFA-deficient glomeruli acccounted for the diminished LTB_4 synthesis. To test this hypothesis, glomeruli were depleted of macrophages using x-irradiation. Glomeruli from irradiated animals also exhibited a marked decrease in LTB_4 synthesis thus corroborating our conjecture.

In recent studies we have been able to show that EFA deficiency prevents the influx of macrophages into the glomerulus that occurs during inflammation (15). Using either anti-glomerular basement membrane antiserum (i.e. nephrotoxic serum or NTS) or aggregated ferritin as an inflammatory stimulus we were able to elicit a 2- to 4-fold increase in glomerular macrophages (Fig. 1). EFA deficiency completely blocked the influx of macrophages into the glomerulus in response to both inflammatory stimuli (Fig. 1). The diminished influx of macrophages into the glomerulus with EFA deficiency did not appear to due to an impairment of chemotactic responsiveness (Table 1). EFA-deficient macrophages responded to chemotactic stimuli equivalently to control macrophages.

TABLE 1. CHEMOTAXIS OF EFA-DEFICIENT AND CONTROL MACROPHAGES [a]

	Chemotactic stimulus		
	ZAS (10%)	PAF (1 nM)	LTB_4 (10nM)
EFA-deficient macrophages	4014±93	418±85	590±89
Control macrophages	3758±116	633±140	518±114

[a]Chemotaxis was assessed using a microchemotaxis chamber method (16). Results are expressed as cells migrating per filter. Abbreviations: ZAS, zymosan-activated serum; PAF, platelet activating factor.

In sum, we have been able to establish that EFA deficiency depletes glomeruli of their resident macrophages. In concert with this depletion we have also observed a decrease in glomerular eicosanoid synthesis, particularly LTB_4. The available data would suggest that the depletion of glomerular macrophages may be the cause of the changes in eicosanoid synthesis. Additionally, we have shown that EFA deficiency impairs the elicitation of macrophages into the glomerulus in the context of inflammation, but does not impair the chemotactic responsiveness of these leukocytes. These observations may provide a basis for understanding how dietary polyunsaturated fatty acid manipulation exerts a beneficial effect in glomerulonephritis. Additionally, these studies may lead to the development of new strategies (both dietary and pharmacologic) to ameliorate immune-mediated glomerulonephritis in man.

ACKNOWLEDGEMENTS

This work was supported by National Institutes of Health grants HL-01313 and DK-37879 (Dr. Lefkowith), and AM-36277 and a Communities Foundation of Texas grant (Dr. Schreiner).

REFERENCES

1. Hurd ER, Johnston JM, Okita JR, MacDonald PC, Ziff M, and Gilliam JN. J. Clin. Invest. 1981;67:476-485.
2. Kelley VE, Ferretti A, Izui S, and Strom TB. J. Immunol. 1985;134:1914-1919.
3. Prickett JD, Robinson DR, and Steinberg AD. J. Clin. Invest. 1981;68:556-559.
4. Andrews BS, Eisenberg RA, Theofilopoulos AN, et. al. J Exp. Med. 1978;148:1198-1215.
5. Yamanaka WK, Clemans GW, and Hutchinson ML. Prog. Lipid Res. 1981;19:187-215.
6. Robinson DR, Prickett JD, Polisson R, Steinberg AD, and Levine L. Prostaglandins 1985;30:51-75.
7. Lefkowith JB and Schreiner G. J. Clin. Invest. 1987;80:947-956.
8. Albrightson CR, Baenziger NL, and Needleman P. J. Immunol. 1985;135:1872-1877.
9. Lovett DH, Resch K, and Gemsa D. Amer. J. Pathol. 1987;129:543-551.
10. Osborne MJ, Droz B, Meyer P, and Morel F. Kidney Int. 1975;8:245-254.
11. Lefkowith JB, Okegawa T, DeSchryever-Kecskemeti K, and Needleman P. Kidney Int. 1984;26:10-17.
12. Smith MJH, Ford-Hutchinson AW, and Bray MA. J. Pharm. Pharmacol. 1980;32:517-518.
13. Lefkowith JB, Morrison AR, and Schreiner GF. J. Clin. Invest. (in press).
14. Lefkowith JB, Jakschik BA, Stahl P, and Needleman P. J. Biol. Chem. 1987;262:6668-6675.
15. Lefkowith JB and Schreiner GF. Clin. Res. 1987;35:565A.
16. Falk W, Goodwin RH, and Leonard EJ. J. Immunol. Methods 1980;33:239-246.

Advances in Prostaglandin, Thromboxane, and Leukotriene Research, Vol. 19, edited by B. Samuelsson, P. Y.-K. Wong, and F. F. Sun, Raven Press, Ltd., New York ©1989.

ROLE OF GTP-BINDING PROTEINS IN PHOSPHOLIPASE C ACTIVATION IN HUMAN PLATELET MEMBRANES

Y. Nozawa, Y. Banno, Y. Yada, K. Yamada and K. Nagata

Department of Biochemistry, Gifu University School of Medicine, Tsukasamachi-40, Gifu 500, Japan

Receptor stimulation has been known to cause the hydrolysis of polyphosphoinositides by activation of phospholipase C (PLC) to produce two intracellular messengers, diacylglycerol and inositol trisphosphate (1,2). Substantial evidence has been accumulating that membrane-associated phospholipase C was activated via guanine nucleotide-binding protein (3-8). However, membrane-bound PLC coupled to receptor activation and its GTP-binding protein(s) have not yet been isolated.

In platelets, the majority of phospholipase C activity is documented to be present in the cytosol (9,10). We demonstrated the presence of phosphatidylinositol 4,5-bisphosphate (PIP_2)-hydrolyzing activity in human platelet membranes (11), suggesting possible involvement of GTP-binding protein(s) in the enzyme activation (12). To gain further evidence for implication of GTP-binding protein in PLC activation of human platelet membranes, we purified PLCs and GTP-binding proteins from human platelet membranes and examined the effects of GTP-binding proteins on the phospholipase C activity in the reconstitution system.

PURIFICATION AND CHARACTERIZATION OF PHOSPHOLIPASE C AND GTP-BINDING PROTEINS FROM HUMAN PLATELET MEMBRANES

About 20 % of the total PIP_2-hydrolyzing activity of the homogenate was found to be associated with the membrane fraction of human platelets (11). Effects of several different nucleotides on the PIP_2-hydrolyzing activity of isolated platelet membranes were examined. The nonhydrolyzable guanine nucleotides GTPγS and Gpp(NH)p were the most potent compound for activation of the enzyme activity. PIP_2-PLC activity in platelet membranes was stimulated by GTPγS in a dose-dependent manner, with a half-maximal stimulation at 6 uM. The stimulatory effects of GTPγS or Gpp(NH)p on the PIP$_2$-PLC activity were reduced in the presence of GDPβS. These results suggest that GTP-binding protein(s) may be involved in guanine nucleotide-induced activation of PIP$_2$-PLC in platelet membranes. In order to assess whether the GTP-induced stimulation of the PLC activity was mediated via GTP-binding protein, we have purified and characterized PLCs and GTP-binding proteins of human platelet membranes.

The membrane-bound PIP$_2$-PLC activity was extracted with 1 % sodium cholate from the residual pellet obtained after 2 M KCl extraction. The cholate extract was applied to a Fast Q-Sepharose column, yielding a single major peak of PIP$_2$-PLC activity eluted between 0.2 M and 0.3 M NaCl. The GTPγS binding activity was coeluted with the peak fraction of PLC activity. As shown in Fig. 1, the PLC activity was separated from the major GTPγS-binding activity peak upon heparin-Sepharose column chromatography. The GTPγS-binding activity went through the heparin-Sepharose column, while the PLC activity was bound to the column. Two activity peaks were obtained; a small broad peak (mPLC-I) eluted between 0.35 M and 0.45 M and a major peak (mPLC-II) between 0.5 M and 0.6 M NaCl. Although the activity to hydrolyze PIP of mPLC-II was no longer enhanced by added GTPγS, addition of the fraction with GTPγS-binding activity caused increase of the PLC activity.

The mPLC-II enzyme solution obtained from heparin-Sepharose column was further purified by succesive chromatographies on Ultrogel AcA-44 column, HPLC ion exchange column (Mono Q), Superose 6-12 combination column, and Superose 12 column. The final preparation of mPLC-II revealed one major protein band migrating at about 61 kDa on SDS-polyacrylamide gel (PAG). The

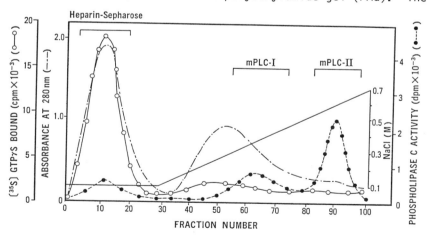

FIG. 1. Heparin-Sepharose column chromatography of mPLCs of human platelets.

procedure achieved 2,700–fold purification of mPLC–II in the particulate fraction of human platelets, with a specific activity of 6.3 umol of PIP$_2$ cleaved/min/mg protein (yield, 0.6 %). The molecular size of purified mPLC–II was estimated to be 63 and 61 kDa by gel filtration on TSK–3000 HPLC column chromatography and by SDS–PAGE, respectively. However, as shown in Fig. 2, the mPLC–II preparation obtained from heparin–Sepharose column chromatography was eluted at position of larger molecular weight (140 – 110 kDa) on the same column, suggesting alteration of the molecular weight during purification procedure. These results lead us to consider that the platelet mPLC–II may be present in an aggregated form of enzyme itself or in association with other component(s) in the crude preparation.

The maximum activity for PIP$_2$–hydrolysis of mPLC–II was obtained at pH 6.5 in the presence of 0.1 % deoxycholate. In the absence of the detergent, PLC activity of mPLC–II was affected by added various lipids. PE, DG and AA were stimulatory but eggPC and the platelet total membrane lipid were inhibitory. The PIP$_2$–hydrolyzing activity was Ca^{2+}– dependent, with a maximal activity at about 10 uM Ca^{2+}, while PI–hydrolysis required milli-molar concentration of Ca^{2+} to obtain a maximum activity. At a physiological concentration of Ca^{2+} (0.1 uM), mPLC–II was capable of hydrolyzing PIP$_2$ about 30–fold higher than PI. The mPLC–II exhibited higher Vmax for PIP than for PI under optimal conditions.

Two GTP–binding proteins serving as specific substrates of islet–activating protein (IAP), pertussis toxin, were purified from the unbound fraction of heparin–Sepharose column by Sephacryl S–300 HR, phenyl–Sepharose, DEAE–Toyopearl 650S, and HCA–100(S) column chromatographies. The major substrate (G–I) was purified to homogeneity as an αβγ–heterotrimeric structure. The molecular weight of the α –subunit was approximately 40 kDa on SDS–PAG. The immunological cross-reactivities of α–subunit between platelet G–I and

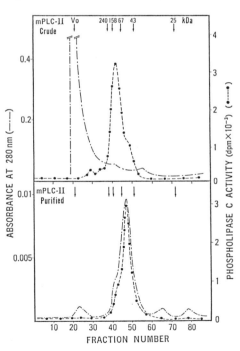

FIG. 2. TSK–3000 column chromatography of crude and purified mPLC–II of human platelets.

brain G-proteins (Gi-1 and Go) were not observed. The analysis of the partial amino acid sequences indicated that the G-I was identical with brain $\alpha40\beta\gamma$, which was recently identified as Gi-2. The minor substrate (G-II) had an α-subunit of 41 kDa on SDS-PAG which was cross-reacted with an antibody raised against rat brain αi.

EFFECTS OF NUCLEOTIDES AND GTP-BINDING PROTEINS ON THE mPLC-II ACTIVITY

As described above, PIP_2-hydrolyzing activity of the isolated platelet membrane was stimulated specifically by GTP or GTPγS. However, the purified mPLC-II enzyme free of GTP-binding protein did not show GTP-specific activation. Some nonspecific increases in PLC activity (10 - 20 % stimulation) were observed for all nucleotides tested. The loss by purification of the responsiveness toward guanine nucleotides suggests that GTP-binding protein is dissociated from PLC.

The PIP_2-hydrolyzing activity of the partially purified mPLC-II fraction from heparin-Sepharose column was enhanced equipotently by addition of rat brain Gi or Go, regardless of the presence or absence of GTPγS. But these GTP-binding proteins failed to induce any increase in PIP_2-hydrolyzing activity of the purified mPLC-II. This may indicate that certain unidentified membrane component(s) interacting with GTP-binding protein could be removed during purification steps or that the reconstitution system employed would not be adequate.

REFERENCES

1. Streb H, Irvine RF, Berridge MJ, et al. Nature 1984;306:67-69.
2. Nishizuka Y. Nature 1984;308:693-698.
3. Cockcroft S, Gomperts BD. Nature 1985;314:534-536.
4. Litosh I, Wallis C, Fain JN. J Biol Chem 1985;260:5464-5471.
5. Gonzales RA, Crews FT. Biochem J 1985;230:799-804.
6. Straub RE, Gershengorn MC. J Biol Chem 1986;261:2712-2717.
7. Ui M. In: Phosphoinositides and Receptor Mechanisms. Alan R. Liss, Inc, 1986;163-195.
8. Cockcroft S. Trends Biochem Sci 1987;12:75-78.
9. Rittenhouse-Simmons SE. J Clin Invest 1979;63:580-587.
10. Billah MM, Lapetina EG, Cuatrecasas P. J Biol Chem 1980;255:10227-10231.
11. Banno Y, Nozawa Y. Biochem J 1987;248:95-101.
12. Banno Y, Nagao S, Katada T, et al. Biochem Biophys Res Commun 1987;146:861-869.

*Advances in Prostaglandin, Thromboxane, and
Leukotriene Research*, Vol. 19, edited by
B. Samuelsson, P. Y.-K. Wong, and F. F. Sun,
Raven Press, Ltd., New York ©1989.

RELATIONSHIP OF INOSITOL PHOSPHOLIPID METABOLISM
TO PHOSPHOLIPASE A_2

Eduardo G. Lapetina and Michael F. Crouch

Molecular Biology Department
Burroughs Wellcome Co., Research Triangle Park, N.C.   27709

Arachidonic acid can be released from membrane
phospholipids of platelets in response to a number of
receptor-mediated signals. The enzyme most responsible for
this activation is phospholipase A_2 (1) and to a lesser
degree 1,2-diacylglycerol lipase (2). In this chapter, we
will describe some of the studies on phospholipase A_2
activation we have carried out and also some other published
work that has helped us understand some of the physiological
control mechanisms of this enzyme.

The importance of phospholipase A_2 in receptor-mediated
platelet activation varies with both the type and the
strength of agonist used. As examples, collagen and
epinephrine are absolutely dependent on the release of
arachidonic acid for stimulation of platelet secretion and
aggregation, whereas thrombin depends on arachidonic acid
release only when used at low concentration; at higher doses
the ability of thrombin to activate platelets is independent
of arachidonic acid metabolites. The most relevant
arachidonic acid metabolites for platelet stimulation are
endoperoxides and thromboxane A_2.

A. INOSITOL TRISPHOSPHATE

It is now thought that upon stimulation of platelets with
an agonist, the initial phospholipid response of the cell is
inositol phospholipid hydrolysis by a phospholipase C (1).
This is followed by the activation of phospholipase A_2 (1).
The sequential nature of these responses has often led to the
conclusion that some products of phosphoinositide hydrolysis
are responsible for phospholipase A_2 activation. (1).

The phosphodiesteratic cleavage of phosphatidylinositol-4,5-bisphosphate yields the two second messenger molecules, inositol trisphosphate (IP3) and 1,2-diacylglycerol (DAG) (3). IP3 has been shown in many cell types, including the platelet, to release intracellular Ca^{2+} stores (3,4). Since it has been clearly established that activation of platelets with the Ca^{2+} ionophore A23187 was able to raise the intracellular Ca^{2+} concentration and also activate phospholipase A_2, a possible link between the two receptor-activated enzymes was established: receptor activation of phospholipase C induced the formation of IP3, which then raised the intracellular Ca^{2+} concentration. This Ca^{2+} signal then directly induced phospholipase A_2 stimulation and release of arachidonic acid.

Support for this concept came from experiments which showed that IP3 would induce thromboxane A_2 formation, in permeabilized platelets and that platelet aggregation and secretion induced by IP3 were sensitive to inhibitors of arachidonic acid metabolism (5,6). Thus, these studies implied that the mobilization of Ca^{2+} by IP3 was sufficient to induce phospholipase A_2 activation.

Despite these results, there are indications that phospholipase A_2 is not primarily under the control of the prevailing Ca^{2+} level in the intact cell. Pollock et al (7) have shown that the activation of phospholipase A_2 by collagen could be accomplished at cytosolic Ca^{2+} levels of around 115 nM, whereas the Ca^{2+} ionophore ionomycin induced a significant release of arachidonic acid only when this compound had elevated the cytosolic Ca^{2+} level to about 1 μM. These results strongly suggested that collagen activated phospholipase A_2 independently of changes in the cellular Ca^{2+} concentration.

Work from our laboratory has also suggested that the same may be true for other agonists (8,9). Alpha-thrombin is a potent agonist for all platelet responses (10,11), including that of phospholipase A_2. Gamma-thrombin is produced by proteolysis of alpha-thrombin, and is a less potent agonist. We have compared the abilities of alpha- and gamma-thrombins, and platelet activating factor (PAF) to stimulate phospholipase A_2 and mobilized cellular Ca^{2+} stores (9). We found that alpha-thrombin elevated the cytosolic Ca^{2+} concentration to about 1 μM, and increased arachidonic acid release by 6-fold (9). Both gamma-thrombin and PAF induced the release of Ca^{2+} stores also, but only to maxima of 350 nM each (9). The peak responses to these two agonists were the same, although gamma-thrombin produced a more sustained response. In contrast, only gamma-thrombin could induce a detectable release of arachidonic acid in our system (9).

Thus, there appeared to be a dissociation of the ability of
an agonist to induce Ca^{2+} mobilization and the activation of
phospholipase A_2. In addition, epinephrine, which alone did
not activate phospholipase A_2, was able to potentiate the
alpha-thrombin-induced release of arachidonic acid (9).
However, we could not detect any potentiation of the peak
release of Ca^{2+} when these two agents were added together
(9).

The reasons for the disparity between the data using IP3
on permeabilized cells to activate phospholipase A_2 and that
of agonists on whole cells are not clear. However, it is
possible that the high concentrations of IP3 required to
activate phospholipase A_2 in permeabilized platelets may
represent non-physiological levels or that the permeabilized
cell is not a realistic model for studying phospholipase A_2
activation.

B. DIACYLGLYCEROL

The other immediate product of phospholipase C activation
is 1,2-diacylglycerol (1,3), which is a known activator of
protein kinase C (12). This enzyme, which can also be
activated by the tumor-promoting phorbol esters,
phosphorylates a major 40 kDa protein substrate in platelets
(1,2). A recent report by Touqui et al (13) implicated the
40 kDa protein in phospholipase A_2 activity. These proteins
are known collectively as 'lipocortins'. Touqui et al
suggested that the 40 kDa protein was a lipocortin, based on
the ability of a monoclonal antibody to inhibit its anti-
phospholipase A_2 activity against renocortin. This antibody
immunoprecipitated a 40 kDa protein phosphorylated in
platelets pretreated with thrombin or phorbol ester (13).
Based on this data, and a previous report that had shown
phorbol esters were able to elicit arachidonic acid release
in the presence of Ca^{2+} ionophores, they suggested that the
40 kDa protein was a lipocortin with intrinsic
antiphospholipase A_2 activity. When cells were stimulated,
protein kinase C phosphorylated this protein, thus reducing
its anti-phospholipase A_2 activity and allowing arachidonic
acid liberation.

We have challenged this proposal by comparing 40 kDa
protein phosphorylation in response to alpha-thrombin with
that of gamma-thrombin and examining the resulting
phospholipase A_2 activation. We found that gamma-thombin,
particularly in the presence of epinephrine, was capable of
stimulating 40 kDa protein phosphorylation to the same degree
as that of alpha-thrombin, but was 6-7 times less potent at
activating phospholipase A_2. That is, we could find no

correlation between 40 kDa protein phosphorylation and stimulation of phospholipase A_2. Pollock et al (7) have further presented evidence that phorbol esters are without effect on phospholipase A_2 in the presence of Ca^{2+} ionophore. Similarly, we could not detect any release of arachidonic acid in response to concentrations of phorbol ester that maximally phosphorylated the 40 kDa protein (unpublished).

C. GTP-BINDING PROTEINS

Thus far, we are left without any convincing evidence for a relationship between the receptor stimulation of phospholipase C and phospholiapse A_2. One may therefore postulate that the receptor may activate these two enzymes by mechanisms that diverge at the receptor level: there may be separate transducing elements from the receptor to each of these enzymes.

There has been a recent flurry of interest in the possibility that receptors control the activity of phospholipase C by first altering the state of a "GTP-binding protein". This class of proteins (or G proteins), first described for their involvement in the adenylate cyclase system, are heterotrimeric. They are composed of alpha, beta and gamma subunits. The beta and gamma subunits are highly homologous, whereas the alpha subunits show a great heterogeneity and appear to convey specificity. Receptors that stimulate cyclase are linked to Gs (the adenylate cyclase stimulatory G protein), whereas those that inhibit adenylate cyclase appear in general to be linked to Gi (inhibitory G protein). The alpha subunit is the GTP-binding component and is thought to be separated from the beta/gamma complex after receptor stimulation. When this occurs, the alpha subunit appears to activate certain processes, such as the stimulation of adenylate cyclase (alpha-s).

It has recently been shown that phospholipase A_2 of mast cells is sensitive to GTP analogs (14) and that inactivation of Gi with pertussis toxin inhibits phospholipase A_2 activation of thyroid cells. In addition, Jelsema and Axelrod (15) have shown that the beta/gamma dimer of G proteins is capable of activating phospholipase A_2 in retinal rod outer segments. In total, these results lend support to the proposal that there may be a direct link between the receptor and phospholipase A_2 via a GTP-binding protein in some cells.

Although the possible contribution for such a G protein involvement in the platelet has not been well examined, we have found evidence that does not support this view, at least for the inhibitory GTP-binding protein Gi. As mentioned above, pertussis toxin is able to inactivate Gi, and this occurs by the toxin-catalyzed ADP-ribosylation of the alpha subunit of Gi (1,10). This acts to inhibit the receptor -GTP-binding protein interaction. When the toxin is introduced to the cell in the presence of radioactively labelled NAD, one can label the ADP-ribosylated Gi, and so obtain a measure of the amount of undissociated Gi that is present in a cell (1,10). If one stimulates platelets with an agonist and dissociates the Gi, it is then no longer a substrate for pertussis toxin-induced ADP-ribosylation, and there is reduced labelling of Gi (10). By this method, one can ascertain if a receptor type is or is not coupled to Gi.

When we did this experiment with alpha-thrombin, we found a potent decrease in the ADP-ribosylation of Gi, indicating dissociation of most of the alpha subunits from the beta/gamma dimers of Gi (10). The same pattern was found for gamma-thrombin, with a decrease in labelling of Gi in the presence of pertussis toxin (10). However, gamma-thrombin is a very weak agonist for phospholipase A_2 (9). These experiments suggest, therefore, that the ability of an agonist to dissociate Gi does not convey an ability to activate phospholipase A_2.

Of course, we have only addressed the question of Gi and know nothing about what these agonists may do to other GTP-binding proteins of the platelet. However, we can conclude with some confidence that the beta/gamma subunits do not contribute significantly to the stimulation of phospholipase A_2 in the activated platelet, since dissociation of Gi would act to supply these within the plasma membrane.

D. SUMMARY

The mechanism by which agonists stimulate phospholipase A_2 of platelets is still much of a mystery. We have presented a discussion that suggests that neither Ca^{2+}, protein kinase C or dissociation of the inhibitory GTP-binding protein Gi is solely responsible for activating this enzyme. We cannot exclude the possibility that there may be some contribution of each pathway for some agonists, and that the contribution may change with agonist concentration or potency. These possibilities await further clarification.

REFERENCES

1. Lapetina EG. J. Putney, Ed. In: Phosphoinositides and Receptor Mechanisms. New York: Alan R. Liss, 1986;271-286.

2. Mahadevappa VG, Holub BJ. Biochem Biophys Res Commun. 1986;134:1327-1333.

3. Berridge MJ, Irvine RF. Nature. 1984;312:315-321.

4. O'Rourke FA, Halenda SP, Zavoico GB, Feinstein MB. J Biol Chem. 1985;260:956-962.

5. Watson SP, Ruggiero M, Abrahams SL, Lapetina EG. J Biol Chem. 1986;261:5368-5372.

6. Authi KS, Evenden BJ, Crawford N. Biochem J. 1986;233:707-718.

7. Pollock WK, Rink TS, Irvine RF. Biochem J. 1986;235:869-877.

8. Crouch MF, Lapetina EG. Biochem Biophys Res Commun. 1986;141:459-465.

9. Crouch MF, Lapetina EG. Biochem Biophys Res Commun. 1988;in press.

10. Crouch MF, Lapetina EG. J Biol Chem. 1988;263:3363-3371.

11. Crouch MF, Lapetina EG. Biochem Biophys Res Commun. 1988;151:178-186.

12. Nishizuka Y. Nature 1984;308:693-697.

13. Touqui L, Rothhut B, Shaw AM, Fradin A, Vergaftig BB, Russo-Marie I. Nature 1986;321:177-180.

14. Okano Y, Yamada K, Yano K, Nozawa Y. Biochem Biophys Res Commun. 1987;145:1267-1275.

15. Jelsema CL, Axelrod J. Proc Natl Acad Sci USA 1987;84:3623-3627.

Advances in Prostaglandin, Thromboxane, and Leukotriene Research, Vol. 19, edited by B. Samuelsson, P. Y.-K. Wong, and F. F. Sun, Raven Press, Ltd., New York ©1989.

REGULATION OF ARACHIDONATE RELEASE BY G-PROTEINS AND PROTEIN KINASE C IN HUMAN PLATELETS

Ichiro Fuse and Hsin-Hsiung Tai

Division of Medicinal Chemistry and Pharmacognosy College of Pharmacy, University of Kentucky, Lexington, KY 40536-0082

A number of platelet agonists such as thrombin, collagen and platelet activating factor are capable of activating platelets and releasing arachidonate and its metabolites (1). However, mechanism and regulation of arachidonate release remain unclear. These platelet agonists are also known to stimulate receptor mediated phospholipase C catalyzed cleavage of phosphatidylinositol-4,5-bisphosphate generating diacyl-glycerol (DG) and inositol-1,4,5-triphosphate (IP_3) as two putative second messengers (2). DG stimulates protein kinase C, whereas IP_3 causes release of Ca^{+2} from internal stores (3,4). Their effects on arachidonate release can be mimicked by a combination of phorbol 12-myristate 13-acetate (PMA) and calcium ionophore A-23187 since those two agents act syner-gistically to elicit arachidonate release (5,6). The precise mechanism by which protein kinase C activation may couple with Ca^{+2} mobilization to stimulate arachidonate release remains to be elucidated.

Agonists induced activation of phospholipase C is also found to be mediated by G-protein (7,8). Whether agonists induced arachidonate release is mediated by the same or different G-protein is not known. The sensitivity of G-proteins to fluoroaluminate and to bacterial toxins provides us valuable tools to explore the involvement of G-proteins in arachidonate release. This paper describes the use of these tools and of agents that activate protein kinases to investigate the role of G-proteins and protein kinases in regulating arachidonate release.

MATERIALS AND METHODS

ATP, CoA, arachidonoyl CoA, phorbol 12-myristate 13-acetate (PMA), calcium ionophore A-23187, L-1-palmitoyl-lyso-phosphatidylcholine (LPC), neomycin, and arachidonic acid were obtained from Sigma. All the phospholipids were purchased from Sedary Research Lab Prostaglandin E_1 (PGE_1), and throm-boxane B_2 (TXB_2) were supplied by the Upjohn Company. [2-^{3}H]

inositol was purchased from the American Radiolabeled
Chemicals, Inc. L-1-[1-^{14}C-palmitoyl]-LPC and [1-^{14}C]arachi-
donic acid were supplied by New England Nuclear. Other bio-
chemicals were obtained as described previously (9,10).
Preparation of [^{3}H]-inositol labeled platelets and
pretreatment of platelets with toxins, neomycin, PMA and PGE$_1$
were carried out as described before (9). Isolation of
[^{3}H]-inositol labeled metabolites was according to the
procedure of Griffin and Hawthorne (11). Radioimmunoassay of
TXB$_2$ was carried out as described by Tai and Yuan (12).
Activities of arachidonoyl CoA synthase and arachidonoyl CoA
lysophosphatide acyltransferase were assayed as previously
reported (10).

RESULTS AND DISCUSSION

The involvement of G-protein(s) in stimulating phospholipase C in platelets has been well documented (7,8). Whether
release of arachidonate from membrane phospholipids is a
consequence of activation of phospholipase C or is induced by
activation of a separated G-protein linked phospholipase A$_2$ is
not clear. We have employed a G-protein modulating agent,
fluoroaluminate (AlF$_4^-$), to explore arachidonate release in
human platelets. AlF$_4$ was found to stimulate the formation
of IP$_3$ and the release of arachidonate determined as
metabolite TXB$_2$ in a time and dose dependent manner. Since
IP$_3$ may mobilize Ca^{+2} and may work in concert with the generated DG to release arachidonate, it is logical to assume that
AlF$_4^-$ induced TXB$_2$ synthesis is attributed at least in part to
phospholipase C activation. Whether there is an alternative
mechanism that can directly activate a separate G-protein
linked phospholipase A$_2$ remains to be determined. Neomycin is
known to bind to polyphosphoinositides and interferes with the
activation of phospholipase C (13). We reason that if release
of arachidonate is solely the consequence of phospholipase C
activation, the addition of neomycin should block AlF$_4^-$
induced arachidonate release. Fig. 1 shows that neomycin at
10 mM inhibited completely the formation of IP$_3$ but affected
only slightly the synthesis of TXB$_2$ induced by AlF$_4^-$. This
observation suggests that an independent G-protein linked
pathway for arachidonate release does exist in platelets.
This suggestion was further supported by the finding that
pertussis toxin exhibited differential inhibition of AlF$_4^-$
induced TXB$_2$ synthesis and IP$_3$ formation as shown in Fig. 1.
Apparently there exists two different G-proteins that are
responsible for respective activation of phospholipase A$_2$ and
C.

Following the release of arachidonate from membrane
phospholipids, two pathways exist for the further metabolism
of arachidonate in platelets. One is concerned with the
oxygenation of arachidonate into TXB$_2$ and 12-HETE, and the

other is related to reactivation of árachidonate and
reacylation of lysophospholipids into membrane phospholipids.
The latter two processes are catalyzed by arachidonoyl CoA
synthase and arachidonoyl CoA lysophosphatide acyltransferase,
respectively.   Since a variety of platelet agonists stimulate

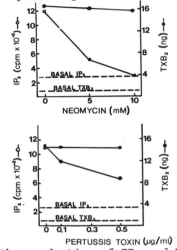

Fig.1: Effect of neomycin and
pertussistoxin on AlF_4^- induced
IP_3 and TXB_2 formation.

-O-, IP_3 -●-, TXB_2

the production of IP_3 and DG in addition to release of
arachidonate. It is very likely that IP_3 may mobilize the
necessary Ca^{+2} to stimulate receptor activated phospholipase
A_2 and subsequent release of arachidonate.   DG may activate
protein kinase C which may inhibit reincorporation of
arachidonate by inactivating arachidonoyl CoA synthase and/or
acyltransferase, and facilitate oxygenation of arachidonate
into biologically potent metabolites.   In fact, the action of
IP_3 and DG in stimulating arachidonate release can be mimicked
by calcium ionophore A-23187 and PMA as reported previously
(5,6).   Therefore, we initiated to examine if platelets
pretreated with PMA might exhibit impairment of arachidonate
uptake into membrane phospholipids. Labeled arachidonate,
linoleate and oleate were respectively incubated with
platelets treated and untreated with 1 μM of PMA.   It was
found that PMA treated platelets took up much less labeled
arachidonate than did untreated platelets. However, no
difference in uptake of labeled linoleate or oleate was
observed between PMA treated and untreated platelets.   These
results suggest that arachidonate is specifically inhibited to
incorporate into phospholipids in platelets activated with
PMA.   To further delineate which of the two enzymes involved
in arachidonate incorporation into phospholipids is affected
by PMA treatment, both enzyme activities in crude homogenates
were determined in treated and untreated platelets. Fig. 2
shows a PMA concentration dependent inhibition of both enzyme
activities in treated platelets.   Inhibition of both enzyme
activities is not likely due to a direct effect of PMA on both

Fig.2: Effect of treatment with increasing concentrations of PMA on arachidonoyl CoA synthase (-●-) and arachidonoyl CoA lysophosphatide acyltansterasc (-O-) activities. Control activities for synthase and transferase are 38 and 39 pmol/min/ 10^8 platelets respectively. Each point is an average of two determinations.

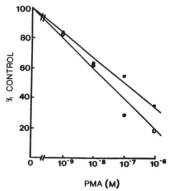

PMA (M)

enzymes since PMA was removed by centrifugation before platelet homogenates were prepared. Similar concentration dependent inhibition of both enzyme activities by another protein kinase C activator, 1-oleoyl-2 acetyl glycerol (OAG) was also observed. These results suggest that protein kinase C activation may directly or indirectly inactivate the enzymes involved in the uptake of the released arachidonate resulting in an increased oxygenation into biologically potent metabolites.

We have also observed that platelets treated with 1.4 uM of PGE_1 before washed platelets were prepared for PMA or OAG treatment did not appear to respond to PMA or OAG as well as untreated platelets. We suspected that PGE_1 might have antagonized the action of PMA or OAG. Therefore, experiments were carried out to test if washed platelets pretreated with PGE_1 would exhibit decrease in both enzyme activities following exposure to PMA. Fig. 3 shows that preincubation of platelets with increasing concentrations of PGE_1 attenuated PMA induced decrease in both enzyme activities.[1] However, pretreatment of platelets with PGE_1 did not impair uptake of arachidonic acid indicating that both enzymes involved in arachidonate incorporation into phospholipids might not be affected by PGE_1 induced activation of protein kinase A.

Fig.3: Effect of PGE, treatment on PMA induced decrease in
arachidonoyl CoA synthase (●) and arachidonoyl CoA
lysophosphatide acyltransferase (-O-) activities. Control
activities for synthase and transferase are 80 and 84
pmol/min/10⁸ platelets respectively, each point is an average
of two determinations.

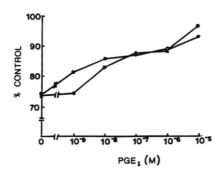

Instead, PGE_1 induced activation of protein kinase A may
render both enzymes unable to be inactivated by protein kinase
C or may interfere with the protein kinase C activation by
PMA. A similar antagonism by PGE_1, on protein kinase C
induced 40K protein phosphorylation has also been observed in
human platelets (14).

In summary, protein kinase C activation induced by DG
which is generated during platelet activation may have
important role of ensuring the released arachidonate to be
further metabolized through cyclooxygenase and lipoxygenase
pathways. This conclusion, if turn out to be applicable to
other systems, has a highly significant physiological
implications, at least concerning the generation of
biologically potent eicosanoids.

ACKNOWLEDGEMENT

This work was supported in part by the NIH grant (HL-32727).

REFERENCES

1. Irvine RT. Biochem. J. 1982, 204:3-16.
2. Nishizuka Y. Science 1984, 225:1365-1370.
3. Kishimoto A, Takai Y, Mori T, Kikkawa V, Nishizuka Y. J.
    Biol Chem. 1980; 255:2273-2276.
4. Streb H, Irvine IR, Bernidge MJ, Schulta I. Nature 1983;
    306:67-69.

5. Mobley A, Tai HH. <u>Biochem. Biophys. Res. Commun.</u> 1985; 130:717-723.
6. Halenda SP, Zavoico GB, Feinstein MB, <u>J. Biol. Chem.</u> 1985; 260:12484-12491
7. Baldassare JJ, Fisher GJ, <u>J. Biol. Chem.</u> 1986; 261:11942-11944.
8. Lapetina EG, Reep BR. <u>Proc. Natl. Acad. Sci., U.S.A.</u> 1987: 84:2261-2265.
9. Fuse I, Tai HH, <u>Biochem. Biophys. Res. Commun.</u> 1987: 146:659-665.
10. Fuse I, Iwanaga T, Tai HH. (Submitted).
11. Griffin HD, Hawthorne JN, <u>Biochem. J.</u> 1978; 176:541-552.
12. Tai HH, Yuan B. <u>Anal Biochem.</u> 1978; 87:343-349.
13. Schacht J. <u>J. Neurochem.</u> 1976; 27:1119-1124.
14. deChaffoy deCourcelles D, Roevens P. Van Belle H. <u>Biochem. J.</u> 1987; 244:93-99.

Advances in Prostaglandin, Thromboxane, and Leukotriene Research, Vol. 19, edited by B. Samuelsson, P. Y.-K. Wong, and F. F. Sun, Raven Press, Ltd., New York ©1989.

BRADYKININ-INDUCED ACTIVATION OF PHOSPHOLIPASE A$_2$ IS INDEPENDENT

OF THE ACTIVATION OF POLYPHOSPHOINOSITIDE-HYDROLYZING

PHOSPHOLIPASE C

Harumi Kaya and Suchen L. Hong

Division of Experimental Medicine, Department
of Medicine, New England Deaconess Hospital,
Harvard Medical School, Boston, Massachusetts 02215

Phosphatidylinositol 4,5-bisphosphate (PIP$_2$) has been implicated as a signal transmitter in many agonist-receptor interactions (1). This role of PIP$_2$ has been based partly on the observations that phospholipase C hydrolysis of PIP$_2$ is one of the earliest events detected in agonist-cell interaction; and that the two products of this hydrolysis, inositol 1,4,5-trisphosphate (IP$_3$) and 1,2-diacylglycerol (1,2-DG), may then regulate cellular responses. IP$_3$ can mobilize intracellular Ca^{2+} and may thereby modulate Ca^{2+} requiring enzymes (1); and 1,2-DG can activate protein kinase C and thus may regulate cellular responses through protein phosphorylation (2).

It is known that the interaction between agonists and a variety of cell types leads to a rapid synthesis of eicosanoids (3). This synthesis results from sudden availability of unesterified arachidonic acid (uAA) arising from the hydrolysis of phospholipids. Phospholipase A$_2$ of various specificities and phospholipase C with specificity toward PI, PIP$_2$ and PC have been suggested to release uAA from phospholipids. It has often been postulated that activation of phospholipase A$_2$ is the result of phospholipase C hydrolysis of PIP$_2$. This postulate seems attractive since IP$_3$ can mobilize Ca^{2+} and since most phospholipase A$_2$ activities are stimulated by Ca^{2+}. Thus several studies, including those using endothelial cells from various sources, have concluded that phospholipase A$_2$ activation results from the activation of PIP$_2$-hydrolyzing phospholipase C. However, this conclusion appears at variance with our findings with porcine endothelial and human umbilical endothelial cells (4,5).

LysoPI was formed very early in these cells after stimulation. Although PIP_2 metabolism was not examined in those studies, the very early lysoPI formation suggested to us that activation of PI-hydrolyzing phospholipase A_2 might be independent of the hydrolysis of PIP_2 by phospholipase C. This contention is supported by the present study.

ACTIVATION AT 37°

We followed the time course of bradykinin-induced activation of PI-hydrolyzing phospholipase A_2 and PIP_2-hydrolyzing phospholipase C in [³H]inositol labeled cells at 37°. As shown in Fig. 1, lysoPI accumulation was detectable by 10 sec, and reached a plateau by 20 to 30 sec. IP_3 accumulation was detectable at 10 sec and reached a maximum at 20 sec. Loss of PIP_2 was detectable at 10 sec. However, no changes in PIP, IP_2 and IP were detected during these early time, although both IP and IP_2 began to accumulated by 2 min. These results indicate that bradykinin-induced activation of PI-hydrolyzing phospholipase A_2 and PIP_2-hydrolyzing phospholipase C are simultaneous.

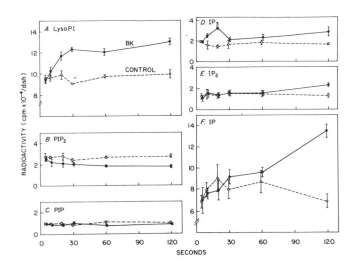

FIG. 1. Time course of bradykinin-induced changes of phosphoinositides and their metabolites at 37° in [³H]inositol prelabeled porcine endothelial cells.

Many studies on the role of PIP_2 in signal transduction in agonist-induced arachidonate and eicosanoid release often monitored only the extracellular levels of these compounds. We believe that the appearance of uAA and eicosanoids in the extra-

cellular medium probably does not accurately reflect the time
course of stimulated phospholipase A_2 activity, because both the
conversion of uAA to eicosanoids and the subsequent release into
the extracellular medium probably require some time. We therefore
monitored the intracellular levels of uAA and eicosanoids in this
study. As shown in Fig. 2, bradykinin–stimulated increase in
intracellular uAA was rapid, comparable to that of lysoPI; it was
detectable at 5 sec and reached a maximum at 30 sec before it
gradually decreased. There was a smaller increase in
intracellular 6-k-PGF$_{1\alpha}$ and PGF$_{2\alpha}$. PA accumulation was much slower
than uAA accumulation, although it continued to increase for at
least 2 min. Essentially no change in 1,2–DG was observed during
the first min; only slight increase was detected by 2 min. No
detectable ^{3}H-containing monoacylglycerol was found. ^{3}H
radioactivity released into the extracellular medium was also
detectable by 10 to 20 sec, but in a smaller quantity than the
intracellular level, and it continued to increase for at least 2
min. These results further support the contention that the
activation of phospholipase A_2 is independent of PIP$_2$ metabolism.

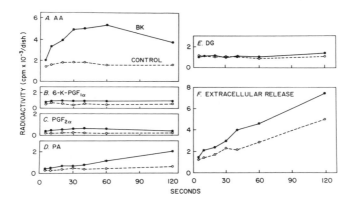

FIG. 2. Time course of bradykinin–induced intracellular and extracellular accumulation of uAA and
eicosanoids in [^{3}H]arachidonate prelabeled porcine
endothelial cells at 37°.

ACTIVATION AT 30°.

We also examined the effect of lower incubation temperature
(30°) on the activation of phospholipase A_2 and phospholipase C
in [^{3}H]inositol prelabeled cells. At 30° bradykinin–stimulated
formation of lysoPI was detectable at 10 sec and reached a
plateau at 60 sec (Fig. 3). However, at this temperature no

significant changes in IP_3 was found. This observation clearly indicates that the activation of PI-hydrolyzing phospholipase A_2 does not depend on the formation of IP_3.

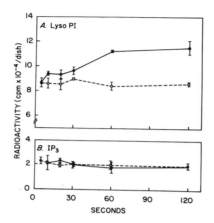

FIG. 3. Changes of lysoPI and IP_3 induced by bradykinin at 30° in [³H]inositol prelabeled porcine endothelial cells. o, with bradykinin (1 uM); o, without bradykinin.

CONCLUSION

The results presented here demonstrate that bradykinin-stimulated phospholipase A_2 activation is independent of activation of PIP_2-hydrolyzing phospholipase C in porcine aortic endothelial cells.

REFERENCES

1. Berridge MJ, Irvine RF. Nature 1984;312:315-321.

2. Nishizuka Y. Nature 1984;308:639-698.

3. Sammuelson B. Harvey Lect 1979;75:1-40.

4. Hong SL, Deykin D. J. Biol. Chem. 1982; 257:7151-7154.

5. Hong SL, McLaughlin NJ, Tzeng CY, Patton GM. Thrombosis Research 1985;38:1-10.

Advances in Prostaglandin, Thromboxane, and Leukotriene Research, Vol. 19, edited by B. Samuelsson, P. Y.-K. Wong, and F. F. Sun, Raven Press, Ltd., New York ©1989.

SUBSTRATE-SPECIFIC FORMS OF PHOSPHOLIPASE A_2 IN HUMAN PLATELETS

Wai Yiu Cheung and Leslie R. Ballou

Department of Biochemistry
St. Jude Children's Research Hospital
Memphis, TN 38101 USA

INTRODUCTION

For some 20 years we have been interested in cellular regulatory mechanisms, with emphasis on certain enzymatic pathways that control the metabolism of intracellular messengers. Initially, we studied the regulatory properties of a cyclic nucleotide phosphodiesterase which catalyzes the hydrolysis of cAMP to AMP, thereby terminating its action. During the course of these studies, we serendipitously discovered calmodulin, the main intracellular Ca^{2+}-receptor in eukaryotes (1,2). Later, our interest was gradually shifted to enzymes in the Ca^{2+}-regulated pathway shown in Fig. 1. It soon became apparent that the cAMP- and the Ca^{2+}-regulated pathways are so functionally and metabolically intertwined that it is oftentimes not practical to

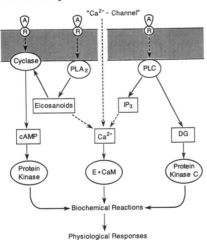

FIG. 1. A schematic rendition of the regulatory pathways for the main cellular messengers. An appropriate agonist could stimulate the adenylate cyclase, PLA_2, or PLC and generate cAMP, eicosanoids, or inositol triphosphate and diacylglycerol, respectively. Although not explicitly indicated, the functions and metabolism of these messengers are often intertwined. For example, the influx of Ca^{2+} or the release of Ca^{2+} from the endoplastic reticulum activates calmodulin, which in turn activates calmodulin-dependent en-zymes, including adenylate cyclase and cyclic nucleotidephosphodiesterase, which catalyze the synthesis and hydrolysis of cAMP, respectively. Stimulation of PLC generates from phosphatidylinositol 4,5-biphosphate two messengers: inositol triphosphate, which releases Ca^{2+} from the endoplasmic reticulum; and diacylglycerol, which activates protein kinase C. Stimulation of PLA_2 by an agonist or by an increase of intracellular Ca^{2+} leads to the release from phospholipids of arachidonic acid, the substrate for all eicosanoids. Eicosanoids usually act on neighboring cells, and are referred to as local hormones. Some eicosanoids stimulate aden-

ylate cyclase, others inhibit it, and some are believed to be Ca^{2+} ionophores. A, agonist; R, receptor; PLA_2, phospholipase A_2; PLC, phospholipase C; cAMP, cyclic AMP; IP_3, inositol 1,4,5-triphosphate; DG, diacylglycerol; CaM, calmodulin; E, CaM-dependent enzyme; E•CaM, enzyme•CaM complex.

speak of one and not the other. Indeed, in many instances the metabolism and functions of eicosanoids, the other class of messengers (usually known as local hormones) mentioned in Fig. 1, are also closely tied in with the two pathways. Eicosanoids are derived from arachidonic acid, which is predominately ester-ified to the second position of phospholipids. The release of arachidonate from phospholipids, catalyzed by phospholipase A_2 (PLA_2), is usually the rate limiting step in eicosanoid biosyn-thesis (3,4).

Several years ago, we began a study on the regulatory pro-perties of PLA_2 from human platelets. Human platelets are easi-ly obtainable in a homogenous state in bulk quantities, and have been used extensively as an experimental model for studying the metabolism of eicosanoids. Since PLA_2 is known to require Ca^{2+} for activity and the effect of Ca^{2+} on many regulatory enzymes are mediated through calmodulin, we first examined if calmodulin affected PLA_2 activity. Using a crude PLA_2 associated with a human platelet membrane fraction, we noted a small stimulation by calmodulin, but when the enzyme was solubilized and partially purified, the stimulation was invariably lost, suggesting that the enzyme, though Ca^{2+}-requiring, is probably not calmodulin-modulated (5). The possibility that a factor conferring respon-siveness to calmodulin was lost in the partially purified PLA_2 preparation, though unlikely, has not been excluded.

One feature about PLA_2 activity in human platelets is that its activity in the crude extract appears insufficient to ac-count for the free arachidonate released from thrombin-activated platelets. An alternative pathway has been proposed in which phosphatidylinositol is converted by a phospholipase C to 1,2-diacylglycerol, which is then acted upon by a diacylglycerol lipase to yield free arachidonate (6). Some investigators have noted, however, that the diacylglycerol cleaved from phospha-tidylinositol by a phospholipase C appeared to be rapidly and quantitatively converted to phosphatidic acid and was not avail-able for the diacylglycerol lipase pathway (7,8). Other inves-tigators have argued that in stimulated platelets a PLA_2 acting on phosphatidylcholine accounted for the release of a majority of the free arachidonate (9). In addition, McKean et al. (10) demonstrated that upon activation by thrombin human platelets rapidly accumulated lysophosphatidylcholine with concomitant loss of phosphatidylcholine, indicating that the release of arachidonate was mediated by PLA_2.

Human platelet PLA_2 activity *in vitro* is inhibited by unsaturat-ed fatty acids

The apparent low level of PLA_2 activity detected in human platelet extract and the *in vivo* evidence that PLA_2 is mainly responsible for generating arachidonate poses a paradox. In an attempt to purify the enzyme for further characterization studies, we noted that the enzyme activity increased more than 10-fold when chromatographed on a DEAE-cellulose column (5). The marked increase of enzyme activity was due to the removal of some inhibitory substances, which were later identified as unsaturated fatty acids endogenous to the enzyme preparation (11). The suppression of PLA$_2$ activity by endogenous unsaturated fatty acids explains its apparent low activity in the platelet extract. We have estimated conservatively that an extract prepared from 10^9 platelets has the potential to catalyze the release of 0.8 n mol of arachidonate per min (5) from phosphatidylcholine (PtdCho) and a larger quantity from phosphatidylethanolamine (PtdEtn) (see Fig. 2 legend), a rate which accounts for much of the *in vivo* formation of arachidonate in response to thrombin stimulation (12).

The level of unsaturated fatty acids present in the platelet extract appears sufficient to inhibit most of the PLA$_2$ activity (11). Although we do not know whether they are accessible to the enzyme *in vivo*, our results indicate that they are associated with the same particulate fraction as the enzyme. This raises an apparently perplexing question. If the PLA$_2$ is inhibited by unsaturated fatty acid *in situ*, how is the inhibition overcome when the platelets are stimulated by various agonists? In stimulated platelets the accumulation of unsaturated fatty acids appears sufficient to inhibit most of the PLA$_2$ activity. Does this constitute a mechanism for feedback control? Indeed, do these findings represent a laboratory phenomenon brought about by mixing the enzyme with the unsaturated fatty acids during the process of homogenization, or do they have some physiological relevance? Answers to these questions may help in understanding the mechanisms regulating PLA$_2$ activity and its role in cellular processes.

PtdCho- and PtdEtn-Specific Forms of PLA$_2$

In our studies on human platelet PLA$_2$, we routinely used PtdCho as a substrate. Some investigators have noted that the enzyme lacks specificity for phospholipid classes (13); others have argued that PtdEtn is the preferred substrate (12,14). In the next series of experiments, we used both PtdCho and PtdEtn to assess PLA$_2$ activities (15). Fig. 2 shows an elution profile

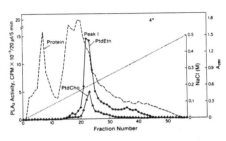

FIG. 2. DEAE-cellulose column chromatography of a particulate fraction of human platelets. The PLA$_2$ activity in the particulate fraction before column chromatography was 0.3 nmol/min for PtdCho and 0.2 mmol/min for PtdEtn. After column chromatography, these activities recovered from Peak 1 increased to 7.1 and 27.5 nmol/min, respectively. From Ballou, DeWitt & Cheung (15).

of PLA$_2$ activity from a DEAE-cellulose column. One major activity peak was observed and it catalyzed the release of arachidonic acid from both PtdCho and PtdEtn. In fact, under our
experimental conditions, the hydrolysis of PtdEtn exceeded that
of PtdCho. The hydrolysis of both substrates could mean that
the enzyme activity peak contained one enzyme which acts on two
substrates or that it contained two distinct forms of enzyme co-
eluted from the column with each form specific for one substrate. Several lines of evidence appear consistent with the
latter interpretation. First, the two activities displayed
different stabilities during storage. Second, the optimal pH
for the hydrolysis of PtdEtn was approximately 7 and that for
PtdCho was 9 or higher. In general, PtdEtn hydrolysis decreased
at a pH above 7, whereas PtdCho hydrolysis increased up to pH 9.
Third, the hydrolysis of PtdCho was Ca^{2+}-dependent, whereas that
of PtdEtn was essentially Ca^{2+}-independent. Fourth, the Km for
PtdCho was 0.6 μM and that for PtdEtn was 7 μM. In the presence
of increasing concentration of nonlabeled PtdCho, the hydrolysis
of labeled PtdCho decreased proportionally, apparently because
both the labeled and unlabeled PtdCho were hydrolyzed indiscrim-
inately at the same catalytic site. Yet, the presence of nonlabeled PtdCho at concentrations up to 10 times greater than
those of labeled PtdEtn did not affect the hydrolysis of PtdEtn.
The finding that the affinity of the enzyme (if it were indeed
one enzyme) for PtdCho was 10-fold higher than that for PtdEtn
and the finding that PtdCho diminished the hydrolysis of PtdCho
but not that of PtdEtn would argue for two separate activity
forms of PLA$_2$. Lastly, and perhaps the strongest evidence that
human platelets contain substrate-specific forms of PLA$_2$ comes
from the observation that under certain conditions, a separate
activity peak specific for PtdEtn (Fig. 3, Left) and another
specific for PtdCho (Fig. 3, Right)) were resolved from the main

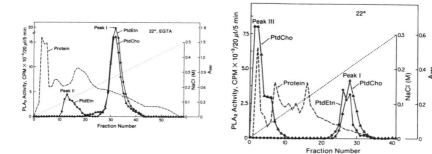

FIG. 3. Isolation of PtdEtn-specific (Left Panel) and PtdCho-specific (Right
Panel) PLA$_2$ from a particulate fraction of human platelets by DEAE-cellulose
column chromatography. PLA$_2$ activity was assayed with either PtdEtn or PtdCho.
From Ballou, DeWitt & Cheung (15).

activity peak that acted on both phospholipids. Unfortunately, the activity of these substrate-specific forms of PLA_2 were highly unstable, making it difficult to isolate and characterize them further.

"PtdIns-Specific" PLA_2 Activity

The existence of two substrate-specific forms of PLA_2 led naturally to a search for a form of the enzyme specific for phosphatidylinositol (PtdIns). In preliminary experiments, we obtained evidence for a soluble enzyme that acted specifically on PtdIns (16). While resolving the reaction products from PtdIns hydrolysis using TLC, we detected a compound corresponding to lysoPtdIns and another that appeared to be slightly more polar than arachidonic acid. Examination of the reaction product by UV spectrophotometry failed to reveal absorption in the UV range. Further analysis by GC/MS indicated the presence of two compounds. The main component displayed a C-value of 19.2, and the fragmentation pattern was identical to that of 14,15-oxido-5,8,11-eicosatrienoic acid (14,15-EET). From the C-value and the mass spectrum we tentatively identified the main component as 14,15-EET. The minor component isolated along with 14,15-EET has not been identified; it could be a degradation product of 14,15-EET, or a secondary reaction product (17).

The enzyme or enzyme system catalyzing the formation of 14,15-EET appears specific for PtdIns; neither arachidonic acid, PtdCho nor PtdEtn served as a substrate. The reaction required Ca^{2+} and was not affected by aspirin, indomethacin or mepacrine. Epoxyeicosatrienoic acids are known to arise from free arachidonic acid in rat liver via a cytochrome P-450 enzyme system referred to as the "epoxygenase pathway." In the liver 4 EETs are formed: 5,6-,   8,9-,   11,12- and 14,15-EET (18).   Human platelets, by contrast, generate apparently only 14,15-EET from PtdIns, by a pathway distinct from the cytochrome P-450 system. Evidence for such a pathway comes from 4 different observations. (1) The production of 14,15-EET was inhibited by carbon monoxide, but the inhibition was readily reversible, in a manner similar to the inhibition by nitrogen; (2) NADPH, a cofactor of cytochrome P-450, did not affect 14,15-EET production; (3) cyanide and SKF 525A, inhibitors of P-450, did not alter 14,15-EET formation; and (4) free arachidonate was *not* a substrate for the formation of 14,15-EET (17).

Whole platelets were labeled with [^{14}C]arachidonic acid in the presence of aspirin, challenged with various agonists, and examined for evidence of 14,15-EET formation. Thrombin induced the formation of 14,15-EET, whereas ionophore A23187 (1 μM), collagen (0.5 mg/ml), epinephrine (10 μM), and ADP (20 μM) were essentially ineffective (17).

Collectively, our findings indicate that human platelets liberate 14,15-EET from the 2-position of PtdIns apparently after epoxygenation of the arachidonyl moiety. The enzyme (or enzyme system) is soluble, Ca^{2+}-dependent, specific for PtdIns, and is insensitive to inhibitors of PLA_2 and cyclooxygenase.

Whether 14,15-EET is formed by one enzyme with two activities, or two distinct enzymes tightly coupled remains unclear. It would appear that two enzymatic steps are necessary: one for epoxidation of the esterified arachidonate and another for its subsequent hydrolysis to liberate 14,15-EET. For simplicity, the enzyme may be tentatively referred to as "epoxygenase-PLA₂".

CONCLUSION

PLA₂'s from snake venom and mammalian pancreas generally lack substrate specificity (19). In contrast, human platelet contains multiple forms of PLA₂ and they appear to be substrate specific. Clearly, multiple forms of PLA₂ afford the cell with distinct regulatory mechanisms for controlling the hydrolysis of various phospholipids and hence are of considerable biological and pharmacological importance. Moreover, the formation of 14,15-EET from PtdIns appears to be a novel process, especially since free arachidonic acid does not serve as a substrate. Further progress in this area will depend on successful purification of each form of PLA₂ and a better understanding of their regulatory properties.

REFERENCES

1. Cheung WY. J Cyclic Nucleic Res 1981;7:71-84.
2. Cheung WY. Science 1980;207:19-27.
3. Samuelsson B. Science 1983;220:568-575.
4. Feinstein MB, Rodan GA, Cutler LA. In: Gordon JL, ed. Platelets in Biology and Pathology, Amsterdam: Elsevier/ North Holland, 1981;437-472.
5. Ballou LR, Cheung WY. Proc Natl Acad Sci 1983;80:5203-5207.
6. Bell RL, Majerus PW. J Biol Chem 1980;255:1790-1792.
7. Brockman MJ, Ward JW, Marcus AJ. J Biol Chem 1981;256: 8271-8274.
8. Lapetina EG, Billah MM, Cuatrecasas P. Nature 1981;292: 367-369.
9. Billah MM, Lapetina EG, Cuatrecasas P. J Biol Chem 1980; 255:10227-10231.
10. McKean ML, Smith JB, Silver MJ. J Biol Chem 1981;256:1522-1524.
11. Ballou LR, Cheung WY. Proc Natl Acad Sci 1985;82:371-375.
12. Broeckman MJ, Ward JW, Marcus AJ. J Biol Chem 1981;256: 8271-8274.
13. Van den Bosch H. Biochim Biophys Acta 1980;604:191-246.
14. Jesse RJ, Cohen P. Biochem J 1976;158:283-287.
15. Ballou LR, Dewitt LM, Cheung WY. J Biol Chem 1986;261: 3107-3111.
16. Cheung WY, Ballou LR. In: Johnson I, ed. A Perspective on Biology and Medicine in the 21st Century, Royal Society of Medicine Services, Ltd. (in press).
17. Ballou LR, Lam BK, Wang PYK, Cheung WY. Proc Natl Acad Sci 1987;84:6990-6994.
18. Oliw EH, Guengerich FP, Oates JA. J Biol Chem 1982;257: 3771-3781.
19. Dennis EA. In: Boyer PD, ed. The Enzymes, Academic Press 1983;16:307-353.

Advances in Prostaglandin, Thromboxane, and
Leukotriene Research, Vol. 19, edited by
B. Samuelsson, P. Y.-K. Wong, and F. F. Sun,
Raven Press, Ltd., New York ©1989.

INHIBITION OF PHOSPHOLIPASE C DEPENDENT PROCESSES by U-73,122

J.E. Bleasdale, G. L. Bundy, *S. Bunting, **F.A. Fitzpatrick,
R.M. Huff, F.F. Sun, and J. E. Pike

The Upjohn Company, Kalamazoo, Michigan 49001
*Dept. of Pharmacological Sciences, Genentech, Inc.
South San Francisco, California 94080
**University of Colorado Health Sciences Center,
Dept. of Pharmacology, 4200 E. 9th Ave., Denver, Colorado 80262

In 1981 the late Don Wallach and Joan Whittier, at Upjohn, began a search for inhibitors of phospholipase A_2. One of the compounds they discovered to be active was a steroidal amine (U-26,384) (N[3-(dimethylamino)propyl]-3-methoxy-N-methylestra 2,5(10)-dien-17β-amine) (Fig. 1). This led us to initiate a chemical program to define structure activity relationships in this series of compounds. The results of these investigations of the phospholipase A_2 (PLA_2) inhibitors will be described in detail in other publications. The subject of this paper is another steroidal amine, U-73,122, that was found to exhibit biological activity that could best be explained not by inhibition of PLA_2, but by inhibition of phospholipase C (PLC).

FIG. 1

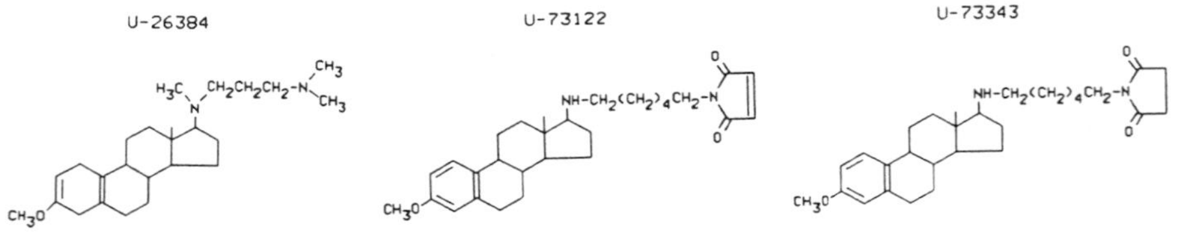

Phosphoinositide-specific (PLC) enzymes are phosphodiesterases which cleave diacylglycerol from phosphatidylinositol (and its derivatives), and are involved in the generation of a variety of biologically active products (1, 2). Elucidation of the various cellular functions of PLC would be facilitated by the availability of a selective PLC inhibitor. As part of a search for PLC inhibitors, compounds were tested for their ability to inhibit agonist-induced aggregation of human platelets. One compound (U-73,122) (1-[6-[[(17 beta)-3-methoxyestra-1,3,5(10)-trien-17-yl]amino]hexyl]-)1H-pyrrole-2, 5-dione) (Fig. 1) proved to be a potent inhibitor of aggregation and had certain unique characteristics.

1. U-73,122 exhibited extremely stringent structure-activity relationships. For example, the closely related structure (U-73,343) (1-[6-[[(17beta)-3-methoxyestra-1,3,5(10)-trien-17-yl]amino]hexyl]-2,5-pyrrolidinedione) (Fig. 1) was essentially inactive as an inhibitor of platelet aggregation.

2. U-73,122 was not an inhibitor of PLA_2 enzymes isolated from either pig pancreas or snake venoms (employing 1-palmitoyl-2[^{3}H]-oleoyl-glycero-3-phosphoethanolamine as the substrate).

3. Inhibition of agonist-induced platelet aggregation was not overcome by the addition of exogenous arachidonic acid and, in fact, U-73,122 was a potent inhibitor of platelet aggregation induced by arachidonic acid.

TABLE 1

INHIBITION BY U-73,122 OF THE AGGREGATION OF HUMAN PLATELETS INDUCED BY VARIOUS AGONISTS

AGONIST	K_i for U-73,122 (µM)
Collagen (1 µg/ml)	1.1
A-23,187 (10 µg/ml)	13
Arachidonic Acid (0.66 mM)	0.95
U-46,619 (1.4 µM) (thromboxane agonist)	2.1
ADP (4 µM)	1.7

Table 1 lists some of the agonists against which U-73,122 inhibited platelet aggregation (K_i all approximately 1µM, except for A-23,187). The inability of exogenous arachidonic acid to overcome the inhibition of platelet aggregation produced by U-73,122 was suggestive that U-73,122 was not simply an inhibitor of PLA_2-dependent mobilization of arachidonic acid, and prompted an investigation of the mechanism by which U-73,122 inhibits arachidonic acid-induced aggregation. Potential sites of inhibition by U-73,122 are outlined in Fig. 2.

Fig. 2

POTENTIAL SITES OF INHIBITION BY U–73,122 OF ARACHIDONIC ACID INDUCED AGGREGATION OF HUMAN PLATELETS

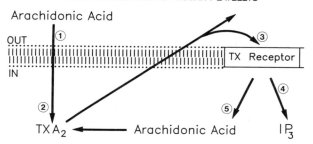

U-73,122 does not appear to inhibit either the uptake of exogenous arachidonic acid or its conversion to thromboxane A_2 (TXA$_2$) (sites 1 and 2) since TXA$_2$ production from exogenous arachidonic acid was unaffected, even though collagen-induced TXA$_2$ production (which requires phospholipase-dependent mobilization of intracellular arachidonic acid) was inhibited by U-73,122. The binding of a thromboxane-receptor antagonist ([3H]-SQ29548) (3) to platelet plasma membranes was also not inhibited by U-73,122 and, therefore, the mechanism of inhibition of platelet aggregation by U-73,122 does not appear to involve an inhibition of the binding of TXA$_2$ to its receptor (site 3). U-73,122 does, however, inhibit aggregation induced by the thromboxane agonist U-46,619 indicating that the inhibitory action of U-73,122 most likely involves inhibition of post-receptor mechanisms (sites 4 and 5).

Experimental evidence in support of this conclusion is as follows: Platelets were pre-labeled for 2 hours with [3H]-inositol and, after washing, they were stimulated with thrombin in either the presence or absence of U-73,122. It was found that the production of 3H inositol-1,4,5-trisphosphate (IP$_3$) was inhibited by U-73,122. In a second set of experiments, the platelets were pre-labeled for 2 hours with [3H]-arachidonic acid, and after washing, they were stimulated with thrombin, with and without U-73,122. It was observed that thrombin-induced mobilization of arachidonic acid from phosphatidylinositol was inhibited by U-73,122. In platelets, agonist-induced generation of IP$_3$ and mobilization of arachidonic acid from phosphatidylinositol are both PLC-dependent processes (4, 5).

Studies with other cell types showed that U-73,122 inhibited the following phenomena:

a. Aggregation of human neutrophils induced by either F-Met-Leu-Phe (FMLP) or platelet activating factor (PAF).

b. A 23,187-induced leukotriene B$_4$ production by neutrophils.

c. A 23,187-induced PAF production by neutrophils.

d. Calcium-dependent generation of IP$_3$ in human erythrocyte ghosts.

e. Phospholipase C activity of human amnion cells (measured as the rate of hydrolysis of [3H]-phosphatidylinositol).

Partially purified amnion PLC was used to characterize the mechanism of inhibition by U-73,122 Hydrolysis of PI (0.5 mm) was inhibited by U-73,122 when the molar ratio of Ca^{2+}:PI was <2; at Ca^{2+}:PI ratios of 4-12 however, U-73,122 increased PLC activity. When Ca^{2+}:PI was >12 (i.e., when PLC activity in this in vitro system was maximal), U-73,122 was without affect. These in vitro effects of U-73,122 on PLC activity can be explained by the model proposed in Fig. 3.

PROPOSED MECHANISM OF THE EFFECT OF U-73122 ON PHOSPHOLIPASE C ACTIVITY

Fig. 3

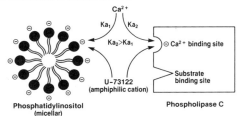

Calcium is suggested to bind with relatively low affinity to the micellar substrate (phosphatidylinositol) and with relatively high affinity to a binding site on the PLC. Binding of Ca^{2+} to the substrate reduces the net negative charge on the micelles and promotes interaction of the PLC with the micelles. At $Ca^{2}:PI>12$, there is sufficient Ca^{2+} to saturate Ca^{2+} binding to substrate and PLC and maximal PLC activity is observed which is unaffected by U-73,122. At $Ca^{2+}:PI$ 4-12, PLC activity declines because of insufficient Ca^{2+} to saturate binding to the substrate. As an amphiphilic cation, U-73,122 substitutes for Ca^{2+} efficiently in interacting with the substrate and thus, under these conditions, U-73,122 increases PLC activity. At $Ca^{2+}:PI<2$, U-73,122 begins to compete with Ca^{2+} for binding to the site on the PLC that must be occupied by Ca^{2+} for expression of PLC activity and, as a result, U-73,122 inhibits PLC activity under these conditions. Stimulation of PLC activity by U-73,122, therefore, appears to be an artifact of the in vitro assay and this explains why only inhibition of PLC activity by U-73,122 is observed in whole cells. The nature of the interaction of U-73,122 with the Ca^{2+}-enzyme site is unclear, but it is reversible and is somehow related to the ability of the maleimide moeity to act as a nucleophilic acceptor, since the succinimide analog, U-73,343 (which is a poorer electrophile) is biologically inactive (Fig. 1).

The results of this investigation support the conclusion that U-73,122 is a selective inhibitor of phospholipase C activity and may be useful in investigations of phospholipase C-dependent cellular processes.

REFERENCES

1. Abdel-Latif, A.A. (1986): Calcium-mobilizing receptors, polyphosphoinositides, and the generation of second messengers. Pharmacol. Rev. 38:227-272.
2. Saltiel, A.R. and Cuatrecasas, P. (1986): Insulin stimulates the generation from hepatic plasma membranes of modulators derived from an inositol glycolipid. Proc. Nat'l. Acad. Sci. (USA) 83:5793-5797.
3. Ogletree, M.L., Harris, D.N., Greenberg, R., Haslanger, M.F. and Nakane, M. (1985): Pharmacological actions of SQ 29,548, a novel selective thromboxane antagonist. J. Pharmacol. Exptl. Therap. 234:435-441.
4. Agranoff, B.W., Murthy, P. and Seguin, E.B. (1983): Thrombin-induced phosphodiesteratic cleavage of phosphatidylinositol bisphosphate in human platelets. J. Biol. Chem. 258:2076-2078
5. Lapetina, E.G. (1985): The relevance of inositide degradation and protein kinase C in platelet responses in Inositol and Phosphoinositides. Metabolism and Regulation (Bleasdale, J.E., Eichberg, J. and Hauser, G. eds.) Humana Press, Clifton, NJ pp. 475-492.

Advances in Prostaglandin, Thromboxane, and
Leukotriene Research, Vol. 19, edited by
B. Samuelsson, P. Y.-K. Wong, and F. F. Sun,
Raven Press, Ltd., New York ©1989.

PROINFLAMMATORY EFFECTS OF PHOSPHOLIPASE A2 (PLA2)

IN SEVERAL IN VITRO AND IN VIVO SYSTEMS

Joseph Chang, Lisa M. Marshall and Richard P. Carlson

Immunopharmacology Division, Wyeth-Ayerst Research
CN 8000, Princeton, New Jersey 08543-8000

INTRODUCTION

It is only within the last 20 years that the importance of phospholipase A2 (PLA2) in the generation of proinflammatory lipid mediators and disease states has been appreciated. PLA2 is ubiquitous in the body and is either membrane associated or secreted. It is not clear whether these two enzyme types are separate and distinct or if they are the same protein residing and acting in different environments. Generally, endogenous PLA2s are reported to have 10-100 fold lower specific activity than the secreted enzymes, even though this may be ascribed to different analytical procedures or relative purity of the enzymes examined. Nonetheless inhibition of PLA2 activity offers an attractive therapeutic approach to the design of novel antiinflammatory agents.

Endogenous Stimulation of PLA2

Various stimuli have been suggested to activate PLA2; angiotensin II, bradykinin, prolactin and thrombin, for example, release arachidonic acid (AA) when added to responsive cells. However, in these studies release of free fatty acids is tacitly assumed to be indicative of PLA2 action. This may or may not be the case since AA can also be derived from non-PLA2 mediated phospholipid hydrolysis. Similarly, while circumstantial evidence suggests that interleukin 1 (IL-1) stimulates PLA2 there has been no direct evidence to support this hypothesis. Our laboratories have now demonstrated that IL-1 induces the activation and secretion of PLA2 from chondrocytes and synovial fibroblasts (1,2). The activation of cell associated PLA2 is rapid and occurs with   new protein synthesis. IL-1 is unique in its ability to induce PLA2 since both IL-2 and IL-3 fail to stimulate PLA2. With time, there is an additional effect with IL-1 where the enzyme is actively secreted into the extracellular medium. It should be noted that other groups have now demonstrated that IL-1 can also induce cyclooxygenase (CO) activity which requires new enzyme synthesis.

Endogenous Inhibition of PLA2

PLA2 is regulated by endogenous inhibitors. This is necessary since cellular PLA2 is required for general membrane lipid remodeling and maintenance and in the release of substrate for conversion to potent lipid mediators. Indeed, antiinflammatory steroids owe their therapeutic actions to the induction of endogenous PLA2 inhibitory peptides termed lipocortins.

While lipocortins are important, regulation of PLA2 may be achieved through different mechanisms. End products such as hydroxyeicosatetraenoic acids (HETEs), free fatty acids (e.g. AA) and platelet activating factor (PAF) can all affect enzyme activity significantly. In fact acid extraction of platelet PLA2 which inactivates these lipids improves PLA2 activity. Low PLA2 activity detected under normal conditions may therefore, be due to HETEs and lipid mediators which are likely to be produced during homogenization of platelets.

Pathobiology of PLA2

Enzyme activity is markedly enhanced in blood, urine or inflammatory exudate fluids during septic shock, rheumatoid arthritis or systemic lupus erythematosis (3). The involvement of PLA2 in the pathophysiology of snake and bee venom toxicity is also well documented. While these studies are indicative of PLA2 action in vivo, the effects of enzymes derived from various non-mammalian and mammalian sources are not well defined. Therefore, our laboratories have initiated several lines of investigation both in vitro and in vivo on the consequences of PLA2 activation and inhibition.

Intradermal injections of 30 µg snake venom PLA2 (Naja. mocambique mocambique) in guinea pig skin resulted in a time- and dose-dependent increase in ^{125}I-BSA protein extravasation into the injected site. Injection of equimolar or greater concentrations of AA did not cause an inflammatory reaction of similar intensity, indicating that other PLA2-derived mediators unrelated to lipoxygenase (LO) or CO products are involved in the inflammatory reaction.

Skin sites, treated with PLA2 for 30 minutes, contained 15-HETE and PGD2 as the major eicosanoids followed by $PGF_{2\alpha}$ with trace amounts of LTC_4 and LTB_4. ^{125}I-BSA accumulation was partially reduced (37-56%) by injection of 100 µM indomethacin, a CO inhibitor; BW755c, a dual 5-LO and CO inhibitor; chlorpheniramine (CHL), an antihistamine; LY-171,883, a leukotriene antagonist or the platelet activating factor (PAF) antagonist, L-652,731 (Table 1). In all cases, injection of drug in the absence of PLA2 did not elicit protein extravasation. Notably a mixture of indomethacin, BW755C, CHL and LY-171,883 was very effective in inhibiting extravasation (75%). Oral administration of ibuprofen (200 mg/kg) or BW 755c (200 mg/kg) two hours before PLA2 challenge resulted in the inhibition of the major CO metabolites or the major LO metabolites present in the skin plugs, respectively. No change in AA metabolite formation was observed when animals were treated with CHL (2 mg/kg, p.o.) alone.

PLA2 also produced a significant concentration dependent (0.03 μg - 3.3 μg PLA2/paw) rise in paw edema. Edema formation was rapid, peaking at 10 minutes reducing slightly between 10 and 20 minutes and persisting over 60-180 minutes. The reaction was principally due to PLA2 action since the edema could be obviated by co-injection with p-bromophenacyl bromide, an irreversible PLA2 inhibitor. Furthermore, injection of other proteins such as bovine serum albumin produced no edema. Phenidone, indomethacin, cyproheptadine or aristolochic acid when co-injected individually with PLA2 all resulted in 25-75% inhibition of PLA2-induced edema formation (Table 1).

Table 1. Characterization of PLA2-Induced Models of Inflammation

Antiinflammatory Drug**	% Inhibition	
	PLA2 Induced Cutaneous Vascular Permeability (Guinea Pig)	PLA2 Induced Paw Edema (Mouse)
PLA2 Inhibitors		
p-Bromophenacyl bromide	80	81
Aristolochic Acid	ND	36
Cyclooxygenase Inhibitor		
Indomethacin	42	25
Lipoxygenase Inhibitors		
BW 755C	29	ND
Phenidone	ND	72
Antihistamines		
Chlorpheniramine	37	ND
Cyproheptadine	ND	75
Other		
Ly 171,883 (LTD4 Antagonist)	56	ND
L -652731 (PAF Antagonist)	37	ND

** Drugs, at concentrations that induced maximal response (10-100 μg/paw or skin plug), were co-injected with PLA2; ND = Not Done

Purified human platelet and synovial fluid PLA2 also produced a marked inflammatory reaction similar to that observed with snake venom PLA2 (FIG. 1). Since the amount of protein injected was several fold less in the human PLA2 enzymes (<50ng/paw) than in the snake venom (0.3μg/paw), the proinflammatory activity of the human PLA2 was considerably greater. Taken together, the data demonstrate that mammalian PLA2s initiate a similar sequence of inflammatory events which are consistent with the proinflammatory role of these enzymes.

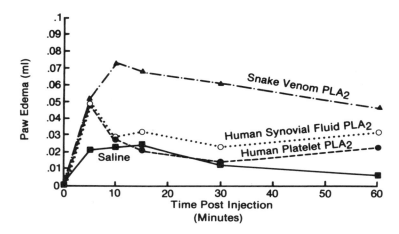

FIG. 1

In summary, we suggest that development and characterization of PLA2 inflammation models accompanied by simultaneous in vitro enzyme studies provide an avenue to identify and characterize novel inhibitors of PLA2. Such inhibitors may offer a novel therapeutic approach to treat a broad spectrum of inflammatory disorders.

BIBLIOGRAPHY

1. Chang J, Gilman SC, and Lewis AJ. J Immunol 1987;136: 1283-1287.

2. Gilman SC, Chang J, Zeigler PR, Uhl J, and Mochan E. Arth Rheum 1985;31:126-130.

3. Bomalaski JS, Clark MA, Crooke ST, Zurier RB. Fed Proc 1985;44:1204.

Advances in Prostaglandin, Thromboxane, and Leukotriene Research, Vol. 19, edited by B. Samuelsson, P. Y.-K. Wong, and F. F. Sun, Raven Press, Ltd., New York ©1989.

PHOSPHOLIPASE A_2 (PLA_2) RELEASE LEUKOTRIENES AND OTHER LIPOXYGENASE PRODUCTS FROM ENDOGENOUS SOURCES

Bing K. Lam and Patrick Y-K Wong

Department of Pharmacology
New York Medical College
Valhalla, New York   10595

Snake venoms contain a number of enzymes and toxins which have profound pathophysiologic effects on experimental animals and man. Some of them are neurotoxic whereas others may be more cytotoxic (1). Mechanisms of neurotoxicity of snake venoms have been extensively studied (2-4), however the adverse effects of snake venoms on the cardiovascular system are less well understood (5). Phospholipase A_2 (PLA_2), a major component of enzymes found in snake venoms, has been proposed to contribute many of these cardiotoxic effects, e.g., it can lyse erythrocytes, induce hypotension (6) and local capillary damage (7), influence the anticoagulant process (8). In addition, PLA_2 has been reported to release thromboxane A_2 and prostaglandin I_2 in rats (6,9) and leukotrienes from isolated perfused guinea pig lung (10). The findings that PLA_2 has a profound effect on the cardiovascular system, suggested that snake venom PLA_2 may affect leukocytes and other blood cells in addition to causing hemolysis. We now report that a PLA_2 isoenzyme of Russelli Vipera venom provokes the generation of leukotrienes and other lipoxygenase products from porcine, human and rat leukocytes.

METHODS AND MATERIAL

PLA_2 isoenzymes were prepared from Russell's viper venom (Sigma Chemical, St. Louis, MO), according to the method of Salach, et al. (11). The isoenzyme with an isoelectric point of 8.8 to 9.0 and molecular weight of 15,000 Da was used in this study.
Porcine leukocytes were isolated from mixed venous blood; rat polymorphonuclear leukocytes from peritoneal exudate of rats fed with eicosapentaenoic acid ethylester (EPA-E) and human leukocytes from human blood buffy coat.
After preincubation of 10-20 x 10^8 leukocytes (10-20 ml) for 5 min at 37°C in a shaking water bath, purified PLA_2 isoenzyme in 0.9% saline was added and the incubation continued for 10 min with continuous shaking. Incubations were terminated by addition of ice cold ethanol followed by immediate

centrifugation at 300 g for 20 min. PGB_2 (2 μg) was added
to the incubation extract as internal standard. After
extraction, the sample was dissolved in 50 μl methanol and
separated by RP-HPLC as described (12). Samples eluted from
HPLC were analyzed by U.V. spectroscopy and by gas
chromatography/mass spectrometry.

RESULTS

Incubation of 1.5 μg/ml (10^{-7}M) of PLA_2 isoenzyme
with porcine leukocytes caused the release of tri-, di- and
mono-hydroxy fatty acids as well as epoxide alcohol derivatives
of AA. Typical experiments yielded a total of twelve fractions
after RP-HPLC separation (Fig. 1). Fraction 1 contained
conjugated trihydroxytetraene identified as lipoxin B (LXB),
8-trans LXB and 14(S)-8-trans-LXB, based on their co-elution
with synthetic standards, U.V. spectra and GC/MS structural
analysis. Details of this identification and structural
elucidation of this group of compounds has been reported

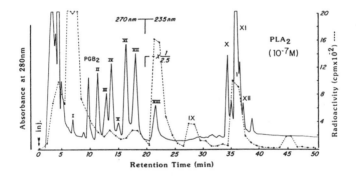

FIG. 1. RP-HPLC chromatograph of sample extract after
incubation of porcine leukocytes with 10^{-7}M PLA_2 under
conditions described under Methods. Materials eluted under
peaks were analysed by U.V. and GC/MS.

previously (12). Fractions II, III and IV contained isomers of
8,15-diHETE as identified by U.V. spectra and GC/MS. In
addition, SP-HPLC and GC/MS analysis revealed that both
fractions II and IV contained on isomer of 5,12-diHETE.
Fraction V showed U.V. λmax of 269 nm and shoulders at 259
and 280 nm. GC/MS revealed that it is an isomer of
5,12-diHETE. Materials eluted under peak VI displayed a U.V.
max of 270 nm with shoulders at 260 and 281 nm. The RP-HPLC
and SP-HPLC retention times as well as U.V. spectra of peak VI

were identical to those of authentic standard LTB_4. Analysis
of peaks VII to XII by U.V. spectrometry and GC/MS revealed that
they contained 14,15-diHETE, 12-HHT, 10-hydroxy-11,12-epoxy-
eicosatrienoic acid, 15-, 12- and 5-HETE, respectively.
Similarly, incubation of PLA_2 with human leukocyte resulted in
the generation of LTB_4, 20-OH-LTB_4, 20-COOH-LTB_4 and
5-HETE (data not shown). When PMN was isolated from peritoneal
exudate of EPA-E-treated rat was incubated with PLA_2, it
generated both LTB_4 and LTB_5 (fig. 2).

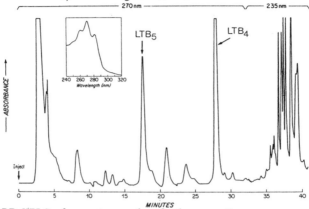

FIG. 2. RP-HPLC chromatograph of the sample extract after
incubation of rat PMN with venom PLA_2. Insert shows U.V.
spectra of materials co-eluted with LTB_4 and LTB_5.

DISCUSSION

Venom PLA_2 isoenzyme is a potent stimulus for the generation of AA metabolites from porcine, human and rat leukocytes as
well as eicosapentaenoic acid metabolites from rat PMN.
The release of large amounts of leukotrienes and other
lipoxygenase products from leukocytes by venom PLA_2 isoenzyme
suggests that endogenously released PLA_2 may play an important
role in inflammation. PLA_2 isoenzymes are released by
macrophages and other leukocytes during cell activation and
platelet aggregation and are present at sites of inflammation
(13-19). More importantly, PLA_2 has also been shown to
mediate inflammatory hyperemia (16). It is likely that
activated leukocytes release granular PLA_2 into the site of
inflammation. AA released by PLA_2 from membrane phospholipids
could be metabolized by either cyclooxygenases to form
prostaglandins or by lipoxygenases to yield leukotrienes and
lipoxins. Prostaglandins affect local vasculature to mediate
signs and symptoms of inflammation, while leukotrienes (i.e.,
LTB_4) recruit leukocytes to the site of inflammation to
further amplify the inflammatory process. The newly discovered
lipoxins could act as intracelluar signals to activate protein

kinase C (20,21) and hence alter cell functions.

In conclusion, our data indicate that PLA_2 isoenzyme isolated from Russell's viper venom is a potent stimulus for synthesis of leukotrienes and other lipoxygenase products in porcine human and rat leukocytes. Furthermore, it suggests that PLA_2 may be involved in the pathophysiology of inflammation. Moreover, the ease of availability of the isoenzyme and its ability to release a wide range of AA metabolites from leukocytes make it a valuable tool for leukotriene and lipoxin research.

REFERENCES

1. Lee CY. In: Cecarelli B, Clementi F, eds. Advances in Cytopharmacology. New York: Raven Press, 1979;1-16.
2. Lee CY. Annu Rev Pharmacol 1972;12:265-284.
3. Ryden L, Gabel G, Eaker D. Int J Peptide Protein Res 1973;5:261-273.
4. Chang CC. In: Lee CY, ed. Handbook of Experimental Pharmacology: Snake Venoms. Berlin: Springer-Verlag, 1979;309-376.
5. Lee CY, Lee SY. In: Lee CY, ed. Handbook of Experimental Pharmacology: Snake Venoms. Berlin: Springer-Verlag, 1979;547-590.
6. Ho CL, Lee CY. Proc Natl Sci Counc ROC, Part B, 1981;5:181-189.
7. Suzuki T, Iwanaga S. In: Erdos ED, eds. Handbook of Experimental Pharmacology: Snake Venoms. Berlin: Springer, 1970;193-197.
8. Boffa MC, Boffa GA. Biochem Biophys Acta 1976;429:839-852.
9. Blackwell GF, Flower RJ, Nykamp FP, Vane JR. Br J Pharmac, 1978;62:70-89.
10. Huang HC. Toxicon, 1984;22:359-372.
11. Salach JI, Turini P, Seng R, Hauber J, Singer TP. J Biol Chem, 1971;246:331-339.
12. Lam BK, Serhan CN, Samuelsson B, Wong PYK. Biochem Biophys Res Commun, 1987;144:123-131.
13. Weissman G, Smolen JE, Korchak HM. N Engl J Med, 1980;303:27-34.
14. Movat HZ. In: Inflammation, Immunity and Hypersensitivity. New York: Harper and Row Publishers, 1984;1-161.
15. Victor M, Weiss J, Klemper MS, Elsbach. FEBS Letters, 1981;136:298-300.
16. Vadas P, Wasi A, Mount HZ, Hay JB. Nature, 1981;293:583-585.
17. Vadas P, Hay JB. Int Arch Allergy Appl Immunol, 1980;62:142-151.
18. Vadas P, Hay JB. Life Sciences, 1980;26:1721-1729.
19. Vadas P, Hay JB. Am J Pathol, 1982;107:285-291.
20. Hansson A, Serhan CN, Haeggstrom J, Ingelman-Sunbert M, Samuelsson B. Biochem Biophys Res. Commun, 1986;134:1215-1222.
21. Nishizuka Y. Nature (Lond), 1984;225:1365-1370.

*Advances in Prostaglandin, Thromboxane, and
Leukotriene Research*, Vol. 19, edited by
B. Samuelsson, P. Y.-K. Wong, and F. F. Sun,
Raven Press, Ltd., New York ©1989.

DIFFERENCES IN n-3 AND n-6 EICOSANOID PRECURSORS

William E.M. Lands

Department of Biochemistry, University of Illinois
at Chicago, Chicago, Illinois 60612

Eicosanoid biosynthesis is suppressed under most normal conditions, and rapid metabolic inactivation of eicosanoids increases the importance of the explosive burst of biosynthesis that occurs when oxygenase activity is stimulated by hydroperoxides (1). Only when the stimulated rate of biosynthesis exceeds the metabolic inactivation would we expect to see the pathophysiological phenomena that are commonly associated with an overproduction of eicosanoids. Cell-cell interactions can accelerate these events by providing the activators (e.g., hydrogen peroxide (2)) that promote a more rapid rate of eicosanoid biosynthesis. By merely slowing the enhanced biosynthetic rate, antagonists can decrease the local pathology without necessarily altering the overall amount of whole-body eicosanoid formed in a 24-hr period.

The n-3 fatty acid, 20:5n-3, is much less able than 20:4n-6 to sustain rapid synthesis of prostanoids in the presence of peroxidase activity (3). This ineffectiveness led to the recognition that n-3 fatty acids could antagonize eicosanoid biosynthesis from 20:4n-6 (4). Because many diseases and disorders are associated with an overproduction of n-6 eicosanoids, there is now a widespread interest in the possible benefits of nutritional supplements of n-3 fats in moderating disorders associated with excessive rates of eicosanoid formation and function (5).

Availability of n-6 eicosanoid precursors is dramatically affected by the conversion of the 18-carbon polyunsaturated fatty acids (PUFA) to the more highly unsaturated 20- and 22-carbon fatty acids (HUFA). All of these acids interact with the different enzymes for phospholipid biosynthesis with 18-carbon PUFA favored in the de novo pathway, the 18-carbon PUFA and 20-carbon HUFA in the retailoring pathway (6), and the 22-carbon HUFA in the CDP ethanolamine:diacylglycerol ethanolaminephosphotransferase pathway (7). However, none of these synthetic paths is reported to discriminate appreciably between n-3 or n-6 acids. The combined effect of fatty acid supply and enzyme specificity maintains a "typical" steady-state composition of acyl chains among the various cellular lipids that are regarded to be hydrolyzed to give non-esterified fatty acids (NEFA), the immediate precursor of eicosanoids (8). The n-3 HUFA are more effective than the n-3 PUFA in antagonizing oxygenation of n-6 HUFA (4).

Investigators often discuss the relative abundance of n-3 and n-6 fatty acids in the phospholipids as an index to possible antagonisms in forming the n-6 eicosanoids. However, a failure to match observed phospholipid compositions with the altered responses requires careful interpretation, because the eicosanoids are formed directly from the NEFA rather than the phospholipids (8). A pulse of dietary 20:4 gave a corresponding pulse of metabolites excreted in the urine in the following 24-hr period (9) without significant effect on the composition of lipid esters. Dietary 18:2n-6 also increased the average daily excretion of prostaglandin metabolites (10), although the response seemed less dramatic due to the need to convert the 18-carbon acid to 20:4n-6. Dietary 18:2n-6 also increased the formation of tumors in experimental models (11,12) while the tissue phospholipids exhibited an increased content of 18:2n-6 and no change in 20:4n-6 (12). Added n-3 acids also modified responses more than expected from the slight change observed in the phospholipid esters (13,14). Apparently, the phospholipid content is not a clear indicator of HUFA accessibility to eicosanoid-forming oxygenases.

The paradox of an apparent change in eicosanoid formation from arachidonate without any evident change in esterified arachidonate led us to reexamine the access of NEFA-20:4 to the active site of the PGH synthase. The pure enzyme has an apparent K_m for 20:4n-6 of about 2 μM. However, cytosolic protein increased this value about 10 nanomoles for each mg protein added (15) suggesting that more than 500 μM 20:4n-6 would be needed for the enzyme to function at half-maximal speed in the presence of native cytosol with its 80-100 mg/protein/ml. This finding indicates that none of the standard kinetic studies of enzyme specificity can approximate the conditions of viscosity, turbidity and protein binding that prevail in vivo, and that subtle differences among n-3 and n-6 acids may be overlooked.

Non-esterified fatty acids are a principal mode of lipid transport in plasma (ca. 500 μM bound to albumin), and we noted total NEFA in liver and heart were 2500 and 700 μM, respectively (16). Within these pools, the corresponding contents of 20:4-NEFA were 310 and 140 μM, much greater than needed to give a maximal velocity with the pure oxygenase and yet the oxygenation remains suppressed in vivo. Thus, we considered whether this large reservoir of NEFA-20:4 was accessible to enzymes other than the oxygenase. Since the ligase reaction is the other

important metabolic step for NEFA, we set out to estimate
how nutritional interventions alter the movement of n-3 and
n-6 acids through cellular acyl-CoA pools. To do this we
developed a new micromethod for quantitating the acyl chain
composition of the acyl-CoA esters (17). Acyl-CoA esters
in liver or heart were only about 100 μM, about one-tenth
as abundant as the NEFA, and they contained large amounts
of 18:0, 18:2 and 20:4 (16).

We noted that the NEFA and acyl-CoA were not altered in
parallel when a changed dietary supply of acids altered the
composition of tissue esters. The mole% of 20:4n-6 was
consistently greater in the acyl-CoA pool than the NEFA,
whereas 20:5n-3 was more abundant in NEFA than the acyl-CoA
(18). When using chow plus corn oil, with only 18:2n-6 as
the dietary PUFA/HUFA, the NEFA and acyl-CoA pools
contained large amounts of 18:2n-6, 14-16 mol% 20:4n-6, and
negligible amounts of n-3 HUFA. This pattern reflected
extensive conversion of 18:2-CoA to 20:4-CoA. However,
when 14% 18:2n-6 was ingested with 15% n-3 HUFA, the
steady-state level of 6% 20:4n-6 in NEFA was accompanied by
7% 20:5n-3 and 17% 22:6n-3. Ratios for the n-3 HUFA/n-6
HUFA were NEFA>acyl-CoA<phospholipid.

n-3/n-6 ratio in HUFA	NEFA	Acyl-CoA	Phospholipid
chow with corn oil	0.1	0.06	0.3
chow with fish oil	5.0	0.5	1.0

With corn oil added to a diet based on sucrose-casein
rather than chow, the rapid conversion of 18:2-CoA to
20:4-CoA led to higher steady-state levels of HUFA-CoA
(18). On the other hand, the low dietary 18:2n-6 with the
fish oil supplement gave lower 18:2-NEFA and 18:2-acyl-CoA,
and the increased n-3 HUFA-CoA appeared to antagonize the
conversion of 18:2-CoA to 20:4-CoA. The amount of n-3
HUFA-CoA (14 mol%) equalled the n-6 HUFA-CoA (15 mol%),
whereas the NEFA had a ratio of 13 (38 mol% n-3 HUFA to
only 3 mol% n-6 HUFA). The different selectivities for
entry and exit from the NEFA pool apparently created ratios
of n-3 HUFA to n-6 HUFA that were higher in NEFA than in
phospholipid.

Thus, further study of the accessiblity of HUFA
precursors and antagonists in the NEFA and acyl-CoA pools
seems warranted. The high ratio in the NEFA pool that is
the immediate precursor of eicosanoids (8) may relate to
the physiological effects that were not well related to the
n-3/n-6 ratios in the esterified lipids. Overall, our
earlier report (8) that phospholipids serve as a reservoir
of eicosanoid precursors needs refocusing to emphasize that
NEFA are the immediate precursors and to acknowledge two
sources of cellular NEFA: hydrolysis of cellular lipids and
entry of nutrient acids.

References

1. Hemler ME, Cook HL, Lands WEM. Arch Biochem Biophys 1979; 193: 340-345.

2. Marshall PJ, Lands WEM. J Lab Clin Med 1986; 108: 525-534.

3. Lands WEM, Byrnes MJ. Prog Lipid Res 1981; 20: 287-290.

4. Lands WEM, LeTellier, PR, Rome LH, Vanderhoek JY. Adv Biosci 1973; 9:15-27.

5. Lands WEM. Fish and Human Health, Orlando: Academic Press, 1986.

6. Hill EE, Husbands DH, Lands WEM. J Biol Chem 1968; 243: 4440.

7. Masuzawa Y, Nakagaway, Waku K, Lands WEM. Biochem Biophys Acta 1982; 713: 185-192.

8. Lands WEM, Samuelsson B. Biochim Biophys Acta 1968; 164: 426.

9. Ramesha CS, Gronke RS, Sivarajan M, Lands WEM. Prostaglandins 1985; 29: 991-1008.

10. Nugteren DH, van Evert WC, Soeting WJ, Spuy JH. Adv Prost Thromb Res 1980; 8: 1793-1796.

11. Ip C, Carter CA, Ip MM. Cancer Res 1985; 45: 1997-2001.

12. Hubbard NE, Erikson KL. Cancer Res 1987; 47: 6171-6175.

13. Lands WEM, Culp BR, Hirai A, Gorman R. Prostaglandins 1985; 30: 819-825.

14. Lee TH, et al. New Eng J Med 1985; 312: 1217-1224.

15. Marshall PJ, Kulmacz RJ, Lands WEM. J Biol Chem 1987; 262: 3510-3517.

16. Masuzawa Y, Prasad MR, Lands WEM Biochim Biophys Acta 1987; 919: 297-306.

17. Prasad MR, Sauter J, Lands WEM. Anal Biochem 1987; 162: 202-212.

18. Prasad MR, Culp B, Lands WEM. J. Biosciences 1987; 11: 443-453.

Advances in Prostaglandin, Thromboxane, and Leukotriene Research, Vol. 19, edited by B. Samuelsson, P. Y.-K. Wong, and F. F. Sun, Raven Press, Ltd., New York ©1989.

THE EFFECTS OF A FISH OIL ENRICHED DIET ON EXPERIMENTALLY-INDUCED AND CLINICAL ASTHMA

Tak H. Lee and Jonathan P. Arm, Dept of Medicine, Guy's Hospital, London SE1 9RT, U.K.

Introduction

The two major types of polyunsaturated fatty acids prominent in marine fish oils are eicosapentaenoic acid (EPA) (20:5,n-3) and docosahexaenoic acid (DCHA) (22:6,n-3). EPA and DCHA competitively inhibit the conversion of arachidonic acid by the cyclooxygenase pathway to prostanoid metabolites (1,2). The endoperoxide and thromboxane A3 derived from EPA are substantially less active than the arachidonic acid derived counterparts in eliciting aggregation of human platelets (3,4). DCHA is not metabolised to any cyclooxygenase product. With respect to the metabolism of EPA and DCHA by the 5 lipoxygenase cascade, EPA is converted to LTB5, LTC5, LTD5 and LTE5 . DCHA is metabolized only to the 7- and 4-hydroperoxy DCHA and their reduction products, 7- and 4-hydroxy DCHA, respectively. LTB5 is substantially less active than LTB4 in a number of pro-inflammatory functions (5-8), but LTC5 and LTC4 are equiactive in constricting non-vascular smooth muscle (9,10). Thus EPA is capable of inhibiting the elaboration of inflammatory mediators by the cyclooxygenase pathway and is metabolized to LTB5 with attenuated biological activity.

Non-esterified EPA but not DCHA inhibits the generation of LTB4 at the level of the epoxide hydrolase. EPA is converted to LTB5 (11). In addition, treatment of monocyte monolayers with EPA at the optimal concentration of 1 ug/ml decreased paf-acether generation (12). LTB4 and paf-acether are pro-inflammatory mediators. The capacity of EPA to inhibit their generation could be considered as an anti-inflammatory effect.

The effects of supplementing the diet with fatty acids derived from fish oil on the 5-lipoxygenase pathway activity of PMN and monocytes have been studied in seven normal human subjects, who supplemented their usual diets for 6 weeks with daily doses of Max EPA containing 3.2 g of EPA and 2.2 g of DCHA (13). The diet increased the EPA content in PMN and monocytes more than seven-fold without changing the quantities of arachidonic acid and DCHA.

When the PMN were activated in vitro with the ionophore A23187, the release of arachidonic acid and its metabolites were reduced by a mean of 37% and the maximum generation of the major 5-lipoxygenase metabolites, including LTB4, was reduced by a mean of 48%. When monocyte monolayers were activated with the ionophore A23187, the release of arachidonic acid and its metabolites was reduced by a mean of 39% and the generation of LTB4 was suppressed by 58%. In addition, the generation of paf-acether was inhibited by approximately 50% (12). The adherence of PMN to endothelial cell monolayers which had been pre-treated with LTB4 was inhibited completely and their average chemotactic response to LTB4 was inhibited by 70% as compared with values determined before the diet was started (13).

The margination of leukocytes to endothelial surfaces is the initial step in the recruitment of cells by a chemotactic stimulus to an inflammatory focus. Thus the impairment of leukocyte function caused by the dietary incorporation of fish oil fatty acids into membrane phospholipids would be expected to be anti-inflammatory. This effect would be amplified by the substantial suppression of the biosynthesis of arachidonic acid-derived metabolites and paf-acether.

Studies in bronchial asthma

Asthma is characterised by airways inflammation, by bronchial hyperresponsiveness to non-specific stimuli, and by episodic and reversible airflow obstruction. Studies in both experimental animals and man have indicated an association between airways hyperresponsiveness and bronchial inflammation. Since airway inflammation may be important in the pathophysiology of bronchial asthma, we have investigated the effects of a fish-oil enriched diet in subjects with mild bronchial asthma (14).Subjects received capsules containing 3.2gm EPA and 2.2 gm DCHA or identical placebo capsules containing olive-oil in a double blind fashion. There was incorporation of EPA into PMN phospholipids from barely detectable amounts prior to treatment to comprising 2.6% of total PMN fatty acids following dietary supplementation with fish-oil. In addition PMN from subjects who had received fish-oil demonstrated a 50% reduction in the generation of LTB (LTB4 and LTB5) in response to calcium ionophore, and a substantial attenuation of their chemotactic responses to FMLP and LTB4. In subjects who had received placebo, the phospholipid content of EPA, LTB4 generation and chemotactic responses of PMN were unchanged. The changes in neutrophil function in subjects who had ingested EPA were not accompanied by changes in airways non-specific responsiveness, or severity of asthma.

Payan et al have studied the effects of EPA in subjects with severe persistent asthma (15). Two groups of six subjects received either 0.1 or 4.0gm of purified EPA a day in a double blind fashion for eight weeks. Both doses of EPA led to a small, but significant generation of LTB5 by PMN and mixed mononuclear leukocytes in response to calcium ionophore, A23187. Only high dose EPA suppressed ionophore induced LTB4 generation by PMN and mononuclear leukocytes. High dose EPA also supressed neutrophil, but not mononuclear leukocyte, chemotaxis to C5a, FMLP and LTB4. Changes in leukocyte function were not accompanied by changes in severity of asthma (16).

The effect of a 6 week fish oil enriched diet containing 3g EPA was studied in 10 patients with aspirin-intolerant asthma (17). Peak flow rates were lower and bronchodilator use was greater during the fifth and sixth week of the fish oil diet than during the control diet. This suggests that a fish oil diet may have a deleterious effect on asthmatic patients with aspirin sensitivity.

We have recently studied the effect of a fish-oil enriched diet on both early and late asthmatic responses to antigen (18). There were no changes in the acute airways response to antigen, but there was a significant attenuation of the late asthmatic response in subjects who had received fish-oil. There were no changes in immediate cutaneous responses to antigen, total serum IgE, or airway responses to histamine in the same subjects. In so far as airways inflammation is believed to be central to the pathophysiology of the allergen-induced late asthmatic response, the attenuation of the late phase reaction by fish oil is consistent with an anti-inflammatory effect.

Conclusions

These studies extend previous observations in normal subjects and demonstrate that a fish-oil enriched diet attenuates PMN functions in subjects with asthma. The associated attenuation of the late asthmatic response to antigen suggests that these alterations in leukocyte function were sufficient to reduce the induction of airways inflammation. The lack of any clinical benefit in subjects with either mild disease (14) or in subjects with severe persistent asthma (16) who are ingesting fish oil may have been due to insufficient time for regeneration of airways epithelium and resolution of the chronic inflammatory response to effect a change in clinical variables. In addition, the ingestion of fish oil may lead to a deterioration of asthma in patients with aspirin-sensitivity.

References
1. Needleman P, Raz A, Minkes N S, Ferendelli A, Sprecher H. Triene prostacyclin and thromboxane biosynthesis and unique biological properties. Proc Natl Acad Sci USA 1979; 76: 944- 8.
2. Corey E J, Shih C, Cashman J R. Docosahexaenoic acid is a strong inhibitor of prostaglandin but not leukotriene biosynthesis. Proc Natl Acad Sci USA 1983; 80:3581 - 4.
3. Dyerberg J, Bang H O, Stofferson E, Moncada S, Vane J R. Eicosapentaenoic acid and prevention of thrombosis and atherosclerosis. Lancet 1978; 2:117-9
4. Whitaker M O, Wyche A, Fitzpatrick F, Sprecher H, Needleman P. Triene prostaglandins: Prostaglandin D3 and eicosapentaenoic acid as potential antithrombotic substances. Proc Natl Acad Sci USA 1979; 76:5919-23.
5. Goldman D W, Pickett W C, Goetzl E J. Human neutrophil chemotactic and degranulating activities of leukotriene B5 (LTB5) derived from eicosapentaenoic acid. Biochem Biophys Res Commun

1983; 117:282 - 8.
6.   Lee T H, Mencia-Huerta J M, Shih C, Corey E J, Lewis R A, Austen K F.   Characterisation and biological properties of 5,12-dihydroxy derivatives of eicosapentaenoic acid including leukotriene B5 and the double lipoxygenase product. J Biol Chem 1984; 259:2383-9.
7.   Terano T, Salmon J A, Moncada S.   Biosynthesis and biological activity of leukotriene B5. Prostaglandins 1984; 27:217-32.
8.   Lee T H, Sethi T, Crea AEG, Peters W, Arm J P, Horton C E, Walport M J, Spur B W. Characterisation of leukotriene B3. Comparison of its biological activities with leukotriene B4 and leukotriene B5 in complement receptor enhancement, lysozyme release and chemotaxis of human neutrophils. Clin Sci. 1988; 74:467-75.
9.   Dahlen S E, Hedqvist P, Hammarstrom S.   Contractile activities of several cysteine-containing leukotrienes in the guinea pig lung strip. Eur J Pharmacol 1982; 86:207-15.
10.   Leitch A G, Lee T H, Ringel E W, Prickett J D, Robinson D R, Pyne S G, Corey E J, Drazen J M, Austen K F, Lewis R A. Immunologically-induced generation of tetraene and pentaene leukotrienes in the peritoneal cavities of menhaden-fed rats. J Immunol. 1984;132:2559 - 64.
11.   Lee T H, Mencia Huerta J M, Shih C, Corey E J, Lewis R A, Austen K F.   Effects of exogenous arachidonic, eicosapentaenoic, and docosahexaenoic acids on the generation of 5-lipoxygenase pathway products by ionophore-activated human neutrophils. J Clin Invest 1984;74:1922-33.
12.   Sperling R I, Robin J L, Kylander K A, Lee T H, Lewis R A, Austen K F.   The effects of N-3 polyunsaturated fatty acids on the generation of platelet-activating factor-acether by human monocytes. J Immunol. 1987; 139: 4186-91.
13   Lee T H, Hoover R L, Williams J D, Sperling R I, Ravalese J, Spur B W, Robinson D R, Corey E J, Lewis R A, Austen K F. Dietary enrichment with eicosapentaenoic and docosahexaenoic acids in human subjects impairs in vitro neutrophil and monocyte function and leukotriene generation. N Engl J Med 1985;312:1217-24
14.   Arm J P, Horton C E, Mencia-Huerta J M, House F, Eiser N M, Clark T J H, Spur B W, Lee T H.   Effect of dietary supplementation with fish oil lipids on mild asthma. Thorax. 1988: 43: 84-92.
15.   Payan D G, Wong Y S, Chernov-Rogan T.   Alterations in human leukocyte function induced by ingestion of eicosapentaenoic acid. J Clin Immunol 1986; 78: 937-42.
16.   Kirsch C M, Payan D M, Wong M Y S et al.   the effect of eicosapentaenoic acid in asthma. Clin Allergy (in press).
17.   Picado C, Castillo J A, Schinca N et al.   Effects of a fish oil enriched diet on aspirin intolerant asthmatic patients: a pilot study. Thorax 1988: 43: 93-97.
18.   Arm J P, Horton C E, Eiser N M, Clark T J H, Lee T H. The effects of dietary supplementation with fish oil on asthmatic responses to antigen. (Abstract) J Allergy Clin Immunol 1988; 81: 57.

Advances in Prostaglandin, Thromboxane, and
Leukotriene Research, Vol. 19, edited by
B. Samuelsson, P. Y.-K. Wong, and F. F. Sun,
Raven Press, Ltd., New York ©1989.

THE EFFECT OF HIGHLY PURIFIED EICOSAPENTAENOIC ACID

IN PATIENTS WITH PSORIASIS

T. Terano, T. Kojima*, A. Seya, E. Tanabe*, A. Hirai,
H. Makuta**, A. Ozawa**, T. Fujita**, Y. Tamura,
S. Okamoto*, and S. Yoshida

2nd Department of Internal Medicine, *Department of Dermatology,
Chiba University School of Medicine, Inohana, Chiba 280, Japan;
**Central Research Laboratory, Nippon Suisan Kaisha,
Kitano-cho, Hachioji, Tokyo 192, Japan

We have been demonstrating the anti-inflammatory effect of
eicosapentaenoic acid (EPA) and shown that EPA ingestion could
reduce the formation of proinflammatory eicosanoids such as PGE_2
and LTB_4 in inflammatory exudates and neutrophils and suppress
the chemotactic activity of neutrophils (1,2). Other investigators have recently reported that fish oil could suppress the
disease activity of chronic inflammatory disorders such as
rheumathoid arthritis and psoriasis (3,4,5). Fish oil contains
both EPA and docosahexaenoic acid (DHA). DHA was reported to
have anti-inflammatory effect although it is weak compared with
EPA (2).
Therefore present study was performed to evaluate the anti-
inflammatory effect of EPA on one of chronic inflammatory
disorders, psoriasis, using highly purified EPA.

STUDY DESIGN

EPA ethylester (EPA-E, 90% pure) without containing DHA at a
daily dose of 3.6 g was administered to 9 patients with chronic
stable psoriasis (male 4, female 5, age 22 to 75) for 3 to 6
months. Patients were instructed to keep their diet and to
continue with their usual topical treatment (mild to moderate
corticosteroids). The severity of skin lesions were rated on 6
points scales for erythema, scaling and thickness every 2 weeks.
Following biochemical parameters were measured at 1, 3 and 6
month after EPA treatment; plasma fatty acid composition by GLC,
eicosanoids formation by A23187 (2 µM) stimulated neutrophils by
RP-HPLC as previously reported (2).
Measurements before and after treatment were compared using a
paired t-test.

RESULTS AND DISCUSSION

The change of skin lesion after EPA treatment was summarized in Fig. 1. Both scaling and erythema had significantly improved 3 month after EPA treatment and this improvement had been maintained until 6 months. Similar and significant improvement was observed in thickness of skin.

Supplementation of EPA caused significant increase in the content of plasma EPA (2.54 ± 0.55, 9.08 ± 0.94, 9.35 ± 0.69 and 10.29 ± 2.74 at 0, 1, 3 and 6 months after EPA ingestion, respectively, mole %, mean $\pm$ SE, $p < 0.01$) without affecting the content of arachidonic acid (AA) and DHA.

EPA treatment decreased the production of LTB_4 and increased the formation of LTB_5 significantly in A23187 stimulated neutrophils shown in Table 1.

Psoriasis is an chronic inflammatory dermatosis in which AA metabolism may play an important role. Increased level of LTB_4 and 12-HETE in the psoriatic plaque was reported.

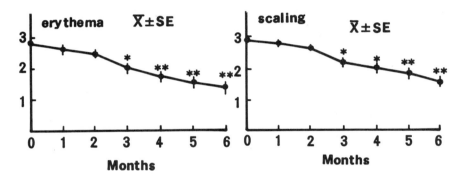

FIG. 1. Effect of EPA treatment on scaling and erythema scores. *$p < 0.05$, **$p < 0.01$

TABLE 1. Effect of EPA on 5-lipoxygenase metabolites formation in A23187 stimulated neutrophils

	LTB_4	LTB_5	5HETE	5HEPE	LTB_5/LTB_4
before	102.3 (13.7)	3.3 (0.51)	202.7 (11.5)	11.5 (3.25)	0.045 (0.01)
after 1M	75.3* (7.74)	12.0** (1.21)	174.0 (9.10)	73.0** (8.91)	0.189** (0.02)
3M	80.3* (7.92)	14.5** (2.77)	196.1 (33.3)	88.7** (7.10)	0.194** (0.02)
6M	71.2* (16.1)	15.0* (3.28)	155.9 (32.8)	81.1* (15.3)	0.240* (0.04)

ng/10^7 neutrophils   mean (S.E.)   *$p < 0.05$, **$p < 0.01$

We demonstrates that highly purified EPA can improve the psoriatic skin lesions over 6 months without any side effects. This clinical improvement by EPA might relate to the reduction of LTB_4 formation and increase in LTB_5 formation in stimulated neutrophils.

The formation of 5HETE (Table 1) and 6-trans-isomers of LTB_4 (data not shown) was not affected by EPA ingestion. These data suggested that EPA, or one of its metabolites such as LTA_5, would suppress the LTA_4 hydrolase resulting in the reduction of LTB_4. Nathaniel et al. (6) reported this possibility in vitro study.

LTB_5 is a weak and partial agonist in activating neutrophils. Interaction between formed LTB_4 and LTB_5 might play a role at inflammatory sites. Therefore the effect of LTB_5 on LTB_4 induced neutrophil activation was investigated. Shown in Fig. 2, LTB_5 itself was far less potent than LTB_4 in inducing β-glucuronidase release and the maximum response to LTB_5 was 60% that of LTB_4. LTB_5 suppressed the enhancement by LTB_4 (2×10^{-8} M) of β-glucuronidase release by 10% and 28%, respectively, at 2×10^{-9} M and 5×10^{-8} M LTB_5. Similar results, although used LTB_5/LTB_4 ratios were higher (10–1000) than ours, were reported by Kragballe et al. in LTB_4 induced activation of human keratinocytes and neutrophils (7). These data suggested that LTB_5 might decrease the response to concurrently present LTB_4 in a competitive manner most likely at receptor site.

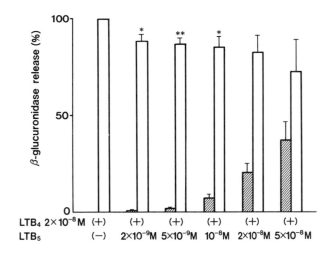

FIG. 2.   Effect of LTB_5 on LTB_4 (2×10^{-8} M) induced β-glucuronidase release in human neutrophils. Each point and bar is the mean and S.E. of 3 separate experiments. Release induced by LTB_4 plus LTB_5 (☐) was compared with that by LTB_5 (▨) alone. *p < 0.05, **p < 0.01

We previously reported that DHA might have also anti-inflammatory effect through the partial retroconversion to EPA and the modulation of membrane characteristics in healthy subjects (2). Therefore the effect of DHA on psoriasis is remained to be clarified.

REFERENCES

1. Terano T, Salmon JA, Higgs GA, Moncada S. Biochem Pharmacol 1986;35:779-785.

2. Terano T, Hirai A, Tamura Y, et al. In Advances in prostaglandin, thromboxane and leukotriene research 17B. New York: Raven Press, 1987;880-885.

3. Ziboh VA, Cohen KA, Ellis CN, et al. Arch Dermatol 1986;122: 1277-1282.

4. Maurice PDL, Allen BR, Barkley ASJ, et al. Br J Dermatol 1987;117:599-606.

5. Bittiner SB, Tucker WFG, Cartwright I, Bleehen SS. Lancet 1988;i:378-380.

6. Nathaniel DJ, Evans JF, Leblanc Y. Biochem Biophys Res Commun 1985;131:827-835.

7. Kragballe K, Voorhees JJ, Goetzl EJ. J Invest Dermatol 1987; 88:555-558.

Advances in Prostaglandin, Thromboxane, and Leukotriene Research, Vol. 19, edited by B. Samuelsson, P. Y.-K. Wong, and F. F. Sun, Raven Press, Ltd., New York ©1989.

MODULATION OF MEDIATOR PRECURSORS BY CHANGES IN

ESSENTIAL FATTY ACID COMPOSITION

W. C. Pickett and C. Ramesha*

Lipid Mediator Laboratory, Lederle Laboratories, Pearl River, NY 10965, USA; *The Syntex Corporation, Palo Alto, CA 94303 USA

Leukotriene (LT) and the Platelet Activating Factor (PAF) have been implicated in fundamental aspects of the inflamatory response. For example, both LTB and PAF actively induce leukocyte margination permitting the emigration of inflammatory cells to the extravasculature (1). Although similar with respect to a number of biological responses, these mediators are structurally diverse. While LTB_4 is derived from the essential fatty acid arachidonate, PAF is an 1-O-alkyl-Lecithin. Recently, however, a number of studies have associated PAF and LTB_4 with a common biosynthetic intermediate.

A direct substrate-product comparison (2) and data from the original structural characterization of PAF (3) indicated that the molecular species of PAF are much more homogenous than the precursor phospholipids (2). That PAF (in inflammatory cells) is derived via a deacylation-reacylation pathway (4,5) requiring arachidonic acid (20:4) has been strenghtened by findings that PAF biosynthesis is inhibited in PMNs depleted of 20:4 (6). One explanation for these findings is the existance of a highly specific alkyl-PLA_2 capable of differentiating 1-0-alkyl-2-20:4-GPC from the mead acid variant, 1-0-alkyl-2-20:3-GPC, generated during essential fatty acid deficiency (EFAD). Pursuant of this possibility, a sensitve assay for the presummed PAF intermediate, 1-O-hexadecyl-2-20:4-GPC, is described below.

METHODS

Isolated phospholipids were hydrolyzed to the 1,2-diglyceride by treatment with phospholipase C (7). The 1,2-diglycerides were immediately dissolved in 100 ul of dry acetonitrile to which 25 ul of

dimethylaminopyridine (1mg/ml) and 100 ul of 1-anthranitrile
(2mg/ml in acetonitrile) was added (FIG. 1).   After 30 min at 60° in a
sealed tube, excess reagent was quenched with 25 ul of methanol and
the solvent was evaporated.   The residue was dissolved in isopropanol
before analysis by reverse phase (C18) high pressure liquid
chromatography.   Typically, retention times of 23 min were obtained
for 1-O-hexadecyl-2-arachidonyl-3-anthroyltriglyceride with 75/25
acetonitrile/isopropanol as the mobile phase pumped at 2 ml/min.
Samples were detected at 261 nm.

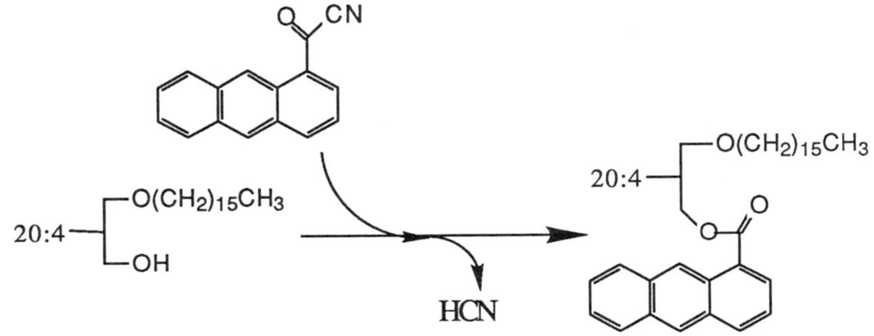

FIG. 1   Formation 1-O-hexadecyl-2-arachidonyl-3-anthroyl-
trigylceride.

RESULTS AND DISCUSSION

Previously we have described a highly sensitive and specific Gas
Chromatographic-Negative Ion Chemical Ionization Mass
Spectrometric method for the analysis of PAF molecular species as
diglycerol-pentaflurobenzoates(7).   When applied to phospholipids
with *sn*-2 fatty acids of normal chain length, these derivatives were
not volatile at temperatures compatible with gas chromatography.
Although the pentaflurobenzoates are well suited for reverse and
normal phase liquid chromatography, the extinction coefficient is
modest.   To enhance sensitivity without sacrificing chromatography,
the anthracene derivative shown in figure 1 was employed.   The
increase in extinction coefficient (>60,000) , allowed the generation
of a dose response curve linear to 20 pg (figure 2). Since the
diglycerides were immediately converted to the anthra diverivative,
there was no sign of acyl migation to the 1,3-digylceride.

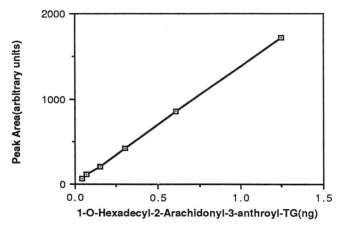

FIG. 3   Dose response curve for 1-O-hexadecyl-2-Arachidonyl-3-anthroyl-triglyceride.

As shown below, diets enriched with fish oil (3 months-10% in Menhadin) or devoid of essential fatty acids (3 months) reduced 20:4 52% and 90% respectively in rat peritoneal PMN. A similar response is seen for 1-O-hexadecyl-2-arachidonyl-GPC.   Depletion of this precursor beyond a critical point in the EFAD cells but not the Menhadin cells may explain the inhibitory effect EFAD on PAF biosynthesis.

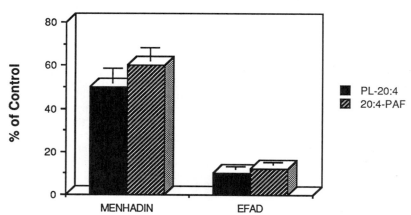

FIG 4.   The effect of EFAD and Menhadin fish oil on 1-O-hexadecyl-2-20:4-GPC(20:4-PAF) and total phospholipid 20:4(PL-20:4) in the rat PMN. The standard deviation of three samples is indicated.

REFERENCES

1. Chang SW, Fedderson CO, Henson PM, Voelkel NF. J Clin Invest 1987;79:1498-1509.

2. Clay KL, Murphy RC, Andress JL, Lynch J Henson P. Biochem Biophys Res Commun 1984;121:815-825.

3. Demopoulos CA, Pinckard RN, Hanahan DJ. J Biol Chem 1979;254:9355-58.

4. Synder F. Med Res Rev 1985; 5:107140.

5. Chilton FN, Ellis JM, Olson SC, Wykle RL. J Biol Chem 1984;259:12014-12019.

6. Ramesha C, Pickett WC. J Biol Chem 1986;261:7592-7595.

7. Ramesha C, Pickett WC. Biomed Environ. Mass Spect 1986;13:107-111.

*Advances in Prostaglandin, Thromboxane, and
Leukotriene Research*, Vol. 19, edited by
B. Samuelsson, P. Y.-K. Wong, and F. F. Sun,
Raven Press, Ltd., New York 1989.

FATTY ACID AND PHOSPHOLIPID SPECIES
COMPOSITION OF RAT TISSUES AFTER A FISH OIL DIET

Norman Salem Jr, Francoise Hullin,
Aron M. Yoffe, John W. Karanian and Hee-Yong Kim

Section of Analytical Chemistry
Laboratory of Clinical Studies, NIAAA, DICBR, ADAMHA
Building 10, Room 3C-218, 9000 Rockville Pike
Bethesda, MD, USA 20892

INTRODUCTION

The lipid composition of animal organs and blood cells is
dependent upon that of the diet. The fatty acyl composition of
mammalian tissues is, in particular, dependent upon the diet
since mammals are not capable of essential fatty acid synthesis
and appear to have a very limited capacity for fatty acid
desaturation and elongation. It has been generally shown that
supplementation of the diet with ω-3 PUFA, such as is found in
fish oil, leads to an increase in $20:5\omega3$ and $22:6\omega3$ and a
decrease in $20:4\omega6$. In order to evaluate the biophysical and
other biological effects of these compositional changes, it is
now important that a more detailed description of their distribution among lipid classes and molecular species within those
classes as well as their localization in biological membranes be
made. This paper will therefore present data concerning our
initial studies of fatty acyl and molecular species differences
between the tissues of rats fed either a corn oil or fish oil
diet.

METHODS

Male, Sprague Dawley rats of 60-70 g weights were obtained from
Taconic Farms. The animals were allowed to acclimate for 7 days
on a commercial rat chow diet. They were then divided into two
groups and one was fed a corn oil- and the other a fish oil-
based diet on an *ad libitum* basis. The basal diet (Teklad) was
similar in composition to that of the AIN-76A (1) except that
sucrose was reduced to 15% and replaced with corn starch, the

Teklad vitamin mix (#40060) was used in place of the AIN mix and calcium carbonate was added at a level of 0.43 wt%. The proportions of mineral mix, vitamin mix, protein and fiber in our diets (10 wt% fat) were each increased by a factor of 1.07 over those of the AIN-76A diet (5 wt% fat), so as to maintain the same ratio of nutrients to calories. The basal diets contained sufficient corn oil to yield a 1% final concentration in order to assure an adequate level of dietary 18:2ω6. The remaining 9% of the lipid was supplied as either microencapsulated corn or fish (menhaden) oil. The fish oil contained 14.5% of 20:5ω3, 8.0% of 22:6ω3, and 8.4% of other ω-3 fatty acids. The corn oil contained 57.5% of 18:2ω6, 0.9% of 18:3ω3 and 26.7% of 18:1. The microencapsulated oils were obtained from the Fish Oils Test Materials Program (DOC/ NIH/ADAMHA) and were a part of a feasibility study. The microencapsulated oils both contained the antioxidants α-tocopherol, γ-tocopherol and TBHQ at levels of 0.2, 0.1 and 0.02 g/kg of diet, respectively.

After 21 days of the dietary regimens, three animals from each group were killed by decapitation and the brains, liver and blood collected. Blood samples were centrifuged and the plasma and erythrocytes were separated. Platelets and red cells were washed in an isotonic buffered saline. Lipids were extracted using the method of Bligh and Dyer (2) and fatty acid methyl esters were formed by reaction with BF_3 in methanol as described by Morrison and Smith (3). Fatty acid methyl esters were analyzed by split mode injection (10:1) onto a 50 m x 0.25 mm OV-351 fused silica capillary column (Analabs) in an HP 5880 gas chromatograph, with helium as carrier gas at a linear velocity of 30 cm/s. The injector, detector and initial oven temperatures were 225, 225 and 200°C, respectively. The oven temperature was raised at a rate of 1°C/min for the first 25 min and thereafter kept constant at 225°C.

RESULTS AND DISCUSSION

After 21 days of these regimens, the average weight gains in the corn oil- and fish oil-fed groups were 101.4 and 97.0 g, respectively. Analysis of the fatty acyl distributions in five different tissues after either a corn oil or fish oil diet shows marked differences in their profiles (table 1). The 20:5ω3 content rose in liver, platelet, erythrocyte and plasma from undetectable or trace levels (< 0.1%) in the corn oil group to the 7.5 to 14.8% range in the fish oil group. There were also marked changes in the 22:6ω3 contents of the fish oil group tissues as they were 3-13 fold higher than those of the corn oil-fed animals. There were also increases in the levels of 22:5ω3 in the peripheral tissues of the fish oil-fed group. These ω-3 PUFAs appear to have replaced the ω-6 PUFAs 18:2ω6 and 20:4ω6 since the levels of these dropped appreciably. Erythrocyte phospholipids were separated and individually analyzed for acyl content. The phosphatidylcholine (PC) and phosphatidylethanolamine (PE) both showed marked increases in 20:5ω3 and

22:6ω3 as well as decreases in 18:2ω6 and 20:4ω6. Most of the 22:5ω3 increase and the 22:4ω6 decrease in the total lipid extract were confined to changes in the PE class. It is often said that the brain is resistant to changes in lipid composition induced by the diet, and this was born out in the present study in that brain composition did not change dramatically as did, for example, the liver. However, brain composition did change and this was reflected mainly as an increase in the 22:6ω3 content (from 11.6 to 14.0%), although 22:5ω3 also increased from 0.1 to 0.6%. There was no 18:3ω3 and only a trace of 20:5ω3 detected in the brains of the fish oil-fed animals. The 22:6ω3 increase was found mainly in the PE and PC with only a slight increase in the PS and no increase in the PI. The 22:5ω3 increased in both the PE and PS; 20:5ω3 reached 0.3 and 0.5% in the PE and PI, respectively, in the fish oil group but was less than 0.01% in the corn oil-fed animal phospholipids.

Table 1. Fatty acyl composition in the total lipid extracts of various tissues in rats after 21 days of either a microencapsulated corn oil or menhaden oil containing diet.

FATTY ACID	PLASMA CORN	PLASMA FISH	ERYTHROCYTE CORN	ERYTHROCYTE FISH	PLATELET CORN	PLATELET FISH	LIVER CORN	LIVER FISH
16:0	19.1	21.0	29.8	32.2	15.3	14.2	22.9	21.4
16:1	1.5	5.1	0.5	1.7	1.5	2.9	1.8	2.6
18:0	8.0	10.4	10.4	9.4	9.0	9.1	14.9	15.3
18:1	18.7	14.3	11.4	12.6	13.6	8.8	12.9	10.8
18:2ω-6	33.9	9.5	13.3	5.8	20.5	5.3	19.4	6.9
18:3ω-3	0.3	0.2	0.03	0.01	0.4	0.2	0.06	0.2
20:4ω-6	13.3	8.9	18.9	11.6	12.2	7.1	18.5	8.9
20:5ω-3	-	14.8	0.08	7.5	-	8.4	0.02	9.1
22:4ω-6	0.5	0.2	2.5	0.3	2.6	0.6	0.9	0.07
22:5ω-6	0.8	0.2	0.9	0.1	0.6	0.2	2.1	0.2
22:5ω-3	0.08	1.8	0.9	4.0	0.3	3.0	0.2	3.7
22:6ω-3	0.5	6.6	1.6	5.0	0.3	2.4	2.0	15.0
Unsat/Sat	2.5	2.0	1.3	1.2	2.3	1.8	1.5	1.6
ω-3/ω-6	0.02	1.2	0.07	0.9	0.03	1.0	0.05	1.7

Changes in the molecular species composition in some phospholipid classes have been analyzed in two different ways. The PC species in the brain, liver and erythrocyte were analyzed by thermospray LC/MS (4) after purification of the lipid classes by TLC. The reconstructed single ion chromatograms displayed in figure 1 show a decrease in the 16:0-18:2, 16:0-20:4 and 18:0-20:4 PC species accompanied by an increase in the 16:0-20:5, 16:0-22:5, 18:0-20:5 and 16:0-22:6 species in the erythrocytes of the fish oil-fed animals in comparison to those of the corn oil-fed group. A qualitatively similar redistribution of PC species was observed in liver and the changes were even more marked than those depicted for the erythrocytes. The brain showed a mild increase in the 16:0-22:6 and 18:0-22:6 PC species but 20:5ω3 species of PC were not observed.

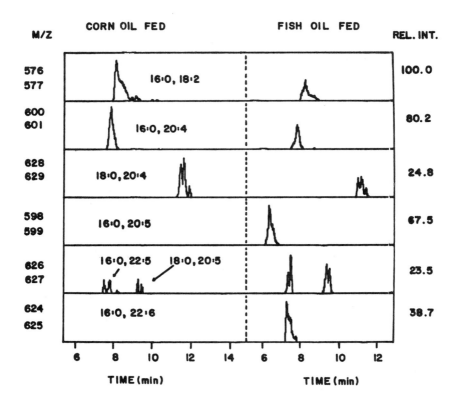

Figure 1. Thermospray LC/MS analysis of the major ω-3 and ω-6 PC species in rat erythrocytes after feeding a corn oil or fish oil diet. Conditions used were: Column, 3 μm Ultrasphere ODS, 0.46 x 7.5 cm; Probe, 142°C; Source, 250°C; Solvents, methanol-0.1 M ammonium acetate-hexane (500:25:25); Flow rate, 1 ml/min.

In the second method of species analysis, RBC PE was derivatized with trinitrobenzenesulfonic acid (TNBS), purified by TLC and subjected to RP-HPLC separation with UV detection at 338 nm. The data thus produced are complex as more than 38 species can be detected (figure 2). It is clear from an examination of these chromatograms that a quite different distribution of PE species is found in the RBC of animals fed these different diets. Current efforts will allow identification of these species and further delineate the topology of PE species changes in the plasma membranes of blood cells.

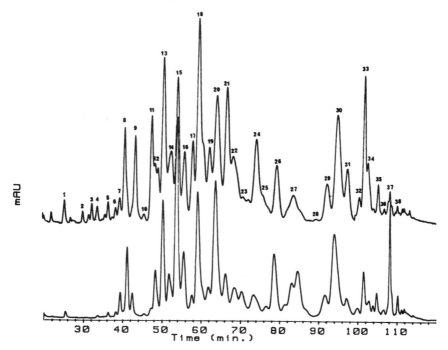

Figure 2. HPLC separation of trinitrophenyl derivatives of erythrocyte phosphatidylethanolamine from rats fed a fish oil (upper trace) or corn oil (lower trace) diet. Conditions used were: Column, 5 μm Axxi-chrom ODS, 0.46 x 25 cm; Oven temp, 40°C; Flow rate, 1 ml/min; Detection, UV at 338 nm; Solvents, (A) 10 mM ammonium acetate (pH 5), (B) methanol; Gradient, 5 min isocratic at 84% B followed by a linear rise to 87% B over the next 15 min, maintain 87% B for 70 min and then a linear rise to 93% B over the final 20 min (110 min analysis time).

1. American Institute of Nutrition Ad Hoc Committee on Standards for Nutritional Studies. J Nutr 1980;110:1726.

2. Bligh EG, Dyer WJ. Can J Biochem Physiol 1959;37:911-917.

3. Morrison WR, Smith LM. J Lipid Res 1964;5:600-608.

4. Kim HY, Yergey JA, Salem Jr N. J Chromatogr 1987;394:155-170.

*Advances in Prostaglandin, Thromboxane, and
Leukotriene Research*, Vol. 19, edited by
B. Samuelsson, P. Y.-K. Wong, and F. F. Sun,
Raven Press, Ltd., New York ©1989.

THE PHYSIOLOGY AND REGULATION OF THE INTESTINAL ABSORPTION AND
TRANSPORT OF OMEGA-3 AND OMEGA-6 FATTY ACIDS

Patrick Tso and Hiroshi Hayashi. Department of Physiology,
Louisiana State University Medical Center, Shreveport, LA 71130

SOURCES OF LUMINAL FATTY ACID

Triglyceride (TG) is the major dietary fat in humans.
Long-chain fatty acids (FA) such as oleate (C 18:1) and
palmitate (C 16:0) are the major FA present. Also present in
the intestinal lumen are long-chain FA of the omega-3 and
omega-6 family. These are mainly derived from diet, bile, or
cells shed from the intestinal mucosa. In humans, it has been
calculated that 11 - 12 g of biliary phospholipid (PL) enters
the small intestinal lumen daily, whereas the dietary
contribution is 1 - 2 g (1). The major FA present in biliary
PL are linoleate and arachidonate (2). When fish are
consumed, there is an increased intake of omega-3 FA, in
particular eicosapentaenoic acid (EPA) and docosahexaenoic acid
(DHA).

LUMINAL DIGESTION OF LIPID

Most of the digestion of TG occurs via pancreatic lipase at
the oil/water interface in the upper small intestine. The
velocity of lipolysis depends on factors which modify the
physicochemical properties of the interface as well as the
surface area (3). Pancreatic lipase acts predominantly at the
1- and 3-ester bonds of TG to release 2-monoglyceride (2-MG)
and free FA (4). Bile salts, at concentrations above the
critical micellar concentration, are potent inhibitors of the
lipolysis of TG, but the pancreas synthesizes another protein
that antagonizes the inhibitory action of bile salts. This
factor has been named colipase (5).

MICELLAR SOLUBILIZATION OF LIPID

Hofmann and Borgstrom have demonstrated that micellar
solubilization is extremely important in the uptake of lipid
digestion products by the small intestine (6). Micellar
solubilization is important because of the presence of an
unstirred water layer which acts as a barrier to the uptake of
FA. The formation of micelles greatly increases the
concentration of FA in the unstirred water layer adjacent to
the intestinal epithelial cell (enterocyte) surface, thereby
markedly enhancing the uptake of FA by the enterocytes.

623

FATTY ACID UPTAKE BY ENTEROCYTES

Although the uptake of most FA is passive (7), this is not true for uptake of linoleate by the enterocytes. Hollander and colleagues have shown that, in the unanesthetized rat, linoleate is absorbed by a concentration-dependent dual mechanism of transport (8). At low physiological concentrations (<1,260 μm), uptake observes saturation kinetics. With higher concentrations (2.5 - 4.5 mM), uptake is predominantly passive. The absorption rate of linoleate is pH dependent and is influenced by the presence of other polyunsaturated FA. When linoleate absorption was studied in rats of different ages, it was found that the ability to absorb linoleate increases dramatically as the animal ages (9). Whether arachidonate uptake behaves in the same way as linoleate is not known. EPA is readily absorbed by the small intestine and the uptake rates of the FA is comparable to that of oleate (10).

METABOLISM OF ABSORBED FATTY ACIDS

Once the FA enter the cell, the major site of metabolism is the endoplasmic reticulum (ER) (11). The mode of transport of these digestion products is presumably simple diffusion. A fatty acid binding protein (FABP) has been described and characterized (12). Ockner and Manning (12) suggest a possible role of FABP in regulating TG biosynthesis by adjusting the amount of FA made available for activation and incorporation into TG. The absorbed 2-MG and FA are reconstituted into TG mainly through the monoglyceride pathway. The enzymes involved exist as a complex called "triglyceride synhetase" (13). The other pathway for the synthesis of TG from the absorbed FA is the α-glycerophosphate pathway. The α-glycerophosphate pathway is particularly important under conditions in which the supply of FA is more abundant than MG. The diglyceride formed from the α-glycerophosphate pathway can also be used in the biosynthesis of phosphatidylcholine (PC) via the Kennedy Pathway (14). When the absorption of arachidonate and linoleate were studied, it was found that a substantial amount of arachidonate was transported into lymph as PL rather than as TG (15). The relative incorporation of arachidonate into PL and TG was dependent on the presence of other lipids in the lipid test meal. Furthermore, the study also demonstrated that linoleate is absorbed into lymph more efficiently than arachidonate.

PACKAGING OF INTESTINAL LIPOPROTEINS

Complex lipids are processed in the endoplasmic reticulum and are then stabilized by the protein and PL coat. The apolipoproteins synthesized by the human small intestine are apo A-I, apo A-II, apo A-IV and apo B. We do not yet know the sequence in which these apolipoproteins are incorporated into lipid-protein droplets within the ER. In the Golgi apparatus, the CM undergo considerable modification. Terminal glycosylation occurs at the Golgi apparatus. The CM are transported in Golgi-derived vesicles and through a process of exocytosis, the CM are externalized into the intercellular space. While the apolipoprotein compositions of CM and VLDL are relatively similar, there is some evidence that these two TG-rich lipoproteins are formed by different pathways and that the CM can be selectively inhibited by the presence of a nonionic hydrophobic surfactant called Pluronic L-81 (16).

FACTORS REGULATING THE TRANSPORT OF INTESTINAL LIPOPROTEINS

Since CM have a surface protein coat, it is possible that the supply of apolipoprotein is rate limiting for its export. As yet the only protein whose biosynthesis seems to be obligatory for the normal transport of CM is apo B. Under normal physiological conditions there is probably an abundant supply of apo B, and thus it is unlikely that the supply of apo B is rate-limiting for intestinal CM transport. O'Doherty, et al. (17) proposed that luminal PC is important for intestinal CM formation and transport. This hypothesis has been confirmed and extended by other studies. Studies by Strauss and Jacob (18) have demonstrated that Ca^{++} is required for the normal transport of CM by the small intestine. The precise role of Ca^{++} in the intestinal CM transport still remains to be elucidated. Microtubules are probably involved in the movement of CM-containing Golgi derived vesicles from the Golgi apparatus to the basolateral membrane. Much work is need to elucidate the various physiologic factors that may regulate the intestinal formation and transport of lipoproteins. Studies by Connors and his associates seem to provide some evidence that the feeding of fish oil over a three week period may have an effect on the ability of the small intestine to absorb lipid (19). In the liver, the consumption of fish oil both in humans and animals results in a significant reduction in the amount of VLDL secreted (20).

REFERENCES

1.   Tso P. Adv. Lipid Res 1985; 21:143-186.

2.   Tso P, Balint JA, Simmonds WJ Gastroenterology 1977; 73:1362-1367.

3.   Desnuelle P Adv Enzymol 1961, 23:129-161.

4.   Borgstrom B Acta Chem Scand 1953; 7:557-560.

5.   Borgstrom B, Erlanson-Albertson C, Wieloch T   J Lipid Res
      1979: 20:805-816.

6.   Hofmann AF.   In: Rommell K, Goebell H, Bohmer R, eds.
      Lipid absorption, biochemical and clinical aspects.
      Lancaster: MTP Press Ltd, 1976; 3-18.

7.   Thomson ABR, Dietschy J.   In: Johnson LR, ed. Physiology
      of the gastrointestinal tract.   New York: Raven Press,
      1981:1147-1220.

8.   Chow SL, Hollander D, J Lipid Res 1979; 20:349-356.

9.   Hollander D, Dadufalza VD, Sletten EG   J Lipid Res 1984;
      25:129-134.

10.   Chen IS, Subramaniam S, Cassidy MM, et al.   J. Nutr 1985;
      115:219-225.

11.   Schiller CM, David JSK, Johnston JM   Biochim Biophys Acta
      1970; 210:489-499.

12.   Ockner RK, Manning JA   J Clin Invest   1974; 54:326-338.

13.   Rao GA, Johnston JM   Biochim Biophys Acta 1966;
      125:465-473.

14.   Johnston JM, Paltouf F, Schiller CM et al.   Biochim
      Biophys Acta 1970; 218:124-133.

15.   Nilsson A, Landin B, Jensen E et al.   Am J Physiol 1987;
      15:G817-G824.

16.   Tso P, Drake DS, Black DD et al.   Am J Physiol 1984:
      247:G599-G610.

17.   O'Doherty PJA, Kakis G, Kuksis A   Lipid   1973; 8:249-255.

18.   Strauss, EW, Jacob JS   J Lipid Res 1981; 22:147-156.

19.   Harris WS, Connor WE   Trans Assoc Am Physicians 1980;
      43:148-155.

20.   Nestel PJ, Connor WE, Reardon MF et al   J Clin Invest
      1984; 74:82-89.

Advances in Prostaglandin, Thromboxane, and Leukotriene Research, Vol. 19, edited by B. Samuelsson, P. Y.-K. Wong, and F. F. Sun, Raven Press, Ltd., New York ©1989.

EFFECT OF ORAL ADMINISTRATION OF HIGHLY PURIFIED EICOSAPENTAENOIC

ACID AND DOCOSAHEXAENOIC ACID ON PLATELET FUNCTION AND

SERUM LIPIDS IN HYPERLIPIDEMIC PATIENTS

A. Hirai, T. Terano, H. Makuta*, A. Ozawa*, T. Fujita*, Y. Tamura, and S. Yoshida

The 2nd Department of Internal Medicine, School of Medicine, Chiba University, Inohana, Chiba 280, Japan; *Central Research Laboratory, Nippon Suisan Kaisha, Kitano-cho, Hachioji, Tokyo 192, Japan

Anti-thrombotic and anti-atherogenic effects of marine lipids rich in ω-3 polyunsaturated fatty acids have been extensively investigated using fish oil concentrate, of which both eicosapentaenoic acid (EPA) and docosahexaenoic acid (DHA) are major constituents (2,3,4). We have manufactured highly purified EPA and DHA in order to perform comparative studies of the supplementation of these two fatty acids in man. In previous healthy volunteer study, we demonstrated that 4 weeks oral ingestion (3.6 g/day) of highly purified EPA ethylester significantly reduced platelet aggregation and thromboxane B_2 (TXB$_2$) production with a concomitant increase in EPA content in platelet phospholipids, while that of highly purified DHA ethylester seemed to be less effective (1). Also in clinical trial study, oral administration (1.8-2.7 g/day) of highly purified EPA has been shown to reduce platelet functions and improve hyperlipidemia in patients with cerebro- and cardiovascular diseases (5). However, it has not determined yet whether orally ingested DHA could affect platelet function and serum lipids in these patients. Therefore, the present study was performed to compare the effect of oral administration of highly purified EPA and DHA on platelet aggregation and serum lipids in hyperlipidemic patients.

MATERIALS AND METHODS

The EPA ethylester (90% pure) and the DHA ethylester (90% pure) used in this study were purified from sardine oil and squid oil, respectively according to the method previously described (1). Each gelatin-coated soft capsule of EPA ethylester (EPA-E) and DHA ethylester (DHA-E) contains 300 mg of EPA ethylester or DHA ethylester, respectively. Twenty-two patients (10 male and 12 female) having Type IIa hyperlipidemia and 15 patients (8 male and 7 female) having Type IIb hyperlipidemia were used in the study. During the experimental period of 8 weeks, the subjects ingested 9 capsule of EPA-E (3.6 g/day) or DHA-E (3.6 g/day).

Venous blood samples were obtained after 12-hr fasting at the beginning of the experiment and at 4 and 8 weeks after the beginning of the start. Fatty acid analysis in total plasma lipids was performed as previously described (4). Platelet aggregation induced by collagen and ADP was measured as previously described (6). Serum levels of total cholesterol, triglycerides, HDL-cholesterol and aproproteins (AI, B and CII) were determined as previously reported (1). Two sample comparisons were made with a paired sample t-test.

RESULTS AND DISCUSSION

After 8 weeks oral administration of EPA-E, a marked increase in EPA content in total plasma lipids (2.9 ± 2.0 mol% to 6.7 ± 2.6, $p < 0.001$) was noted. In addition, content of docosapentaenoic acid (DPA) significantly increased (0.7 ± 0.1 to 1.2 ± 0.4, $p < 0.001$), while content of DHA did not change (4.2 ± 1.1 to 4.0 ± 1.3). There was no significant change in content of AA (3.8 ± 1.0 to 4.2 ± 0.9). This result is in agreement with our previous data (1), and suggests that orally ingested EPA could be elongated to DPA, while further desaturation of DPA to DHA could not be observed in man. In contrast, after 8 weeks oral administration of DHA-E, not only DHA content, but also EPA content in plasma total lipids were significantly increased. This result indicates that orally ingested DHA could be retroconverted to DPA *in vivo* as previously described (4).

Platelet aggregation induced by threshold dose and low-dose of collagen (0.5 and 0.75 µg/ml) was significantly decreased by EPA-E administration ($65.8 \pm 11.3\%$ to $35.1 \pm 26.4\%$, $p < 0.01$, 65.6 ± 16.4 to 46.4 ± 25.2, $p < 0.05$, 73.4 ± 18.3 to 59.5 ± 23.7, $p < 0.05$). Platelet aggregation induced by ADP (threshold dose and 1 µM) was significantly decreased (71.1 ± 8.0 to 45.5 ± 24.0, $p < 0.05$, 44.4 ± 26.8 to 23.4 ± 17.2, $p < 0.05$). The present results were in agreement with those of previous studies in healthy subjects (6) and in patients with cerebro- and cardiovascular diseases (5). Thus oral administration of EPA-E may have beneficial effects by reducing platelet aggregability in hyperlipidemic patients. In contrast, after DHA-E administration, platelet aggregation induced by threshold dose of collagen showed no significant change (57.5 ± 9.2 to 45.8 ± 22.5). Only 0.75 µg/ml collagen-induced platelet aggregation was significantly decreased (53.2 ± 28.2 to 45.8 ± 28.9, $p < 0.05$). Platelet aggregation induced by threshold dose of ADP was significantly decreased (63.1 ± 9.6 to 49.7 ± 15.4, $p < 0.05$), while ADP (1 and 2 µM)-induced platelet aggregation showed no significant change. Similar changes were observed in previous healthy volunteer study (1). These results in the present study, it could be posturated that orally administered EPA and DHA may have anti-aggregatory effect in hyperlipidemic patients, though

DHA may be much less potent.

After oral administration of EPA-E, a significant decrease in serum total cholesterol was observed at 4 weeks in patients of Type IIa hyperlipidemia (245.8 ± 20.7 mg/dl to 217.4 ± 15.5, $p < 0.05$) and at 8 weeks in patients of Type IIb hyperlipidemia (248.9 ± 35.9 to 233.1 ± 33.7, $p < 0.05$). In patients of Type IIb hyperlipidemia, a marked decrease in serum triglycerides in concomitant with a significant increase in HDL-cholesterol was observed at 4 and 8 weeks (284.3 ± 104.7 to 205.4 ± 66.6, $p < 0.05$, and to 192.1 ± 68.0, $p < 0.05$, 38.5 ± 11.4 to 42.4 ± 14.9, $p < 0.05$ and to 42.1 ± 9.9, $p < 0.05$). A significant decrease in serum apo-protein AI, B and CII was observed in patients of Type IIb hyperlipidemia. Similar changes in serum lipid profile were observed after EPA-E administration in previous patient study (5). Thus oral administration of EPA-E produced favorable changes in serum lipid profile in hyperlipidemic patients both of Type IIa and Type IIb. After 8 week oral administration of DHA-E, a significant decrease in serum total cholesterol was observed both in patients of Type IIa and Type IIb hyperlipidemia (242.2 ± 31.6 to 225.0 ± 5.4, $p < 0.05$ and 246.0 ± 35.2 to 233.3 ± 33.1, $p < 0.05$). In patients of Type IIb hyperlipidemia, a marked decrease in serum triglycerides in concomitant with a significant increase in HDL-cholesterol was observed at 4 and 8 weeks (257.1 ± 86.0 to 197.0 ± 45.1, $p < 0.05$ and to 209.5 ± 68.1, $p < 0.05$, 42.1 ± 11.0 to 50.3 ± 8.6, $p < 0.05$, and to 47.6 ± 9.1, $p < 0.05$). A significant decrease in serum apoprotein B and CII was noted. The present results first and clearly demonstrated that oral administration of DHA could improve serum lipid profile in patients of Type IIa and Type IIb hyperlipidemia.

In conclusion, EPA and DHA in marine lipids may have beneficial effects in the prevention and the treatment of thrombotic cardio-vascular disorders by the reduction of platelet aggregability and the improvement of serum lipid profile, though DHA seems to be less potent.

REFERENCES

1. Hirai A, Terano T, Takenaga M, et al. Ad. in Prostaglandin, Thromboxane, and Leukotriene Research, vol 17, New York: Raven Press, 1987;838-845.

2. Nestel PJ, Connor WE, Reardon MF, Connor S, Wong SH, Boston R. J Clin Invest 1984;74:82-89.

3. Phillipson BE, Rothrock DW, Connor WE, Harris WS, Illingworth DR. N Engl J Med 1985;312:1210-1216.

4. Sanders TAB, Sullivan DR, Reeve J, Thompson GR.
   Arteriosclerosis 1985;5:459–465.

5. Tamura Y, Hirai A, Terano T, Yoshida S, Takenaga M, Kitagawa H.
   Jpn J Circ 1987;51:471–477.

6. Terano T, Hirai A, Hamazaki T, Kobayashi S, Fujita T, Tamura Y,
   Kumagai A. Atherosclerosis 1983;46:321–331.

*Advances in Prostaglandin, Thromboxane, and
Leukotriene Research*, Vol. 19, edited by
B. Samuelsson, P. Y.-K. Wong, and F. F. Sun,
Raven Press, Ltd., New York ©1989.

NATURAL AND UNNATURAL PROSTAGLANDINS
VIA THE THREE-COMPONENT COUPLING SYNTHESIS

R. Noyori, A. Yanagisawa, H. Koyano, and M. Suzuki

Department of Chemistry, Nagoya University,
Chikusa, Nagoya 464, Japan

Among various strategies for prostaglandin (PG) chemical synthesis, the three-component coupling process, _viz._, consecutive linking of the two side chains to the five-membered cyclenone unit is obviously the most attractive. Some years ago we realized

a convergent one-pot construction of the PG framework by the organocopper-mediated conjugate addition of the ω side-chain unit to a protected (R)-4-hydroxy-2-cyclopentenone followed by trapping of the enolate intermediate by α side-chain alkyl iodides (1,2). Transmetalation using triphenyltin chloride at the enolate stage serves as key operation for the successful three-component coupling synthesis. As illustrated in Scheme I, the 5,6-didehydro-PGE_2 derivatives of type **1** are convertible to a wide variety of naturally occurring PGs by the controlled hydrogenation of the acetylenic linkage and stereoselective reduction of the 9-keto function, if necessary. Appropriate selection of the protective groups of the 11- and 15-hydroxyl groups allows reversal of the oxidation state at the 9 and 11 positions, leading to D series of PGs.

A short synthesis of PGI_2 (prostacyclin, **5**) from the versatile intermediate **2** has been accomplished as shown in Scheme II (2). The α-selective (≥99%) reduction of the cyclopentanone unit is best effected by reduction with the (R)-BINAL-H reagent (3) or L-Selectride. The resulting acetylenic alcohol **3** undergoes intramolecular alkoxypalladation with a Kharasch Pd(II) complex and subsequent reductive removal of the Pd moiety leads to the protected PGI_2 (**4**) having 5Z configuration in a stereo-defined manner. Deprotection of **4** completes the synthesis of **5**.

Scheme I. General Synthesis of Prostaglandins

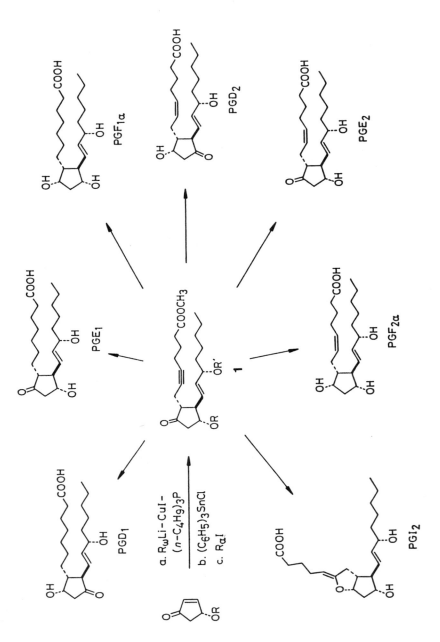

Scheme II. Synthesis of Prostacyclin

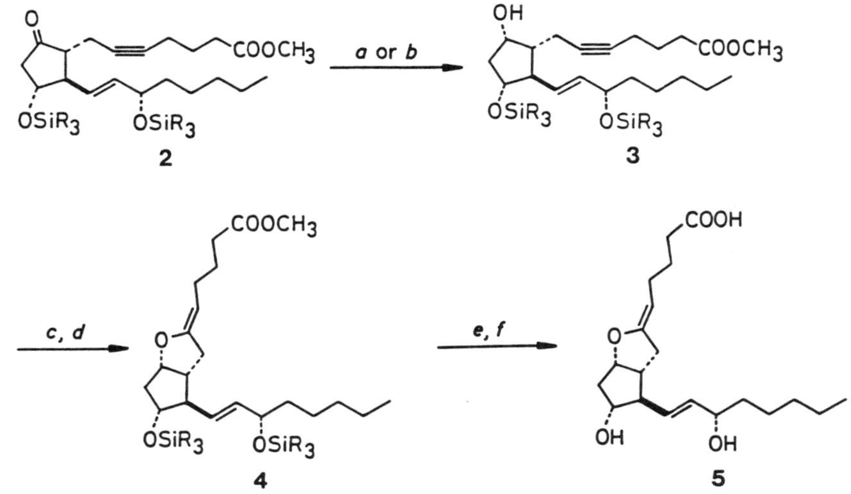

SiR$_3$ = Si(CH$_3$)$_2$-t-C$_4$H$_9$

(a) (R)-BINAL-H, -100 to -78 °C; (b) L-Selectride, -100 to -78 °C; (c) bis(benzonitrile)palladium(II) dichloride, -78 to -28 °C; (d) ammonium formate, -78 °C; (e) tetrabutylammonium fluoride; (f) sodium hydroxide.

Scheme III outlines an efficient synthesis of isocarbacyclin (**10**) (4), one of the most potent and stable analogues of PGI$_2$ (**5**). The cyclopentanone **2** is first converted to the methylene-cyclopentane **6** by a Zn-CH$_2$Br$_2$-TiCl$_4$ mixed reagent, which in turn is transformed to the 9α-hydroxymethyl compound **7** via stereoselective hydroboration. The oxidation-silylation procedure gives the silyl alcohol **8**. Organotin chemistry or a photochemical deoxygenation procedure allows generation of free radicals from the alcohol derivatives, causing the cyclization to give the allyl-silane **9**. Deblocking of the 11- and 15-hydroxyls, regiospecific protodesilylation of the allylsilane, and alkaline hydrolysis of the ester group realize the synthesis of **10**.

Scheme III.   Synthesis of Isocarbacyclin

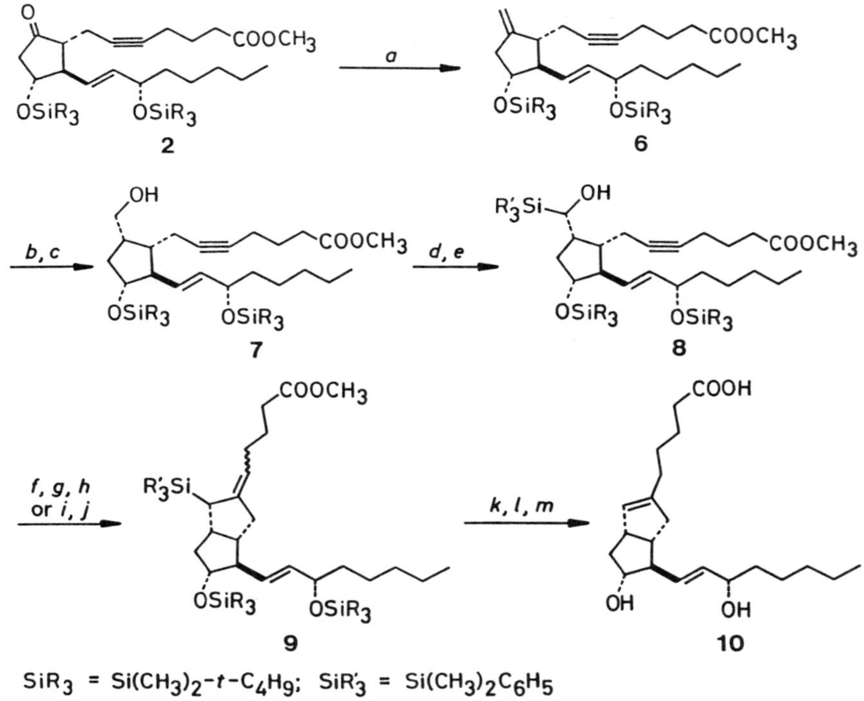

SiR$_3$ = Si(CH$_3$)$_2$-t-C$_4$H$_9$; SiR$_3'$ = Si(CH$_3$)$_2$C$_6$H$_5$

(a) zinc-dibromomethane-titanium(IV) tetrachloride, 0 °C; (b) 9-BBN, 0 °C; (c) hydrogen peroxide, sodium hydroxide, 0 °C; (d) pyridinium dichromate; (e) dilithium cyanobis(dimethylphenyl-silyl)cuprate, -78 °C; (f) LDA, carbon disulfide, HMPA, 0 °C; (g) methyl iodide, 0 °C; (h) tributyltin hydride, di-tert-butyl peroxide, 80 °C; (i) m-trifluoromethylbenzoyl chloride, DMAP; (j) hν, N-methylcarbazole, magnesium perchlorate; (k) perchloric acid, 18 °C; (l) trifluoroacetic acid, -78 to -20 °C; (m) sodium hydroxide.

REFERENCES

1. Suzuki M, Yanagisawa A, Noyori R. J Am Chem Soc 1985; 107:3348.
2. Suzuki M, Yanagisawa A, Noyori R. J Am Chem Soc 1988; 110 (in press).
3. Noyori R. Tomino I, Tanimoto Y, Nishizawa M. J Am Chem Soc 1984; 106:6709-6716.
4. Shibasaki M. Torisawa S. Ikegami S. Tetrahedron Lett 1983; 24:3493-3496.
5. Suzuki M, Koyano H, Noyori R. J Org Chem 1987;52:5583-5588.

Advances in Prostaglandin, Thromboxane, and
Leukotriene Research, Vol. 19, edited by
B. Samuelsson, P. Y.-K. Wong, and F. F. Sun,
Raven Press, Ltd., New York ©1989.

CHEMICAL SYNTHESES OF TRIOXILINS

J.R. Falck, Sun Lumin, Pendri Yadagiri, and Dong-Soo Shin

Departments of Molecular Genetics and Pharmacology,

University of Texas Southwestern Medical Center,

Dallas, Texas   75235   USA

The intramolecular rearrangement (1) of 12(S)-hydroperoxyeicosatetraenoic acid leads to a mixture of 8(R/S)-hydroxy-11(S),12(S)-epoxyeicosa-5Z,9E,14Z-trienoic acid (Hepoxilin A_3) and 10(R/S)-hydroxy-11(S),12(S)-epoxyeicosa-5Z,8Z,14Z-trienoic acid (Hepoxilin B_3) whose exact constitutions have been confirmed by total synthesis (2). Hepoxilin A_3 and B_3 can be transformed further to trioxilins (1), i.e., diastereomeric triols arising from hydration at C(9)/(11) and at C(12), respectively.

Arachidonate metabolites of the hepoxilin/trioxilin pathway have been implicated as mediators of neural signal transduction in <u>Aplysia</u> (3) and as insulin secretagogues (4). Related metabolites of homologous fatty acids have been reported (5), although generally their stereochemistries remain obscure. To expedite biological evaluation and to clarify structure assignments, it was deemed essential to develop versatile and unambiguous routes to the isomeric trioxilins utilizing readily available, chiral precursors.

SYNTHESES

Protected methyl furanoside <u>2</u>, obtained from <u>1</u> (70%) by a standard sequence (Scheme I), was oxidized to the corresponding aldehyde and condensed with the β-oxido ylide of 2(S)-hydroxydeca-4Z-en-1-yltriphenylphosphonium chloride <u>6</u> to give <u>3</u> (52%). Benzoylation, acidic hydrolysis, and homologation with 4-carboxybutyl Wittig reagent <u>7</u> furnished differentially protected triol <u>4</u> which afforded methyl 8(S),9(R),12(S)-trihydroxyeicosa-5Z,10E,14Z-trienoate <u>5</u> (62%).

Scheme I

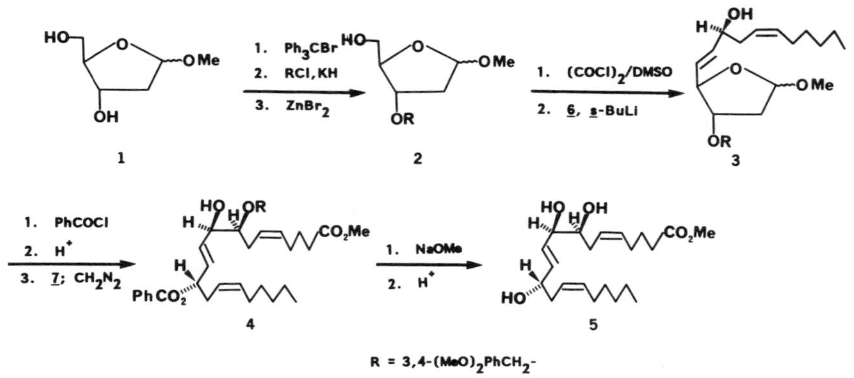

R = 3,4-(MeO)$_2$PhCH$_2$-

Mitsunobu inversion (6) of **4** and deprotection as described above yielded **8** (52%). Diastereomeric triols **9**-**11** were derived likewise from intermediates in Scheme I.

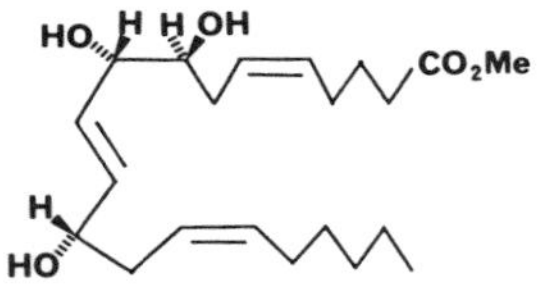

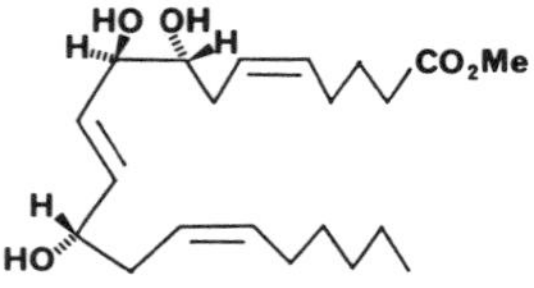

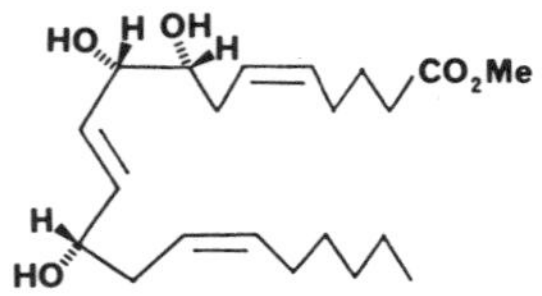

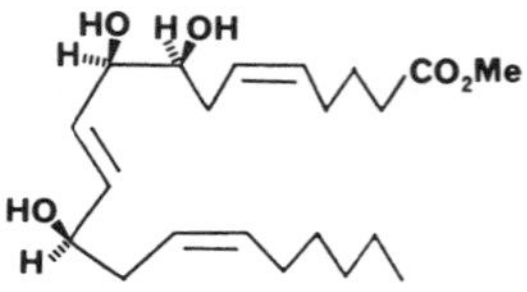

Access to the other regioisomeric trioxilins began with pyranoside **12** (Scheme II). Selective protection as **13** (72%), Swern oxidation, and olefination using 7-carbomethoxyhepta-3Z-en-1-ylidenetriphenylphosphorane **17** gave rise to **14** (93%)

which was transformed to 15 (55%) by acidic lactol hydrolysis and Wittig condensation. Deprotection of 15 gave methyl 10(R),11(R),12(R)-trihydroxyeicosa-5Z,8Z,14Z-trienoate 16 (74%).

Scheme II

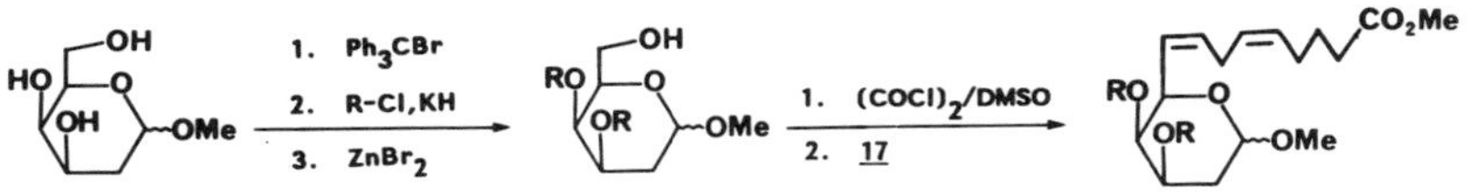

12 13 14

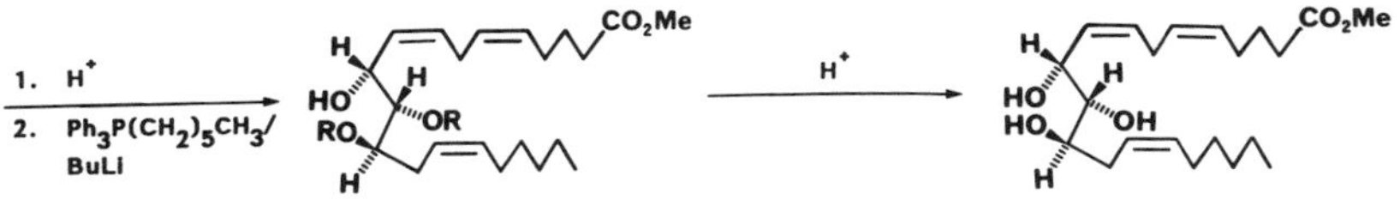

15 R = 3,4-$(MeO)_2PhCH_2$- 16

Stereochemical inversion of 15 at C(10) by the Mitsunobu procedure followed by routine deprotection evolved 18 (30%) along with 8,11,12-triol 19, the result of allylic transposition, isolated as a mixture of C(8) isomers.

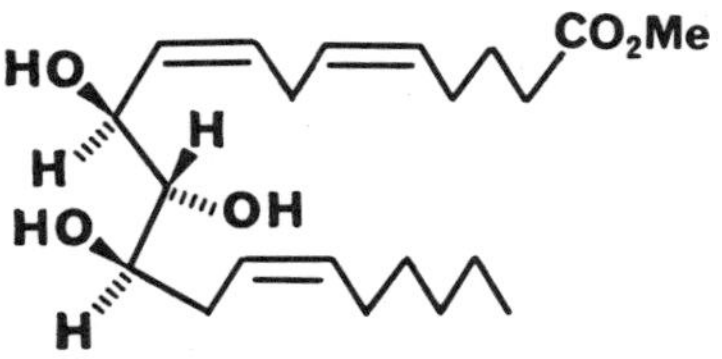

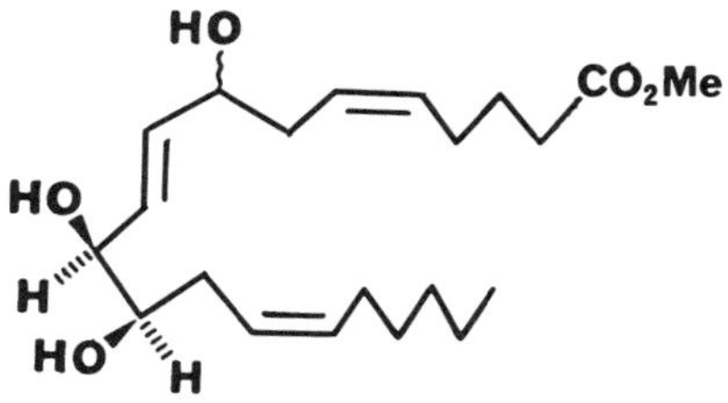

18 19

Preliminary pharmacological study revealed that the free acid of **18** was a potent in vitro stimulus of substance P release from chick dorsal root ganglia cells in culture, whereas its C(10) isomer **16** was inactive at the same dose (Dr. Michael Vasko, UT Southwestern, personal communication).

REFERENCES

1. Pace-Asciak, C.R. J. Biol. Chem. 1984; 259:8332-8337.

2. Corey, E.J., Su, W-g. Tetrahedron Letters 1984; 25: 5119-5122. Corey, E.J., Kang, J., Laguzza, B.C., Jones, R.L., ibid. 1983; 24:4913-4916.

3. Piomelli, D., Feinmark, S.J., Schwartz, J.H. Society for Neuroscience 17th Annual Meeting, New Orleans, Louisiana, Nov. 16-21, 1987: Abstract No. 169.11, p. 598.

4. Pace-Asciak, C.R., Martin, J.M., Corey, E.J. Prog. Lipid Res. 1986; 25: 625-628.

5. Kato, T., Yamaguchi, Y., Ohnuma, S.-I., Uyehara, T., Namai, T., Kodama, M., Shiobara, Y. Chem. Lett. 1986; 577-580. Powell, W.S., Funk, C.D. Prog. Lipid Res. 1987; 26: 183-210. Holland, D.L., East, J., Gibson, K.H., Clayton, E., Oldfield, A. Prostaglandins 1985; 29: 1021-1029.

6. Mitsunobu, O. Synthesis 1981; 1-28.

Advances in Prostaglandin, Thromboxane, and Leukotriene Research, Vol. 19, edited by
B. Samuelsson, P. Y.-K. Wong, and F. F. Sun,
Raven Press, Ltd., New York ©1989.

SYNTHESIS OF METHANOLEUKOTRIENE A₄ ANALOGS AND THEIR PHARMACOLOGICAL ACTIVITIES

A. Hazato, S. Kurozumi, T. Ohta, A. Ohtsu, Y. Nagyu, K. Komoriya,
H. Fujiwara*, and R. Mori[†]

Teijin Institute for Bio-Medical Research, Hino, Tokyo 191, JAPAN.
*Department of Ophthalmology, Kawasaki Medical School, Kurashiki, Okayama
710, JAPAN.
[†]Deparment of Virology, Kyushu University, Fukuoka 812, JAPAN.

Leukotriene A₄(LTA₄) is the first metabolite of arachidonic acid (AA) by 5-lipoxygenase (5-LO), which is converted into LTs responsible for inflammatory, allergic, and immunological reactions (1). 5,6-Methano-LTA₄ is a chemically stable analog of LTA₄ synthesized by Nicolaou et al. and was found to be an inhibitor of 5-LO as well as a weak inhibitor of cyclooxygenase (CO) in masto-cytoma P-815 cells(2). Since 5,6-methano-LTA₄ has an unstable triene structure in the molecule and is considered to be unsuitable for the use as a pharmaceut-ical, we synthesized an analog TEI-8005 having a stable naphthalene moiety with the 5,6-methano-side chain instead of the triene. This compound showed a similar inhibitory activity to that of the parent compound of 5,6-methano-LTA₄ (3). In vitro inhibitory profile of AA cascade by TEI-8005 was dependent on the experimental systems used (3,4).

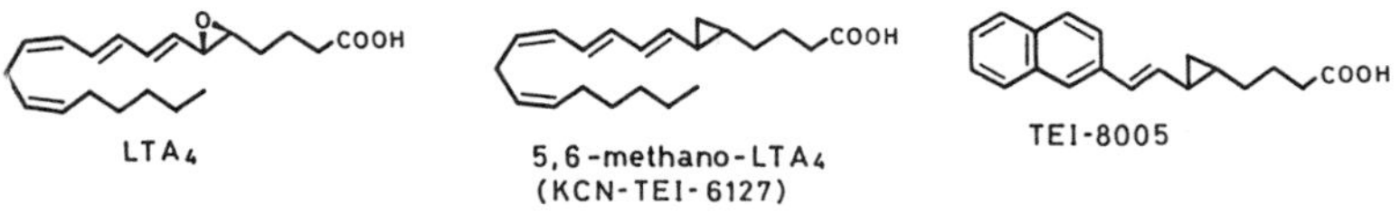

Fig.1. Leukotriene A₄ and its related compounds.

We have studied further on the synthesis of derivatives of TEI-8005, and investigated on the inhibitory activities of LO using in vitro and in vivo systems to assess detailed pharmacological profile of these compounds.

SYNTHESIS

Chemical synthesis of TEI-8005 and its related compounds are shown in Fig.2. 2-Bromomethylnaphthalene was converted into the corresponding phosphonate, which was coupled with the cyclopropanealdehyde under Wittig-Horner condition to give the ester TEI-8001. Hydrolysis of the ester gave the acid TEI-8005, and this was amidated with methyl o-aminobezoate to give the amide TEI-1338. Reduction of the acid(TEI-8005) followed by the condensation with 3,4-dimethoxycinnamic acid gave the ester TEI-1345.

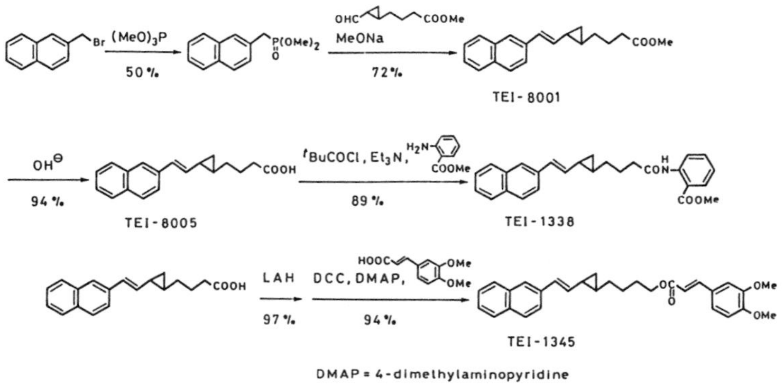

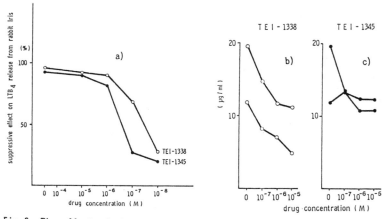

DMAP = 4-dimethylaminopyridine

Fig. 2. Synthesis of TEI-8005 and its related compounds.

IN VITRO STUDIES

Rabbit iris tissue is a good LTB₄ releasing system and we investigated the effect of the parent compound TEI-8005 on the LTB₄ release from the iso-lated tissue. Ten minites after the isolation, TEI-8005 at $10^{-4} \sim 10^{-5}$M sig-nificantly suppressed the formation of LTB₄, while indomethacin had no effect under the same condition. Similarly, new analogs of TEI-1338 and TEI-1345 also showed potent inhibitory effect on LTB₄ formation from the tissue in a dose dependent manner(Fig. 3-a)(5).

Fig. 3. The effect of the drug on LTB₄ release from rabbit iris tissue (incubation, 37°C, 5 min., n=3), and from human whole blood (10^{-5}M calcium ionophore).

These potent LTB₄ inhibitory activities were also observed using human whole
blood (6). Both TEI-1338 and TEI-1345 inhibited LTB₄ formation from human
whole blood stimulated by 10^{-5}M calcium ionophore(Fig. 3-b and 3-c).

There are some reports that virus formation or growth is affected by the
metabolites of AA cascade, and some flavonoids are reported to inhibit Aujesky
virus and herpes simplex type 1 virus (HSV-1) formation in vitro (7). Thus we
investigated on the HSV-1 growth in HEL or Vero cells in the presence of the
new lipoxygenase inhibitors. By the treatment of TEI-8005 at the concentration
of 10 μg/ml, HSV-1 of strain KOS growth was inhibited (10~46% inhibition),
and at the concentration of 20 μg/ml of the drug, there was observed a slight
damage for the host cells (data not shown). Another lipoxygenase inhibitor
TEI-1338 showed the similar inhibitory effects (70~90% inhibition) in both
HEL and Vero cells at the concentration of 5~10 μg/ml. These observations
seemed to be new findings and suggested that LO metabolites might participate
in the HSV-1 growth.

Since LTB₄ stimulates the chemotaxis of leukocytes, we investigated the
effect of TEI-8005 on the leukocytes chemotaxis comparing with known anti-
inflammatory drugs such as aspirin, indomethacin, dexamethasone, and a lipoxygenase inhibitor of NDGA. On the leukocytes chemotaxis in response to zymosan-activated serum, AA, and LTB₄, the compound at 30~100 μM showed the significant inhibitory activities (detailed data not shown).

IN VIVO STUDIES

As mentioned above, the naphthalene derivatives were observed to inhibit
LTB₄ formation or relase in several in vitro systems. Then these lipoxygenase
inhibitors were studied on their anti-iflammatory activity by in vivo models
focusing on the topical dosage of the drugs. Studies on the effects of the

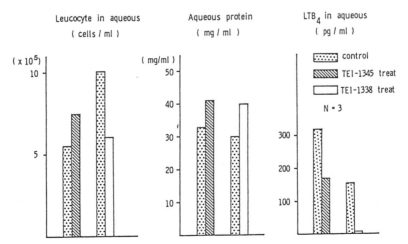

Fig. 4. The effect of drugs on endotoxin-induced endophthalmitis.

drugs to the endotoxin-induced endophthalmitis in rabbits were carried out. Eye inflammation was caused by the challenge of lipopolysaccharide from E. coli ($5\mu g/50\mu l$ saline) into the rabbit vitreous body. The drugs were applied to the one side eyes of rabbits as 0.38% oil droplets 3 times before the challenge. After 20 hr, LTB_4 formation (pg/ml), leukocyctes accumulation (cells/ml) in aqueous humor, and aqueous humor protein content (mg/ml) were determined. The inhibitor of TEI-1338 significantly reduced leukocyctes accumulation as well as LTB_4 formation in aqueous humor, while aqueous protein was not affected. The compound TEI-1345 was less effective than TEI-1338 in these experiments (Fig. 4).

To acertain the ocular distribution of TEI-1338, the drug level was determined after 5 times applications of 0.1% oil suspension of the drug to the rabbit eye. After 2 hours, there was observed the distribution of TEI-1338 mainly to the cornea, conjunctiva, and choroid-retina (data not shown).

In a typical systemic inflammation model induced by carrageenin in rats, oral administration of TEI-8005 (1~3mg/kg) suppressed the foot pad edema formation (ca.30~40% inhibition) with relatively shorter duration of action (1~3hr) than ordinary nonsteroidal anti-inflammatory drugs such as ibuprofen or indomethacin, while TEI-1338 (1~3mg/kg, p.o.) showed no effect in this model.

CONCLUSION

Several derivatives of methanoleukotriene A₄ analogs were synthesized, and their pharmacological activities were investigated by *in vitro* and *in vivo* systems of arachidonic acid cascade. These studies on the naphthalene derivatives suggested that topically applied lipoxygenase inhibitors may be useful in preventing some part of the inflammatory process in ocular tissues by inhibiting LTs and/or prostaglandins formations.

REFERENCES

1. Zor U, Naor Z, Kohen F, Advances in Prostglandin, Thronboxane, and Leukotriene Research, Vol.16, New York: Raven Press, 1986.
2. Koshihara Y, Murota, Petasis NA, Nicolaou KC, Febs Letters 1982; 143: 13~16.
3. Ohta T, Ohtsu A, Hazato A, Kurozumi S, Prostaglandins, Leukotrienes and Med. 1985; 19: 279~281.
4. Bazan HEP, Reddy STK, Bazan NG, Abstr. of 6th Internatl. Conf. on Prostaglandins and related compounds, Florence Italy; 1986: pp374.
5. The compound TEI-1338 showed no effect on *in vitro* prostaglandin synthesis in the ocular tissue whereas TEI-8005 showed a dual inhibitory activity on both LT and PG formation (4).: private communication from prof. Bazan.
6. Greles P, Arnout J, Coene MC, Deckmyn H, Vermylen J, Biochem. Biophys. Res. Comm. 1986; 137: 334~342.
7. Beladi I, Musci I, Pusztai R, Bakay M, et al., Stud. Org. Chem. 1981; 11: 443~450. (Chem. Abstr., 1983; 98: 200P).

Advances in Prostaglandin, Thromboxane, and Leukotriene Research, Vol. 19, edited by
B. Samuelsson, P. Y.-K. Wong, and F. F. Sun,
Raven Press, Ltd., New York ©1989.

STRUCTURAL ANALYSIS OF SULFIDO-PEPTIDE LEUKOTRIENES:
APPLICATION TO THE DESIGN OF POTENT AND SPECIFIC ANTAGONISTS
OF LEUKOTRIENE D_4

Robert N. Young

Merck Frosst Canada Inc., P.O. Box 1005
Pointe Claire-Dorval, Québec, Canada, H9R 4P8

INTRODUCTION

The sulfido-peptide leukotrienes LTC_4, LTD_4 and LTE_4
collectively account for the activity known as slow-reacting
substance of anaphylaxis (SRS-A) and are some of the most
potent spasmogenic agents known.[1]
These leukotrienes exert their effects through specific
receptors found on a variety of tissues and cell types and in
human lung LTC_4, LTD_4 and LTE_4 are thought to act through
a single common receptor on which LTD_4 is the most potent
agonist.[2] The potent biological activities of the
leukotrienes together with their demonstrated release from lung
tissues under a variety of physiologically relevant conditions
has lead to the hypothesis that an effective LTD_4 receptor
antagonist will be a useful therapeutic agent particularly for
the treatment of asthma.
Many research groups have investigated through synthesis
the structure activity relationships of the leukotriene,
analogs and isomers, thus providing a body of knowledge from
which one can develop a representation of the important
interactions of LTD_4 with its receptor.[3] Molecular
modelling studies have also been used in attempts to define
minimum energy conformations of leukotrienes that they might
present to the receptor.[4]

Development of an LTD_4 Receptor Model

Evaluating these data, we have been able to derive a model
of the LTD_4 receptor which has allowed the rational analysis
of interaction of known antagonists with the receptor and thus

predict structural modifications which would improve potency.

The model we have derived can be represented thusly: (see Figure 1) 1) The receptor presents a flat lipophilic region on which the polyene chain of LTD_4 is arrayed in a generally extended planar conformation with the terminus of the chain binding in a lipophilic pocket. Planarity is most critical in the region of the 7,8 double bond. 2) The binding of the cysteinyl-glycine unit likely involves both hydrogen bond and ionic interactions and the acid is probably ionized in the receptor. These postulates are supported by evidence that the conversion of the glycine acid to an amide or cyclic diketo-piperazine leads to a ten-fold loss in activity.[3] 3) The C-1 carboxyl group binds through H-bonds and is likely <u>not</u> ionized in the receptor (as the primary amide analog is equipotent). 4) The C-5 hydroxyl group binds to the receptor sufficiently strongly to impart stereospecific recognition of both the relative and absolute stereochemistry at C-5 and C-6 of LTD_4.

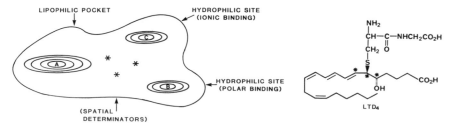

Fig. Conceptualized LTD_4 Receptor

Applications of the Model to the Design of LTD_4 Antagonists

Using this model we were able to hypothesize that antagonists such as FPL-55712 (1) fit in the receptor such that the chromone system occupies the cysteinyl-glycine binding site and that the rest of the molecule binds with the propyl chain in the lipophilic pocket and with the hydroxy acetophenone unit involved in an adventitious hydrogen bond with some unit on the receptor normally not involved with binding of LTD_4 itself. This extra binding might then make up to some degree for the lack of a second carboxyl group to bind in the second polar binding site. This suggested that such a chromone might act as an antagonist equivalent of cysteinyl-glycine a hypothesis that was supported by the preparation leukotrienes incorporating a 2-carboxychromone at C-6 which were indeed quite potent antagonists (e.g. compound 2, IC_{50} 100 nM vs [^{3}H]-LTD_4 on guinea-pig lung membrane).

In the end, important constraints of chemical and metabolic stability and biological half-life lead to the development of compounds such as the orally active L-649,923[5] (3) which has shown activity as an LTD_4 antagonist in man.[6]
Considering our hypothesis for the binding of FPL-55712 and L-649,923 in the LTD_4 receptor, it was logical to suggest that addition of a second polar chain should enhance receptor binding and therefore biological potency. Comparison of L-649,923 with LTD_4 suggested that a second chain could be added at the benzylic position and a number of such derivatives were prepared which showed significant increases in potency (eg compound 4, IC_{50} 180 nM vs 900 nM for L-649,923) lending further support to our receptor model.

$\underline{3}$: R = OH

$\underline{4}$: R =

Development of L-660,711 (7)

The ultimate utility of this receptor model has been its application in the development of L-660,711, one of the most potent LTD_4 antagonists known. Large scale screening of the Merck sample collection allowed the initial discovery of significant activity of 2-(2-(3- pyridyl)ethenyl)quinoline (IC_{50} = 3 μM). We surmized that these structures occupied the central flat lipophilic binding site in the LTD_4 receptor and that binding could be enhanced by adding lipophilic components and acid chains in appropriate positions. The observation of enhanced activity by introduction of polarity into the meta-position of phenyl analogs lead to the preparation of the 7-chloro-3'-carboxypropyloxyphenyl analog (compound 5, Table I) which showed excellent intrinsic activity. The addition of a second acid chain was explored and this lead to the preparation of the bis-mercaptopropionic acid thioacetal (compound 6, Figure 3) which showed another ten-fold increase in potency. Finally, L-660,711 (7) was derived by preparation of the mono-N,N-dimethyl amide derivative. In keeping with our receptor model, this monoamide derivative is equipotent with the diacid analog. This compound shows excellent potency on a variety of tissues and has been developed in preference due to its superior in vivo profile (Zamboni et al this meeting). In that L-660,711 embodies the planar lipophilic component with extended conjugation, coupled with two polar chains one ionizable, the other not, it represents the type of structure predicted to be required for potent activity by our receptor model.

It is indeed gratifying that L-660,711 also has the in vivo profile of oral activity, long half-life and lack of toxicity which have allowed it to be developed for clinic evaluations which are now ongoing.

IC_{50} vs [^{3}H]-LTD$_4$
(guinea-pig lung)

5: R = OCH$_2$CH$_2$COOH	19 nM
6: R = CH(CH$_2$CH$_2$COOH)$_2$	1.5 nM
7: R = CH(CH$_2$CH$_2$COOH)(CH$_2$CH$_2$CONMe$_2$) (L-660711)	0.9 nM

Table 1 : Styrylquinoline LTD$_4$ Antagonists

CONCLUSIONS

Based on a growing body of knowledge on structure activity relationships and physical studies of sulfido-peptide leukotrienes, their analogs and on specific antagonists, a model of the LTD$_4$ receptor has been evolved which has proved useful in designing novel and potent LTD$_4$ receptor antagonists.

REFERENCES

1. Samuelsson B. Science (Washington, D.C.) 1983;220:568-575.

2. Buckner CK, Krell RD, Laravusa RB, et al. J Pharmac Exp Ther 1986;237:558-562.

3. For a recent review see: Rokach J, Guindon Y, Young RN, et al. In: Apsimon J ed. The total synthesis of natural products, Vol 7, New York; Wiley-Interscience, 1988, 141-274.

4. Herron DK, Bollinger NG, Harper RW, "The Three-Dimensional Shape of Leukotriene D$_4$", Xth International Congress of Pharmacology, Sydney, Aug. 23-28, 1987, abstracts of the meeting.

5. Jones JR, Young RN, Champion E, et al. Can. J Physiol Pharmacol 1986;64:1068-1075.

6. Barnes N, Piper PJ, Costello J J Allergy Clin Immunol 1987;79:816-821.

Advances in Prostaglandin, Thromboxane, and Leukotriene Research, Vol. 19, edited by B. Samuelsson, P. Y.-K. Wong, and F. F. Sun, Raven Press, Ltd., New York ©1989.

Leukotriene D4 (LTD4) Antagonists: Structure Activity Relationships of Stable Phenylsubstituted Leukotriene Analogs.

A. von Sprecher, W. Breitenstein, A. Beck, W. Anderson, M.A. Bray and F. Märki

Research Department, Pharmaceuticals Division, CIBA-GEIGY Ltd., CH-4002 Basel, Switzerland

INTRODUCTION

Replacement of the 1-carboxylic group in the eicosanoid chain of LTD4 by a methyl group produces the LTD4 antagonist "1-Methyl-LTD4" (1) (1,2). A representative of this "METHYL PRINCIPLE" is CGP 34 064A (2). In addition to LTD4 antagonism in vitro and in vivo, CGP 34 064A is also active as an inhibitor of phospholipase A2 (PLA2) from human neutrophils in vitro. Importantly CGP 34 064A displays 5R, 6S stereochemistry in contrast to the 5S, 6R configuration of LTD4.

"1-Methyl-LTD4" **1**

CGP 34 064A **2**

In view of the poor chemical stability and short duration of action in vivo, CGP 34 064A is not suited for further development. It is likely that this lack of stability is due to the conjugated triene system in the lipophilic part of this molecule. Integration of these double bonds into a phenyl nucleus leads to stable phenylsubsituted LT analogs.

STRUCTURE ACTIVITY RELATIONSHIPS

Table 1 shows three stable phenylsubstituted LT analogs. The ortho and meta substituted preparations 3 and 4 are equally active as antagonists of LTD4 with IC50 values of 0.78 μM and 0.62 μM for inhibiting LTD4 induced contractions of the guinea pig ileum in vitro. Both compounds are active in vivo at -15 min. when applied as an aerosol (For compound 4 > 0.1 means that a 0.1% solution of the preparation inhibits the LTD4 induced bronchospasm by 45%). The IC50 value of 2.6 μM of compound 5 indicates that para substitution is not preferred in this series of LT analogs. The duration of action of these chemically stable compounds still is not satisfactory as a 1% solution of the ortho substituted preparation 3 applied 1 hour prior to challenge only weakly inhibits the bronchoconstriction.

TABLE 1

Stable Phenylsubstituted LT-analogs: Substitution Pattern

	LTD₄(1 µg/ml) Antagonism Guinea-pig Ileum IC₅₀ (µmol/l)	Inhibition of LTD₄ Induced Bronchoconstriction, Guinea-pig (0.3 µg/ml aerosolised LTD₄) IC₅₀ (% aerosol)		Phospholipase A₂ Inhibition Human Neutrophils IC₅₀ (µmol/l)
		−15 Min	−60 Min	
3	0.78	0.19	>1	5
4	0.62	>0.1	–	9.5
5	2.6	–	–	~6

Table 2 indicates, that the chromone carboxylic acid (compound 3) represents the best sulfur side chain in terms of LTD₄ antagonism for these stable phenylsubstituted LT analogs. Other heterocycles, like quinoline carboxylic acids (6), imidazole carboxylic acids (7) and aminothiadiazoles (8) are less potent than the chromone derivative *in vitro*. The cysteinylglycine and the simple propionic acid substitutions give compounds 9 + 10 which are also less potent than compound 3.

TABLE 2

Sulfur Side Chain

R	LTD₄(1 µg/ml) Antagonism Guinea-pig Ileum IC₅₀ (µmol/l)	Inhibition of LTD₄ Induced Bronchoconstriction, Guinea-pig (0.3 µg/ml aerosolised LTD₄) IC₅₀ (% aerosol)		Phospholipase A₂ Inhibition Human Neutrophils IC₅₀ (µmol/l)
		−15 Min	−60 Min	
3	0.78	0.19	>1	5
6	~6.9	–	–	4.5
7	3.2	–	–	–
8	∅ 6.4	–	–	–
9 −CH₂CHCONHCH₂COONa | NHCOCF₃	2.0	–	–	11
10 −CH₂CH₂COONa	2.6	–	–	10

Table 3 shows the influence on the biological activity of the replacement of the methyl group by other substituents. In vitro there are only minor differences with IC_{50} values between 0.78 and 1.3 µM. However in vivo the methyl derivative 3 is the only compound showing reasonable in vivo activity with an IC_{50} value of 0.19% applied 15 min. prior to challenge. In contrast 0.1% solutions of the carboxylate 11, the fluoro- and the chloro-compounds (12 + 13) are inactive.The methylderivative 3 is also the best inhibitor of PLA_2 activity from human neutrophils in vitro with an IC_{50} of 5 µM. The carboxyderivative 11, with an IC_{50} of 45 µM, shows only weak PLA_2 inhibitory activity.

TABLE 3

Stable Phenylsubstituted LT-analogs:
Replacement of Methyl

R	LTD_4(1 µg/ml) Antagonism Guinea-pig Ileum IC_{50} (µmol/l)	Inhibition of LTD_4 Induced Bronchoconstriction, Guinea-pig (0.3 µg/ml aerosolised LTD_4) IC_{50} (% aerosol)		Phospholipase A_2 Inhibition Human Neutrophils IC_{50} (µmol/l)
		−15 Min	−60 Min	
3 −CH_3	0.78	0.19	>1	5
11 −COONa	1.20	Ø 0.1	–	45
12 −CH_2F	1.30	Ø 0.1	–	10
13 −CH_2Cl	1.14	Ø 0.1	–	5.5
−CF_3	1.10	–	–	–

Our previous studies (1) have shown that the double bonds in the lipophilic part of the LT analogs are important for the antagonistic activity. For this reason we have synthesized phenylsubstituted LT analogs containing one double bond. As expected the additional double bond improves the biological activity with IC_{50} values of 0.11 µM in vitro and 0.025% applied -15 min. prior to LTD_4 challenge in vivo for compound 14 in comparison to compounds 3, 4 and 5 (Table 1). Again preparation 14 with the unnatural 5R, 6S configuration is more active than compound 15 with the 5S, 6R stereochemistry of LTD_4.

Instead of stabilizing the lipophilic chain of a LT analog the phenyl nucleus may be built into the polar region of the eicosanoid chain. In general these compounds are more active and have a prolonged duration of action in comparison to the corresponding preparations without phenyl bridging. The racemic chromone derivative 16 is a potent LTD4 antagonist in vivo. Applied as an aerosol 15 min. prior to challenge with LTD4 a 0.016% solution inhibits the LTD4 induced bronchospasm in the guinea pig by 50%. With the pure enantiomers the usual pattern is found. Compound 17 displaying the 1R, 2S configuration is six times more active in vitro (IC50: 0.11 μM), than the enantiomer 18 with the 1S, 2R configuration of the native LT's. The comparison of methyl versus carboxyl in this series also favours our "methyl-principle". The carboxy derivative 19 shows only weak antagonist activity with an IC50 of 2.8 μM (approximately one tenth of the activity of the corresponding methyl derivative 16).

16
17 1R,2S
18 1S,2R

19

CONCLUSIONS

The application of the "methyl principle" together with phenylsubstitution in the eicosanoid chain leads to LT antagonists with a longer duration of action and better chemical stability in comparison to LT analogs containing the natural backbone. These LT analogs not only block the action of LTD4 at the receptor level, but also potentially block the biosynthesis of the leukotrienes by inhibiting phospholipase A2.

REFERENCES

1. von Sprecher , A., Ernest, I., Main, A., Beck, A., Breitenstein, W., Märki, F. and Bray, M.A. (1987): In: Advances in Prostaglandin, Thromboxane, and Leukotriene Research, Vol. 17, edited by B. Samuelsson, R. Paoletti, and P.W. Ramwell, pp. 519-525. Raven Press New York.

2. von Sprecher, A., Beck, A., Lang, R.W., Anderson, W., Bray, M.A. and Märki, F., (1988): In: Annals of the New York Academy of Sciences, Vol. 524, edited by R. Levi and R.D. Krell, pp. 438-441.

Advances in Prostaglandin, Thromboxane, and Leukotriene Research, Vol. 19, edited by
B. Samuelsson, P. Y.-K. Wong, and F. F. Sun,
Raven Press, Ltd., New York ©1989.

QUINONE DERIVATIVES: SYNTHESIS AND STRUCTURE-ACTIVITY RELATIONS OF
A NOVEL CLASS OF EICOSANOID ANTAGONISTS, AA-2414 AND ITS ANALOGS

Shinji Terao

Chemistry Laboratories, Central Research Division, Takeda Chemical
Industries, Ltd., 17-85, 2-Chome, Juso-honmachi, Yodogawa-ku,
Osaka, 532, Japan

Our continuing efforts on new synthetic and pharmacologic
searches for quinone derivatives have been carried out by assuming
that quinones might play a significant role in living cells not
only as antioxidants and scavengers of active oxygen species (AOS)
but also as lipoxygenase inhibitors related to the redox
properties (1-2).

In these studies, we discovered another new pharmacologic
activity of the quinone derivatives, AA-2414 and its analogues.
It was concluded that biologic effects are mainly based on the
TXA_2/PGH_2 receptor antagonistic action (3-4).

DRUG DESIGN AND CHEMISTRY

Generally, quinones are easily reduced in living cells to their
hydroquinones, which are sulfonated or gluculonized to form
conjugates. To prevent metabolic inactivation and conjugation, we
designed molecules having a bulky substituent on the quinone ring
and/or on the a-position of the side chain (3-4). Reactions of
hydroquinones 1 with benzyl alcohols 2 in the presence of a Lewis
acid as catalyst, followed by ferric chloride oxidation of the
resulting hydroquinones gave the corresponding quinone derivatives
3 in good yields. Most of the desired quinone compounds were
easily prepared by this method (Fig. 1).

BIOLOGIC RESULTS AND DISCUSSION

The compounds synthesized here were evaluated for their effects on tests of IgG_1-mediated bronchoconstriction in actively

sensitized guinea-pigs and agonist-induced bronchoconstriction in guinea-pigs, and on the test of U-44069-induced contraction of the rabbit aorta in vitro as shown in Table 1. The results are summarized as percent inhibition at various doses. The potency of the compounds in vivo depended on the number of methylene groups. The highest potency appeared in AA-2414 with five methylene groups. As for the quinonyl moiety, 3,5,6-trimethyl-1,4-benzoquinon-2-yl group appeared to be more effective when compared with compounds with the same number of methylene groups. Interestingly, the compound with methoxy groups in the quinone moiety had a very low activity.

The biologic effects on the substituents of the phenyl group were examined. The compounds with substituents at the para position were generally better than those with substituents at the ortho or meta position, and the compounds with fluorine or methyl group at the para position were as active as AA-2414.

The effects of terminal groups (X) were investigated. It was found that the compounds with methoxycarbonyl, aminocarbonyl, hydroxymethyl, or methyl as X had significant activity in tests in vivo, but in tests in vitro the compounds with groups other than the carboxyl group were significantly less active. It was found that the carboxyl group is essential for the assay in vitro.

On the basis of the structural similarity of AA-2414, TXA_2, and CV-4151 (5) and the biologic data, we postulated that the potent antiasthmatic effects were mainly based on the receptor antagonistic action of TXA_2/PGH_2. To prove this assumption, optical active compounds of AA-2414 were prepared by optical

Table 1. Pharmacologic Effects of ω,ω-Phenylquinonylalkanoic Acids

Compd	R	n	G.p. Bronchoconstrn. IgG$_1$-mediated %inhibn 20	5mg/kg	LTD$_4$-induced %inhibn 5mg/kg	Rabbit Aorta Contrn. U-44069-induced %inhibin 10^{-5}	10^{-6}	10^{-7}M
a	Me	2	37			0		
b	Me	3	80**	2		24		
c	Me	4	52			63		
AA-2414	Me	5	89**	91**	94**	99	99	49
e	Me	6	78	18		98	0	
f	Me	7			86**	94	0	
g	Me	8	64			41		
h	MeO	5	22			0		
i		5	80		79**	100	99	20

resolution using two optical phenylethylamines. p-Bromoanilide of the (+)-isomer was determined to be the R-(+)-configuration by X-ray crystallographic analysis. Each optical isomer and AA-2414 were tested for their biologic effects (Table 2). The R-(+)-isomer and AA-2414 showed very potent inhibitory effects, whereas the S-(-)-isomer was much less active. The latter effect might result from 2% contamination of the active compound. These data suggested that AA-2414 is a non-prostanoid TXA$_2$/PGH$_2$ receptor antagonist, since no antagonistic actions on the receptors of LT or PAF were observed.

Table 2. Comparison of Pharmacologic Effects of AA-2414 and its Optical Isomers (Dose, mg/kg, p.o.)

Compd	% Inhibition of Bronchoconstriction (G.P.) IgG$_1$-mediated 20	5	1.25	0.31	0.08	LTD$_4$-induced 1.25	0.31	0.08
AA-2414	89**	91**	77**	58**	24	90**	89**	31
R-(+)-		80**	85**	85**	12	93**	75**	72**
S-(-)-	65*	27	NT			NT		

Very interestingly, AA-2414 showed highly potent inhibitory effects on platelet activating factor(PAF)-induced broncho-constriction in guinea pig (po) and on PGD_2-, $PGF_{2\alpha}$-, and $9\alpha,11\beta$-PGF_2-induced constriction of the guinea-pig tracheal trips in vitro (Table 3). These widely inhibitory effects might be expressed as the eicosanoid antagonistic action from these assays. Moreover, as matter of course, these quinone compounds also showed both 5-lipoxygenase inhibitory and AOS scavenging activities.

Table 3. Effect of AA-2414 on Agonist-induced Constractions
of Tracheal Strips in Guinea-pigs

Agonist	pA_2	% Maximum	N
U-46619	7.69 ± 0.11	100	5
PGD_2	7.20 ± 0.09	100	6
$9\alpha,11\beta$-PGF_2	7.79 ± 0.29	100	6
$PGF_{2\alpha}$	5.71 ± 0.28	100	3

It is concluded that AA-2414, a non-eicosanoid compound, is a novel, highly potent, orally active, and long-lasting eicosanoid antagonist. Thus, this compound posesses a variety of pharma-cologically beneficial effects and is under clinical investigations for the treatment of asthma, allergy, and other diseases.

REFERENCE

1. Yoshimoto,T.,Yokoyama,C.,Ochi,K.,Yamamoto,S.,Maki,Y.,Terao,S., and Shiraishi,M.(1982): Biochim.Biophys.Acta,713: 470.

2. Shiraishi,M.and Terao,S.(1983): J.Chem.Soc.Perkin Trans.I,1591.

3. Shiraishi,M.,Kato,K.,and Terao,S.(1988): submitted to J.Chem. Soc.Perkin Trans.I.

4. Shiraishi, M., Kato, K., Terao, S., Ashida, Y., Terashita, Z., and Kito,G.(1988): submitted to J.Med.Chem.

5. Kato,K.,Ohkawa,S.,Terao,S.,Terashita,Z.,and Nishikawa,K.(1985): J.Med.Chem.28:287.

Advances in Prostaglandin, Thromboxane, and Leukotriene Research, Vol. 19, edited by B. Samuelsson, P. Y.-K. Wong, and F. F. Sun, Raven Press, Ltd., New York ©1989.

STABLE 9β- OR 11α-HALOGEN-15-CYCLOHEXYL-PROSTAGLANDINS WITH HIGH AFFINITY TO THE PGD$_2$-RECEPTOR [1]

K.-H. Thierauch, C.-St. Stürzebecher, and E. Schillinger
Institute of Pharmacology

H. Rehwinkel, B. Radüchel, W. Skuballa, and H. Vorbrüggen*
Institute of Medicinal Chemistry

Research Laboratories of Schering AG,
Berlin (West) and Bergkamen,
Federal Republic of Germany.

PGD$_2$ is a chemically rather labile, ubiquitously occuring, natural prostaglandin formed from PGH$_2$ by PGD$_2$-synthetase, which inhibits aggregation of human-, sheep- and horse platelet rich plasma [2] and can be a vasodilator as well as an ateriolar constrictor if given intraarterially in sheep [3]. In man after i.v. infusion PGD$_2$ causes facial flushing and nasal congestion with little or no effects on platelets and blood pressure at the concentrations studied [4]. In dogs, PGD$_2$ increases lung resistance and pulmonary arterial pressure, which might be due to the conversion of PGD$_2$ into 11ß-PGF$_2$ [5] or its isomers [6].

We [7] and others [8] had earlier discovered that the replacement of the 9-keto group in PGE$_2$-type prostaglandins by halogens leads to chemically stable PGE$_2$-analogues with high affinity to the PGE$_2$-receptor like 9-desoxy-9ß-chloro-16,16-dimethyl-PGF$_2$α, nocloprost [9], a new potent cytoprotective drug for the treatment of stomach ulcers without <u>any</u> systemic side effects on oral application in man.

These results encouraged us to try to synthesize chemically stable PGD$_2$-analogues, with halogens replacing the 11-keto group and further modification of the lower side chain. Among the numerous analogues synthesized only the 11-desoxy-11α-chloro-16,17,18,19,20-pentanor-15-cyclohexyl derivative (ZK 111 298) and even more so the corresponding 11α-fluoro analogue (ZK 115 886) showed pronounced affinity to the PGD$_2$-receptor.

The synthesis of the 11α-chloro compound started (Scheme 1) with the conversion of the 11α-hydroxyl group in the 9,15-dibenzoylated PGF$_2$α-analogue 1 with Zn(OTs)$_2$ acc. to Galynker and Still [10] to give the 11ß-tosylate 2. Subsequent reaction with LiCl in DMF at 65°C to 3 followed by removal of the protecting groups afforded a 38 % overall yield of the analogue 4 (ZK 111 298), which has a competing factor of 12 i.e. binds to the PGD$_2$-receptor approximately 1/10 as well as PGD$_2$.

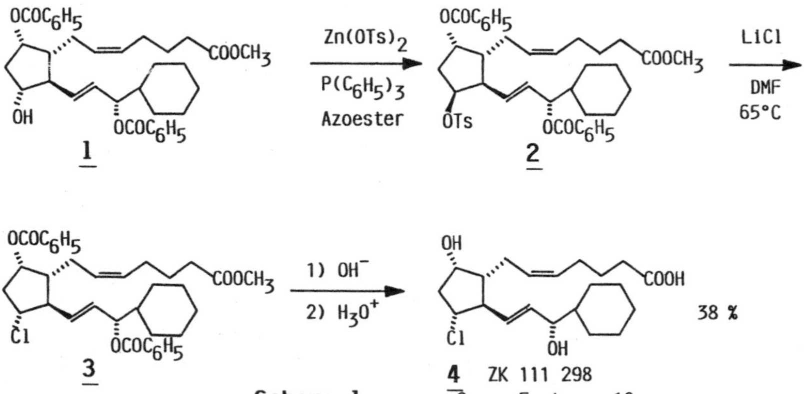

Scheme 1

4   ZK 111 298
Comp. Factor = 12

The synthesis of the corresponding 11α-fluoro compound (Scheme 2) turned out to be much more difficult. After some experimentation it was discovered that the t-butyl-dimethylsilyl protection group for the 9α- and 15α-hydroxyl groups was best suited and survived treatment of the free 11ß-hydroxyl groups with DAST. Thus, reaction of the bis-silylated 11α-tosylate 5 with KNO2 in DMSO 11) afforded the 11ß-hydroxyl-compound 6, which on treatment with DAST at -70°C gave the desired 11α-fluoro compound 7 in 25 % yield and about 35 % of the corresponding 11,13-diene. Removal of the protecting groups in 7 furnished a 12 % overall yield of the free 11α-fluoro compound 8 (ZK 115 886), which has a competing factor for the PGD2-receptor of 4.

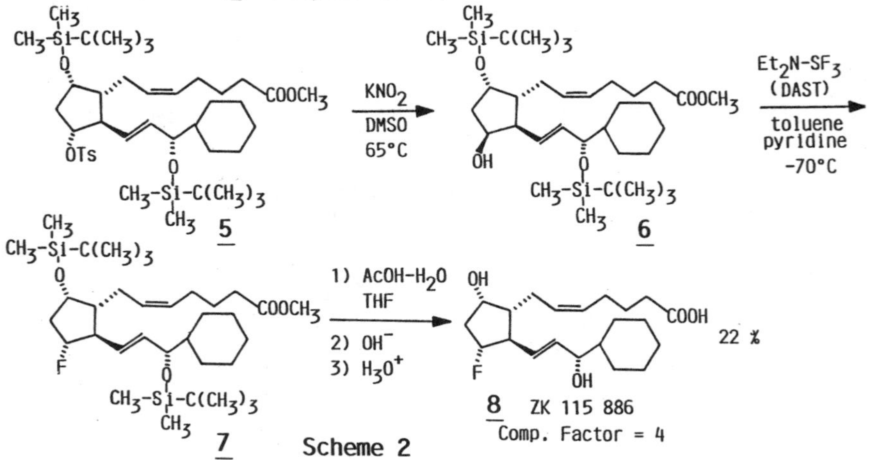

8   ZK 115 886
Comp. Factor = 4

Scheme 2

Since the 15-cyclohexyl moiety thus seems to dramatically enhance the PGD2-character in 11α-halogen-prostaglandins as in 16,17,18,19,20-tetranor-15-cyclohexyl-PGD2 12) and in the hydantoin-derivative BW 245 C 13), we wondered whether the corresponding 9-halogen-16,17,18,19,20-pentanor-15-cyclohexyl-prostaglandins might also possess PGD2-like qualities.

Starting from the protected PGF$_2\alpha$-analogue 9 (Scheme 3) with a free 9α-hydroxy group, reaction with DAST and subsequent removal of the protection groups gave a 20 % overall yield of the free 9ß-fluoro compound 10 (ZK 112 151), which has a competing factor to the PGD$_2$-receptor of 1.2.

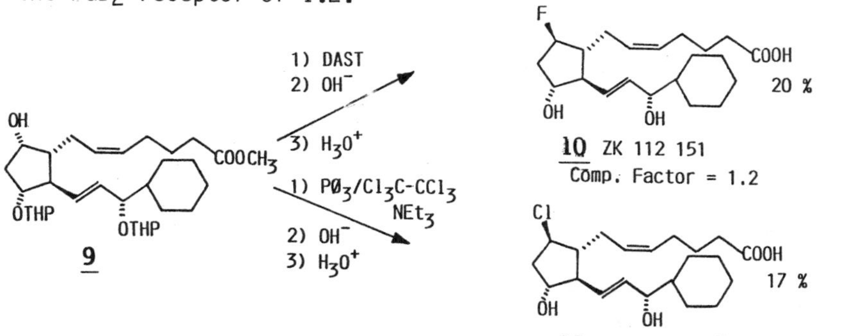

F

1) DAST
2) OH⁻
3) H$_3$O⁺

COOH
20 %

10 ZK 112 151
Comp. Factor = 1.2

OH

COOCH$_3$

1) PØ$_3$/Cl$_3$C-CCl$_3$
   NEt$_3$
2) OH⁻
3) H$_3$O⁺

ÖTHP   ÖTHP
9

Cl

COOH
17 %

Scheme 3

11 ZK 110 841 (mp 53-55°C)
Comp. Factor = 0.5

The corresponding crystalline 9ß-chloro compound 11 (ZK 110 841), which is readily available from 9 with a 17 % overall yield by treatment with triphenylphosphine-dichloride in the presence of triethylamine and subsequent removal of the protecting groups, shows a competing factor to the PGD$_2$-receptor of 0.5. Thus 11 (ZK 110 841) binds twice as well to the PGD$_2$-receptor as PGD$_2$ and furthermore does not bind to the PGE$_2$-receptor. Due to its biological potency, ease of preparation and its crystalline state, 11 (ZK 110 841) was chosen as our prototype of a chemically stable PGD$_2$-analogue to be further investigated and characterized.

On Scheme 4 some of the biological results are summarized obtained up to now with our ZK 110 841.

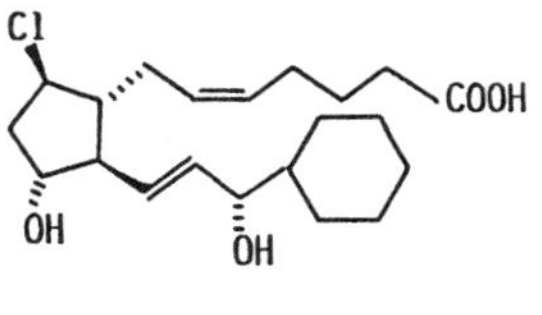

Cl

COOH

ZK 110 841 (mp 53-55°C)

OH   ÖH

- Receptor binding: PGD$_2$-receptor   comp. factor = 0.5 (PGD$_2$ = 1) ·
                     PGE$_2$-receptor   no competition

- Stimulates cAMP formation in human platelets to twice basal level at 5 ·10⁻⁸ mol/l

- Hypotensive in SHR on i.v. infusion at 30 µg/kg/min for 20 min

- Hypotensive for up to 40 min in conscious rats (acc. to Weeks) on oral application of 4 mg/kg

- No antiproliferative effect on cultured human glioma cells in culture [Westphal et al., Acta Neurochir. 83, 56 (1986)]

Scheme 4

The lack of antiproliferative effects of 11 [14) is probably due to its chemical stability, since no ready formation of an α,ß-unsaturated 5-ring-ketone [15) is possible.

Concerning potential clinical applications of these new chemically stable PGD2-analogues a recent pertinent patent application [16) describes the use of PGD2 and its analogues including BW 245 C for the treatment of ocular hypertension and glaucoma.

REFERENCES

1. The full paper has been submitted for publication.

2. Whittle BJR, Moncada S, Vane JR, Prostaglandins 1978;16:373-388.

3. Jones RL, Acta biol. med. germ. 1978;37:837-844.

4. Heavey DJ, Lumley P, Barrow SE, Murphy MB, Humphrey PPA, Dollery CT, Prostaglandins 1984;28:755-767.

5. Pugliese G, Spokas EG, Marcinkiewicz E, Wong PYK, J. Biol. Chem. 1985;260:14621-14625.

6. Wendelborn DF, Seibert K, Roberts II LJ, Proc. Natl. Acad. Sci. USA 1988;85:304-308.

7. Loge O, Radüchel B, Naunyn Schmiedeberg's Arch. Pharm., Suppl. 1984;325:R33.

8. Arroniz CE, Gallina J, Martinez E, Muchowski JM, Velarde E, Rooks WH, Prostaglandins 1978;16:47-64.

9. Drugs of the Future 1986;11:660-662.

10. Galynker I, Still WC, Tet. Letters 1982;23:4461-4464.

11. Radüchel B, Synthesis 1980;292-295.

12. Tynan SS, Andersen NH, Wills MT, Harker LA, Hanson SR, Prostaglandins 1984;27:683-696.

13. Town MH, Casals-Stenzel J, Schillinger E, Prostaglandins 1983;25:13-28.

14. Westphal M, Neuss M, Herrmann HD, Acta Neurochir. (Wien) 1986;83:56-61.

15. Fukushima M, Kato T, Ota K, Arai Y, Narumiya S, Hayaishi O, Biochem. Biophys. Res. Comm. 1982;109:626-633.

16. Res. Develop. Corp. Jap., Europ. Patent Appl. 253094, May 5, 1987.

Advances in Prostaglandin, Thromboxane, and
Leukotriene Research, Vol. 19, edited by
B. Samuelsson, P. Y.-K. Wong, and F. F. Sun,
Raven Press, Ltd., New York ©1989.

SYNTHESIS AND IN VITRO EFFECTS ON PLATELETS AND VASCULAR SMOOTH MUSCLE OF S-145, A NOVEL THROMBOXANE RECEPTOR ANTAGONIST

M. Narisada, M. Ohtani, F. Watanabe, K. Uchida, H. Arita,
M. Doteuchi, M. Ueda, K. Hanasaki, H. Kakushi, K. Otani,
S. Hara, and M. Nakajima

Shionogi Research Laboratories, Shionogi & Co., Ltd.,
Fukushima-ku, Osaka 553, Japan

Thromboxane A_2 (TXA$_2$), an inducer of platelet aggregation and vasoconstriction as well as bronchoconstriction, may be a mediator in several ischemic diseses. S-145, (±)-5Z-(3-*endo*-phenylsulfonylamino-[2.2.1]bicyclohept-2-*exo*-yl)heptenoic acid (**7a**), its derivatives at the sulfonyl residue **7b-t**, and its stereoisomers (+)-**7a**, (−)**7a**, **10**, **12**, and **15** were synthesized and examined for their in vitro inhibitory activity against responses induced by TXA$_2$-related substances. Compound **7a**, which was designed based on the idea that U-shaped analogs of sultroban, 4-(2-phenylsulfonylaminoethyl)phenoxyacetic acid, may be good TXA$_2$ receptor antagonists, was found to be a potent, selective TXA$_2$ receptor antagonist against aggregation of platelets and contraction of vascular smooth muscle.

SYNTHESIS

Synthesis of the sulfonyl amino derivatives are depicted in Scheme 1 and 2. *exo*-Allylketone **2**, prepared from (dl)-nor-camphor[1]) was converted into **3** by reduction of a mixture of the corresponding oximes with lithium aluminum hydride, followed by benzyloxycarbonylation. Trans configuration of the side chains in **3** was confirmed based on its proton NMR signal at $\delta = 3.53$ ($J = 7.4$ and 4.0 Hz). Cleavage of olefin in **3** by peracid epoxydation, followed by periodic acid oxidation, gave **4**. Wittig reaction of **4** with the reagent, prepared from δ-carboxyl-butyl, triphenylphosphonium bromide and dimsyl sodium, followed by treatment with diazomethane, yielded mostly the desired **5Z**. Deprotection of benzyloxycarbonyl group in **5Z** with trifluoroacetic acid afforded the amine as its trifluoroacetate **6**. Sulfonylation of **6** with suitable sulfonylating agents, followed by saponification gave **7a** and its derivatives **7b-t**.

Isomers with different stereochemistry at the junction of the side chains were also synthesized. A key intermediate **9** was prepared from

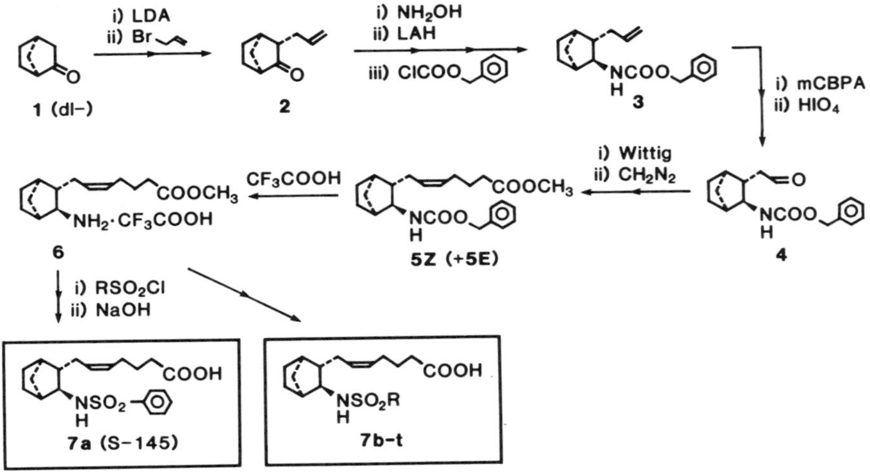

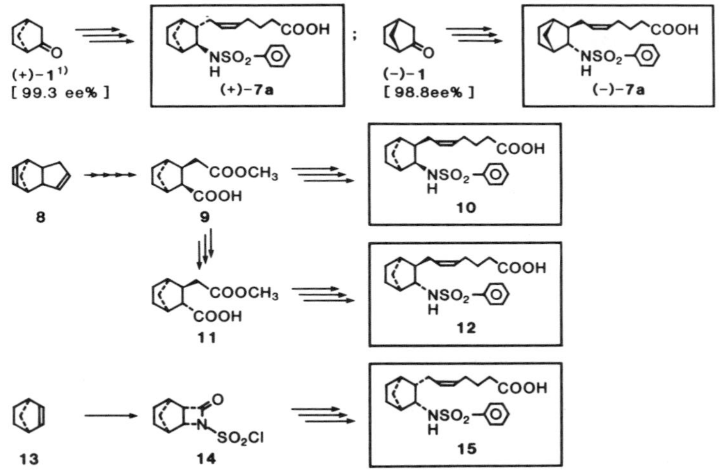

i) LDA
ii) Br

1 (dl–)

2

i) NH₂OH
ii) LAH
iii) ClCOO

3

i) mCBPA
ii) HIO₄

CF₃COOH

COOCH₃

NH₂·CF₃COOH

6

i) Wittig
ii) CH₂N₂

COOCH₃

NCOO

5Z (+5E)

NCOO

4

i) RSO₂Cl
ii) NaOH

COOH

NSO₂

7a (S-145)

COOH

NSO₂R

7b-t

(+)-1 [99.3 ee%]

COOH

NSO₂

(+)-7a

;

(–)-1 [98.8ee%]

COOH

NSO₂

(–)-7a

8

COOCH₃
COOH

9

COOH

NSO₂

10

COOCH₃
COOH

11

COOH

NSO₂

12

13

14

SO₂Cl

COOH

NSO₂

15

8 by the following procedures: selective hydrogenation, oxidative cleavage of the resulting olefin in the cyclopentene ring, anhydride formation, and methanolysis. Formal epimerization of the *endo*-carboxyl group to the *exo*-one afforded 11. Sulfonylation after Curtius rearrangement of the carboxyl group and extension of the acetic acid

side chain in **9** and **11** gave **10** and **12**, respectively. Compound **14** obtained by cycloaddition to **13** was similarly modified to **15** after hydrolysis of its β-lactam ring.

BIOLOGICAL ACTIVITY

In vitro activity of the obtained compounds are given in Table 1. IC_{50} values are listed for aggregation of rabbit PRP (platelet-rich plasma) induced by arachidonic acid, aggregation of rat washed platelets induced by collagen, and contraction of rat thoracic aorta induced by U-46619. Effects of the modification of the structure of the ω-side chain appear to depend upon lipophilicity of the sulfonylamino residues and the location of the phenyl group in the ω-side chain. Thus, IC_{50} values for **7a** are the lowest followed by those for **7c**, **7d**, and **7b**, in this order. The values for **7a** are also lower than those for each of its isomers in the side chain stereochemistry **10**, **12**, and **15**. (+)-Enantiomer **7a** exhibits lower IC_{50} values than **7a**, while (−)-**7a** has significantly higher values.

TABLE 1. In vitro activity

Compd[a]	Preparation R	Rabbit PRP IC_{50} (μM)[b]	Rat washed platelets IC_{50} (nM)[c]	Rat thoracic aorta IC_{50} (nM)[d]
7a	phenyl	1.0	2.9	1.4
7b	benzyl	113	26	111
7c	2-phenylethyl	8.2	3.7	3.4
7d	3-phenylpropyl	14	10.9	10.9
7e	*methyl*	640	370	1580
7f	*n*-hexyl	13.3	19	17.2
7g	*p*-methylphenyl	0.5	2.4	0.7
7h	*o*-methylphenyl	6.2	4.3	3.7
7i	*m*-methylphenyl	1.7	5.6	3.2
7j	*p*-ethylphenyl	4.6	3.3	1.5
7k	*p*-(n-hexyl)phenyl	800	14.5	--
7l	2-naphtyl	1.1	2.7	2.7
7m	*p*-diphenyl	200	6.0	9.8
7n	*p*-hydroxyphenyl	0.5	4.0	--
7o	*p*-methoxyphenyl	1.7	3.9	--
7p	*p*-nitrophenyl	1.4	8.9	--
7q	*p*-fluorophenyl	0.6	2.9	--
7r	p-chlorophenyl	0.3	2.9	--
7s	*p*-oxycarbonylphenyl	800	>1000	--
7t	*p*-dimethylaminophenyl	7.1	52	--
(+)-**7a**		0.6	1.8	0.49
(−)-**7a**		7.4	13.4	15.3
10		43	4.1	18
12		9	2.9	5.9
15		18	11	19

[a] Corresponding sodium salts dissolved in aqueous solutions were measured.
[b] Aggregation induced by 500 μM of arachidonic acid.
[c] Aggregation induced by 4 μg/mL of collagen.
[d] Contraction induced by 30 nM of (15*S*)-hydroxy-11,9-epoxymethanoprosta-5*Z*,13*E*-dienoic acid (U-46619).
[e] Synthesis of (+)-enantiomer has recently been reported, independently.[3]

TABLE 2. Pharmacological profile of inhibitory activity of S-145

Preparation		Ligand/Inducer	(μM)	IC_{50} (nM)
Human washed platelets	Binding	[^{3}H]-U46619	0.012	3
		[^{125}I]-PTAOH[a]	0.0002	3
	Aggregation	Arachidonic acid	6	2
		U46619	0.5	7.7
		Collagen	2 μg/ml	4.5
		ADP, primary	4	>1000
		Thrombin	0.2 unit/ml	>1000
	TXB2 synthesis	Thrombin	2 units/ml	>10000
Rat thoracic aorta	Contraction	U46619	0.03	1.4
		KCl	50000	>1000
		Norepinephrine	1	>1000
		Angiotensin II	0.1	>1000
		Serotonin	10	>1000
Cat coronary artery	Contraction	U46619	0.1	2.5
Human PRP	Aggregation	Arachidonic acid	500	250
		U46619	4	340
		Collagen	0.5 μg/ml	240
		ADP, secondary	2-3	80

[a] [^{125}I]-(5Z,15ξ)-9α,11α-dimethylmethano-13-aza-15-hydroxy-16-(3-iodo-4-hydroxy-phenyl)-17,18,19,20-tetranor-11a-carbathrombo-5-enoic acid.

Substituent effects are indicated by the values for **7g-t**. Compounds with substituents of limited structure at the *p*-position, **7g**, **7n**, **7o**, **7p**, **7q**, and **7r**, exhibit the lowest IC_{50} values. Note, however, the high values for **7k**, **7m**, and **7s**.

From the pharmacological profile of the inhibitory activity of **7a** shown in Table 2, **7a** was concluded to be a potent, selective TXA₂ receptor antagonist on platelets and vascular smooth muscle. This compound might be useful as a drug for treatment of various TXA₂-related diseases and also as a reagent for studying the pharmacological roles of TXA₂.

ACKNOWLEDGMENT

The authors are grateful to Professor M. Fujiwara and Associate Professor S. Narumiya of the Department of Pharmacology, Faculty of Medicine, Kyoto University, for their helpful discussion and for supplying us with the data of the binding experiments.

REFERENCES

1. Barraclough P. *Tetrahedron Lett* 1980; 21: 1897-1900.

2. Irwin AJ, Jones JB. *J Am Chem Soc* 1976; 98: 8476-8481.

3. Furuta K, Hayashi S, Miwa Y, Yamamoto H. *Tetrahedron Lett* 1987; 28: 5841-5844.

*Advances in Prostaglandin, Thromboxane, and
Leukotriene Research*, Vol. 19, edited by
B. Samuelsson, P. Y.-K. Wong, and F. F. Sun,
Raven Press, Ltd., New York ©1989.

DEVELOPMENTS OF TXA$_2$ ANTAGONISTS

Nobuyuki Hamanaka

Minase Research Institute, Ono Pharmaceutical Co., Ltd.
Shimamoto, Mishima, Osaka 618, Japan

Thromboxane A$_2$ is well known to play a very important role in
cardiovascular system and is proposed to be an origin of some
kinds of deseases, e.g., angina and thrombosis. Therefore, TXA$_2$
antagonist is of great importance in order to develop a therapeutic agent for these deseases.

We had already reported some effective antagonists, ONO-11120,
1 (1) and ONO-3708, **2** (2). ONO-11120 showed potent antagonistic
activities, however, this compound is hardly insoluble in water.
Therefore, we introduced an amide grouping to improve this dis-
advantage and obtained ONO-3708.

ONO-3708 showed marked inhibitory effects on platelet aggregation induced by 10^{-6}M of STA$_2$ (3) and on smooth muscle constriction induced by 10^{-6}M of U-46619. Distinct features of ONO-
3708 are as follows.
(1) Several pharmacological studies proved that ONO-3708 does not
    show any agonistic properties.
(2) The effects of ONO-3708 were cleared in less than 30 min.
    after discontinuation of infusion, which was proved to be due
    to rapid metabolization in blood.
Therefore, ONO-3708 is proposed to be a useful agent for an
urgent treatment which demands a transient effect. However,
second feature of ONO-3708 is the less effective by oral
administration.

1   **2** (0.45 µM)

To realize our second subject, development of an orally
active and long lasting TXA$_2$ antagonist, we carried out the
following modification on ONO-3708.
First, the carboxylic amide grouping was replaced by sulfonic
amide grouping to improve the susceptibility of the former amide

to hydrolysis. This modification not only provided an orally active TXA$_2$ antagonist, but afforded such a restriction that the sulfonyl admie moiety should bear an aromatic ring to retain a potent antagonistic activities, as seen in the compound 3. For example, the compound 3 shows potent inhibitory activities against human platelet aggregation and against aortic constriction.

Second, the pinane ring system seen in the compounds 1, 2, and 3, was transformed to the other ring system in which the sulfonyl amide moiety was conserved. Among a variety of ring systems we prepared, so far, bicyclo [2.2.1] heptane ring system seen in the compound 4 produced very potent and persistent antagonistic activities, and, hence, the compound 4 was adopted as a template for further modifications. For example, i.v. administration 100 µg/kg of the compound 4 suppresses STA$_2$ induced pressor response with long duration, and oral administration persistently inhibited platelet aggregation (ex. vivo) and pressor response (in vivo) induced by STA$_2$. Marked progress were gained in this modification, however, the compounds 3 and 4 showed unfavorable transient agonistic activities.

Before further modification to eliminate these adverse effects from the template 4, a careful conformational analysis on the structure of the compound 4 was carried out by observation of nuclear overhauser effect and double resonance method of nuclear magnetic resonance spectroscopy. This study afforded the evidence that the compound 4 was existed in two preferred conformers, 4a and 4b, and also showed a spacial arrangement of the amide moiety and a-side chain is rather fixed.

The compounds 5 and 6, which were prepared to fix the orientation of both moieties based on the second evidence, were unexpectedly not potent antagonists, although these two derivatives were very nicely overlapped with the template 4, structurally.

Finally, modification on the side chain was carried out. When the position of the ring system was slidden to the adjacent carbon toward the carboxylic acid terminal, not only a comparable potent antagonistic activity was retained as seen in the compounds 7, 8, and 9, but a very interesting result for assuming the spacial arrangement of TXA$_2$ receptor was obtained.

Absolute configuration of the compound 4, which is twice more potent than its dl-mixture, is reflected in the derivative 7, which is, however, 10 times less potent than the enantiomeric isomer 9, of which absolute configuration is opposit to the template 4, consequently.

These modification on ONO-3708 described here provided a derivative 9 which is 10 times more potent than ONO-3708, however, the unfavorable agonistic activities could not be completely eliminated.

We still continue to develop a TXA$_2$ antagonist freed from the adverse effects.

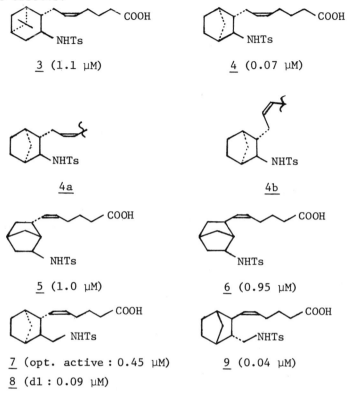

3 (1.1 µM)   4 (0.07 µM)

4a   4b

5 (1.0 µM)   6 (0.95 µM)

7 (opt. active : 0.45 µM)   9 (0.04 µM)

8 (dl : 0.09 µM)

inhibition of human platelet aggregation induced by STA$_2$(IC$_{50}$)

REFERENCES

1. Katsura M, Miyamoto T, Hamanaka N, et al. 1983;11:351.

2. Suga H, Hamanaka N, Kondo K, et al. Adv. Prostaglandin Thromboxane Leukotriene Res 1987;17B:799.

3. Ohuchida S, Hamanaka N, Hayashi M. 1983;39:4263,4269.

Advances in Prostaglandin, Thromboxane, and Leukotriene Research, Vol. 19, edited by B. Samuelsson, P. Y.-K. Wong, and F. F. Sun, Raven Press, Ltd., New York ©1989.

STEREOCHEMISTRY-ACTIVITY STUDIES IN

6-KETO-PROSTAGLANDIN-E1 (6-KETO-PGE1) ANALOGS

Katsuhiro Imaki, Masanori Kawamura, Yoshinobu Arai,
Yoshiki Sakai, and Takashi Muryobayashi

Minase Research Institute, Ono Pharmaceutical Co., Ltd.,
Shimamoto, Mishima, Osaka 618, Japan

Ornoprostil (17S,20-dimethyl-6-Keto-PGE1 methyl ester; trade name: RONOK) has been launched in Japan as an oral therapeutic drug for a gastric ulcer in 1987 (1).

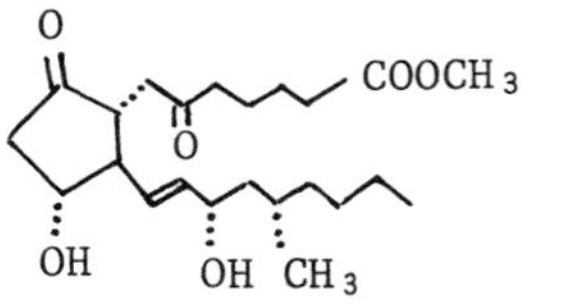

Structural features of this compound are as follows.
1) Being an analog of 6-Keto-PGE1.
2) Comprising a methyl group at C-17 position with S-absolute configuration.

Fig. 1 Structure of Ornoprostil

The configuration of methyl group at C-17 position has remarkable influence on a biological activity because R-isomer shows little efficacy. This result encouraged us to investigate the relationships between biological activities and stereochemistry of alkyl substituent on ω side chain of 6-Keto-PGE1 in more detail. It is potentially interesting to note whether a separation of the agonist activities of 6-Keto-PGE1, especially in anti-aggregating and vasodilator actions, can be acheived by this kind of approach. For this purpose, we have synthesized several 6-Keto-PGE1 analogs having an alkyl cyclopentane ring ir ω side chain in which two new chiral centers at C-16 and C-18 position were incorporated. Furthermore, these ω side chains were also applied to carbacyclin series.

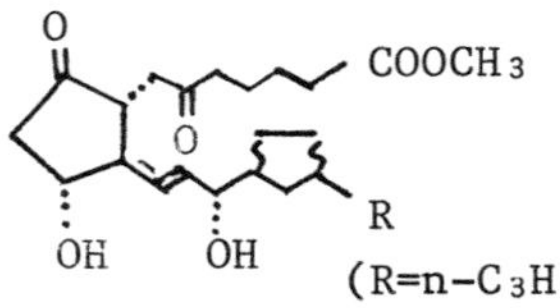

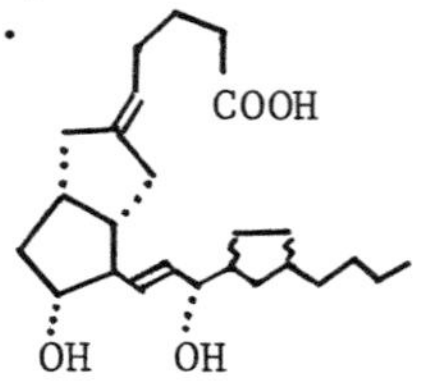

Fig. 2 Structures of synthesized 6-Keto-PGE1 and carbacyclin analogs

CHEMISTRY

Key intermediates, the optically active phosphonates, were prepared from optically active cyclopentanone carboxylic acid (2) as shown in Figure 3. 6-Keto-PGE1 and carbacyclin analogs were synthesized respectively using these phosphonates according to well known method mentioned by Hayashi et al., (3, 4, 5).

Fig. 3 Synthesis of optically active Phosphonates

1) t-BuOH,DCC 2)NaBH₄ 3)CH₃SO₂Cl

HOOC ⟨⟩=O S-form

4) R₂CuLi (R=n-C₃H₇,n-C₄H₉)

5) (MeO)₂PCH₂Li   and

$(MeO)_2PCH_2C$ — R (S,S)

$(MeO)_2PCH_2C$ — R (S,R)

As above

HOOC···⟨⟩=O R-form

and

$(MeO)_2PCH_2C$ (R,S) R

$(MeO)_2PCH_2C$ (R,R) R

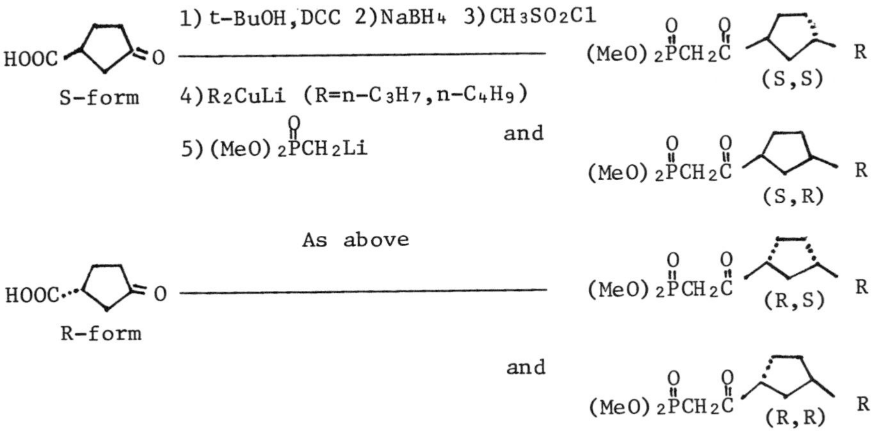

RESULTS AND DISCUSSION

The structure and biological activities of 6-Keto-PGE₁ and carbacyclin analogs are shown in Table 1.

1) Introduction of alkyl cyclopentane ring to 6-Keto-PGE₁ uniformely enhanced the agonist activity. n-Propyl group as alkyl moiety produces more potent agonist activities in all stereoisomers than n-butyl group.

2) The absolute configuration at C-16 position of 6-Keto-PGE₁ analogs has remarkable influence in potency of both agonist activities. 16S-isomers exhibited more potent activity, whereas 16R - isomers showed less activity. On the other hand, the C-18 configuration has relatively less influence in their potency. These results seem to indicate that the binding models of 6-Keto-PGE₁ analogs to the receptor on platelet and blood vessels are very similar each other. A quite similar tendency was observed in carbacyclin analogs. This result seems to be reasonable because it has been previously shown that 6-keto-PGE₁ and prostacyclin act through the same receptor (6).

Table 1.   Relative potency and selectivity of 6-Keto-PGE₁ and carbacyclin analogs on anti-aggregating and hypotensive activities.   Potency was compared with PGE₁ (taken as 1).

	Absolute configuation (C-16,C-18)	a) Inhibition rat platelet aggregation	b) Dog B.P	c) Selectivity ratio Agg/B.P
PGE₁		1	1	1
	S.S	230.0	43.0	5.3
	S.R	128.0	21.0	6.0
	R.S	29.4	11.0	2.6
	R.R	36.4	12.0	3.0
	S.S	99.6	14.5	6.8
	S.R	28.4	8.0	3.0
	R.S	11.1	2.5	4.4
	R.R	21.3	4.6	4.6
	S.S (ONO-1579)	506.0	24.5	20.6
	S.R	76.9	14.9	5.4
	R.R	26.3	5.1	5.1
	S.S	9.4	0.9	10.4
	S.R	5.8	0.5	11.6
	R.S	1.3	0.05	26.0
	R.R	2.2	0.20	11.0

a) Inhibition of ADP-induced platelet aggregation was evaluated in rat platelet rich plasma.
b) Vasodilation activity was assessed as the ability to decrease mean arterial blood pressure in anaesthetised dogs.
c) Selectivity ratio indicates the ratio of anti- aggregating activity versus hypotensive activity.

3) We could not find out interesting tendency in selectivity between anti-aggregating activity and hypotensive activity among these isomers.

4) A series of free acids corresponding to 6-Keto-PGE₁ methyl ester analogs uniformely showed remarkable increase in both agonist activities. Among these compounds, 16S,18S-isomer

(refered as to ONO-1579) showed dramatically high potency in anti-aggregating activity. It seems that this potent activity of ONO-1579 may be caused by high degree of affinity to the receptor on platelets, however we can not clearly visualize the binding mode of this agonist to the receptor. In conclusion, we could find out the potent agonist of 6-Keto-PGE$_1$, however, we could not achieve the separation of its agonist activities by our present approach.

REFERENCES

1. Sochynsky R., Hardcastle J., eds. "Pharmaproject" Vol. 7, Prostaglandin (H4B), V&O Publication Ltd., (Surrey), 1986.
2. Toki K., Bull. Chem. Soc. Japan, 1957; 30:450.
3. Hayashi M., Arai Y., Wakatsuka H., et al., J. Med. Chem., 1980; 23:525-535.
4. Johnson R.A., Lindoln F.H., Thompson J.L., Nidy E.G., Mizsak S.A., and Axen U., J. Ame. Chem. Soc., 1977; 99:4182-4184.
5. Konishi Y., Kawamura M., Arai Y., and Hayashi M., Chemistry Letters, 1979; 1437-1440.
6. Samuelsson B., Paoletti R., Ramwell P.W. eds. Advances in Prostaglandin, Thromboxane, and Leucotriene Research, Vol. 17. New York:Raven Press , 1987;474-478.

Advances in Prostaglandin, Thromboxane, and Leukotriene Research, Vol. 19, edited by B. Samuelsson, P. Y.-K. Wong, and F. F. Sun, Raven Press, Ltd., New York ©1989.

SYNTHESIS OF 15-*cis*-(4-*n*-PROPYLCYCLOHEXYL)-16,17,18,19,20-

PENTANOR-9-DEOXY-6,9α-NITRILOPROSTAGLANDIN F_1 METHYL ESTER

(OP-2507), A NOVEL ANTI-CEREBRAL ISCHEMIC AGENT

S. Iguchi, Y. Miyata, H. Miyake, Y. Arai, T. Okegawa, and A. Kawasaki

Minase Research Institute, Ono Pharmaceutical Co., Ltd., Shimamoto, Mishima, Osaka 618, Japan

In the research for stable mimics of PGI_2, many analogs have been synthesized in which the unstable enol-ether linkage is replaced by a more stable grouping (1). One target molecule of this type was the nitrogen-containing PGI_2, 9-deoxy-6,9α-nitrilo-PGF_1 methyl ester (2). In order to increase the bioactivity, we have carried out the modification of its ω-chain, and have found that the highest anti-cerebral ischemic activity was obtained when a *cis*-4-*n*-propylcyclohexane ring was introduced at C_{15}.

We have evaluated the activity of a novel, stable PGI_2 analog 15-*cis*-(4-*n*-propylcyclohexyl)-16,17,18,19,20-pentanor-9-deoxy-6,9α-nitrilo-PGF_1 methyl ester (OP-2507), on the acute cerebral ischemic edema using the middle cerebral artery occlusion model in cats (3). In addition, OP-2507 was highly potent in its effect on cerebral energy metabolites in hypoxic mice, and also significantly prolonged the time of the gasping movement in complete ischemia in mice (4).

Herein we describe the total synthesis of OP-2507. The crucial step in this synthesis was the stereoselective preparation of methyl *cis*-4-propylcyclohexanecarboxylate (**2**) which was converted to the phosphonate **4** and applied for the construction of ω-chain. At first, the catalytic hydrogenation of methyl 4-(1-propylidene)

OP-2507

cyclohexanecarboxylate using many kinds of the commercially available catalysts did not afford the satisfactory *cis*-selectivity: 2 was obtained in a slight excess over its *trans* isomer.

The catalytic hydrogenation of methyl 4-*n*-propylbenzoate(1) utilizing the common catalysts, Raney Ni or Pd/C, led predominantly to the undesired *trans*-isomer (*cis/trans*, 1/5). Various catalysts were tried to use in vain in this hydrogenation involving Ir-black, IrCl(CO)(PPh₃)₂, RuCl₃, PdCl₂(PPh₃)₂, and (C₅H₅)₂Ni. After the extensive trials had given unsatisfactory *cis*-selectivity, we found that *cis*-selective hydrogenation could be achieved by use of a catalytic amount of commercially available dimer of chloro-(1,5-cyclooctadiene)rhodium [RhCl(COD)]₂, hydrogen (50 atm), hexane as an organic phase and a buffer solution at pH 7.6 containing a quaternary salts as a phase-transfer catalyst at room temperature. 1 was converted smoothly to the desired methyl *cis*-4-*n*-propylcyclohexanecarboxylate (2) and its *trans*-isomer (the ratio, 84/16). The both isomers could be separated cleanly by column chromatography on silica gel.

Chart 1. Catalytic Hydrogenation of Methyl 4-*n*-Propylbenzoate

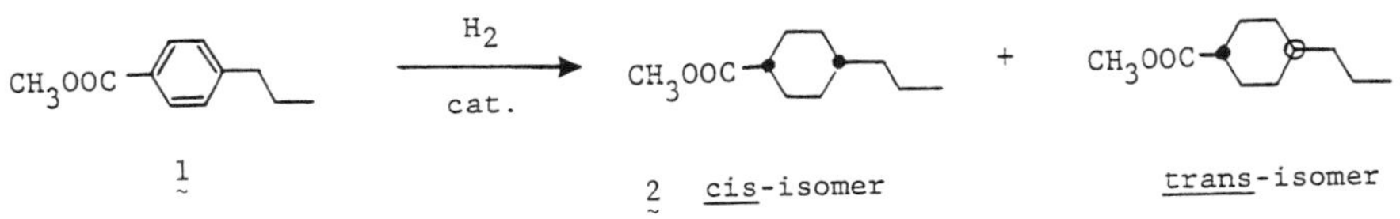

Catalyst	*cis/trans* ratio
[RhCl(COD)]₂	5.3/1.0
Pd/C	1.0/5.1
Raney Ni	1.0/5.3

The treatment of the *cis*-ester 2 with the anion derived from dimethyl methylphosphonate and *n*-butyllithium in tetrahydrofuran (THF) at -70°C gave the *cis*-phosphonate in 84% yield without isomerization at the cyclohexane ring according to the NMR analysis and TLC mobility.

The synthetic route to OP-2507 is straight-forward as shown in Chart 2. The ω-chain was introduced by the Wadsworth-Emmons reaction of the aldehyde 3 (5) with the anion derived from the *cis*-phosphonate (4) and sodium hydride in THF at room temperature in 81% yield. After the removal of the tetrahydropyranyl (THP) group in the enone 5 with 65% aqueous acetic acid and THF at 45°C the resulting C₁₁-hydroxy enone 6 was reduced stereoselectively with diisobutyl aluminum 2,6-di-*tert*-butyl-4-methylphenoxide(6) in toluene at -78°C to furnish the 15α-alcohol 7 in 69% yield accompanied with the undesired 15β-alcohol in 13% yield after easy column chromatography on silica gel. The diastereoselective reduction of the enon 6 with (S)-binaphthol-EtOH-LiAlH₄ in THF at

Chart 2. Synthetic Route to OP-2507

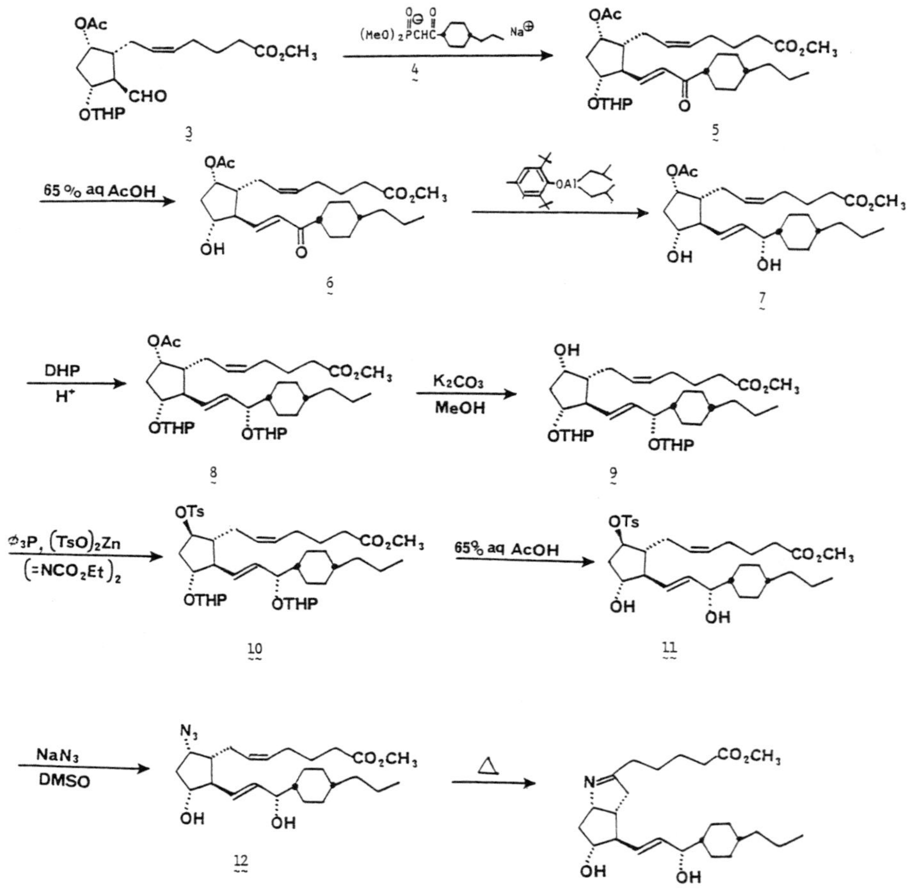

−78°C proceeded very slowly and the more than half of the enone remained in a period of 18 h although the stereoselectivity was fairly good (15α/15β-alcohol, 96/4). Sodium borohydride reduction of 6 afforded a 1:1 mixture of 15α- and 15β-alcohols. Tetrahydropyranylation of the two hydroxy functions in the 15α-alcohol 7 with dihydropyran in methylene chloride in the presence of a catalytic amount of p-toluenesulfonic acid gave the bisTHP compound 8 quantitatively. The compound 8 was treated with anhydrous potassium carbonate in methanol at room temperature to produce the C₉-alcohol 9 in 85% yield.

The ring-closure to produce the cyclic imine was carried out by the known method (2) utilizing a slight improvement of tosylation with the inversion at C₉. Tosylation of 9 with the inversion at C₉ was accomplished by the Still method (7) using zinc tosylate, diethyl azodicarboxylate, and triphenylphosphine in benzene to furnish the $C_9\beta$-tosylate 10 in 74% yield. After the removal of the THP groups in 10 with p-toluenesulfonic acid in methanol, displacement of the tosylate 11 by sodium azide in dimethylsulfoxide at 40°C for 14 h gave the azide 12, which underwent intramolecular cycloaddition with loss of nitrogen on heating in toluene at 70°C for 16 h to the final OP-2507 in 73% yield after column chromatography on silica gel.

By using a sequence of reactions similar to that described for the synthesis of OP-2507, the *trans*-isomer of 2 was led to the final *trans*-OP-2507, whose biological activity was 1/10 of that of OP-2507.

REFERENCES

1. Aristoff PA, Adv Prostaglandin Thromboxane Leukotriene Res 1985;14:309-324.

2. Bundy GL, Baldwin JM. Tetrahedron lett 1978;1731-1734.

3. Terawaki T, Takakuwa T, Iguchi S, et al. Europ J Pharmacol (submitted).

4. Masuda Y, Ochi Y, Ochi Y, et al. 1986;123:335-344.

5. Hayashi M, Arai Y, Wakatsuka H, et al. J Med Chem 1980; 23:525-535.

6. Iguchi S, Nakai H, Hayashi M, Yamamoto H. J Org Chem 1979; 44:1363-1364.

7. Galynker I, Still WC. Tetrahedron Lett 1982;23:4461-4464.

Advances in Prostaglandin, Thromboxane, and Leukotriene Research, Vol. 19, edited by B. Samuelsson, P. Y.-K. Wong, and F. F. Sun, Raven Press, Ltd., New York ©1989.

RS-5186, A NOVEL, LONG-ACTING THROMBOXANE SYNTHETASE INHIBITOR

Keiichi Matsuda, Shigeru Ushiyama, Tomiyoshi Ito*, Fumitoshi Asai*, Takeshi Oshima*, Toshihiko Ikeda**, Akihiko Nakagawa**,*Atsusuke Terada† and Mitsuo Yamazaki

New Lead Res. Labs., Biological Res. Labs.*, Analytical and Metabolic Res. Labs.**, Medicinal Chemistry Res. Labs.† Sankyo Co., Ltd., Shinagawa, Tokyo 140, Japan

RS-5186, sodium 6-[2-[2-(1H)-imidazolyl] methyl-4,5-dihydrobenzo(b)thiophene]carboxylate, is a novel and selective TXA_2 synthetase inhibitor synthesized in our Research Laboratories. The purpose of the present study was to investigate its profile for the inhibition of TXA_2 production and to compare its potency and duration with those of reported TXA_2 synthetase inhibitors, OKY-046, CV-4151 and dazoxiben.

RS-5186

Effect of RS-5186 on TXA_2 synthetase

RS-5186 inhibited human and rabbit platelet microsomal TXA_2 synthetase with IC_{50} of 6 nM and 13 nM, respectively (Table 1). The inhibitory activity of RS-5186 was more potent than those of CV-4151, OKY-046 and dazoxiben in both human and rabbit microsomal enzymes.

TABLE 1. Inhibitory effect of RS-5186 and other TXA_2 synthetase inhibitors on human and rabbit platelet microsomal TXA_2 synthetase

Enzyme source	IC_{50} (nM)			
	RS-5186	CV-4151	OKY-046	Dazoxiben
Human	6	20	300	620
Rabbit	13	39	38	106

The enzyme activity was assayed by the method of Greenwald et. al. (1).

Effects on blood prostanoid production

Oral administration of RS-5186 to beagle dogs at doses of 0.1 and 1 mg/kg markedly reduced the serum concentration of TXB_2 with sustained duration of action (Fig. 1A). A complete suppression continued over 8 hr after dosing and the suppression lasted more than 24 hr. The suppression of CV-4151 and OKY-046 was less potent than that of RS-5186 throughout the course of the treatment. Intravenous administration of RS-5186 at doses of 0.1–10 mg/kg reduced the serum TXB_2 concentration with long duration of action as shown in Fig. 1B. Serum PGD_2, PGE_2 and 6-keto $F_{1\alpha}$ were enhanced after the administration. Similar results were obtained with rabbits and rats.

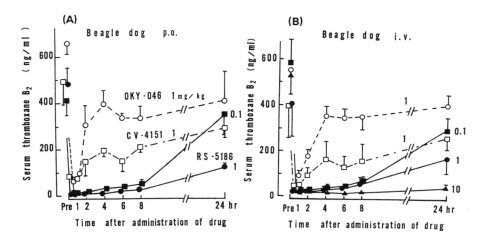

FIG. 1.   Effect of oral (A) and intravenous (B) administration of RS-5186 and other TXA_2 synthetase inhibitors on serum TXB_2 concentration in beagle dogs (n = 4). The blood samples were allowed to clot at 37° for 90 min and the serum TXB_2 were radioimmunoassayed.

Suppression of arachidonate (AA) - induced sudden death

Oral administration of RS-5186 (1 mg/kg) completely protected against AA-induced sudden death of rabbits at 1 hr after dosing and this complete protection sustained over 8 hr (Table 2). The ED_{50} of RS-5186 1 hr after the administration was calculated to be 0.12 mg/kg. CV-4151 and OKY-046 were effective at 1 hr after dosing, but were almost ineffective at 8 hr.

TABLE 2.   Effect of oral administration of RS-5186 and other TXA_2 synthetase inhibitors on sudden death induced by AA-injection in rabbits.

Group	Time before AA-injection	
	1 hr	8 hr
	survivors/total	survivors/total
Vehicle	0/4 (0 %)	0/6 (0 %)
RS-5186	4/4 (100)	6/6 (100)
CV-4151	4/4 (100)	1/6 (17)
OKY-046	4/4 (100)	0/6 (0)

Sodium arachidonate (1.4 mg/kg) was injected intravenously to rabbits. RS-5186 and other compounds (1 mg/kg) were administered orally 1 or 8 hr before AA-injection.

Blood concentration and the metabolite of RS-5186

Concentrations of RS-5186 in plasma, platelets and blood cells were determined after oral administration of ^{14}C-RS-5186 (1 mg/kg) to rabbits. As shown in Fig. 2, plasma level of RS-5186 was rapidly increased after the administration. Platelet RS-5186 level was maximum at 2 hr and the concentration was much higher than that of plasma or other blood cells (erythrocytes and leukocytes). The high RS-5186 level in platelets lasted over 24 hr. This rapid incorporation and long sustainment in platelets may explain the potency and long duration of pharmacological activities of RS-5186. The acyl-glucuronides of RS-5186 were found in bile, but only a small amount of RS-5186 metabolites was detected in blood and urine.

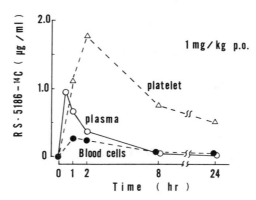

FIG. 2.   RS-5186-^{14}C concentration in rabbit blood (1 mg/kg, p.o.)

Effect on myocardial ischemia

Acute myocardial infarction model was produced in rabbits by coronary occlusion for 60 min and reperfusion for 3 hr. RS-5186 was administered intravenously at a dose of 2 mg/kg 30 min before the occlusion. Infarct size was determined by a TTC staining. Myeloperoxidase activity in the infarcted region was measured by the method of Mullane et al. (2), to estimate the neutrophil infiltration. The infarct size of no-drug control was $23.5 \pm 3.1\%$ (n = 8) and was reduced to $10.3 \pm 3.6\%$ (n = 5) (p < 0.01) by RS-5186. This drug also decreased the myeloperoxidase activity of infarct region; control (n = 8) 714 ± 123 units/g tissue vs RS-5186 group (n = 5) 343 ± 77 units/g tissue, (p < 0.05). The myeloperoxidase activity of non-infarcted rabbit heart was 1.4 units/g tissue. RS-5186 was reported to have beneficial effects in the myocardial infarction model in dogs (3).

Toxicity and tachyphylaxis

In acute toxicity studies, RS-5186 showed LD_{50} of 2.8 and 2.7 g/kg, p.o., for male and female Swiss albino mice respectively, and 1.9 g/kg, p.o. for male Fischer rats. Neither obvious toxicity nor adverse side effect was observed in the successive oral administration up to 300 mg/kg, daily for 5 weeks to Sprague-Dawley rats and beagle dogs. No significant tachphylaxis or rebound phenomenon was observed during or after successive administration of this compound to dogs for 7 days (0.1 mg/kg, p.o.).

CONCLUSION

RS-5186 is readily absorbed by oral administration and exhibits a potent and long-lasting activity in vivo without any adverse side effects, therefore this compound may prove to be of significant usefulness in diseases where TXA_2 is involved.

REFERENCES

1. Greenwald, J.E., Wong, L.K., Rao, M., Bianchine J.R. and Panganamala, R.V. Biochem. Biophys. Res. Commun., 1978; 84: 1112–1118.

2. Mullane, K.M., Kraemer, R. and Smith, B. J. Pharmacol. Methods, 1985; 14: 157–167.

3. Toki, Y., Hieda, N., Okumura, K., Hashimoto, H., Ito, T., Ogawa, K. and Satake, T. Arzneim-Forsh., 1988; 38: 224–227.

Advances in Prostaglandin, Thromboxane, and Leukotriene Research, Vol. 19, edited by
B. Samuelsson, P. Y.-K. Wong, and F. F. Sun,
Raven Press, Ltd., New York ©1989.

ENZYME IMMUNOASSAY OF THROMBOXANE B$_2$ USING
IMMOBILIZED HAPTEN AND ENZYME AMPLIFICATION

Pamela Houtz and Hsin-Hsiung Tai

Division of Medicinal Chemistry and Pharmacognosy
College of Pharmacy, University of Kentucky,
Lexington, KY 40536-0082

Determination of eicosanoid concentrations in biological
fluids has been performed by various methods notably radioimmunoassay (RIA)(1) and gas chromatography-mass spectrometry
(2). The ease and sensitivity of RIA have rendered this
analytical method a popular practice in research endeavors.
However, RIA poses some problems in radioactive contamination,
waste disposal and instability of labeled antigen of high
specific activity. Attempts to develop non-isotopic immunoassays notably enzyme immunoassay (EIA) have increased. One
major draw back is that non-isotopic immunoassays generally
possesses lower sensitivity. This aspect was recently improved by using enzymes of high turnover number (3) or employing highly sensitive enzyme assays (4,5).
We have attempted to improve EIA of hapten by using
immobilized hapten instead of conventional immobilized antibodies. This approach proves to be more feasible and greater
advantage when antiserum of low titer is used. In this paper
we describe the development of EIA for TXB$_2$ by immobilizing
TXB$_2$ after conjugation with polylysine. The rapidity and
sensitivity of the assay are further enhanced by using enzyme
amplification technique. Current sensitivity of EIA for TXB$_2$
is at least comparable or even better than that of RIA.

MATERIALS AND METHODS

Prostaglandins and thromboxane B$_2$ (TXB$_2$) were obtained
from the Upjohn Company. 1-ethyl-3-(3-dimethylaminopropyl)
carbodiimide (EDC), P-nitrophenyl phosphate, diethanolamine,
A-23187, phorbol 12-myristate 13 acetate (PMA), p-iodonitro-
tetrazolium violet (INT), Tween 20, NADP$^+$, yeast alcohol
dehydrogenase, diaphorase, anti-rabbit IgG horse radish
peroxidase conjugate, anti-rabbit IgG alkaline phosphatase
conjugate and polylysine (M.W. 15,000) were purchased from the
Sigma Chemical Company. TXB$_2$ antibodies were produced as
described previously (6). Flat bottom polyvinyl chloride
microtiter plate was obtained from the Dynatech Lab.
Conjugation of TXB$_2$ to Polylysine, Egg Albumin and Bovine
Serum Albumin -- Six hundred µg of polylysine, egg albumin, or
bovine serum albumin was dissolved in 0.4 ml of H$_2$O and the pH

was adjusted to 5.5. One hundred µg of TXB$_2$ in 0.1 ml of H$_2$O
was added. Conjugation was initiated by adding 1.5 mg of EDC
in 0.1 ml of H$_2$O. The mixture was stirred at room temperature
for one hour followed by 4°C for 15 hours. The mixture was
applied to a Sephadex G-25 column (1x20 cm) equilibrated with
water. The void volume fraction was collected, lyophilized
and stored at -20°C.

Immobilization of TXB$_2$ on Microtiter Plate and Immunoassay
Procedure -- TXB$_2$ polylysine conjugate (90 µg TXB$_2$ equivalent
with 80 ng polylysine) in 0.2 ml of coating buffer (0.1M
carbonate/bicarbonate buffer, pH 9.6) was dispensed in each
well. Control wells received 0.2 ml of polylysine (80 ng) in
coating buffer. After one hour incubation at 37°C, the plates
were washed two times with 0.25 ml of washing buffer (20 mM
Tris-HCl, pH 7.5 containing 0.14M NaCl, 2.7 mM KCl and 0.05%
Tween 20) in each well. Subsequently, each well received 0.25
ml of blocking buffer (1% Tween 20 in coating buffer) and the
plates were allowed to incubate at 37°C for one hour. The
plates were washed twice as described above. TXB$_2$ standards
or samples containing TXB$_2$ in 0.1 ml of phosphate buffered
saline were respectively added to each well in duplicates
followed by adding appropriately diluted TXB$_2$ antiplasma or
normal plasma in 0.1 ml of phosphate buffered saline containing 1% BSA. The assay mixture was mixed and incubated at 37°C
for one hour before washing the wells twice with washing
buffer. Two hundred µl of appropriately diluted anti-rabbit
IgG-alkaline phosphatase or anti-rabbit IgG-horse radish
peroxidase was added to each well and the mixture was incubated at 37°C for one hour before washing the plates three times.
Two hundred µl of alkaline phosphate substrate (17 mM
p-nitrophenyl phosphate and 5 mM MgCl$_2$ in 1M diethanolamine
buffer, pH 9.8) or horse radish peroxidase substrate (4 mM
o-phenylene diamine and 8 mM H$_2$O$_2$ in 50 mM sodium acetate
buffer, pH 5.0) was added to each well and the absorbance at
405 nm or 490 nm respectively for phosphatase or peroxidase
was measured after 30 min to 2 hours of incubation as described above. The non-specific reading shown in wells
containing normal serum was subtracted from reading of other
wells and the standard curve was constructed and the concentration in each sample determined.

Enzyme Amplification System -- Sensitivity of the above
phosphatase system can be greatly increased by using the
enzyme cycling system as described by Self (7). Briefly,
NADP$^+$ was used as substrate for alkaline phosphatase. The
product, NAD$^+$, formed was used to initiate alcohol dehydrogenase catalyzed reaction. The NADH produced was used to
reduce INT to formazan (λmax 495 nm) catalyzed by diaphorase
and NAD$^+$ was regenerated and continued to initiate another
cycle of oxidation/reduction resulting in an amplified formation of formazan. The amplified substrate system contained:
A, 0.2 mM NADP$^+$ and 1mM MgCl$_2$ in 50 mM diethanolamine buffer,

pH 9.5; B, 0.55 mM INT, 0.4 mg/ml alcohol dehydrogenase and
0.4 mg/ml diaphorase in 25 mM sodium phosphate buffer, pH 7.2
containing 4% ethanol. Both alcohol dehydrogenase and
diaphorase were devoid of any endogenous NAD$^+$ by incubating
each enzyme solution (4 mg/ml) with 1% charcoal (200 µl per ml
of enzyme solution) for 30 min at room temperature. After
centrifugation at 3,000 rpm for 5 min, the clear supernatant
was removed and diluted 10 fold with 25 mM sodium phosphate
buffer, pH 7.2. If the amplification system was used with the
above EIA system, 65 µl of the A solution was added to each
well and incubated for 15 min at room temperature before
adding 175 µl of the B solution. Absorbance at 495 nm was
measured after 5 min to one hour incubation of the amplified
substrate system.
Radioimmunoassay of TXB$_2$ - RIA of TXB$_2$ was carried out as
described previously (6).
Stimulation of Human Platelets with A-23187 or A-23187 plus
PMA - Human platelets were prepared as described earlier (8).
Platelet suspension (2x10^8/ml) was stimulated with increasing
concentrations of A-23187 alone or with 0.1 µM PMA at 37°C for
5 min. The reaction was terminated with 30 µl of lN HCl
followed by neutralization with 40 µl 1 M Tris base. The
mixture was diluted with immunoassay buffer for EIA and RIA.

RESULTS AND DISCUSSION

Conventional EIA relies on the immobilization of antibodies on
the solid phase either directly or indirectly. This procedure
requires antibodies of higher titer and may require isolation
of IgG molecules for direct immobilization. Antibodies of low
titer may not be suitable for this type of EIA as discussed by
Parsons (9). Therefore, we initiated a different approach by
immobilizing the hapten on the solid phase. Since TXB$_2$ is not
readily adsorbed by microtiter plate, we have conjugated TXB$_2$
to three different proteins to enhance immobilization.
Among polylysine, bovine serum albumin and chicken egg albumin
conjugates, TXB$_2$-polylysine conjugate provides the most
desirable properties of EIA as shown in Fig. 1.
Sharp completion between TXB$_2$ and TXB$_2$-polylysine for TXB$_2$
antibodies was clearly observed. This might be due to less
steric hindrance for TXB$_2$-polylysine conjugate to bind to
antibodies and better competition by TXB$_2$ for binding. The
amount of TXB$_2$- polylysine conjugate needed for coating was
determined by using a series of diluted antibodies and varying
the amount of conjugate coated on the plate. A non-saturable
amount of conjugate giving a reasonable reading (e.g. 1.0) of
absorbance in a relatively short time of incubation (10-30
min) was chosen for coating the plate. Similarly, the
dilution of antibodies should be such that reasonable reading
of absorbance is reached within 30 min. We have employed both
anti-rabbit IgG alkaline phosphatase conjugate and anti-rabbit

IgG horse radish peroxidase conjugate to "light up" the
absorbed primary TXB₂ antibodies. Both enzyme conjugates can
be used with desirable sensitivity as shown in Fig. 2.

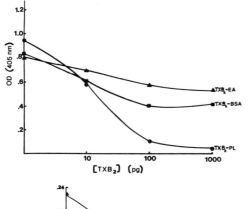

Fig.1:
Comparision of EIA
of TXB₂ using
different protein
conjugate to
immobilize TXB₂.

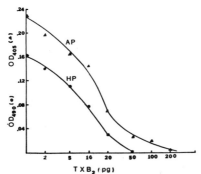

Fig.2:
Comparison of EIA
of TXB₂ using
different enzyme
marker.
Alkaline
ph-osphatase (AP),
Horseradish
peroxidase (HP)

In most cases we have employed phosphatase conjugate for our
studies since it gives higher absorbance reading.
    If the assay needs to be increased in sensitivity and
rapidity, enzyme amplification system can be included in EIA
using phosphatase marker. The system exploits the fact that
phosphatase catalyzed dephosphorylation of NADP⁺ generates
NAD⁺ which can be used to oxidize ethanol by alcohol dehydrogenase and the NADH so produced can reduce INT to produce
colored formazan by diaphorase. The resulting NAD⁺ can
initiate another cycle of oxidation/reduction giving amplified
signal of colored formazan. The only requirement of using
amplified substrate system is that both alcohol dehydrogenase
and diaphorase should be devoid of NAD⁺. Commercially available enzymes have been contaminated with different amount of
NAD⁺. Removal of this contamination by treating the enzyme
preparation with charcoal as described in the Method Section
is highly desirable. Fig. 3 indicated that the color development can be greatly facilitated by the addition of the enzyme
amplification system as opposed to regular addition of
p-nitrophenyl phosphate as a substrate. Although the sensi-

tivity did not appear to increase significantly by using the
amplification system as indicated in Fig. 3, a separate
experiment using greatly reduced amount of TXB_2-polylysine
conjugate and antibodies should increase the sensitivity of
the assay.

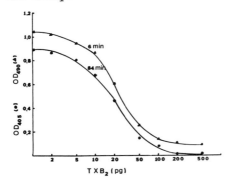

Fig.3:
EIA of TXB_2 with and
without enzyme
amplification system.
(EAS)
▲,with EAS
●,without EAS

Since non-amplified system gives better sensitivity than
the previously developed RIA (6), we have used this system to
assay TXB_2 content in biological samples. Validation of the
EIA was performed. Both EIA and RIA gave comparable results
as indicted in Fig. 4. Calcium ionophore A-23187 dose dependently stimulated platelets to release TXB_2. This
stimulation was further enhanced by the addition of PMA (data
not shown). This confirms our previously finding using RIA
as an assay method (8).

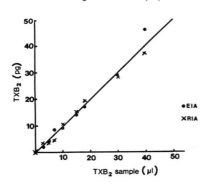

Fig.4:
Determination of TXB_2
in a biological
sample (platelet
suspension after
stimulation with 1 μM
of A-23187) using
EIA and RIA.
●, EIA
✗, RIA

The limitation of using EIA as opposed to using RIA is that the EIA assay systems appears to be more affected by the proteins present in the biological samples than does the RIA assay system. We have observed that studies on stimulation of platelets with collagen requires purification of the samples by solvent extraction before EIA can be performed. Simple purification of eicosanoids from biological fluids by Sep-Pak cartridge has been reported (10). With the advent of a sensitive EIA for TXB_2, many routine determinations of TXB_2 can be performed with a faster pace using microtiter plate and automated EIA reader. The EIA we developed should be readily applicable to the development of EIAs for other eicosanoids and haptens. All the reagents are commercially available except for polylysine conjugate and the preparation of which is as simple as preparing the conjugate for injection. We believe that the procedure developed herein should be of great value in future EIA development particularly when immobilization of antibodies may lose their avidity and/or low titers of antibodies are produced.

ACKNOWLEDGEMENTS

This work was supported in part by NSF grant (DMB-8417093)

REFERENCES

1. Granström E, Kindahl H. Adv Prostaglandin Thromboxane Res. 1978; 5:119-210.
2. Green K, Hamberg M, Samuelsson B, Smigel M, Trölich JC. Adv. Prostaglandin Thromboxane Res; 5:39-94.
3. Pradelles P, Grass J, Maclouf J. Anal. Chem. 1985; 57:1170-1173.
4. Swada M, Inagawa T, Frolich JC. Prostaglandins 1985: 29:1039-1048.
5. Hsu IC, Yolken RH, Harris CC. Methods Enzymol. 1981; 23:383-394.
6. Tai HH, Yuan B. Anal. Biochem. 1978: 87:343-349.
7. Self CH. J. Immunol. Methods 1985; 76:389-393.
8. Mobley A, Tai HH. Biochem. Biophys. Res. Commun. 1985; 130:717-723.
9. Parsons GH. Methods Enzymol. 1981; 73:224-239.
10. Powell WS. Methods Enzymol 1982; 86:467-477.

Advances in Prostaglandin, Thromboxane, and
Leukotriene Research, Vol. 19, edited by
B. Samuelsson, P. Y.-K. Wong, and F. F. Sun,
Raven Press, Ltd., New York ©1989.

A SIMPLE PURIFICATION METHOD FOR QUANTITATION OF
EICOSANOIDS, IN BIOLOGICAL SPECIMENS BY GAS
CHROMATOGRAPHY/SELECTED ION MONITORING

H.Miyazaki[1], K.Watanabe[1], T.Sakurai[2],
K.Yamashita[1], M.Ishibashi[1], and F.Nakayama[2]

1) Research Laboratories, Pharmaceuticals Group,
Nippon Kayaku Co., Ltd., 3-31-12 Shimo, Kita-ku,
Tokyo 115 Japan, 2) Department of 1st Surgery,
School of Medicine, Kyushu University, 3-1-1,
Imade, Azuma-ku, Fukuoka, 812, Japan.

Gas chromatography/selected ion monitoring (GC/SIM)
has been widely used for quantitation of trace
amounts of eicosanoids in biological specimens as
the most reliable method owing to its excellent
selectivity and sensitivity of detection. However,
it has been recognized that some impurities were
contaminated into a peak appeared selected ion
recording. For this problem, a number of
improvements of analytical procedures involving
pre-instrumental and instrumental steps have been
carried out.
In this presentation, we describe a simple
purification method for quantitation of eicosanoids
in biological specimens by GC/SIM.
Urine was collected over 24 hours from healthy male
volunteers who had not taken asprin or any other
drugs in the previous ten days and had been stored
at -20°C until analysis.
Mucosal cells or muscle tissue of dog gall bladder
was washed with an ice cold saline containing 3 μM
indomethacin and 30 μM AA861 and homogenated in an
alcohol solution containing the above cyclooxygenase
and lipoxygenase inhibitors.
After centrifugation at 6,500 x g for 15 min at
4°C, the supernatant was collected and the solvent
was evaporated under reduced pressure. The residue
was dissolved with 15% ethanol solution and adjusted
to pH 3 with diluted hydrogen chloride. Adequate
amounts of $[^2H_8]$-leukotriene-LTB$_4$, $[^2H_4]$-prostaglandin
(PG) E$_2$, $[^2H_5]$-PGF$_{2\alpha}$, $[^2H_4]$-TXB$_2$, $[^2H_4]$- and
$[^{18}O_2]$-6-keto PGF$_{1\alpha}$ were added to the sample.
The sample was extracted and purified by the present
method described in TABLE 1.
The preparation of the derivatives with
dimethylisopropylsilyl (DMUPS) imidazole and the

conditions of GC/SIM in low and high resolution modes were as described previously. (2,3)

TABLE 1. Extraction, and purification of 11-dehydro-TXB$_2$ from human urine

---

1. Add [$^{18}O_3$]-11-dehydro-TXB$_2$ to 1 ml of urine aliquot and adjust at pH 2.8.
2. Apply to Clin Elute Column, elute in ethyl acetate.
3. Evaporate to dryness.
4. Dissolved the residue in 15% ethanol.
5. Apply to SEP-PAK C$_{18}$ Column, wash with 15% ethanol, and n-hexane, and elute in ethyl acetate.
6. Evaporate to dryness.
7. Derivatize as the methyl ester (ME) with diazomethane at room temperature for 60 min. and evaporate to dryness.
8. Dissolved the residue in n-hexane-ethyl acetate (2:1).
9. Apply to silica gel column, wash n-hexane-ethyl acetate (2:1), and elute in n-hexane-ethylacetate (1:1).
10. Evaporate to dryness.
11. Derivatize as the ME-DMiPS ether with DMiPS imidazole at 60°C for 60 min.
12. Apply to Sephadex LH-20 column elute in n-hexane-chloroform-methanol (10:10:1) and evaporate to dryness.
13. GC-SIM

FIG. 1a. shows selected ion recordings of 11-dehydro-TXB$_2$ and its [$^{18}O_3$] variant in the eluate of ethyl acetate-methanol (99:1) from silica gel column when the HPLC extract from urine was obtained by the conventional purification procedure for radio immunoassay of eicosanoids using the combination of SEP-PAK and μ-Bondapak columns(4). The analysis was achieved by elevation of mass spectrometric resolution from 3,000 to 12,000 and utilization the programming GC mode as shown in FIG. 1b.

Selective purification for 11-dehydro-TXB$_2$ from human urine was achieved by changing the elution mixture from ethyl acetate-methanol (99:1) to n-hexane-ethyl acetate (1:1) as shown FIG. 2.

The present technique was applied to quantitation of LTB$_4$, 6-keto PG F$_{1\alpha}$, PGE$_2$, PGF$_2$ and TXB$_2$ in

a)
LOW RESOLUTION MODE (M/ΔM=3,000)

b)
HIGH RESOLUTION MODE (M/ΔM=12,000)

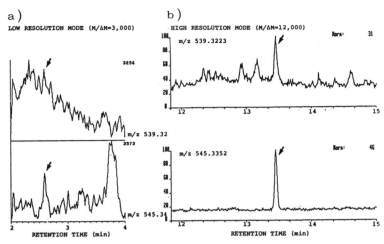

FIG. 1. Selected ion recordings of 11-dehydro-TXB$_2$ ME-DMiPS ether derivative and its [^{18}O$_3$] variant in the eluate of ethyl acetate (99:1) from silica gel column obtained from the HPLC extract from human urine a) low and b) high resolution modes.

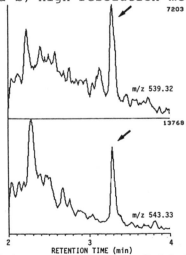

FIG. 2. Selected ion recordings of 11-dehydro-TXB$_2$ ME-DMiPS ether derivative and its [^{18}O$_3$] variant in n-hexane-ethyl acetate (1:1) by the present method in low resolution (M /ΔM=4,000) mode.

muscal cells and muscle tissue of dog gall bladder.

A highly selective purification for LTB_4 from gall bladder was achieved by the combination of washing of n-hexane-ethyl acetate (3:1) and elution of the same solvents (2:1) from silica gel column.

The present purification method provided an isotope effect on the elution of $[^2H_4]$-6-keto-$PGF_{1\alpha}$ methyl ester in n-hexane-ethyl acetate (1:1) and the corresponding 6-keto $PGF_{1\alpha}$ derivative in ethyl acetate-methanol (99:1) from silica gel column, which indicates that the present technique is very powerful.

Thus, this phenomenon disappeared by the use of $[^{18}O_2]$ variant.

In conclusion, the present technique made it possible to quanify the trace amounts of eicosanoids in biological specimens without any disturbance of endogenous substances by CG/SIM in low resolution mode.

REFERENCES

1) Strife R.J., Murphy R.C, <u>Prostaglandins,</u>

   <u>Leukotrienes Med</u>, <u>13</u> 1 (1984)

2) Miyazaki H, Ishibashi M, Itoh M, Yamashita K.

   <u>Biomed. Mass Spectrom.</u>, <u>11</u> 377 (1984)

3) Ishibashi M, Watanabe K, Yamashita K, Miyazaki H.

   In: Gaskell S.J ed, <u>Mass Spectrometry in</u>

   <u>Biomedical Research</u>, Wiley, Chichester 1986 p.423

4) Shono F, Yokota K, Horie K. Yamamoto S,

   Yamashita S, Yamashita K, Watanabe U, Miyazaki H.

   <u>Anal. Biochem.</u>, <u>168</u> 284 (1988)

Advances in Prostaglandin, Thromboxane, and Leukotriene Research, Vol. 19, edited by B. Samuelsson, P. Y.-K. Wong, and F. F. Sun, Raven Press, Ltd., New York ©1989.

RADIOIMMUNOASSAY OF 11-DEHYDRO-THROMBOXANE B$_2$

USING MONOCLONAL ANTIBODY

Y. Hayashi, F. Shono, S. Yamamoto, *K. Yamashita, *K. Watanabe, and *H. Miyazaki

Department of Biochemistry, Tokushima University School of Medicine, Kuramoto-cho, Tokushima 770, and *Research Laboratories, Pharmaceutical Division, Nippon Kayaku Co., Kita-ku, Tokyo 115, Japan

Recently 11-dehydro-thromboxane (TX)B$_2$ has been identified as a major metabolite of infused TXB$_2$ in human. The compound is now considered as an appropriate analytical parameter to follow the endogenous synthesis of TXA$_2$, because it has a longer life than TXB$_2$ in the circulating blood and its amount is not influenced artificially in the blood-sampling procedures (1). We attempted to prepare a monoclonal antibody against 11-dehydro-TXB$_2$ by the hybridoma technique. This method requires only a very small amount of antigen and allows an unlimited supply of antibody of the same specificity and affinity.

A female BALB/c mouse was immunized four times each with 5.5 μg of 11-dehydro-TXB$_2$ conjugated to bovine serum albumin. Spleen cells were fused with myeloma cells (SP2/0-Ag14) using 50% poly-ethylene glycol-1000 (2). Antibody-producing hybridomas were screened and cloned twice. The hybridoma cells were grown in the peritoneal cavity of mouse. The antibody in the ascites fluid was collected with ammonium sulfate at 50% saturation, and was further purified by the use of a protein A-Sepharose column.

Fig. 1 shows a calibration curve of 11-dehydro-TXB$_2$ determined by radioimmunoassay using the monoclonal antibody. The IC$_{50}$ value was 90 fmol (33 pg).

11-Dehydro-TXB$_2$ can exist either as a lactone or as an open form depending on the pH of the medium (3). At pH values higher than 4, the compound occurs predominantly as an open form. Assuming that the antibody recognizes either of the two forms, the dependency of the antigen-antibody reaction on pH was tested with different buffers of various pH values. ^{3}H-11-Dehydro-TXB$_2$ methyl ester prepared as described below was preincubated at each pH at 25°C for 24 h prior to the addition of the antibody. Incu-bation of the antibody with the radioligand was continued at the same pH, and the immunoprecipitation was performed at pH 7.4. The EC_{50} values of the antibody were plotted against the pH value as shown in Fig. 2. The antibody showed a higher affinity above neutral pH, indicating that the antibody recognizes the open form of 11-dehydro-TXB₂. Such a pH-optimum was not seen in the expe-

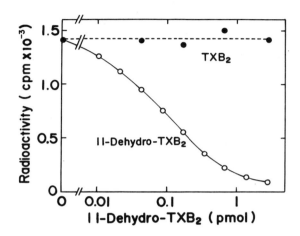

FIG. 1. Calibration curve of 11-dehydro-TXB₂.

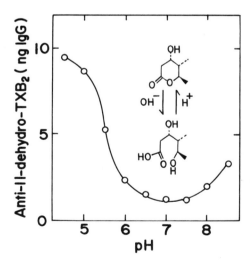

FIG. 2. Dependency of immunoreaction on pH. The amount of antibody which gave 50% of maximum binding (EC_{50}) was plotted against the pH value in which the antigen had been preincubated for 24 h.

riments with anti-PGF$_{2\alpha}$ antibody as a control.

Affinity of the antibody for 11-dehydro-TXB$_2$ was calculated by Scatchard plots of the binding data with ^{3}H-11-dehydro-TXB$_2$ methyl ester. Association constant was 6.5 x 10^9 M^{-1}. Cross-reactivity of the antibody with other eicosanoids and their metabolites was examined in the presence of the standard amount of ^{3}H-11-dehydro-TXB$_2$ methyl ester. TXB$_2$ (Fig. 1), 2,3-dinor-TXB$_2$, PGB$_2$, PGD$_2$, PGE$_2$, PGF$_{2\alpha}$, 6-keto-PGF$_{1\alpha}$, 15-keto-PGF$_{2\alpha}$, 13,14-dihydro-15-keto-PGE$_2$ and 13,14-dihydro-15-keto-PGF$_{2\alpha}$ showed cross-reactivities of less than 0.05%.

When we prepared the antibody, ^{3}H-11-dehydro-TXB$_2$ was not available. Therefore, we prepared 11-dehydro-TXB$_2$ methyl ester as a heterologous ligand using ^{3}H-methyl iodide (85 Ci/mmol) by the method of Moonen et al. (4). The labeled compound was well separated from the unlabeled 11-dehydro-TXB$_2$ by reverse-phase HPLC.

The standard assay condition by the use of our monoclonal antibody and ^{3}H-radioligand is as follows. Authentic 11-dehydro-TXB$_2$, labeled antigen and the sample to be tested were preincubated separately at pH 7.4 at 24°C for 48 h in order to complete a hydrolysis of the lactone form. Then, the standard solution or the sample to be tested (100 μl) was mixed with 0.8% gelatin (50 μl), and incubated with ^{3}H-labeled antigen (100 μl) and the antibody (100 μl) at 4°C for 16 h. The procedures using polyethylene glycol were essentially as described for PGE$_2$ (5).

We applied the radioimmunoassay to determine the amount of 11-dehydro-TXB$_2$ in human urine. Urine was applied to a Sep-Pak C$_{18}$ column, and the crude extract was further purified by reverse-phase HPLC. When the amount of the purified material was raised, the value of 11-dehydro-TXB$_2$ determined by the radioimmunoassay increased in a linear fashion. Radioimmunoassay was also carried out with a given amount of the purified extract, to which various known amounts of authentic 11-dehydro-TXB$_2$ were added. A good correlation was observed between the added and the measured 11-dehydro-TXB$_2$. Validity of the radioimmunoassay of 11-dehydro-TXB$_2$ was examined by gas chromatography-selected ion monitoring (GC-SIM). Various known amounts of 11-dehydro-TXB$_2$ were added to a given amount of the purified urinary extract, and the mixtures were assayed by GC-SIM. A good correlation was observed between the added and the measured amounts of 11-dehydro-TXB$_2$. By extraporation, 11-dehydro-TXB$_2$ content in the urine was estimated to be 1.43 pmol/ml by GC-SIM, and this value was not far from the value of 0.90 pmol/ml determined by our radioimmunoassay.

REFERENCES

1. Westlund P, Granström E, Kumlin M, Nordenström A
    Prostaglandins 1986;31:929-960.

2. Goding JW J Immunol Methods 1980;39:285-308.

3. Kumlin M, Granström E Prostaglandins 1986;32:741-767.

4. Moonen P, Klok G, Keirse MJNC Prostaglandins 1985;29: 443-448.

5. Shono F, Yokota K, Horie K, et al. Anal Biochem 1988;168: 284-291.

Advances in Prostaglandin, Thromboxane, and Leukotriene Research, Vol. 19, edited by
B. Samuelsson, P. Y.-K. Wong, and F. F. Sun,
Raven Press, Ltd., New York ©1989.

Derivatization of prostaglandins to corresponding anilides and analysis by HPLC

J. Knospe, T. Herrmann, D. Steinhilber and H.J. Roth

Pharmaceutical Institute, University of Tuebingen, Auf der Morgenstelle 8, D-7400 Tuebingen, F.R.G.

Analysis of Prostaglandins (PG's) by HPLC requires derivatization, since PG's show no UV-absorbance and no fluorescence. Anodic oxidation of PG's starts not until applied potentials above + 1.6 Volts [1]. So, PG's are electrochemically inactive at potentials employed for electrochemical detection (EC). In general, EC allows very sensitive detection of oxidisable compounds [2]. Therefore, we strived for this mode of detection of PG's. A new derivatization method was developed for PGE_2, $PGF_{2\alpha}$, PGD_2, TXB_2 and $6K\text{-}PGF_{1\alpha}$, leading to electrochemically active 4-methoxyanilides (ME) or 2,4-dimethoxyanilides (DI), respectively. Moreover, the anilides offer the possibility of UV-detection owning a UV-maximum at 249 nm. Both detection systems allowed reliable quantification of PG's in the investigated concentration range; EC offered significant lower detection limits compared with UV-detection. A new internal standard, 16,16-dimethyl-PGE_2, was used in this assay. TXB_2 produced by thrombin treated platelets was determined by this method.

Materials and methods

The HPLC system consisted of a Waters 730 data module, a Waters 590 pump, a Waters U6K-injector, a Waters 481 UV-detector and a Waters 460 electrochemical detector, thin-layer cell, equipped with a glassy carbon working-electrode. Constant sensivity of the working electrode was ensured by treating the surface as described in [3].The reference electrode was an Ag/AgCl electrode (filling: 3M LiCl in 65 % aqueous methanol). The PG-derivatives were separated by reversed-phase HPLC (column: Nucleosil C-18; 250 x 4.6 mm I.D.; particle size: 5 μm) using two different solvent systems depending on the applied mode of detection. Eluent A (UV-detection) was acetonitrile-water (42:58 v/v) adjusted to pH 3.5 with trifluoroacetic acid (TFA). Eluent B (EC) was acetonitrile-methanol-water (35:22:43 v/v/v), supplemented with $LiClO_4$: 0.5 g/l. The pH was set to 4.1 using TFA.

Derivatization reaction

To a methanolic PG solution (10-100 μl) various amounts of an aqueous 0.02 M 4-methoxyaniline-HCl (ME-HCl) or 2,4-dimethoxyaniline-HCl (DI-HCl) solution and an ethanolic 0.125 M 1-ethyl-3-dimethylaminopropylcarbodiimide-HCl (EDC) solution, containing 1.5% pyridine (v/v), were added, so that the final concentrations of reagents in the reaction mixture were:
ME-HCl,DI-HCl: 1.8×10^{-3} M
EDC 2.2×10^{-2} M
Pyridine   0.27 % (v/v)

The reaction mixture was shaked in a waterbath for one hour (37°C). Excess of reagent was removed according to [4].

The extraction of PG's produced by washed platelets (of 10 ml EDTA-blood) which had been incubated with 5 U of thrombin for 5 min (37°C) was done using Baker C-18 columns [5].

Results

The varying characteristics in electrochemical and UV-response of the derivatives (DI and ME) were investigated:

	halve-wave potential	ϵ 249 nm in methanol	chosen mode of detection
DI-derivatives	1.02 V	10300	EC
ME derivatives	1.12 V	14000	UV

Best separation of PG's is achieved by using an eluent consisting of an acetonitrile-water mixture [6]. It was used for the separation of the ME-derivatives (Fig. 1). A pH of 3.5 of the eluent presents a compromise between the response of ME-6K-PGF$_{1\alpha}$ and that of ME-TXB$_2$ (Fig.2). The response of the other ME-PG's was not significantly influenced by varying the pH of the mobile phase.

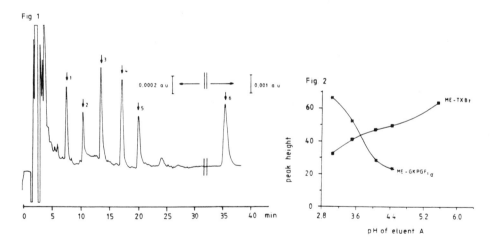

Fig. 1: Chromatogram of ME-derivatives of PG's: eluent A; flow-rate: 1 ml/min.; UV-detector: 249 nm; peaks: 1 = 6K-PGF$_{1\alpha}$, 2 = TXB$_2$, 3 = PGF$_{2\alpha}$, 4 = PGE$_2$, 5 = PGD$_2$, 6 = 16,16-dimethyl-PGE$_2$; approximately 10 ng each, internal standard 100 ng;

Fig. 2: Effect of the pH of the eluent A on the response of ME-6K-PGF$_{1\alpha}$($\star$) and ME-TXB$_2$($\blacksquare$); 40 ng were injected;

The advantages of using eluent B in EC are discussed in [4]. The DI-derivatives were detected at a potential of + 1.10 V. The response, resulting at this potential, was improved by the addition of an electrolyte to the eluent. A sufficient amount of LiClO$_4$ was 0.5 g/l eluent. Typical chromatograms are presented in Fig. 3 and 4.

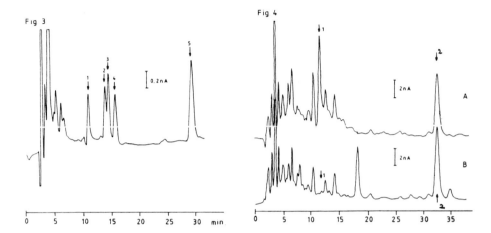

Fig. 3: Chromatogram of DI-derivatives of PG's: eluent B; flow rate: 1 ml/min.; detector potential: 1.10 V (vs. Ag/AgCl); peaks: 1 = TXB$_2$, 2 = PGF$_{2\alpha}$, 3 = PGE$_2$, 4 = PGD$_2$, 5 = 16,16-dimethyl-PGE$_2$; approximately 2.5 ng each, internal standard 5 ng;

Fig. 4: Chromatograms of TXB$_2$ (DI-derivative) produced by thrombin treated platelets: A in the absence of indomethacin; B in the presence of 1 x 10^{-4} M indomethacin; One tenth (10μl) of the eluate containing the PG-derivatives was injected on column; eluent B; flow-rate: 1 ml/min.; peaks: 1 = TXB$_2$, 2 = internal standard;

Preparation of calibration graphs were carried out in the presence of a constant amount of internal standard.

	derivatized amounts of PG's	injected amounts of PG's
DI-derivatives	10 - 100 ng	1 - 10 ng
ME-derivatives	50 - 1000 ng	10 - 200 ng

Equations for calibration graphs and correlation coefficients (r):
The equation is defined as: $y = ax + b$

1. DI-derivatives

y = peak height in nA; x = amount of eicosanoid in ng;

eicosanoid	RT	equations	r
TXB$_2$	11.27	y = 0.152 x - 0.054	0.99879
PGF$_{2\alpha}$	14.34	y = 0.206 x + 0.039	0.99915
PGE$_2$	14.99	y = 0.255 x + 0.053	0.99893
PGD$_2$	16.21	y = 0.159 x + 0.037	0.99828

2. ME-derivatives

y = peak area x 1000 a.u. at 249 nm;

x = amount of eicosanoid in ng;

eicosanoid	RT	equations	r
6K-PGF$_{1\alpha}$	7.88	y = 7.305 x - 9.612	0.99967
TXB$_2$	10.81	y = 2.520 x + 14.132	0.99635
PGF$_{2\alpha}$	14.02	y = 9.437 x + 13.342	0.99991
PGE$_2$	17.55	y = 10.341 x + 25.569	0.99997
PGD$_2$	20.39	y = 6.500 x + 17.286	0.99947

Detection limits based on a peak height versus baseline noise ratio of 5:1:

	detection mode	amount of PG's	used eluent for determination
DI-derivatives	EC	45-75 pg	B
ME-derivatives	UV	1.2-2.2 ng	A

Remarks

This work is part of a doctoral thesis.

(J.Knospe, ref.: H.J. Roth;)

References

1) Herrmann, T., ref.: Roth, H.J., doctoral thesis, 1988

2) Stulic, K., Pacakova, V. (1984): Crit. Rew. Anal. Chem., 14: 297-351

3) Herrmann, T., Steinhilber, D., and Roth, H.J. (1987): J. Chromatogr., 416: 170-175

4) Knospe, J., Steinhilber, D., Herrmann, T., and Roth, H.J. (1988): J. Chromatogr., 442: 444-450

5) Luderer, J.R., Riley, D.L., and Demers, L.M. (1983): J. Chromatogr., 273: 402-409

6) Powell, W.S. (1985) Anal. Biochem., 148: 59-69

Advances in Prostaglandin, Thromboxane, and Leukotriene Research, Vol. 19, edited by B. Samuelsson, P. Y.-K. Wong, and F. F. Sun, Raven Press, Ltd., New York ©1989.

Determination of HETEs by HPLC and electrochemical detection

T. Herrmann, D. Steinhilber, O. Morof and H. J. Roth

Pharmaceutical Institute, University of Tübingen, Auf der Morgenstelle 8, D 7400 – Tübingen

HETEs are arachidonic acid metabolites formed by the 5-, 12- and 15-lipoxygenase pathways [1,2]. Since only trace amounts are released by biological sources, there is a need to develop a convenient method for the determination of small amounts of these compounds. Recently, we reported that the combination of HPLC and subsequent electrochemical detection (ED) proves to be a highly sensitive method for the determination of readily oxidizable compounds such as leukotriene B_4 (LTB_4) [3] and lipoxins [4]. Here, we describe a similar, highly sensitive method for the HETEs and structurally related 12-HHT. This method allows the determination and separation of eicosanoids by HPLC-ED after solid phase extraction of human polymorphonuclear leukocytes(PMNL) and platelets using C_{18}-disposable columns. Our chromatographic conditions combine low background current with high electrochemical response.

EXPERIMENTAL

The HPLC equipment consisted of a Waters Assoc. 460 electrochemical detector with a thin-layer glassy carbon electrode assembly, a 481 variable wavelength UV detector, a 590 pump and a U6K injector. Both detector outputs were displayed simultaneously on a Waters M 730 data module. All potentials were measured against a Ag/AgCl reference electrode filled with 3 M LiCl in 65% methanol. The surface of the electrode was treated as previously described [3,4]. 5-, 12-, 15-HETE, 12-HHT were purchased from Paesel (Frankfurt, FRG), methanol (Chromasolv^R) from Riedel de Haën (Seelze, FRG) water was distilled just before use. All other chemicals used were of analytical grade. The separations were carried out on a column (250 x 4.6 mm I.D.) packed with Nucleosil^R C_{18} (particle size 5 μm) A flow-rate of 1.0 ml/min was used. Preparation of biological extracts from human PMNL was done as descibed previously [3,4].

RESULTS AND DISCUSSION

Fig. 1 shows the peak areas of 5-, 12-, 15-HETE and 12-HHT as a function of the applied oxidation potential. The half-wave potentials ($E_{1/2}$) are listed in Tab. I and show only small differences. It can, therefore, be concluded that the position of the diene unit and allylic hydroxyl group in the backbone, responsible for the resolution on C_{18} columns, exerts no influence on ED. Also the lack of the isolated double–bond does not affect the ED. For these reasons 12-HHT was chosen for further experiments.

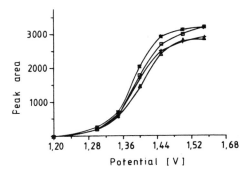

Fig. 1. Dependence of the electrochemical response on the applied potential (V, vs. Ag/AgCl) for 5-HETE [□] , 12-HETE [△], 15-HETE [+], 12-HHT [*], (10 ng each).

To investigate the influence of electrolytes on ED, various concentrations of $LiClO_4$ and two different acids (TFA and H_2SO_4) were tested at pH value 5 and 3. In subsequent experiments a potential of +1.5 V was chosen to illustrate the dependence of the peak area on the specific conductivity, as a measure of the ionic strength of the mobile phase at different concentrations of $LiClO_4$ (0, 1, 10, 20 or 50 mM). At a constant pH, the current rose with an increase in the concentration of lithium perchlorate. Therefore, a sensitive method for the detection of 12-HHT with a lower background current was established at a specific conductivity above 500 $\mu S/cm$. At this conductivity, H_2SO_4 with $LiClO_4$ seems to have little advantage over TFA for lower background current. For trace determinations a mobile phase containing 0.5 mmol/l H_2SO_4 and 1 g/l $LiClO_4$ and an oxidation potential of +1.50 V were chosen. Tab. II lists the equations for calibration graphs and correlation coefficients (r) for 5-, 12-, 15-HETE and 12-HHT under these conditions. Fig. 2 represents a chromatogram of 12-HHT, 15-HETE and 5-HETE. Using an extremely refined mobile phase, the background current could be reduced to 52 nA. The detection limits, based on signal-to-noise ratio of 3 : 1, are shown in Tab. I.

Tab. I lists the half-wave potentials $E_{1/2}$ of the HETEs and 12-HHT and detection limits at a detector potential of + 1.5 V. Mobile phase; methanol - water (75:25, v/v); H_2SO_4, 0.05 g/l; $LiClO_4$, 1 g/l.

Eicosanoid	5-HETE	12-HETE	15-HETE	12-HHT
$E_{1/2}$	+1.40 V	+1.40 V	+1.39 V	+1.38 V
Detection limit UV	1000 pg	1000 pg	1000 pg	1000 pg
Detection limit ED	100 pg	100 pg	110 pg	80 pg

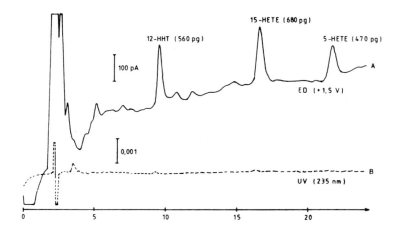

Fig. 2: HPLC-ED/UV chromatograms of 12-HHT, 15-HETE and 5-HETE. Eluent, methanol-water (75:25, v/v) containing 0.5 mmol/l H_2SO_4 and 1 g/l $LiClO_4$; flow rate 1 ml/min; electro-chemical detector + 1.5 V (vs. Ag/AgCl); "response time", 5 s; "filter", 2; background current, 52 nA; UV detector was set at λ = 235 nm.

Tab.II: Equations for calibration graphs and correlation coefficients (r) for 5-, 12-, 15-HETE and 12-HHT. The equation is defined as $y = ax + b$, were y is the peak area and x is the amount of sample (pg).

Eicosanoid	Range [pg]	Equation	r
5-HETE	100 – 4700	y = 0.330 x - 0.42	0.9998
12-HETE	100 – 5500	y = 0.275 x + 0.001	0.9997
15-HETE	110 – 6800	y = 0.298 x - 8.22	0.9997
12-HHT	80 – 5600	y = 0.284 x + 1.8	0.9999

An extract of PMNL was chosen to demonstrate the detectability of 5-HETE by this new method, and an extract of platelets was used for 12-HHT and 12-HETE. Thus, Fig. 5 shows HPLC-ED profiles of such an extract and the numbers indicate the retention times of the standards. An UV-detector (λ = 235 nm) displayed corresponding peaks too. As an internal standard, we are considering a compound that would be oxidized in the same manner and separate quite well from the HETEs or 12-HHT. Hydroxy metabolites from other precursors might fulfil the requirements to be used as internal standard and to exclude the inter-assay variability caused by the electrode performance .

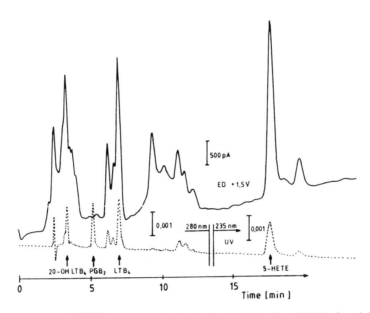

Fig. 3. Chromatograms of PMNL extract using electrochemical detection (full line) and UV detection (dotted line). Eluent, methanol-water (76:34, v/v), TFA 1 mM, LiClO₄ 1 g/l; ED: + 1.5 V (vs. Ag/AgCl); UV detection λ = 280/235 nm.

CONCLUSIONS

In summary, we report here studies of a new method of detection for 5-, 12-, 15-HETE and 12-HHT. The HPLC-ED approach provides a rapid and sensitive method of estimation, without a need for derivatization. For sensitive determination a low background current is necessary. Since the ED is 10 times more sensitive than UV detection, it could serve as a powerful tool in the analysis of activities of the lipoxygenase pathways in biological assays.

References

1. Samuelsson, B. (1983): *Science*, 220: 568.

2. Hamberg, M., Samulsson, B. (1974): *Proc. Natl. Acad. Sci. U.S.A.*, 71: 3400.

3. Herrmann, T., Steinhilber, D., and Roth, H. J. (1987): *J. Chromatogr.*, 416: 170.

4. Herrmann, T., Steinhilber, D., Knospe, J., Roth, H. J. (1988): *J. Chromatogr.*, 428: 237.

Subject Index